KERN'S CARDIAC
CATHETERIZATION
HANDBOOK

KERN'S CARDIAC CATHETERIZATION HANDBOOK

7th Edition

Editors

Paul Sorajja, MD, FACC, FAHA, FSCAI
Director, Center for Valve and Structural Heart Disease
Minneapolis Heart Institute
Abbott Northwestern Hospital
Minneapolis, Minnesota

Michael J. Lim, MD
Co-Director, Center for Comprehensive Cardiovascular Care (C4)
Director, Division of Cardiology
Professor of Internal Medicine
Jack Ford Shelby Endowed Professor in Cardiology
Director, Cardiac Catheterization Laboratory
Director, Cardiovascular Diseases and Interventional Cardiovascular
    Diseases Fellowship Programs
Saint Louis University School of Medicine
St. Louis, Missouri

Morton J. Kern, MD, MSCAI, FAHA, FACC
Professor of Medicine
University of California
Chief of Medicine
Long Beach Veterans Health Care System
Long Beach, California

ELSEVIER

Elsevier
1600 John F. Kennedy Blvd.
Ste 1800
Philadelphia, PA 19103-2899

Notice

Practitioners and researchers must always rely on their own experience and knowledge in evaluating and using any information, methods, compounds or experi-
ments described herein. Because of rapid advances in the medical sciences, in
particular, independent verification of diagnoses and drug dosages should be made.
To the fullest extent of the law, no responsibility is assumed by Elsevier, authors,
editors or contributors for any injury and/or damage to persons or property as a
matter of products liability, negligence or otherwise, or from any use or operation
of any methods, products, instructions, or ideas contained in the material herein.

Previous editions copyrighted 2016, 2011, 2003, 1999, 1995, and 1991.

Library of Congress Control Number: 2019941298

Executive Content Strategist: Robin Carter
Content Development Specialist: Angie Breckon
Publishing Services Manager: Shereen Jameel
Project Manager: Radhika Sivalingam
Book Designer: Ryan Cook

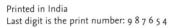

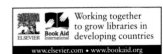

Working together
to grow libraries in
developing countries

www.elsevier.com • www.bookaid.org

Printed in India
Last digit is the print number: 9 8 7 6 5 4

I thank my wife, Margaret, and daughter, Anna Rose,
who are the ever-stronger systole of my life.

Morton J. Kern

Inspiration and Foundation starts with family–
thanks to my wife, Kerri, and children, Parker and
Taylor. May all who read and learn from these pages
remember that our patients are somebody's family and
deserve everything we would do for our own.

Michael J. Lim

To my loving daughters, Natali and Amalin,
who inspire me every day.

Paul Sorajja

List of Contributors

Subhash Banerjee
VA North Texas Healthcare System and University of Texas
Southwestern Medical Center
Dallas, Texas

Barry A. Borlaug, MD, FACC
Consultant, Cardiovascular Diseases
Cardiology
Professor of Medicine
Mayo Medical School
Director, Circulatory Failure Research
Cardiology
Mayo Clinic
Rochester, Minnesota

Emmanouil S. Brilakis, MD, PhD
Director
Cardiac Catheterization Laboratories
Minneapolis Heart Institute
Minneapolis, Minnesota
Professor
Internal Medicine
University of Texas Southwestern Medical Center
Dallas, Texas

Charles E. Chambers, MD
Professor of Medicine and Radiology
Heart and Vascular Institute
Penn State, Hershey Medical Center
Hershey, Pennsylvania

Adnan K. Chhatriwalla, MD
Medical Director, Structural Intervention
Cardiology
Saint Luke's Mid America Heart Institute
Associate Professor
Medicine
University of Missouri-Kansas City
Kansas City, Missouri

Joaquin Cigarroa, MD
Heart and Vascular Institute
Penn State, Hershey Medical Center
Hershey, Pennsylvania

Douglas Emmet Drachman, MD
Director of Education
Division of Cardiology
Massachusetts General Hospital
Boston, Massachusetts

Scott Ferreira, MD, MSE
Assistant Professor
Internal Medicine/Cardiology
Saint Louis University
St. Louis, Missouri

Michael Forsberg, MD
Assistant Professor of Medicine
Cardiology
Saint Louis University
Staff Physician
Cardiology
John Cochran VA Medical Center
St. Louis, Missouri

Santiago Garcia
Interventional Cardiologist
Minneapolis Heart Institute at Abbott Northwestern Hospital
Minneapolis, Minnesota

Joerg Herrmann
Associate Professor of Medicine
Division of Cardiovascular Diseases
Mayo Clinic
Rochester, Minnesota

Navin K. Kapur, MD
Interventional Cardiologist
The Cardiovascular Center
The Molecular Cardiology Research Institute
Tufts Medical Center
Boston, Massachusetts

Morton J. Kern, MD, MSCAI, FAHA, FACC
Professor of Medicine
University of California, Irvine
Orange, California
Chief of Medicine
Long Beach Veterans Health Care System
Long Beach, California

Andrew J.P. Klein, MD, FACC, FSCAI
Interventional Cardiology, Vascular and Endovascular Medicine
Piedmont Heart Institute
Atlanta, Georgia
Adjunct Professor of Medicine
Cardiology
Saint Louis University School of Medicine
St. Louis, Missouri

Chad Kliger, MD, MS
Director, Valve and Structural Heart Center
Cardiothoracic Surgery
Lenox Hill Hospital, Northwell Health
New York, New York

Michael J. Lim, MD
Jack Ford Shelby Endowed Professor of Cardiology
Center for Comprehensive Cardiovascular Care
Saint Louis University
St. Louis, Missouri

Ali A. Mehdirad, MD, FACC
Professor of Medicine
Director of Electrophysiology Service
Division of Cardiology
Saint Louis University
St. Louis, Missouri

Pranav M. Patel, MD
Chief of Cardiology Director, Cardiac Catheterization Laboratory
Associate Director, Cardiovascular Medicine Fellowship
Assistant Professor of Medicine Division of Cardiology
University of California, Irvine
Orange, California

Paul Sorajja, MD
Senior Consulting Cardiologist
Minneapolis Heart Institute
Abbott Northwestern Hospital
Minneapolis, Minnesota

Preface

The techniques of cardiac catheterization, coronary angiography, and cardiovascular percutaneous interventions (PCIs) have evolved dramatically during the last 25 years. The change in standard vascular access for coronary angiography to a "radial first" approach has been nothing short of a revolution, improving patient comfort and safety. This advance has not negated the need to become expert in large vessel femoral and axillary artery access for structural interventions and left ventricular support device insertions. These advances allow us to take on higher complexity coronary and structural procedures in today's laboratories. Modern cardiac catheterization and interventions are a marvel!

From its inception, *Kern's Cardiac Catheterization Handbook* has been dedicated to providing a simple and straightforward guide to the basics of cardiac catheterization. The novice fellow, nurse, student, or industry support teams will find the information in this introduction to the catheterization laboratory central to understanding the safe performance of the procedures. In addition, we have updated the section on percutaneous coronary revascularization for a large variety of patients with both simple and complex coronary stenoses or occlusions. Percutaneous coronary revascularization for chronically occluded diseased vessels is a feat that was probably never imagined by Dr. Gruentzig, the pioneer of PCI. We can only imagine how he would view percutaneous structural heart interventions such as transaortic valve replacement.

Mastery of the complex catheterization laboratory technology and techniques begins with a clear understanding of the basics. It should also be emphasized that a team effort whereby everyone involved functions in a safe and coordinated manner is essential. As with the earlier editions, the purpose of the 7th edition of *Kern's Cardiac Catheterization Handbook* is to provide a basic, practical explanation of the methods used to acquire diagnostic information and to complete the therapeutic interventional procedures. We hope nurses, technologists, students, physician trainees, physicians in practice, and anyone needing to know what catheterization is all about will find the book easy and enjoyable to use.

What's New in this Edition?

As interventional cardiology continues to evolve, it is always important to have operators working in the laboratory contribute their insights to the teaching of the techniques. It is for this reason that Dr. Michael Lim from Saint Louis University and Dr. Paul Sorajja from the Minneapolis Heart Institute have taken the helm for this edition of the handbook. Their in-laboratory experience and practical knowledge of complex procedures have made the substantial revisions to structural heart disease interventions the most valuable updates.

The 7th edition is refreshed and as up-to-date as any handbook can be. In Chapter 1, we kept the focus on procedural indications, patient evaluation and preparation, strategies for teamwork, function of the imaging system, basic pharmacology, and credentialing requirements. Descriptions of how the procedure should flow, which steps should be learned first, how to approach patients undergoing this often-frightening test, how to be part of the catheterization laboratory team, and similar work matters are presented.

The technique of vascular access (Chapter 2) remains among the most critically important areas, with radial artery access for coronary angiography and intervention strongly emphasized. Multiple techniques for large vessel, large bore sheaths are also described in more detail. The diagnosis and management of complications including periprocedural bleeding, is updated.

Chapter 3, Coronary Angiography and Ventriculography, focuses on imaging projections, anomalous arteries, ventriculography, and clinical application of fractional flow reserve (FFR), intravascular ultrasound (IVUS), and optical coherence tomography (OCT). Radiation safety, the generation of the radiographic image with the use of modern flat-panel image detectors, and issues related to radiographic contrast media are highlighted.

Hemodynamic data and best methods of signal acquisition and interpretation are described in Chapter 4. This chapter is especially relevant as more operators and teams become involved with valve interventions. In Chapter 5, Dr. Subhash Banerjee, Andrew Klein and and Dr. Doug Drachman give a new view of peripheral vascular intervention, explaining the diagnosis and management of peripheral vascular disease including the role of adjunctive noninvasive testing, and a synopsis of state-of-the-art peripheral interventional therapies.

The chapter on electrophysiologic testing and device use in the catheterization laboratory (Chapter 7) has been updated with new modalities of remote guidance of electrophysiology catheters and electrophysiologic arrhythmia ablations. For individuals working in electrophysiology laboratories and fellows entering this area while in training, this section provides an excellent basic framework for understanding when and how these very specialized procedures should be used.

Coronary intervention has advanced with high-risk patients and special working groups dedicated to teaching operators the appropriate methods for these complex patients. Chapters 6 and 8 are dedicated to operators taking on high-risk patients, including those with chronic total occlusions, a specialty within a specialty. Chapter 8, High-Risk Cardiac Catheterization, describes the potential complications and strategies to minimize their occurrence. Approaches for advanced hemodynamic support in the periprocedural period are highlighted, including pharmacologic management, intraaortic balloon pump (IABP) use, and percutaneous ventricular assist devices.

Chapter 9, Special Techniques, provides a detailed description of current areas of catheterization laboratory research, with an emphasis on their clinical relevance. Techniques described include sophisticated methods for assessing coronary flow, vessel histology, and ventricular function.

Chapter 10, Research Techniques have undergone revision to provide the latest information on pressure volume loops, assessment of coronary physiology and exercise hemodynamics.

Chapter 11 addresses quality in the catheterization laboratory. The understanding of quality systems and its metrics, appropriate professional documentation, and risk management in the cardiac catheterization laboratory are critical to good operations.

Our goal for this handbook is to provide a state-of-the-art and plain-spoken resource for use in the cardiac catheterization laboratory. Each edition is an achievement that is only made possible with the help of many colleagues, teachers, and mentors. These individuals have taught us not only the practice but also the importance of inquiry and humility, while having the privilege to care for patients in the cardiac catheterization laboratory and beyond. We are deeply indebted to these individuals, many of whom continue to teach us both in and out of the catheterization laboratory.

Morton J. Kern
Michael J. Lim
Paul Sorajja

Dedication and In memoriam

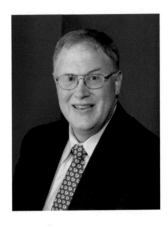

In June, 2019, Charles E. Chambers, MD, MSCAI, a devoted physician and master in the field of interventional cardiology passed away at the age of 64. Dr. Chambers was the 38th president of SCAI, from 2014-2015, and practiced medicine at the Hershey Medical Center of the Penn State University College of Medicine where he served as the Director of Cardiac Catheterization Laboratories since 1994 and Professor of Medicine and Radiology since 2002.

Dr. Chambers' contributions to SCAI (and to this review book, see Chapter 11) were remarkable and significant. Over the course of more than 25 years, he served with distinction on the Board of Trustees and numerous committees including the nominating committee, ethics committee, and political action committee. He also served as the SCAI representative to the National Quality Forum. Dr. Chambers served as chair of the SCAI Cath Lab Survey Committee, the precursor to the SCAI Quality Improvement Committee, and chair of SCAI's Public Relations and Laboratory Performance Standards committees. During his presidency, Dr. Chambers furthered SCAI's quality mission through founding the SCAI Cath Lab Leadership Boot Camp, which debuted in 2014. The Boot Camp is aimed at standardizing and strengthening the training provided to those in cath lab leadership positions.

Dr. Chambers' commitment to the hazards and risks of interventional cardiology is well-documented in many publications, and he served on the editorial board of the Catheterization and

Cardiovascular Interventions journal authoring or co-authoring multiple position papers for the Society in the area of quality improvement, infection control, and radiation safety. In addition, Dr. Chambers served on the writing committee for numerous health care policy statements and expert consensus documents.

In 2006, Dr. Chambers received the F. Mason Sones, Jr. Award from SCAI recognizing his dedication to education and quality of care. In 2015, Dr. Chambers was named a Master of SCAI (MSCAI) for his commitment to excellence throughout his career and his commitment to the highest levels of clinical care, innovation, publication, and teaching.

As noted by the current SCAI President Ehtisham Mahmud, MD, FSCAI, "Charlie spent his entire career caring for and serving others and made enormous contributions to the field of interventional cardiology. His vision, guidance, and commitment to SCAI and our specialty are greatly appreciated and cannot be overstated. He guided our Society through turbulent waters, and he will be missed tremendously."

Dr. Chambers embodied the ideals and values that SCAI hopes to instill in each of its members, and with great sadness, we say good-bye to a friend and physician of the highest caliber. We, the editors and authors of this Cardiac Catheterization Handbook, 7th edition, dedicate this page to Charlie.

Contents

Video Contents

The Cardiac Catheterization Laboratory

MORTON J. KERN

Cardiac catheterization is the insertion and passage of small plastic tubes (catheters) into arteries and veins to the heart to obtain x-ray images (angiography) of coronary arteries and cardiac chambers and to measure pressures in the heart (hemodynamics). The cardiac catheterization laboratory performs angiography to obtain images not only of coronary arteries to diagnose coronary artery disease but also to look for abnormalities of the aorta, pulmonary, and peripheral vessels. In addition to providing diagnostic information, the cardiac catheterization laboratory performs catheter-based interventions (e.g., angioplasty with stent implantation, now called *percutaneous coronary intervention* [PCI]) or catheter-based treatments of structural heart disease (e.g., transaortic valve replacement [TAVR]) for both acute and chronic cardiovascular illness. Table 1.1 lists procedures that can be performed with coronary angiography. Figure 1.1 shows common vascular access routes for cardiac catheterization.

Indications for Cardiac Catheterization

Cardiac catheterization is used to identify atherosclerotic coronary or peripheral artery disease, abnormalities of heart muscle (infarction or cardiomyopathy), and valvular or congenital heart abnormalities. In adults, the procedure is used most commonly to diagnose coronary artery disease. Other indications depend on the history, physical examination, electrocardiogram (ECG), cardiac stress test, echocardiographic results, and chest radiograph. Indications for cardiac catheterization are summarized in Table 1.2.

Table 1.1

Procedures That May Accompany Coronary Angiography.[a]

Procedure	Comment
1. Central venous access	Used as IV access for emergency medications (femoral, internal jugular, subclavian) or fluids, temporary pacemaker (pacemaker not mandatory for coronary angiography)
2. Hemodynamic assessment	
a. Left heart pressures	Routine for nearly all studies (aorta, left ventricle)
b. Right heart pressures	Not routine for coronary artery disease, combined pressures; mandatory for valvular heart disease; routine for CHF, right ventricular dysfunction, pericardial diseases, cardiomyopathy, intracardiac shunts, congenital abnormalities
3. Left ventricular angiography	Routine for nearly all studies; may be excluded with high-risk patients, left main coronary or aortic stenosis, severe CHF, renal failure
4. Internal mammary artery selective angiography	Not routine unless used as coronary bypass conduit
5. Femoral angiography	Routine for femoral arterial access assessments before closure device
5a. IC/IV/sublingual NTG	Useful during coronary angiography and intracoronary device manipulations
6. Aortography	Routine for aortic insufficiency, aortic dissection, aortic aneurysm, with or without aortic stenosis; routine to locate bypass grafts not visualized by selective angiography, anomalous coronary origin
7. Cardiac electrophysiologic studies	Arrhythmia evaluation, conduction tract catheter ablation procedures
8. Interventional and special techniques	Coronary stents, rotoblator, etc. FFR/CFR/IVUS for lesion assessment
	TAVR, Balloon valvuloplasty (see Chapter 6, Interventional Cardiology Procedures)
	Myocardial biopsy
	Transseptal or left ventricular puncture
9. Arterial closure devices	Available to reduce access site bleeding

CFR, Coronary flow reserve; CHF, congestive heart failure; FFR, fractional flow reserve; IC, intracoronary; IV, intravenous; IVUS, intravascular ultrasound imaging; NTG, nitroglycerin; TAVR, transaortic valve replacement.
[a]See Table 1.2 for indications.

RIGHT HEART CATHETERIZATION

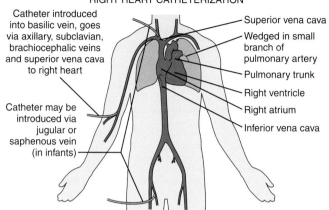

Catheter introduced into basilic vein, goes via axillary, subclavian, brachiocephalic veins and superior vena cava to right heart

Catheter may be introduced via jugular or saphenous vein (in infants)

Superior vena cava

Wedged in small branch of pulmonary artery

Pulmonary trunk

Right ventricle

Right atrium

Inferior vena cava

LEFT HEART CATHETERIZATION

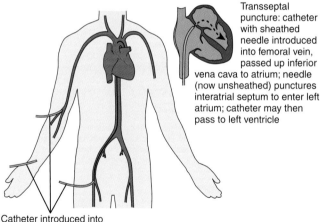

Transseptal puncture: catheter with sheathed needle introduced into femoral vein, passed up inferior vena cava to atrium; needle (now unsheathed) punctures interatrial septum to enter left atrium; catheter may then pass to left ventricle

Catheter introduced into brachial, radial, ulnar (and rarely axillary), or femoral artery and passed retrograde via aorta to left ventrical

Fig. 1.1   Vascular access routes for cardiac catheterization (also see Chapter 2). Radial and femoral arteries are the most common approaches for coronary angiography.

Table 1.2

Indications for Cardiac Catheterization.	
Indications	**Procedures**
1. Suspected or known coronary artery disease	LV, COR
a. New-onset angina	LV, COR
b. Unstable angina	LV, COR
c. Evaluation before a major surgical procedure	LV, COR
d. Silent ischemia	LV, COR
e. Positive exercise tolerance test	LV, COR
f. Atypical chest pain or coronary spasm	LV, COR, vasomotor stimuli
2. Myocardial infarction	LV, COR, PCI
a. Unstable angina postinfarction	LV, COR, PCI
b. Failed thrombolysis	LV, COR, PCI
c. Shock	LV, COR, RH, LV support
d. Mechanical complications (ventricular septal defect, rupture of wall or papillary muscle)	LV, COR, RH, pacemaker, LV support
3. Sudden cardiovascular death	LV, COR, R + L
4. Valvular heart disease	LV, COR, R + L, ±AO
5. Congenital heart disease (before anticipated corrective surgery or ASD/PFO closure)	LV, COR, R + L, ±AO
6. Aortic dissection	AO, COR
7. Pericardial constriction or tamponade	LV, COR, R + L
8. Cardiomyopathy	LV, COR, R + L, ±BX
9. Initial and follow-up assessment for heart transplant	LV, COR, R + L, BX

AO, Aortography; *ASD,* atrial septal defect; *BX,* endomyocardial biopsy; *COR,* coronary angiography; *LV,* left ventriculography; *PCI,* percutaneous coronary intervention; *RH,* right heart oxygen saturations and hemodynamics (e.g., placement of Swan-Ganz catheter); *R + L,* right and left heart hemodynamics; ±, optional.

Elective Procedures

For most patients, diagnostic cardiac catheterization is performed as an elective procedure. It should be deferred if the patient is not prepared either psychologically or physically.

Urgent Procedures

If the patient's condition is unstable because of a suspected cardiac disorder, such as acute myocardial infarction, catheterization must proceed. In the event of decompensated congestive heart failure (CHF) in patients with acute unstable coronary syndromes, rapid medical management is needed. Although a patient must be able to lie flat for easy catheter passage, patients with acute

> **Box 1.1   Contraindications to Cardiac Catheterization.**
>
> **Absolute Contraindications**
>
> Inadequate equipment or catheterization facility
>
> **Relative Contraindications**
>
> Acute gastrointestinal bleeding, anemia
> Anticoagulation (or known, uncontrolled bleeding diathesis)
> Electrolyte imbalance
> Infection and fever
> Medication intoxication (e.g., digitalis, phenothiazine)
> Pregnancy
> Recent cerebrovascular accident (<1 month)
> Renal failure
> Uncontrolled congestive heart failure, high blood pressure, arrhythmias
> Uncooperative patient

cardiac decompensation may benefit more from aggressive management in the catheterization laboratory where intubation, left ventricular (LV) mechanical support devices, and vasopressors can be instituted rapidly before angiography, and a rapid decision made for revascularization.

Contraindications

Contraindications to cardiac catheterization include fever, anemia, electrolyte imbalance (especially hypokalemia predisposing to arrhythmias), and other systemic illnesses needing stabilization (Box 1.1). The clinical necessity of cardiac catheterization should also be carefully considered when the diagnostic information or therapeutic intervention from the procedure would not meaningfully impact the management of a patient.

Complications and Risks

For diagnostic catheterization, an analysis of the complications in more than 200,000 patients indicated the incidences of risks: death, ~0.2%; myocardial infarction, ~0.05%; stroke, ~0.07%; serious ventricular arrhythmia, ~0.5%; and major vascular complications (thrombosis, bleeding requiring transfusion, or pseudoaneurysm), ~1% (Box 1.2 and Table 1.3). Vascular complications occurred most often when the brachial approach was used and least when the radial approach was used. Risks are increased in well-described subgroups (Box 1.3).

Box 1.2   Complications of Cardiac Catheterization.

Major

Cerebrovascular accident
Death
Myocardial infarction
Ventricular tachycardia, fibrillation, serious arrhythmia

Other

Aortic dissection
Cardiac perforation, tamponade
Congestive heart failure
Contrast reaction (anaphylaxis, nephrotoxicity)
Heart block, asystole
Hemorrhage (local, retroperitoneal, pelvic)
Infection
Protamine reaction
Supraventricular tachyarrhythmia, atrial fibrillation
Thrombosis, embolus, air embolus
Vascular injury, pseudoaneurysm
Vasovagal reaction

Table 1.3

Incidence of Major Complications of Diagnostic Catheterizations.

Procedure-Related Complications in Patients Without STEMI		
	PCI Patients Without STEMI (*n* = 787,980)	Diagnostic Catheterization Only Patients Without STEMI (*n* = 1,091,557)
Complications (%)		
• Any adverse event	4.53	1.35
• Cardiogenic shock	0.47	0.24
• Heart failure	0.59	0.38
• Pericardial tamponade	0.07	0.03
• CVA/stroke	0.17	0.17
• Total strokes that were hemorrhagic	15.6	9.16
• New requirement for dialysis	0.19	0.14
In-Hospital Mortality:		
• Non–risk-adjusted	0.65	0.72
• Non–risk-adjusted excluding CABG patients	0.62	0.60
• CABG performed during admission	0.81	7.47

Table 1.3

Incidence of Major Complications of Diagnostic Catheterizations. (Continued)		
Procedure-Related Complications in Patients Without STEMI		
	PCI Patients Without STEMI ($n = 787,980$)	**Diagnostic Catheterization Only Patients Without STEMI** ($n = 1,091,557$)
CABG Status		
• Salvage/emergency	0.01/0.17	0.01/0.27
• Urgent/elective	0.47/0.16	5.27/1.92
CABG Indication		
• PCI failure without clinical deterioration	0.26	
• PCI complication	0.14	
Bleeding Complications (%)		
• Any bleeding event within 72 hours of procedure	1.40	0.49
• Any other vascular complication requiring treatment	0.44	0.15
• RBC/whole-blood transfusion	2.07	N/A

From Dehmer GJ, Weaver D, Matthew T, et al. A contemporary view of diagnostic cardiac catheterization and percutaneous coronary intervention in the United States. A report from the CathPCI Registry of the National Cardiovascular Data Registry, 2010 through June 2011. *J Am Coll Cardiol.* 2012;60:2017-2031.

CABG, Coronary artery bypass graft; *CVA*, cerebrovascular accident; *N/A*, not applicable; *PCI*, percutaneous coronary intervention; *RBC*, red blood cell; *STEMI*, ST-segment elevation myocardial infarction.

Box 1.3   Conditions of Patients at Higher Risk for Complications of Catheterization.[a]
Acute myocardial infarction
Advanced age (>75 years)
Aortic aneurysm
Aortic stenosis
Congestive heart failure
Diabetes
Extensive three-vessel coronary artery disease
Left ventricular dysfunction (left ventricular ejection fraction <35%)
Obesity
Prior cerebrovascular accident
Renal insufficiency
Suspected or known left main coronary stenosis
Uncontrolled hypertension
Unstable angina

[a]See also Chapter 8, High-risk Catheterization.

Catheterization Laboratory Data

Information gathered during the cardiac catheterization can be divided into two categories: hemodynamic and angiographic. Electrophysiologic data are discussed in Chapter 7. The term *cineangiography* describes the x-ray examination of cardiac structures from the era when film was the recording medium. Use of this term (i.e., cine) persists even though the images are now acquired and stored electronically on digital computer imaging media (e.g., CD-ROM) rather than on celluloid film. The digital cineangiogram provides anatomic information about the chambers of the heart and the coronary arteries. Hemodynamic information is recorded from catheters inside the heart and consists of pressure tracings processed and stored in a digital format and cardiac output and blood oxygen saturation measurements.

Preparation of the Patient
Consent for the Procedure

Consent may be obtained by the operator or his or her assistant but is usually obtained by a physician. The person obtaining consent should do the following:

1. Explain in simple terms what procedure will take place, for what reason each step of the procedure will occur, the roles of the team performing the procedure, and what is expected to be learned from the test.

2. Explain the risks for routine cardiac catheterization. Major risks include stroke, myocardial infarction, and death (usually less than 1 in 1000). Minor risks include vascular injury, allergic reaction, bleeding, hematoma, and infection. If PCI is anticipated, consent for this should be obtained and options should be discussed in advance of the procedure such as medical therapy, stenting, or coronary bypass surgery.

3. Explain any portions of the study used for research and the associated risks (e.g., electrophysiologic study—perforation, arrhythmia [<1:500]; pharmacologic study—varies depending on drug and study duration; intracoronary imaging or sensor-pressure wire study—spasm, myocardial infarction, embolus, dissection [<1:500]).

4. Provide the necessary information and explanation but do not overwhelm the patient. It is good practice to include the family when explaining what will happen and possible outcomes.

After explaining all aspects of the cardiac catheterization for informed consent, it is important to remember that the final decision to undergo the procedure is always the patient's. Informed consent entails a shared decision-making process, in which there is a two-way exchange of pertinent information. This information allows the patient (and family) to make a fully informed decision based on his or her expectations, risks of the procedure, and choice of alternatives. If the patient is reluctant to have the catheterization, the procedure can be deferred until the referring physician speaks to the patient to clarify why the procedure is necessary. A reluctant patient should never sign the consent form. When possible, the family should be present when the procedure is discussed. This approach encourages a cooperative and generally sympathetic appreciation of the procedure, the risks, and expected outcome.

Communication With Patients: A Nonmedical Person's Understanding

The clinician establishes rapport and builds the patient's confidence by listening and explaining. The procedure should be discussed with the patient in terms that he or she can understand. The purpose of the procedure should be clear such as "to look at the arteries in the heart" (coronary arteries) and "to examine the heart muscle" (ventricular function). Simple terms are best so that the patient can grasp the concepts. The clinician should explain what small catheters are (plastic tubes similar in size to spaghetti) and that they will be used to put x-ray contrast media ("dye") into the arteries supplying blood to the heart. Explain that the procedure is *not* painful because the arteries are generally not sensitive to the passage of the small catheters. The heart muscle may be weakened (infarcted) in certain areas, and the way to identify this weakness is to take x-ray pictures of the "main pumping chamber" (i.e., the left ventricle). This example of a simple, forthright explanation facilitates the operator team–patient relationship so that confidence in the operator and team performing the procedure is established.

Laboratory Atmosphere: The Patient's Confidence Builder

1. In the laboratory, a confident, professional attitude should be adopted by all personnel at all times. Straightforward routine communication should occur quietly and without alarming tones. Patients should be addressed directly, by name, to let them know what their instructions are, as opposed to requests or communications to co-workers.

2. The circulating team members should be confident, reassuring, and professional in every respect. The patient feels helpless and is tuned in to all types of stimuli (especially verbal).

3. Extraneous conversation is distracting for the patient and the operators. This is especially true when the patient is draped in a manner that does not allow him or her to see his or her surroundings. In the laboratory, all players should be in the game; that is, focused on the patient's needs and safety, which become paramount goals.

4. Communication with the patient (and family) before, during, and after the procedure ensures a satisfied and well-cared-for individual. Communication among the team members in a professional, courteous, and quiet tone builds patient confidence and helps the procedure go smoothly.

5. Factory worker attitudes of "another coronary" or "another ST-segment elevation myocardial infarction" (STEMI) should be avoided. Each procedure is potentially life threatening and should be undertaken seriously and with concern as if each patient were a family member.

6. Cardiac catheterization is stressful to the patient and the operator team. This stress should be minimized by thoughtful preparation and professional attention to detail. Practical notes for the new operator include the following:

   a. Immediately before the catheterization in the laboratory, a brief reiteration of the history ensures that no interval change has occurred since the last interview.

   b. A reexamination of the patient's ECG is essential.

   c. A brief examination of the patient (checking heart sounds, breath sounds, and carotid and peripheral pulses) should be routine immediately before and after cardiac catheterization. No patient should be studied without the operator's full understanding of the clinical conditions and results of previous catheterizations and other pertinent laboratory data.

When on the catheterization table, the patient remembers two major potentially painful points of a case: (1) the initial introduction of the local anesthetic (and sometimes radial sheath introduction) and (2) any discomfort experienced after the study has been completed. Such discomfort usually occurs while the operator or nurse is holding the femoral puncture site. If the local anesthetic injection is performed too quickly or if the arterial closure or compression after the procedure is difficult or painful, the patient will remember that the physician who performed the catheterization "hurt me." The period between the two events is often forgotten (thanks to premedication), but these two points should be kept in mind as the major new-operator take-home messages. Patients cannot discern the operator's skill or level of accomplishment during the procedure, but they judge the operator (and the team) on the manner and care they receive at the beginning and end of the study. Skill and accomplishment during the procedure are essential, and these are developed during the new operator's training period.

7. General catheterization orders:

· Before catheterization, preferably the preceding night, precatheterization orders should be written.

· All medications and procedural premedications should be tailored to the patient and timing of the catheterization. If the patient is using long-acting insulin (neutral protamine Hagedorn [NPH]), the dose should be reduced by 50% and the patient should not eat breakfast. The patient should be watched carefully for hypoglycemic reactions (e.g., shaking, confusion, slurred speech).

· A more recent suggestion to avoid dehydration and increased chance of contrast-induced nephropathy is to permit or encourage the patient to drink water before the procedure and confine the nothing-by-mouth (NPO) orders to solid foods or dairy products before the procedure.

8. Patients should wear their glasses and dentures in the laboratory to make communication easier.

In-Laboratory Preparations and the Time-Out

The staff of the cardiac catheterization laboratory is responsible for patient preparation before the start of the procedure. On the patient's arrival in the laboratory, a staff member should review a brief checklist to ensure that all preprocedural requirements have been met. A sample checklist follows:

· Check the patient's ID band and known allergies.

· Check laboratory results (key tests: hemoglobin, platelet count, electrolytes including blood urea nitrogen, creatinine).

· Check blood pressure, all pulses (arms and legs), and baseline ECG.

· Anticoagulant status: Check the international normalized ratio (INR) and partial thromboplastin time (PTT) and, if on heparin, the activated clotting time (ACT).

· Recheck childbearing potential (patient may need β-human chorionic gonadotropin level).

- Verify that the proper paperwork has been copied and filled out for the procedure and confirm that the consent form has been signed.
- Assess the patient's understanding of the procedure and answer the patient's questions.
- Check that the oral airway forms for the procedure are signed and in the chart. If not, make arrangements for their completion before the procedure.
- Check that the intravenous (IV) line is secure and patent.
- Check that the patient has ingested nothing solid by mouth before the procedure.
- Check whether premedications were given as ordered.
- Start documentation of the precatheterization condition and note any physical deficits (abnormal neurologic examination, bruising, or bleeding sites).

Cautionary Note

The cardiac catheterization laboratory, like any operating area in a hospital, has potential injury risks to both patients and staff. Common risks of any operating room are listed in Table 1.4. Good sense and proven work routines help the laboratory take precautions against accidents. Specific situations in which patient-related accidents should also be considered and attended to include the transfer and centering of the patient on the table and removing any sharp or hard-edged objects from contact with the patient.

Table 1.4

Safety Hazards.	
Safety Hazards in the Catheterization Laboratory	**Person at Risk**
Ionizing radiation, electricity, impact with stationary equipment	Staff, patient
Blood products, microorganisms	Staff, patient
Pharmaceutical agents	Patient
Chemical solvents, acids, bases, cleansers	Staff
Ergonomic injury (lifting in awkward positions, working in tight spaces, slipping on wet floors)	Staff
Falls from table, gurney, floor	Patient (possibly staff during rescue attempt)

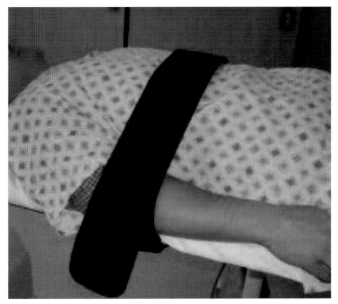

Fig. 1.2 Strap for holding patient on catheterization table. Despite restraints, patient should be closely attended to while the potential of falling is present. (Reprinted with permission from *Cath Lab Digest*. Copyright HMP Communications.)

One unresolved issue is how to protect patients from falling or rolling off the catheterization table and whether all patients should be restrained on the catheterization laboratory table (Fig. 1.2). Patients who are at high risk of falls include high body mass index (BMI) patients, those who cannot follow simple instructions, or patients who are agitated or uncooperative. Patients who cannot keep their arms at their sides, or keep their legs or body still on the table, are also at high risk. These are the same patients who may fall during transfer on or off the catheterization table. There is no formal algorithm for deciding who is truly at high risk. All laboratories use operator and nurse judgment at the time of the procedure. Table restraints are not always effective in preventing falls off the catheterization table. It is good practice that during the time-out and after the administration of conscious sedation, all patients should be assessed for their fall risk.[1]

After all precatheterization requirements have been fulfilled, the patient may be taken to the angiographic suite and the technical preparations can be completed.

Catheterization Suite Preparations

Before the start of the catheterization procedure, the staff performs the following tasks:

1. Establish ECG monitoring. The ECG should be considered the first of the two major lifelines. The heartbeat is monitored for rate and rhythm during the entire procedure. It is the responsibility of the staff to place the electrodes and lead wires in such a fashion that a quality trace is obtained. Care must be taken that the electrodes and lead wires do not interfere with the movement of the x-ray and cineangiographic unit. All leads should be secure, and a good signal should be present before the application of sterile drapes; it is difficult to reach under the sterile drapes to reattach loose lead wires once the procedure has begun. Radiolucent leads permit complete 12-lead ECG monitoring but are more prone to breakage than heavier cable leads.

2. Establish IV access. The second lifeline is IV access for routine medications and fluids as well as for emergency resuscitation measures. Without good IV access, emergency drugs to counteract vagal or allergic reactions will not be effective. When the patient is in the laboratory, the nurse or physician may identify the need for additional sedation or analgesia before the start of the procedure. The IV line is also important for hydration after cardiac catheterization.

Caution must be exercised when premedicating elderly patients. If meperidine (Demerol), fentanyl, or morphine is used, a narcotic antagonist, such as naloxone (Narcan), should be available. Flumazenil (a benzodiazepine antagonist) should also be available if diazepam (Valium) or midazolam (Versed) is used.

The Time-Out

In any catheterization laboratory, preparations can be hectic, perhaps even frantic at times. This frenetic pace can cause problems, important steps can be missed, and patient safety can be compromised. As part of procedural safety, every patient coming to the laboratory must be assessed for his or her suitability for conscious sedation and potential complications of the catheterization procedure. Every laboratory is required to perform a

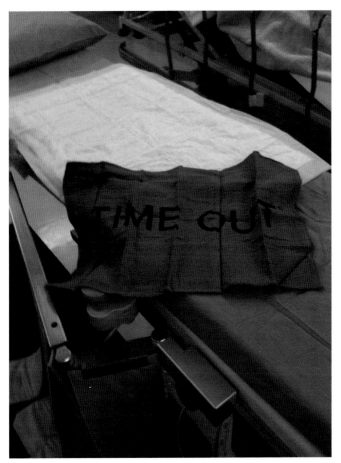

Fig. 1.3 The time-out towel is a reminder to conduct a safety check before proceeding with the procedure. (Reprinted with permission from *Cath Lab Digest*. Copyright HMP Communications.)

preprocedure safety review, called the *time-out* (Fig. 1.3). In the time-out before sedation, the team verifies the right patient is in the room, the right procedure is going to be performed, the right operative site will be used, and whether the patient has renal failure, allergies, or is being treated with anticoagulants so that the team has no concerns about whether to proceed. At this time, the team agrees to proceed and then specifies what analgesia and sedation dose will be given. Time-out is a Joint Commission requirement.

When Should the Time-Out Occur?

The time-out, the immediate preprocedure pause, must occur in the location where the procedure is to be performed (catheterization laboratory suite). The time-out may precede anesthesia or it may occur in the operating room after the patient is anesthetized (participation by the patient is not expected in surgical procedures but is recommended for catheterization laboratory procedures) but just before starting the procedure. In some laboratories, a second time-out is done before the PCI after completion of the diagnostic portion of the study.

Who Should Participate in the Time-Out Process?

The time-out must involve the entire operative team. At a minimum, this includes the catheterization laboratory operator, their assistant, any anesthesia provider, and the circulating nurse. Participation with active (out-loud) verbal communication by all members of the team is required. ("I concur" is the proper acknowledgment.) In particular, if there is concern about a possible error, no one should be afraid to speak up to protect the patient. Even when there is only one person doing the procedure, a brief pause to confirm the correct patient, procedure, and site is appropriate. It is not necessary to engage others in this verification process if they would not otherwise be involved in the procedure.

The out-loud verbal acknowledgment is also an important safety behavior at other times for instructions given during the procedure and received by the circulating team. Active acknowledgment of orders eliminates confusion, redundant requests, and frustration.

The Reverse Time-Out or "I Need 2 Minutes"

The time-out before the procedure is a routine safety requirement. However, another kind of time-out is sometimes needed when the case goes too fast. This is especially true with overeager fellows and catheterization laboratory attending physicians who sometimes want to work so fast that they outstrip the ability of the catheterization laboratory team to keep up with their demands or become confused by conflicting or changing orders from the operators. Whenever this happens, anyone working in the laboratory can call a time-out, which is stated out loud as "I need 2 minutes." The operators should stop and take a breath. This gives the person (and the team) who called time-out a couple of minutes of uninterrupted time for them to get everything caught up and correct. For example, when the circulating nurse is asked, "Please give the patient NTG, give me a JR4 6 F, set the injector at 12 for 36, and show me the ECG…," it is clear that this is too much to do quickly enough for the smooth operation of the laboratory, and the nurse should call for a 2-minute time-out. The called 2-minute time-out is the request back to the operators to give the nurse, technician, or team 2 minutes to get all the steps, equipment, or setup going and correctly brought together. During complex procedures, the nurse can say, "I need 2 minutes to do xyz." Everyone will hear and should understand. The operators will relax and wait for the team to catch up. Of course the called time-out would not be appropriate if there were a critical situation in which the patient could not wait for an emergency drug or other life-sustaining intervention (e.g., LV support device or an intraaortic balloon pump [IABP] insertion).

Sterile Preparations

Cardiac catheterization occurs in an operating room environment, and all preparations for the procedure must be performed using aseptic technique, with personnel in scrubs, protective hats, masks, and gowns. Some laboratories do not require masks during the back-table setup.

Vascular Access Site Preparation

The most common vascular access sites are the right groin for the femoral approach and the right wrist for the radial artery approach. Of course, the left-side arteries are also available when needed. The usual sterile preparation begins by clipping the area of hair and vigorously applying an antiseptic solution. Shaving should be avoided because of micro-lacerations or abrasions breaking the skin barrier to infection.

During patient preparation, the staff should always be aware of the patient's need for privacy. Curtains in the viewing area should be drawn. The patient should be kept covered as much as possible. In addition, procedure rooms are typically cold; every effort should be made to keep the patient warm and comfortable.

Sterile Field Preparation and Patient Draping

Staff members assigned to assist the physician in the procedure put on hair and shoe covers and a surgical face mask and wash hands and forearms as a surgical scrub. They then put on a sterile surgical gown and gloves. An equipment stand is prepared in a sterile fashion to hold all the catheters and other equipment to be used during the procedure. At this time, a circulating staff member opens the sterile packaged catheters and necessary equipment not included in the sterile catheter laboratory pack is taken from a circulating nurse by the scrub nurse or technician. A sterile drape is placed over the patient, starting at the patient's upper chest and extending to the foot, covering the entire examination table. Special arm boards and drapes are used for radial procedures.

It is important for all personnel to understand sterile techniques to avoid accidentally contaminating any sterile fields. As a basic rule, no unsterile object may be passed over a sterile field. A sterile gown and gloves, rather than gloves alone, should be worn when preparing the back table and patient, especially for team members who are very short or wide or whose body may accidentally contact the sterile areas. When moving around a crowded angiographic room, all personnel should be careful to avoid bumping into or passing hands or arms over the sterile tray, table, or patient drapes. Personnel should not walk between the sterile table or equipment tray and the patient. Avoid touching the ends of catheters, extension tubes, or syringe tips in a sterile field or the exposed power injector syringe tip.

Rules for Observers in the Laboratory

Some hospitals have policies that limit nonhospital personnel from being in the catheterization laboratory without prior consent of the patient. Any observers in the angiographic room should respect the professional atmosphere and keep extraneous conversation to a minimum. Observers should adhere to the policy of the laboratory and wear scrubs or paper gowns and a lead apron as protection against scattered radiation. Observers should avoid sterile fields and should be aware of the precautions necessary for protection from blood and other body fluids.

No one but catheterization laboratory personnel should ever manipulate or adjust any device, equipment, or medication system in the laboratory. To prevent observers who are not laboratory personnel from becoming overly enthusiastic and attempting to assist the nurses or physicians, they should never be given sterile gloves. This is important to avoid potential liability for the laboratory, hospital, and staff.

Conscious Sedation for Invasive Cardiac Procedure

The purpose of conscious sedation is to minimize patient anxiety, discomfort, and pain associated with the procedure. The following criteria define conscious sedation:

1. The patient at no time loses protective reflexes.
2. The patient retains the ability to maintain an open airway continuously without help.
3. The patient responds appropriately to verbal and physical stimulation.

If the patient can no longer do the things listed, the sedative technique evolves to deep sedation or general anesthesia. At this point, the monitoring and care of the patient must be elevated to avoid an adverse outcome.

A conscious sedation protocol has four major components: (1) preprocedural baseline assessment, (2) drug dosage and administration, (3) patient monitoring, and (4) postprocedure monitoring and assessment and discharge criteria.

Preprocedural Assessment

Before the administration of sedative agents, the patient should have a complete assessment of his or her current physical condition. The clinician should pay particular attention to any preexisting conditions that would put the patient at risk for an adverse outcome if sedatives are administered. A preprocedural evaluation should include a review of the major organ systems, the time and type of the last oral intake, a history of drug and alcohol use, a history of smoking, and a history of previous experience with sedative agents.

Preprocedural fasting is the rule. Sedative agents may impair airway reflexes, placing the patient at increased risk for aspirating gastric contents. For elective procedures, these risks can be minimized by allowing sufficient time for gastric emptying before the procedure. The patient should be NPO for solids and nonclear liquids after midnight or at least 8 hours before the start of the procedure. Clear liquids may be appropriate 1 to 3 hours before the procedure, depending on the type and dose of the sedative agent to be used.

Physical Examination and Airway Assessment

An airway assessment should be part of the preprocedural routine. Most preprocedural checklists include the Mallampati classification, which is used to predict the ease of intubation. Mallampati scoring is as follows:

Class 1: full visibility of tonsils, uvula, and soft palate

Class 2: visibility of hard and soft palate, upper portion of tonsils, and uvula

Class 3: soft and hard palate and base of the uvula are visible

Class 4: only hard palate is visible

A high Mallampati score (class 4) is associated with more difficult intubation and a higher incidence of sleep apnea. Factors associated with difficult airway management also include:

1. A history of sleep apnea, snoring, or stridor
2. Dysmorphic jaw or facial features
3. Advanced rheumatoid arthritis
4. A short neck with limited extension caused by obesity, mass, or injury
5. Mouth or jaw irregularities or deformities, including loose or capped teeth or dentures.

American Society of Anesthesiologists Physical Status Classification

The American Society of Anesthesiologists Physical Status Classification (Table 1.5) is helpful in determining the patient's eligibility for conscious sedation. It uses a 1 to 5 classification range, with 1 being a healthy patient and 5 being a moribund patient. Procedural sedation is appropriate for patients in classes 1, 2, and

Table 1.5

American Society of Anesthesiologists Physical Status Classification.	
Class	**Description**
1	A healthy patient (e.g., varicose veins in an otherwise healthy patient)
2	A patient with mild systemic disease that in no way interferes with normal activity (e.g., controlled hypertension, controlled diabetes, chronic bronchitis)
3	A patient with severe systemic disease that is not incapacitating (e.g., insulin-dependent diabetes, angina, pulmonary insufficiency)
4	A patient with severe systemic disease that is a constant threat to life (e.g., cardiac failure, major organ insufficiency)
5	A moribund patient who is not expected to survive for 24 hours with or without surgery (e.g., intracranial hemorrhage in coma)

3. Patients in class 4 and higher are better suited for general anesthesia. There are several contraindications to conscious sedation that include:

1. Recent (<2 hour) ingestion of large food or fluid volumes
2. A physical class 4 or greater
3. A lack of support staff or monitoring equipment
4. A lack of experience/credentialing on the part of the clinician.

Monitoring Parameters

Level of Consciousness. The patient's level of consciousness should be assessed often before and during the procedure. The level of consciousness can be assessed by the patient's response to verbal commands or to light tactile stimulation. Once aroused, the patient should respond appropriately to verbal commands. The nurse or operator can assess this easily by periodically talking to the patient and listening to his or her response. When the patient's only response is reflex withdrawal from painful stimuli, deep sedation is evident, and special care must be taken to ensure patency of the airway, proper ventilation, and hemodynamic stability.

Pulmonary Ventilation. Pulmonary ventilation can be monitored by the observation of spontaneous respiratory activity or, when possible, auscultation of breathing sounds. During certain invasive procedures, direct monitoring of the respiratory rate is often difficult because of sterile drapes and equipment.

Oxygenation. Continuous assessment of the patient's blood oxygen saturation by pulse oximetry should be a part of any conscious sedation monitoring and assessment protocol. This monitor is only a tool and not a replacement for direct observation of the patient. There can be a 1-minute delay between the onset of hypoxia and the decrease in the monitor reading.

    End-tidal carbon dioxide monitoring measures exhaled carbon dioxide and is most commonly used in intubated patients receiving mechanical ventilation, but it is also used in nonintubated patients undergoing moderate or deep sedation. The measurement of end-tidal carbon dioxide (E_tCO_2), called *capnography*, is useful as an adjunct to other monitoring methods in detecting hypoventilation before pulse oximetry indicates oxygen desaturation. It is a more sensitive gauge of hypoventilation than visual observation. In procedural sedation, side-stream capnography equipment usually consists of sampling probes to measure gases from the nose and sometimes the mouth. Additional oxygen can be administered through the same cannula.

The Practice Guidelines for Sedation and Analgesia by Non-Anesthesiologists published by the American Society of Anesthesiologists (ASA) outlines the following areas for patient monitoring during moderate or deep sedation states: "During moderate or deep sedation, the adequacy of ventilation shall be evaluated by continual observation of qualitative clinical signs and monitoring for the presence of exhaled carbon dioxide unless precluded or invalidated by the nature of the patient, procedure, or equipment." The ASA amended its Standards for Basic Anesthetic Monitoring to include mandatory exhaled dioxide E_tCO_2 monitoring during both moderate and deep sedation to its existing requirement.[2]

Sedative agents may cause arrhythmias and hypotension. Although continuous ECG monitoring is performed during preprocedural patient preparations, blood pressure should also be monitored often at 1- to 2-minute intervals during the onset of sedation and 5- to 10-minute intervals during the procedure. Hemodynamics should return to baseline before discharge.

The Aldrete Scoring System (Table 1.6) can be used to assess the effects of sedation on the patient's major systems (neurologic, respiratory, and circulatory). A score of 0, 1, or 2 is given for level of activity, level of consciousness, respiratory ability, blood pressure, and color.

Table 1.6

Aldrete Scoring System				
Score	Activity	Respiration	Circulation	Conscious-ness	Color
2	Able to move four extremities	Able to breathe deeply and cough	BP ±20% of baseline	Fully alert and answers questions	Normal pink
1	Able to move two extremities	Limited respiratory effort (dyspnea)	BP ±20% to 50% of baseline	Arousable	Pale, dusky, blotchy
0	Not able to control any extremities	No spontaneous respiratory effort	BP >50% of baseline	Failure to elicit response	Frank cyanosis

BP, Blood pressure.

Table 1.7

First-Line Drugs for Conscious Sedation.				
Drug	Dose	Max	Onset (min)	Duration (min)
Morphine (narcotic analgesic)	1–2 mg	10 mg or 0.15 mg/kg	1–2	30–60
Meperidine (narcotic analgesic)	10–20 mg	100 mg or 1.5 mg/kg	1–2	20–40
Fentanyl (narcotic analgesic)	25 µg	200 µg or 3 µg/kg	1	10–15
Midazolam (sedative, amnesic)	0.5–1.0 mg	5–10 mg or 0.1 mg/kg	1–3	15–30

Drugs for Conscious Sedation

First-line drugs and dosages for conscious sedation are listed in Table 1.7.

Postprocedure Monitoring and Discharge Criteria

Patients who receive conscious sedation should be monitored for 1 to 2 hours before discharge. During this time the patient should be assessed and monitored with the same parameters used in the preprocedural assessment. When the patient returns to baseline, discharge is appropriate. The following discharge criteria should be met before the patient is sent back to the floor or home:

1. The Aldrete score has returned to baseline (summed Aldrete scores of 9 or 10).
2. At least 2 hours have elapsed since the last dose of sedative agents.
3. Vital signs have returned to baseline.
4. Ventilation (respiratory rate and oxygen saturation) has returned to baseline.
5. The patient is mentally alert, and all protective reflexes are intact.

Outpatients who are being discharged to home should be able to ambulate appropriately for their age and condition. An escort should be available, and the patient should be instructed about not driving a motor vehicle for an appropriate period.

Postcatheterization Check-Up

The operator should check on the patient several hours after the procedure. Vital signs should be normal. Low blood pressure is usually a result of diuresis and responds to normal saline. Tachycardia with low blood pressure indicates blood loss until proven otherwise. The arterial access site should be checked for pain and hematoma. The operator should check the groin site and distal pulses in legs or the wrist for loss of pulse. Urine output should be >30 mL/h. Low urine output may reflect unsatisfactory volume replacement or early onset of contrast-induced renal failure. A cool or painful extremity requires immediate assessment to determine whether thrombus, spasm, or vasoconstriction is responsible for arterial occlusion. Limb ischemia, including the arm for radial cases, or an enlarging hematoma requires urgent consultation with a vascular surgeon, repeat angiography, and at times an urgent return to the catheterization laboratory.

Angiogram Review

To provide the patient and family with an understanding of the coronary artery disease or other findings, a preliminary schematic diagram of the heart and coronary arteries can be provided. A similar diagram should be put in the chart to help others understand the findings. A catheterization instruction book is helpful and may contain a blank standard diagram (Fig. 1.4). The booklet explains the catheterization procedure and the possible meaning of various findings on the coronary angiogram. In some cases, reviewing the actual coronary cineangiograms with the patient and family members may be helpful. After discharge, the patient may wish to see the angiograms to understand the disease better and to ask questions and receive answers specifically with regard to future treatment (after the operator discusses the findings and plans with the referring or primary care physician). Taking the time to explain the findings by referring directly to the diagram or cineangiographic film is rewarding. "No one ever took time to explain my heart problem this way, and now I understand what is wrong" is a frequent comment. The risk of a patient becoming alarmed or depressed after viewing the cineangiogram has not been borne out by experience with thousands of patients and their families. The additional burden of taking the time to show the angiograms to the patient is worth the effort. In some busy laboratories, this approach may not be feasible, but with images on disks, almost every laboratory has an open computer to share the angiograms with the patient. The operator should always discuss the findings and possible recommendations with the primary

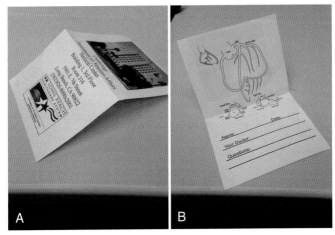

Fig. 1.4   Diagram for patient after cardiac catheterization. (A) Name and contact information of practitioner is included. (B) Details of angiogram are drawn on figure. (Reprinted with permission from *Cath Lab Digest.* Copyright HMP Communications.)

physician first because catheterization is principally a consultative service.

Special Preparations for Cardiac Catheterization

Table 1.8 lists conditions that require special preparations.

Contrast Media Reactions

The Committee on Safety of Contrast Media of the International Society of Radiology reported that in more than 300,000 patients the overall incidence of adverse reaction was 5% or less. Adverse reactions were found in 10% to 12% of patients with a history of allergy and in 15% of patients with reported reaction on previous x-ray examination. From these reports, major reactions do not tend to recur on reexamination, whereas minor reactions are more likely to be repeated. There are three types of contrast allergies (Box 1.4): (1) cutaneous and mucosal manifestations, (2) smooth muscle and minor anaphylactoid responses, and (3) cardiovascular and major anaphylactoid responses. Management of contrast reactions is summarized in Table 1.9.

Table 1.8

Conditions Requiring Special Preparations	
Condition	**Management**
1. Allergy	1. Allergy
a. Prior contrast studies	a. Contrast premedication
b. Iodine, fish	b. Contrast reaction algorithm
c. Premedication allergy	c. Hold premedication
d. Lidocaine	d. Use Marcaine (1 mg/mL)
2. Patients receiving anticoagulation (INR >1.5)	2. Defer procedure
	a. Vitamin K$^+$, 10 mEq/h
	b. Fresh frozen plasma
	c. Hold heparin
	d. Protamine for heparin
3. Diabetes	3. Hydration to increase urine output >50 mL/h; metformin held 48 hours; if renal insufficiency, postpone catheterization and consider urgency and risks of lactic acidosis
a. NPH insulin (protamine reaction)	
b. Renal function (prone to contrast-induced renal failure)	
c. Metformin usage	
4. Electrolyte imbalance (K$^+$, Mg^{2+})	4. Defer procedure, replenish, or correct electrolytes
5. Arrhythmias	5. Defer procedure, administer antiarrhythmics
6. Anemia	6. Defer procedure
	a. Control bleeding
	b. Transfuse
7. Dehydration	7. Hydration
8. Renal failure	8. Limit contrast
	a. Maintain high urine output
	b. Hydrate

INR, International normalized ratio; *NPH,* neutral protamine Hagedorn.

Box 1.4   Anaphylactoid Reactions to Contrast Medium.

Cutaneous and Mucosal

Angioedema
Flushing
Laryngeal edema
Pruritus
Urticaria

Cardiovascular

Arrhythmia
Hypotension (shock)
Vasodilation

Smooth Muscle

Bronchospasm
Gastrointestinal spasm
Uterine contraction

Table 1.9

Anaphylactoid Reaction Prophylaxis for Emergency Percutaneous Coronary Intervention			
Medication	**Dose**	**Route**	**Mechanism**
Standard Agents			
Methylprednisolone or	80–125 mg	IV	Antiinflammatory
Dexamethasone or	16 mg	IV	Antiinflammatory
Solu-Cortef	100 mg	IV	Antiinflammatory
Cimetidine	300 mg	IV	H_2 blockage
Benadryl	25–50 mg	IV or PO	H_1 blockage

Modified from Klein LW, Sheldon MW, Brinker J, et al. The use of radiographic contrast media during PCI: a focused review. A position statement of the Society of Cardiovascular Angiography and Interventions. *Cath Cardiovasc Intervent.* 2009;74:728–746.

Major reactions involving laryngeal or pulmonary edema are often accompanied by minor, or less severe, reactions. Although some reactions to a pretest contrast dose may be violent (but rarely life threatening), pretesting has been found to be of no value in determining who will have an adverse reaction.

Full emergency resuscitation equipment and a trained team should always be available for any patient receiving contrast media. Nonionic, low-osmolar ionic, or iso-osmolar contrast media have replaced ionic high-osmolar contrast media to minimize the possibility of adverse events related to contrast media (e.g., allergic reaction or contrast-induced nephropathy).

Patients reporting allergic reactions to contrast media should be premedicated with prednisone and diphenhydramine (Benadryl). The routine for the laboratory may vary, but common dosages include 60 mg of prednisone the night before and 60 mg of prednisone the morning of the procedure, with 50 mg of oral Benadryl given at the time of call to the catheterization laboratory. Pretreatment with corticosteroids to alleviate reactions to IV contrast media has been found to be helpful in reducing all types of reactions except those characterized predominantly by hives. Premedication may not completely prevent the occurrence of adverse reactions. Routine treatment of patients with prior allergic reactions with an H_2 blocker (e.g., cimetidine) does not appear to have any benefit. Patients with known prior anaphylactoid reactions to contrast dye should be pretreated with steroids and an H_2 blocker.

Protamine Reactions

Although protamine is used widely for reversing systemic heparinization after cardiac catheterization, major reactions simulating anaphylaxis can occur, albeit rarely. Minor protamine reactions may appear as back and flank pain or flushing with peripheral vasodilation and low blood pressure. Major reactions involve marked facial flushing and vasomotor collapse, which may be fatal. Patients taking NPH insulin have an increased sensitivity to protamine. The incidence of major protamine reactions in NPH insulin-dependent diabetics is 27% compared with 0.5% in patients with no history of insulin use. Diabetic patients receiving NPH insulin and patients with allergies to fish should not be given protamine after cardiac catheterization. If use of protamine is necessary for these patients, it should be administered cautiously in anticipation of a major reaction.

Contrast-Induced Renal Failure (Contrast-Induced Nephropathy)

Patients with diabetes or renal insufficiency or patients who are dehydrated from any cause are at risk of contrast-induced renal failure. Advance preparations to limit contrast-induced renal failure include hydration and maintenance of large-volume urine flow ($\geq$200 mL/h). These patients should be hydrated intravenously the night before the procedure. After the catheterization procedure, IV fluids should be continued liberally unless intravascular volume overload is a problem. Furosemide (Lasix), mannitol, and calcium channel blockers are not helpful in reducing contrast-induced renal failure (Box 1.5). In the recovery area and medical floor, the patient's urine output should be monitored. If output falls and is not responsive to increased IV fluids, renal insufficiency should be suspected. A consultation with a nephrologist may be helpful. Nonionic or low-osmolar contrast agents have a lower

---

Box 1.5   Pharmacologic Prophylaxis for Contrast-Induced Nephropathy.

Detrimental

Furosemide
Mannitol
Endothelin receptor antagonist

Ineffective

Fenoldopam
Dopamine
Calcium channel blockers

Atrial natriuretic peptide
L-Arginine

Merits Further Study

Theophylline
Statins
Ascorbic acid
Prostaglandin E_1

Modified from Stacul F, Adam A, Becker CR, et al. Strategies to reduce the risk of contrast-induced nephropathy. *Am J Cardiol.* 2006;98(suppl):59K–77K.

incidence of contrast-induced nephropathy than ionic agents. Suggested contrast media limits are 5 mL of contrast per kilogram body weight/SCr (serum creatinine, mg/dL) maximum dose of 300 mL.

Insulin-Dependent Diabetic Patients

For patients taking subcutaneous insulin (NPH, regular), an overnight fast with their normal dose of insulin could cause hypoglycemia. The dose of NPH insulin should be decreased by 50% for patients coming to the catheterization laboratory when they are NPO in the early morning. Remember that patients receiving NPH insulin are at higher risk of protamine reactions.

Diabetic Patients Using Metformin

Metformin (Glucophage) is an analog of phenformin, an oral anti-hyperglycemic agent that was withdrawn from the market because of the risk of lactic acidosis. Rare cases of metformin-associated lactic acidosis have been reported in diabetic patients with chronic renal insufficiency. Contraindications and precautions in the product literature state the following:

> *Parenteral contrast studies with iodinated materials can lead to acute renal failure and have been associated with lactic acidosis in patients receiving Glucophage. Therefore in patients in whom any such study is planned, Glucophage should be withheld for at least 48 hours before and 48 hours subsequent to the procedure and reinstituted only after renal function has been reevaluated and found to be normal.*

Metformin is contraindicated in patients with renal dysfunction, as determined by elevated serum creatinine levels. There is no evidence that withholding metformin for 48 hours before a contrast procedure in patients with normal renal function provides any clinical benefit.

Guidelines for Use of Metformin and Iodinated Contrast Material (Adopted from the University of Kentucky)

A. Elective procedures

1. If renal function is normal (serum creatinine <1.5 mg/dL), contrast material may be administered parenterally without discontinuing metformin before the study. The patient should be hydrated.

2. After the study, the patient should consult with their physician before resuming metformin. In most cases, the patient may resume metformin after 48 hours unless there is evidence of

acute renal failure or the patient is at high risk of renal failure related to:

   a. Low cardiac output

   b. Hypovolemia

   c. Contrast administration (<72 hours) or excess contrast load >3 mg/kg

   d. Cyclosporine therapy

  3. If renal function is abnormal (serum creatinine ≥1.5 mg/dL), the contrast study should be postponed for patients who have received metformin within 48 hours.

B. Emergency procedures

  1. If renal function is normal, the study may proceed as with elective procedures.

  2. If renal function is abnormal, the relative risks versus benefits must be considered and the following precautions taken:

   a. Discontinue metformin.

   b. Hydrate the patient during and after the procedure (IV saline 1 mL/kg/h).

   c. Increase urine output (if possible).

   d. Minimize the volume of low-osmolality contrast material.

   e. Monitor renal function closely after the procedure.

   f. If acute renal failure occurs after the procedure, do not resume metformin.

   g. Monitor the patient for signs of lactic acidosis (e.g., abdominal pain, obtundation, hypotension, hypercapnia) when metformin is resumed. Arterial blood gas analysis and measurement of plasma lactate, glucose, and ketones (including β-hydroxybutyrate dehydrogenase) confirm the diagnosis. Early hemodialysis may be needed.

Team Approach to Cardiac Catheterization

Physician Viewpoint

A new person in the cardiac catheterization laboratory should observe the variety of catheterization procedures for at least 10 consecutive cases. This observation period gives the new member of the catheterization team a chance to appreciate the timing, rhythm, and recurrent steps that are required of each member as an integral part of the laboratory. Each laboratory has an individual routine that may vary among operators. No one laboratory routine is best, but learning the routine and joining the team smoothly are important first steps.

The new operator-in-training learns that the attending physician is ultimately responsible for all aspects of the procedure and must check each step of the procedure to ensure accuracy and safety. A similar approach can be recommended for new nurses and technicians.

Learning the Routine Overview

1. The patient is seen by a member of the cardiac catheterization team, indications for the procedure are discussed, risks are explained, consent is obtained, special preparations are made, and orders and chart notes are written.

2. The patient arrives in the laboratory, greeted by the nurses, moved from a holding area into the angiographic suite, and prepared and draped in a sterile fashion. The physician may or may not participate with the nurses in the draping.

3. Arterial and venous access is obtained depending on the patient's clinical problem and the routine of the laboratory.

4. Right-sided heart catheterization, coronary angiography, and left-sided ventriculography are performed as indicated by the clinical situation with the appropriate hemodynamic and angiographic measurements. PCI may proceed ad hoc if the patient has consented in advance.

5. At the conclusion of data collection, angiographic study, and possible intervention, the catheters are removed.

6. For femoral access procedures, hemostasis may be obtained in the laboratory with a vascular closure device (VCD). Alternatively, the patient may be transferred to the holding area where the sheath is pulled, and hemostasis is obtained with manual compression. The patient is returned to his or her room. For 5-F to 6-F femoral sheaths, recovery usually requires 4 hours or more of bed rest. For procedures using sheaths of 5 F or less or procedures in which hemostasis is obtained with a VCD, 1 to 2 hours of bed rest with 4 hours of observation before discharge is usually sufficient.

7. For radial artery access and hemostasis, the patient can sit in a reclining chair and after premedication has worn off can be discharged (usually within 2 to 3 hours).

8. Several hours after the procedure, a member of the catheterization team checks the patient's arterial access site(s), identifies (and treats) any problems that may have occurred, and presents

the preliminary findings again to the patient and family after discussion with the referring physician. Unless the operator is also the primary care physician, the catheterization team should discuss results and management options with the patient's primary care physician before taking the patient's treatment into their own hands.

9. Preparations for discharge (that day or the following morning) or for further procedures are made after the attending and referring physicians have reviewed the cardiac catheterization data.

Nurse and Technician Viewpoint: The Catheterization Team

The composition of a catheterization team varies among laboratories. The smallest functioning unit would consist of a physician, an assisting physician or nurse, a nurse circulator or recording technician assigned to the laboratory, and a nurse outside the laboratory able to assist. For more specialized procedures, the team is increased appropriately.

Personnel are trained specifically to provide technical support necessary for the safe performance of cardiac catheterization procedures. Several disciplines are called on to provide this support. Each member of the team assumes an important role during the procedure.

Personnel and Functions

1. A circulating nurse or technologist must be capable of assisting the physician in all aspects of care of the patient, including routine cardiovascular emergency care.

2. A scrub nurse or technologist is needed at the x-ray table to assist the operating physician with all equipment and supplies used in catheterization. This person assists in the exchanging of catheters and other specialized maneuvers.

3. A radiologic technologist is trained in x-ray principles related to cardiovascular procedures, cineangiography, fluoroscopy, and the use of power contrast injectors and digital cineangiographic imaging systems.

4. A monitoring and recording technologist is responsible for monitoring and recording the ECG and hemodynamic data and keeping the physician apprised of changes in cardiac pressures and rhythms. The technician must be able to interpret pressure and ECG waveforms and operate all physiologic recording equipment.

Rule for Success: Communication in the Catheterization Laboratory

Communication between team members is critical. Communication at the beginning of the day with team members will improve efficiency. Keeping the physician informed about the status of the procedure will enhance their ability to manage time and minimize delays in arriving at the laboratory. Likewise, communication from the physician to the staff will assist their ability to move patients into and out of the laboratory to satisfy the needs of the numerous operators and types of procedures and to manage the availability of special equipment.

Communication at the table during the procedure will also improve efficiency. The informed team can prepare the equipment, anticipate catheter and pharmacologic needs, and shorten the time to set up. By letting the team know where the operator is in the procedure, the next steps can be anticipated. The recording technologists appreciate these announcements for documentation. The staff should be "in the game," watching and listening to be ready to get the needed supplies without undue delay. On the other hand, communication from the room back to the table improves efficiency by clearly acknowledging requests from the operating table, reducing redundant and unnecessary repetition of orders. Clear and open two-way communication, especially under critical portions of procedures, also leads to improved safety through error reduction and timely performance of the catheterization. Pointers are:

1. The physician as well as the staff set the tone of communication in the laboratory, like a pilot with the "right stuff": cool, clear, and confident.

2. Orders from the table should be acknowledged clearly by those designated to carry out the order. Just as military efficiency is built on this rule, so should that of the well-run laboratory. It is disturbing to request medications and supplies and not know whether someone has heard the request and is attending to it.

3. Repeat orders to reduce errors.

4. When at the table, announce what the "table" is doing. For example, "Left Jud going up…,", which the recording person then acknowledges.

Optimal Staffing and Cross Training of Personnel

Not every case of coronary angiography requires all of the previously mentioned people to be present. In most laboratories, three assistants are required for most catheterization procedures: One person is scrubbed and assists the physician at the table; one person is not scrubbed and circulates in the room, providing patient care (nurse responsibilities) and procuring any supplies that are needed during the procedure; and one person performs the duties of recording technician and radiologic technologist by selecting proper cineangiographic programs and hemodynamic recording functions as required.

Cross-training of the individuals in the catheterization laboratory helps maintain morale and confidence in each job described. Cross-training also means that each individual in the laboratory is competent to start up the laboratory and assist in operation on an emergency 24-hour basis when needed.

Cardiopulmonary Resuscitation

All members of the catheterization team should be fully trained in cardiopulmonary resuscitation (CPR) and the use of defibrillators. In some laboratories, advanced cardiovascular life support (ACLS) training and biannual renewal of certification is required. An algorithm for CPR in the catheterization laboratory is presented in Chapter 8.

The Catheterization Laboratory and Code Team Interaction

The practice of calling and running a code in the catheterization laboratory varies depending on the hospital type, staff composition and experience, and leadership of the catheterization laboratory nurses and physicians. The type of assistance brought to a code in the catheterization laboratory may also depend on the hospital type and staffing, hospital policy, and whether the code occurs during weekend or off hours.

Who's in Charge in the Catheterization Laboratory?

The physician performing the procedure is in charge of directing the care of the patient at all times. Whether the patient is experiencing ventricular tachycardia/ventricular fibrillation (VT/VF) or hypotension from tamponade, cardiogenic shock, or hypovolemia (from bleeding or anaphylaxis), the attending catheterization laboratory physician calls the shots. However, conventional critical care theory and practice state that the code leader should be responsible for nothing besides the resuscitation efforts. The cardiologist performing an emergency PCI on a patient in full arrest may not be the best person to monitor and decide whether and when drugs such as lidocaine should be given, CPR held , and so on. On the other hand, most cardiologists would never want to be told by a code leader that CPR cannot be held for a minute to obtain vascular access, or that CPR efforts should cease. Most now agree that joint decision-making is necessary.

The attending physician may recognize that the best person to intubate his patient is an anesthesiologist or an experienced pulmonary or emergency room physician. When the situation becomes critical and the physician in charge requests more help to manage the patient's airway or perform chest compressions, the quickest way to get this help may be to call a code. Alternatively, the laboratory may have an airway emergency system that activates the anesthesiologist on call for immediate airway help. The catheterization laboratory team will continue to manage the patient while waiting for anesthesia or the emergency room physicians. In the laboratory, the patient's ventilatory needs can temporarily be managed with bag mask ventilation. Hemodynamic support will be maintained with the administration of ACLS medications and defibrillation as indicated. After intubation, it remains very helpful to have respiratory therapy (RT) technicians support the airway placement and ventilator management. RT technicians are usually key members of most code blue teams.

Upon arrival of the code team in the laboratory, the attending physician should identify the problem to the code team, ask for the appropriate person to help with the problem (usually ventilation), and continue to direct the code. If the physician cannot attend to all of these aspects, they should designate a code leader and return to the management of the interventional cardiac procedure. The designated code team leader and the person who will be in charge must be announced to the laboratory team as they continue to work with the patient still undergoing the procedure. In airline safety parlance, despite whatever the emergency, "someone still has to fly the plane."

Patient Viewpoint

Teaching Before the Procedure

Most patients undergoing cardiac catheterization have vague and often confused ideas of how the procedure is performed. They know little regarding what information will be provided about their cardiac status. Procedural patient teaching is important to allay fears and to provide optimal patient care, cooperation, and satisfaction.

The teaching should start at the time the patient enters the hospital. The nurse on the floor should provide information on what the patient can expect while being cared for on the floor before and after the cardiac catheterization. Topics such as diet, medications, IV therapy, and postprocedural bed rest should be discussed.

The nurse should explain step-by-step how the procedure is performed, how long it will take, and what the patient should expect regarding sensations and discomfort associated with the procedure. A prepared booklet (sometimes with a videotape) explaining the procedure should be given to the patient to read before the procedure. This booklet reinforces the verbal teaching done by the nurse (e.g., the steps of the catheterization, breath holding, and types of equipment that the patient will see). When possible, the nurse should see the patient first. The information given by the nurse may stimulate questions that the patient can ask when the physician arrives to speak to the patient. Some laboratories may not have the resources to send a staff member to do this type of teaching. If that is the case, the floor nurse should be well versed in catheterization laboratory techniques to provide adequate patient teaching.

The physician's role in patient education should focus on four areas. First, the physician should make clear to the patient why the procedure is being performed. Second, the patient should be told what information the cardiac catheterization will provide. Third, the patient should be told which treatment options are available when a diagnosis is made. Fourth, the physician should discuss the possible risks and potential complications of the procedure. The risks, benefits, and alternatives to cardiac catheterization should be discussed with the patient and family. After this has been done, the physician obtains the written informed consent from the patient. The physician has the final patient responsibility. It is neither the nurse's nor the technician's job to obtain consent.

Teaching in the Laboratory

Teaching should continue when the patient has arrived in the catheterization holding area. The team members should introduce themselves and explain their jobs. A staff member should orient the patient to the x-ray suite and explain briefly the function of the various pieces of equipment. While in the laboratory, the patient should be encouraged to communicate freely with the staff and physician. It is important that the patient inform the staff of any pain or discomfort during the procedure.

Patients are often overwhelmed by the mere thought of such an invasive procedure and may have difficulty digesting all of the information that will be given. Teaching sessions should be limited to 10 to 15 minutes, with important points stressed two or three times. A well-informed patient is less anxious, and this makes the procedure much easier and more comfortable for the patient, the physician, and staff members.

Team Teaching and Conferences

The educational experience of the staff and physician is enhanced by a daily or at least a weekly cardiac catheterization conference. These conferences emphasize to the physicians and technical staff the relationship of clinical data to the hemodynamic and angiographic data. Review of data and discussion of various therapies (e.g., medicine, surgery, and PCIs) provide an excellent opportunity to learn from colleagues who share cases of educational value. With the complexity of an anticipated procedure, such as TAVR, an organized heart team of the various participating disciplines become critical to good planning and good outcomes.

Equipment in the Catheterization Laboratory

Figures 1.5 to 1.7 show the catheterization laboratory and equipment (also see Chapter 3 for more detail).

Fluoroscopic Imaging System

A high-resolution, image-intensifying television system with digital cineangiographic capabilities is the eyes of the cardiovascular laboratory. The fluoroscopic image comes from a C-arm, which is a semicircular support with the x-ray tube at one end and the image intensifier at the other. Rotation of the C-arm allows viewing over a wide range of different angles. The patient is placed in the center of the semicircle that can be moved 180 degrees around the patient as needed to visualize the heart. Two C-arms, side-by-side, are called *biplane* and, when used with a double monitoring system, can provide visualization of the heart from two different angles at the same time. The fluoroscopic and physiologic recorders have sets of display television monitors.

X-Ray Table

The patient is positioned on a special table that is easily panned under the fluoroscopes during angiography. The tables have bearings and brakes activated by hand controls at the end or side of the table. The table extends from its base to permit the under table

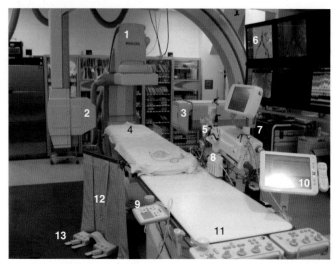

Fig. 1.5   Equipment components of the cardiac catheterization laboratory: *1*, Fluoroscope anterior-posterior (AP) tube, AP projection; *2*, fluoroscope, lateral x-ray generator; *3*, fluoroscope, lateral front panel image intensifier; *4*, patient table; *5*, contrast media power injector; *6*, display screen, fluoroscopy, hemodynamic, intravascular ultrasound (IVUS) imaging, and fractional flow reserve (FFR) measurement; *7*, crash cart; *8*, pressure transducer holder and oximeter; *9*, touch panel control for IVUS/FFR; *10*, touch panel control for x-ray system; *11*, positioning control for x-ray table and fluoroscope; *12*, wedge shield under table; *13*, foot pedal control for x-ray fluoroscope.

tube to cover a large area of the patient during the imaging examination. Patient weight limits for cardiac catheterization laboratories are set to prevent damage to the table machinery that has free-floating tabletop bearings permitting translation in the horizontal, vertical, and tilting directions. For cardiac catheterization laboratories in the United States, weight limits for minimum, mean, and maximum patient weights have been reported to be 160 kg, 198.9 kg, and 250 kg (350 lb, 437.5 lb, and 550 lb, respectively). At least three to five patients per hospital per year are rejected for being over their laboratory's weight limit.

Physiologic Hemodynamic Recorder

In addition to observing and recording images of the heart during catheterization, it is necessary to observe and record the ECG and

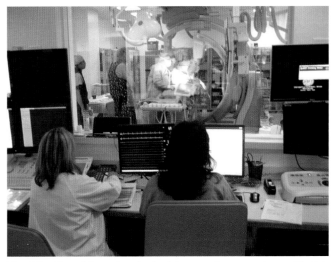

Fig. 1.6 View of the catheterization laboratory from control room. Multiple monitoring screens for hemodynamic recording, intravascular ultrasound (IVUS) imaging, fractional flow reserve (FFR), and procedure documentation are in front of the nurse and technician.

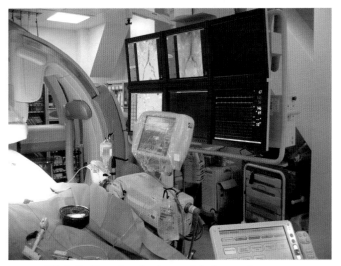

Fig. 1.7 View of contrast power injector monitor screen.

various blood pressures within the cardiovascular system. A reliable ECG and pressure monitoring system is essential for the safety of the patient and collection of hemodynamic information.

Contrast Power Injector

A high-pressure contrast media injector is needed to administer a large bolus of contrast media into the left ventricle (10–20 mL/s), pulmonary arteries (10–25 mL/s), or aortic arch (40–60 mL/s). When properly set and flushed, the power injector can be used to inject contrast media into the coronary arteries (3–8 mL/s). Some injector systems also incorporate a pressure transducer and have replaced traditional manifolds with stopcocks.

Crash Cart and Defibrillator

Every cardiovascular laboratory is equipped with an emergency crash cart near the x-ray table. The crash cart contains emergency drugs, oxygen, airways, suction apparatus, and other emergency equipment.

A defibrillator should be charged and ready for use during a procedure. The defibrillator must be tested daily and kept at close range for prompt use. Electrode gel, temporary pacemakers, and new electrode patches should be on every cart.

Sterile Equipment and Supplies

The angiographer works from a sterile pack or tray that contains the various supplies needed to perform the procedure. The pack contains syringes and needles, local anesthetic, basins for flushing solutions, small drapes and towels, clamps, scalpels, pressure manifolds, and connecting tubing (Fig. 1.8). These trays may be made up at the hospital or prepackaged by various suppliers.

Training Requirements
Cardiovascular Technologist Training Requirements in Cardiac Catheterization

Cardiovascular technology is a field recognized by the American Medical Association. The cardiovascular technologist specializing in invasive cardiovascular technology is a health care professional who, through the use of specific high-technology equipment and at the direction of a qualified physician, performs procedures on patients leading to the diagnosis and treatment of congenital and acquired heart disease and peripheral vascular

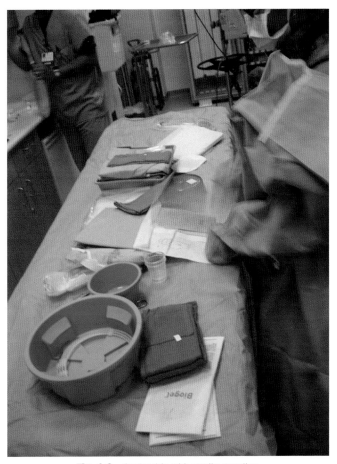

Fig. 1.8 Back table with sterile supplies.

disease. The technologist is proficient in the use of physiologic analytical equipment during diagnostic and therapeutic procedures. The cardiovascular technologist is trained in advanced life support techniques because the patient population under study is often at increased risk of cardiopulmonary arrest. The technologist, through established methodology of diagnostic examinations, creates a database from which a correct anatomic and physiologic diagnosis may be developed for each patient. The invasive cardiovascular technologist is a highly specialized diagnostician of the various presentations of cardiovascular disease. A list of procedures performed in the catheterization laboratory is provided in Appendix A.

Scope of Practice

The invasive cardiovascular technologist performs diagnostic procedures involving patients in the invasive cardiovascular laboratory (and coronary care and medical-surgical intensive care environments, if needed). The technologist may also assist a qualified physician in the performance of procedures in specialized clinics. The duties of the technicians and nurses in the laboratory often cross over but everyone should review the particular scope of their practice (i.e., what they can and cannot do alone and under the direction of a physician) within the specific hospital and laboratory. Nurses, unlike technologists, are the only people who are responsible for administration of medications and patient monitoring unless specific provisions are made to the contrary.

The scope of practice in any laboratory can also be divided into tasks performed by the nurse/technician without direct physician supervision, tasks performed with remote physician supervision (e.g., VCD), tasks with direct supervision (e.g., critical procedures, such as seating an angiographic catheter), and tasks that should be performed only by physicians (e.g., PCI and use of complex devices). For catheterization laboratories, there is no gold standard of practice patterns across the nation. Local practice establishes catheterization laboratory standards. The scope of what can be done in the catheterization laboratory comes from several important interacting competencies and laws:

1. Nurse/technician individual competence
2. Physician competence
3. Hospital policies
4. Health care regulatory laws, the most important of which is that it is illegal to practice medicine without a license.

Nurse/technician duty requirements can be viewed as tasks within the three stages of the catheterization experience:

1. Preprocedure setup and preparation
2. Critical procedures (the angiogram, hemodynamic study, and percutaneous intervention)
3. Postprocedure care (including access site management)

1. Preprocedure duties: These consist of checking clinically important aspects related to the patient entering the laboratory (consent, laboratory tests, indications, complicating conditions such as drug or food allergies, pulses and records of prior procedures with their associated problems, or access or contrast reaction). The nurse/technician should be knowledgeable, able to communicate clearly and sympathetically, and compulsive enough to collect this information to protect the patient from medical misadventure.

   Once in the room and on the table, nurse/technician duties include IV access, groin preparation, ECG monitoring, and hemodynamic setups. Preprocedural and intraprocedural medication knowledge and administration are critical. All personnel in the laboratory should be familiar with the scope of these activities. Critical procedures begin with the arterial puncture.

2. Critical procedures: Because physicians are responsible for everything that happens during the critical procedures, their competence is always on the line. The physician's trust in the laboratory personnel also is part of this competence. The transfer of critical procedures to competent technicians requires time, effort, education, and physician trust. The variations on these components form the standard of practice in the laboratory for that particular case.

   a. Noncritical tasks of critical procedures: (A noncritical task during a critical procedure means that the task is not required to be done by a physician and generally is not life threatening. But remember that anything done wrong or poorly in the laboratory can potentially be life threatening.) These tasks include performing angiography, contrast injection during angiography, and hemodynamic studies (pulling back catheters during hemodynamic recording is a noncritical task of a critical procedure). For PCI, passing angioplasty guidewires falls into the task category of critical procedure (needing direct physician supervision). Angioplasty balloon inflation is a noncritical task performed by an assistant or the operator. For special devices such as intraaortic balloon pumps, LV mechanical Impella pumps, rotoblators, AngioJets, thrombus aspiration systems, cutting balloons, filter wires, and so forth, concentrated expertise is required. These device tasks are critical procedures and fall to the physician. However, in some laboratories, physician experience (and selected device competence) with an infrequently used device may be less than that of the nurses/technicians working with the numerous other physicians on a daily basis.

b. What should be the scope of practice in this situation? The physician selecting the device is still responsible for all aspects of its use and complications. The nurse/technician and the laboratory itself will be at risk should they take on the placement and use of a specialty device with which the physician is not entirely competent, comfortable, and certified. These activities fall outside the scope of nurse/technician practice. Assistance with these critical procedures is needed, but solo or direct performance by a trained technician, even with direct supervision, is questionable, mainly for the reasons that this is part of the practice of cardiovascular medicine and the ethically difficult explanation of complications should they occur.

A physician who is not comfortable with a special technique or procedure required in the course of a catheterization should not be performing a critical procedure that may require this technique. For example, if a physician is not comfortable with a filter wire and has not achieved competence in the device use, the filter wire should not be placed by a technician requiring that person to perform the critical placement and recovery. If a complication occurs, who takes the responsibility?

3. Postprocedure duties: For vascular closure, the physician is responsible for arterial closure either by compression or a closure device. Manual/mechanical access site compression is usually delegated to the staff with indirect physician supervision (indirect supervision indicates that the physician is in the area but not immediately in the room). However, in some laboratories, the nurses/technicians are trained on VCD, certified (and trusted) by the physician and hospital policy, and permitted to close the artery alone, often with the physician in the control room (i.e., they are indirectly supervised).

Emergency Life Support

The cardiovascular technologist is proficient in basic life support techniques as recommended by the American Heart Association as follows:

1. Techniques of CPR, cardioversion, or defibrillation;
2. Management of the airway, including orotracheal and nasotracheal intubation and bag-mask ventilation;
3. Proficiency in the preparation and delivery of emergency medications by means of IV line placement and IV infusion, including cardioactive medications at the request of a qualified physician.

Preparation, Inventory, Maintenance, and Sterile Techniques

The invasive cardiovascular technologist is proficient in the preparation of the patient for all procedures and for the maintenance, inventory, stocking, and sterile preparation of all equipment, parts, catheter devices, and room preparations for each procedure:

1. Information and support to the patient before, during, and after each procedure, including sterile preparation of the patient.
2. Cleaning, packaging, and sterilization of all sundry catheterization trays and ancillary area equipment.
3. Maintenance of the sterile field during such procedures.
4. Preparation, recording, interpretation, and filing of all procedural protocols and reports.
5. Ordering all disposable supplies necessary for each procedure.
6. Retrieval of data regarding individual patients and disease entities for clinical and research purposes.

Equipment Used in the Invasive Cardiovascular Laboratory

The invasive cardiovascular technologist is proficient in the operation and maintenance of all diagnostic and therapeutic equipment used for procedures, including electrical safety for each piece of equipment. The equipment listed is neither all-inclusive nor exclusive to the various types and brands of equipment used in the cardiovascular laboratory areas.

1. Physiologic equipment
   a. ECG/pressure recorder/analyzer (with computer interfaces)
   b. Pressure transducers
   c. Electrocardiographic interfaces
   d. Cardiac output thermodilution computer
   e. Blood gas and oxygen content and saturation analyzer
2. Angiographic equipment
   a. Cineangiography operations
   b. Digital imaging interfaces
   c. Contrast media pressure injector
3. Temporary pacemakers
   a. External and transvenous pacemakers
   b. Connecting cables

4. Left ventricular support devices
   a. intraaortic balloon pumps
   b. LV catheter support pumps (e.g., Impella)
   c. cardiopulmonary bypass systems (e.g., TandemHeart, ECMO)
   d. consoles
5. Emergency (code) cart equipment
   a. medications
   b. defibrillator

Medications Used in Coronary Angiography

This section describes common medications used in the cardiac catheterization laboratory. It is not intended to be all-inclusive, and the reader is encouraged to review the doses, indications, contraindications, and side effects in more detail. A list of the medications commonly used is provided in Box 1.6.

Box 1.6   Medications Used in the Cardiac Catheterization Laboratory.[a]

Inotropic Agents

Digitalis: 0.125 to 0.25 mg IV >4 hours apart
Dobutamine: 2 to 10 µg/kg/min IV drip
Dopamine: 2 to 10 µg/kg/min IV drip
Epinephrine: 1:10,000 IV

Antiarrhythmic Agents, Anticholinergic Agents, β-Blockers, Calcium Blockers

Adenosine: 5 to 12 mg IV bolus
Amiodarone: 150 mg IV × 10 min (15 mg/min)
Atropine: 0.6 to 1.2 mg IV
Diltiazem: 10 mg IV
Esmolol: 4 to 24 mg/kg IV drip (β-blocker)
Lidocaine: 50 to 100 mg IV bolus; 2 to 4 mg/min IV drip
Propranolol: 1 mg bolus; 0.1 mg/kg in three divided doses (β-blocker)
Verapamil: 2 to 5 mg IV; may repeat dose to 10 mg (calcium channel blocker)

Analgesic Agents, Sedatives

Diazepam: 2 to 5 mg IV
Diphenhydramine: 25 to 50 mg IV
Meperidine: 12.5 to 50 mg IV

Box 1.6   Medications Used in the Cardiac Catheterization Laboratory. (Continued)

Morphine sulfate: 2.5 mg IV
Naloxone: 0.5 mg IV

Anticoagulants

Heparin: 2000 to 5000 U IV; 1000 U/h IV drip; 40–70 U/kg for PCI
Bivalirudin bolus: 0.75 mg/kg with infusion of 1.75 mg/kg/h

Antiplatelet Agents

Clopidogrel: 600 mg loading with 75 mg daily PO
Prasugrel: 60 mg loading with 10 mg daily PO
Ticagrelor: 180 mg with 90 mg q 12 h PO loading
IV Abciximab: 0.25 mg/kg IV bolus given 10 to 60 minutes before PCI with
    a continuous infusion of 0.125 µg/kg/min (to a maximum of 10 µg/min)
    for 12 hours
IV Eptifibatide: Patients >120 kg, maximum bolus of 22.6 mg with infusion
    of 15 mg/h; patients with renal impairment (CrCl <50 mL/min) should
    receive the standard 180 mcg/kg loading dose followed by infusion at
    1 mcg/kg/min
IV Tirofiban: High-dose bolus 25 mcg/kg over 3 minutes with 0.15 mcg/kg/
    min for up to 18 hours; in patients with CrCl ≤60 mL/min, give 25 mcg/
    kg over 3 minutes and then 0.075 mcg/kg/min

Vasodilators

Nitroglycerin: 1/150 sublingual 100 to 300 µg IC
Nitroprusside: 5 to 50 µg/kg/min IV

Vasoconstrictors

Metaraminol: 10 mg in 100 mL saline, 1 mL IV
Phenylephrine: 0.1 to 0.5 mg bolus, 100 to 180 µg/min IV drip
Norepinephrine: 1:10,000 IV, 1 mL doses IV

CrCl, Creatinine clearance; *IC,* intracoronary; *IV,* intravenous; *PCI,* percutaneous coronary intervention; *PO,* orally.

[a]The list is not meant to be all-inclusive nor to exclude emergency life-support techniques or standards.

Anticoagulation and Antiplatelet Agents for Cardiac Catheterization

Heparin

The appropriate doses of heparin and measurement of satisfactory anticoagulation for catheterization are dependent on the clinical needs. For routine diagnostic procedures from the radial approach, some suggest 40 to 70 U/kg. Heparin is satisfactory for patients in whom a prolonged (>20 minute arterial time) catheterization procedure is anticipated or in whom prior clinical indications for use of heparin exist (e.g., acute coronary syndromes [ACSs] with patients on glycoprotein [GP] IIb/IIIa blockers, thrombotic tendency, known severe peripheral vascular disease, and/or embolic phenomenon on previous study). For most femoral procedures, additional heparin (beyond that included in heparinized flush solutions) is omitted from routine left-sided heart catheterization when the procedure is performed in a timely manner.

Heparin reversal with protamine sulfate should be reserved for patients without fish allergy or previous use of NPH insulin. Low-molecular-weight heparin has replaced unfractionated heparin in some circumstances and is partially reversible with protamine.

Warfarin

While warfarin is not given in the catheterization laboratory, the management of patients receiving warfarin undergoing cardiac catheterization is a common problem because of the increased risk of procedure-related bleeding. In a patient with an elevated international normalized ratio (INR), femoral access is potentially associated with an increased risk of bleeding and access site complications, especially after PCI. This issue is not as great a concern when using radial artery access.

In general, cardiac catheterization should not proceed until the INR is <1.8 but the appropriate level is specific to the local hospital practice. The cessation of warfarin and potential clotting problems must be balanced against increased bleeding risks during the procedure. Annala and colleagues reported on 258 patients on warfarin therapy in two centers with extensive experience in uninterrupted warfarin and in one center with a policy of preprocedural warfarin pause (Annala et al. 2008). Radial artery access was used 56% of the time in the uninterrupted warfarin group and 60% of the time in the controlled warfarin pause group. There was no difference between the two groups in access site bleeding complications (1.9% vs. 1.6%) or major cerebrovascular or cardiovascular events (0.4% vs. 0.8%). The heparin-bridged patients had higher INR levels than the uninterrupted warfarin group (2.3 vs. 1.9) and had higher access site bleeding complications (1.7% vs. bridging therapy of 8.3%). Access site complications were more common in the supratherapeutic anticoagulant group with INRs >3 (9.1% vs. 1.5%, $P<0.05$).

If necessary and in experienced centers, access coronary angiography during uninterrupted therapeutic warfarin anticoagulation can be performed safely, especially from the radial approach. However, concern will always exist about potential bleeding, not only at the access site but also from cardiac perforation and venous or arterial vascular injury, or from spontaneous retroperitoneal bleeding.

Some laboratories use the following strategy. For patients who must remain on warfarin for strong clinical indications, catheterization is performed with the INR between 1.5 and 2, thus achieving continued therapy without excessive risk. If the INR must be maintained between 2 and 3, the radial artery access is considered as the first approach, or femoral access is performed with accurate (lower rather than higher) puncture and anticipation of using a secure vascular closure device. Of course, the traditional approach of heparin as a bridging therapy after stopping warfarin until the INR is <1.8 and then proceeding to catheterization, while less than optimal, can still be useful.

Bivalirudin (Angiomax)

Bivalirudin is a direct thrombin inhibitor that can be used in place of heparin, particularly for ACSs with a reduced bleeding risk. Bivalirudin is a synthetic peptide that is potent, highly specific, and reversibly inhibits both circulating and clot-bound thrombin. It also inhibits thrombin-mediated platelet activation and aggregation.

Because it has a rapid onset and a short half-life, while not binding to red cells or plasma proteins (other than thrombin), bivalirudin has a predictable antithrombotic response. For patients at risk for heparin-induced thrombocytopenia (HIT)/heparin-induced thrombocytopenia and thrombosis syndrome (HITTS), bivalirudin is the preferred anticoagulant. In clinical studies, bivalirudin demonstrated consistent positive outcomes in patients with stable *angina*, unstable angina (UA), non–ST-segment elevation myocardial infarction (NSTEMI), and STEMI undergoing PCI in major randomized trials.

Bivalirudin should be administered with optimal antiplatelet therapy (aspirin plus clopidogrel, prasugrel, or ticagrelor). Bivalirudin has class-I recommendations in multiple national guidelines.

Dosing recommendations for ACS procedures: Administer bolus 0.75 mg/kg with infusion of 1.75 mg/kg/h. If patient proceeds to PCI, an additional bolus of 0.5 mg/kg of bivalirudin should be administered before the procedure and the infusion increased to 1.75 mg/kg/h for the duration of the procedure. Bivalirudin should be continued for 2 to 4 hours post-PCI. For active ACS after 4 hours, additional bivalirudin may be given at a rate of 0.2 or 0.25 mg/kg/h for up to 20 hours, if needed. Although bivalirudin activity is not directly related to the activated clotting time (ACT), the ACT should be measured after administration to assess whether the patient received the drug.

For patients proceeding to coronary artery bypass graft (CABG) surgery off-pump, an IV infusion should be continued until the time of surgery. Immediately prior to surgery, a 0.5 mg/kg bolus should be administered followed by a 1.75 mg/kg/h infusion for the duration of the surgery. For patients proceeding to CABG surgery on-pump, bivalirudin should be continued until 1 hour prior to surgery and then discontinued.

Bivalirudin dosing in patients with renal impairment should include a reduction in the infusion dose. In patients with moderate or severe renal impairment or if a patient is on hemodialysis, the infusion should be reduced to 0.25 mg/kg/h. No reduction in the bolus dose is needed.

Antiplatelet Drugs

There are six classes of antiplatelet drugs that have different mechanisms of action and potency effects and thus can function synergistically. Administration of combinations of antiplatelet drugs is common, weighing the risk of bleeding against the benefit of preventing stent thrombosis. Antiplatelet drug classes are:

- cyclooxygenase inhibitors (Aspirin)
- adenosine diphosphate (ADP) receptor inhibitors (clopidogrel [Plavix], prasugrel [Effient], and ticlopidine [Ticlid])
- phosphodiesterase inhibitors (cilostazol [Pletal])
- GP IIb/IIIa receptor inhibitors (abciximab [ReoPro], eptifibatide [Integrilin], and tirofiban [Aggrastat])
- adenosine reuptake inhibitors (dipyridamole [Persantine])
- cyclopentyl triazolo-pyrimidines (CPTPs) (ticagrelor [Brilinta])

Oral Antiplatelet Agents for Percutaneous Coronary Intervention (Other Than Aspirin)

- Clopidogrel, a thienopyridine, is the most commonly used adjunctive antiplatelet agent. This drug class affects the ADP-dependent activation of platelet aggregation and adhesion through platelet IIb/IIIa receptor, a GP responsible for platelet linkage to fibrinogen and von Willebrand factor (VWF), resulting in platelet-platelet attachment (fibrinogen) and platelet–vessel wall adhesion VWF, respectively. Doses are commonly a loading dose (300 or 600 mg) followed by 75 mg daily.

· Prasugrel is a second-generation antiplatelet agent. Like clopidogrel, it is a prodrug that is metabolized to an active component before binding to a specific platelet receptor ($P2Y_{12}$) to block platelet activity. Prasugrel is more efficiently metabolized than clopidogrel and is a more effective platelet inhibitor. The TRITON-TIMI 38 trial of ACS patients undergoing PCI found that prasugrel reduced recurrent myocardial infarction (10% vs. 7%; $P<0.001$) and stent thrombosis (2.4% vs. 1.1%; $P<0.001$) compared with clopidogrel but at the cost of increased bleeding in the prasugrel group (2.4% vs. 1.8% for clopidogrel, $P = 0.03$). Those with previous stroke or transient ischemic attack should not receive prasugrel because of excessive risk of intracranial hemorrhage. Mean steady-state inhibition of platelet aggregation was about 70% after a 60 mg loading dose followed by 3 to 5 days of dosing at 10 mg daily. The cost of prasugrel relative to clopidogrel was economically feasible because of a lower rate of rehospitalization involving PCI.

· Ticagrelor is the first drug in a new class of the antiplatelet agents called CPTPs, which are chemically distinct from thienopyridines. Like prasugrel, clopidogrel, and ticlopidine, ticagrelor blocks ADP receptors of subtype $P2Y_{12}$ but in a reversible fashion. Ticagrelor does not need hepatic activation, which reduces drug interactions. When compared with clopidogrel in the PLATO trial, ticagrelor had few cardiovascular-related deaths, myocardial infarction, or stroke (10% vs. 12%) without an increase in major bleeding and with a significant reduction in both cardiovascular death (4.0% vs. 5.1%, $P = 0.001$) and myocardial infarction (5.8% vs. 6.9%, $P = 0.005$) with no difference in stroke (1.5% vs. 1.3%, $P = 0.22$). Unlike other antiplatelet agents, ticagrelor reduced cardiovascular death in ACS patients whether an invasive or noninvasive course was planned. Contraindications for ticagrelor include active pathological bleeding and a history of intracranial bleeding, and reduced liver function and combination with drugs that strongly influence activity of the liver enzyme CYP_3A_4, because the drug is metabolized via CYP_3A_4 and excreted via the liver. The loading dose is 180 mg PO (two 90 mg tablets) and then 90 mg PO twice daily. Administer with aspirin, initial loading dose of 325 mg, and then maintenance dose of aspirin of 75 to 100 mg/day; *do not* exceed aspirin dose of 100 mg/day (see Black Box Warnings on drug labels).

Intravenous Antiplatelet Agents

IV antiplatelet GP IIb/IIIa receptor blockers (abciximab [ReoPro], eptifibatide [Integrilin], and tirofiban [Aggrastat]) are the most potent and most effective agents because they inhibit platelet activation at a final common receptor, the GP IIb/IIIa receptor. Because of the IV-only administration, these agents are limited to intra- and post-PCI procedure periods.

Abciximab (ReoPro) is a GP IIb/IIIa receptor antagonist and potent platelet aggregation inhibitor mainly used during and after PCI to prevent coronary thrombosis. It was developed as an antibody to the c7E3 mouse. Abciximab binds to the vitronectin ($\alpha v\beta 3$) receptor found on platelets and vessel-wall endothelial and smooth muscle cells. Abciximab has a short plasma half-life as a result of its strong affinity for its receptor on the platelets. Abciximab is contraindicated in patients with:

- active bleeding
- recent (within 6 weeks) surgery, trauma, gastrointestinal (GI) or genitourinary (GU) bleeding
- cerebrovascular accident (CVA) within 2 years or CVA with a significant residual neurological deficit
- bleeding diathesis
- use of oral anticoagulants (<7 days) unless prothrombin time is $\leq 1.2 \times$ control
- thrombocytopenia (<100,000 cells/μL)
- intracranial neoplasm, arteriovenous malformation, or aneurysm
- severe uncontrolled hypertension
- known hypersensitivity to murine proteins
- presumed or documented history of vasculitis

Platelet aggregation gradually returns to normal about 96 to 120 hours after discontinuation of the drug. The recommended dose of abciximab in adults is a 0.25 mg/kg IV bolus administered 10 to 60 minutes before the start of PCI, followed by a continuous IV infusion of 0.125 μg/kg/min (to a maximum of 10 μg/min) for 12 hours. Patients with unstable angina not responding to conventional medical therapy and who are planned to undergo PCI within 24 hours may be treated with an abciximab 0.25 mg/kg IV bolus followed by an 18- to 24-hour IV infusion of 10 μg/min, concluding 1 hour after the PCI.

Eptifibatide (Integrilin), another GP IIb/IIIa inhibitor, is a cyclic heptapeptide derived from rattlesnake venom and reversibly binds to platelets. Eptifibatide has a short half-life. The recommended adult dose is an IV loading dose of 180 µg/kg over 1 to 2 minutes immediately after diagnosis, followed by continuous IV infusion of 2 µg/kg per minute until either hospital discharge or initiation of coronary artery bypass grafting, or for up to 72 hours. At least 4 hours before discharge, all local or systemic bleedings should have been controlled and terminated. Patients weighing >120 kg should receive a maximum bolus of 22.6 mg followed by a maximum infusion rate of 15 mg/h. Patients with renal impairment evidenced by creatinine clearance (CrCl) <50 mL/min should receive the standard 180 mcg/kg loading dose followed by infusion at 1 mcg/kg/min.

Tirofiban (Aggrastat) is another GP IIb/IIIa inhibitor with a rapid onset and short duration of action after proper IV administration. Coagulation parameters return to normal 4 to 8 hours after the drug is withdrawn. A high-dose bolus regimen is IV administration of 25 mcg/kg over 3 minutes and then 0.15 mcg/kg/min for up to 18 hours. In patients with CrCl ≤60 mL/min, give 25 mcg/kg over 3 minutes and then 0.075 mcg/kg/min. The duration of therapy can be up to 18 hours.

Coronary Vasodilators

Nitroglycerin

Nitroglycerin, a safe and short-acting drug, is the most commonly used drug during coronary angiography and ventriculography. Nitroglycerin dilates both the coronary and peripheral arteries as well as the venous beds. Nitroglycerin can be given through the sublingual, IV, intracoronary, or intraventricular route. Sublingual (or oral spray) nitroglycerin (0.4 mg) is often given before coronary angiography. Exceptions include patients in whom coronary spasm is suspected (hold until after diagnosis is made) and patients with hypotension (<90 mm Hg systolic pressure or right ventricular [RV] infarction). In patients with documented coronary spasm, sublingual or intracoronary nitroglycerin is given to eliminate coronary spasm. In patients with unstable angina, IV infusions of nitroglycerin of up to 250 µg/min with a systolic blood pressure of 90 mm Hg are permissible. In patients with elevated LV end-diastolic pressure from ischemia or CHF, intraventricular or IV boluses of 200 µg of nitroglycerin reduce LV end-diastolic pressure and are appropriate before and after ventriculography. Intracoronary nitroglycerin in doses of 50, 100, and 200 mcg modestly increases coronary blood flow without a marked reduction in pressure. With doses of more than 250 mcg, hypotension without further increases in coronary blood flow may be evident. Care should be used to avoid inducing hypotension when administering nitroglycerin to patients with known or suspected severe aortic stenosis, significant left main coronary artery (LMCA) narrowing, or hypertrophic obstructive cardiomyopathy.

Nitroglycerin should not be given to patients taking sildenafil (Viagra) or similar medicines for erectile dysfunction treatment because of the potential for severe hypotension. Be sure to ask patients about this before assuming that they do not take sildenafil or similar medication.

Calcium Channel Blockers

Calcium channel blockers dilate vascular smooth muscle and reduce heart muscle contractility, and some agents block atrioventricular nodal conduction. Calcium channel blockers are used to reduce peripheral vascular resistance, decrease blood pressure, block coronary spasm, and increase coronary blood flow. Acute use in the cardiac catheterization laboratory is limited to treating arrhythmias and no-reflow of coronary interventions or to treat radial artery spasm when the transradial approach is used. Because of variable absorption, sublingual administration is not recommended. Doses for calcium channel blockers are as follows: diltiazem, 30 to 60 mg orally, 10 mg IV; and verapamil, 120 mg orally, 2.5 to 5 mg IV (for coronary no-reflow, give an intracoronary bolus of verapamil, 200 µg, repeated for two to four doses if needed).

Adenosine

Adenosine IV is used for breaking supraventricular tachycardia (SVT) and is the drug of choice for intracoronary induction of maximal hyperemia for coronary vasodilator reserve.

For SVT, doses of 6 to 12 mg IV bolus are commonly used. For inducing coronary hyperemia for fractional flow reserve (FFR) measurements, 140 µg/kg/min given via IV or adenosine given via intracoronary (50–100 mcg for the right coronary artery [RCA] and 100 to 200 µg for the left coronary artery [LCA]) produces optimal results. For laboratories with no or limited FFR experience for lesion assessment, IV adenosine is recommended because it is weight-based, simple, and free of operator hands and interference. IV adenosine infusions produce sustained hyperemia after 1 to 2 minutes. Adenosine hyperemia lasts less than 60 seconds after drug administration is ended.

Nitroprusside

Nitroprusside is a potent, short-acting IV arterial vasodilator used to treat aortic insufficiency, mitral regurgitation, hypertensive crisis, and CHF. Administered doses range from 10 to 100 μg/min and must be monitored by direct arterial pressure measurement.

For coronary no-reflow or for induction of intracoronary hyperemia when adenosine is not available, a 50- to 100-μg bolus of nitroprusside can be used and repeated as needed.

Coronary Vasoconstrictor (for Provocation of Coronary Spasm Only)

Ergonovine was used to provoke coronary vasospasm in patients with chest pain syndromes and normal or near-normal coronary angiograms. Ergonovine malate is no longer manufactured in the United States. Some investigators have used methylergonovine, but little is reported with this agent. Intracoronary acetylcholine produces coronary vasoconstriction in patients with propensity for spasm or in those with endothelial dysfunction. It should be reserved for laboratories with a particular interest in this problem and most often under a research protocol.

Peripheral Vasoconstrictor for Transient Hypotension

Phenylephrine, an alpha-receptor agonist, is used as a vasopressor to increase the blood pressure in unstable patients with hypotension. Phenylephrine works by peripheral vasoconstriction and has the advantage of not being an inotropic (contractility increase) or chronotropic (heart rate increase) drug. Phenylephrine increases the blood pressure without increasing the heart rate or contractility. Rarely, reflex bradycardia may accompany the blood pressure increase. This response is especially useful if the heart is already tachycardic and/or cardiomyopathy is present. Phenylephrine is administered at 0.2 mg/dose (range: 0.1 to 0.5 mg/dose) every 10 to 15 minutes as needed (initial dose should not exceed 0.5 mg). The IV infusion rate is 100 to 180 mcg/min initially. The usual maintenance dose is 40 to 60 mcg/min. The elimination half-life of phenylephrine is about 2.5 to 3 hours.

Anticholinergics for Vagal Reactions

Atropine

Atropine is used to block vagally-induced slowing of the heart rate and hypotension. IV doses of 0.6 to 1.2 mg can be given immediately and reverse bradycardia and hypotension within 2 minutes. In elderly patients and patients who have pacemakers, the heart rate may not slow during vagal episodes in which the only manifestation is low blood pressure. This low blood pressure can be alleviated by the administration of IV atropine and normal saline. In the rare patient in whom IV access is not immediately available, intraaortic atropine can be administered. Vasoconstrictors are reserved for persistent hypotension after recovery of heart rate.

Antiarrhythmic Drugs

Lidocaine

Lidocaine is an antiarrhythmic drug used to block or to reduce the number of ventricular extra systoles. In rare circumstances, lidocaine can be administered as an IV bolus of 50 to 100 mg before ventriculography if a stable and quiet catheter position within the left ventricle cannot be obtained. In patients in whom myocardial ischemia develops during cardiac catheterization or angioplasty, lidocaine for frequent ventricular ectopy is indicated. An IV bolus of 50 to 100 mg followed by a 1 to 2 mg/min infusion is usually satisfactory.

Amiodarone

Amiodarone is used to treat poorly controlled atrial fibrillation and VT. In the catheterization laboratory, amiodarone is indicated for recurrent ventricular fibrillation or recurrent hemodynamically unstable VT. The loading dose is 150 mg IV over 10 minutes (15 mg/min) and then 360 mg IV over the next 6 hours (1 mg/min), followed by 540 mg IV over the next 18 hours (0.5 mg/min). After the first 24 hours, a maintenance IV infusion of 720 mg/24 h (0.5 mg/min) is continued.

In the catheterization laboratory, amiodarone has been associated with bradycardia, hypotension, arrhythmias, heart failure, heart block, sinus arrest, and edema. Amiodarone may reduce hepatic or renal clearance of certain antiarrhythmics (especially flecainide, procainamide, and quinidine). Use of amiodarone with other antiarrhythmics (especially mexiletine, propafenone, quinidine, disopyramide, and procainamide) may induce torsades de pointes. Amiodarone should be used cautiously with antihypertensives, β-blockers, and calcium channel blockers because of increased cardiac depressant effects and slowing of sinoatrial node and atrioventricular conduction. Amiodarone may potentiate anticoagulant response with the a possibility of serious or fatal bleeding. The warfarin dose should be decreased by 33% to 50% when amiodarone is initiated.

Amiodarone is contraindicated in cardiogenic shock, second-degree or third-degree atrioventricular block, and severe sinoatrial node disease resulting in preexisting bradycardia unless a pacemaker is present.

Cardiac Inotropic Agents

Dopamine

Dopamine is a potent vasoconstrictor. It is most commonly used in the treatment of severe hypotension, bradycardia, and cardiogenic shock. Its effects, depending on dosage, include an increase in sodium excretion by the kidneys, an increase in urine output, an increase in heart rate, and an increase in blood pressure. At a dose of 2 to 10 μg/kg/min, dopamine acts through the sympathetic nervous system to increase heart muscle contraction force and heart rate, thereby increasing cardiac output and blood pressure. At a dose of 10 to 20 μg/kg/min, dopamine also causes vasoconstriction that further increases blood pressure. However, higher doses can produce negative side effects, such as cardiac arrhythmias.

Dobutamine

Dobutamine is a potent inotropic agent with no peripheral vasoconstrictor effects. It increases cardiac contractility (inotropy) and is especially useful in patients with low cardiac output or CHF. Dobutamine administration should be started at a low rate (0.5 to 1.0 mcg/kg/min) and titrated by the patient's response, including systemic blood pressure, urine flow, frequency of ectopic activity, heart rate, pulmonary capillary wedge pressure, and cardiac output. Dobutamine may be used in conjunction with a potent vasodilator, such as nitroprusside, in patients with markedly elevated filling pressures and poor cardiac output.

Norepinephrine (also Known as Levophed)

Norepinephrine is a neurotransmitter synthesized from dopamine. It is released from the adrenal medulla into the blood as a hormone. It activates the sympathetic nervous system via binding to adrenergic receptors when it is released from noradrenergic neurons. Norepinephrine is a potent vasopressor for patients with critical hypotension. It is given intravenously and acts on both α_1 and α_2 adrenergic receptors to cause vasoconstriction. Its effects are often limited to an increase in blood pressure through the increase in peripheral vascular resistance. At high doses, and especially when it is combined with other vasopressors, it can lead to limb ischemia and limb death. Norepinephrine is mainly used to treat patients in vasodilatory shock states, such as septic shock and neurogenic shock, and has shown a survival benefit over dopamine. Doses of norepinephrine begin at 2 to 4 mcg/min for an initial bolus with a maintenance dose of 1 to 12 mcg/min.

Epinephrine

Epinephrine (1:10,000) is a naturally occurring catecholamine that stimulates cardiac function. It is administered only during cardiac emergencies. This medicine increases heart rate and blood pressure immediately, sometimes to very high levels. Epinephrine should be reserved for patients needing cardiac resuscitation, patients in whom refractory hypotension is present and not responding to peripheral vasoconstrictors, or patients with anaphylactic reactions. Transthoracic administration of epinephrine through a long needle is no longer performed. IV or intraarterial administration of 1 mL of 1:10,000 dilution can increase systemic pressure transiently during hypotension to a safe level until IV vasopressors have been prepared. This dose of epinephrine has a duration of action of 5 to 10 minutes. For management of cardiac arrest, an IV dose of 1:10,000 (0.1 mg/mL) solution at 0.1 to 1 mg (1 to 10 mL), repeated every 5 minutes, as necessary, is recommended. Alternatively, in intubated patients, epinephrine can be injected via the endotracheal tube directly into the bronchial tree at the same dose as that for IV injection.

Environmental Safety in the Catheterization Laboratory

The cardiac catheterization laboratory is a potentially hazardous area if proper safety measures are not followed. There is the constant risk of exposure to radiation, blood and other body fluids, and infectious diseases, such as hepatitis and tuberculosis. Laboratory-specific environmental safety plans reduce the risk associated with this environment.

The invasive cardiovascular technologist is responsible for the radiation protection of patients and laboratory personnel in cooperation with the hospital radiation safety officer. Electrical hazard protection is also maintained through the technologist and the biomedical engineering department.

Blood, Blood-Borne Viruses, and Body Fluids

Occupational exposure to blood and other body fluids is a serious concern for personnel working in the cardiac catheterization

Table 1.10

Catheterization Laboratory Blood Exposure Hazards.	
Procedure	**Exposure**
IV therapy	Needle stick, blood-to-skin contact
Local anesthesia administration	Needle stick
Arterial puncture	Needle stick, splashing of blood
Catheter insertion or exchange	Splashing of blood to skin, mucous membrane contact
Catheter flushing	Splashing of blood to skin, mucous membrane contact
Catheter removal and groin	Splashing of blood to skin, mucous compression membrane contact
Contact with soiled linen or equipment	Needle stick, splashing of blood to skin, mucous membrane contact

IV, Intravenous.

laboratory. The Occupational Safety and Health Administration (OSHA) published blood-borne pathogen standards in the Federal Register in 1991. The standard outlines specific guidelines that must be followed to protect employees from occupational exposure (Table 1.10 lists hazards in the catheterization laboratory).

Hepatitis B virus (HBV) and human immunodeficiency virus (HIV) are two blood-borne viruses that pose a risk to health care workers. These viruses have been found in blood, semen, vaginal secretions, tears, saliva, cerebrospinal fluid, amniotic fluid, breast milk, body cavity fluids, and urine. Blood and equipment contaminated with blood and bloody saline flush solutions pose the greatest risk to cardiac catheterization laboratory personnel.

Transmission of blood-borne viruses can occur when contaminated body fluids come in contact with the skin by needles or through an open sore or small cut or contact with the eyes or other mucous membranes.

Universal and Standard Precautions

The goal of the exposure control plan is to isolate the health care worker from these hazards. Universal precautions are an infection control technique in which all blood and body fluids are treated as if they are contaminated. The universal precautions technique should be incorporated in the specific exposure control plan for the cardiac catheterization laboratory.

Standard precautions are designed to reduce the risk of transmission of microorganisms from recognized and unrecognized sources of possible infection. Standard precautions incorporate the major features of universal precautions for blood and body fluid and body substance isolation that are designed to reduce the risk of transmission of pathogens from moist body substances. Standard precautions apply to blood, all body fluids, secretions, and excretions, regardless of whether they contain visible blood, broken skin, and mucous membranes.

In addition to standard precautions, the guidelines recommend transmission-based precautions for patients known or suspected to be infected or colonized with highly transmissible or epidemiologically significant pathogens. The three types of transmission-based precautions are (1) airborne, (2) droplet, and (3) contact precautions.

In the past, it was rare to have a patient with a known transmissible disease scheduled for elective catheterization. Interventional procedures have expanded the indications for cardiac procedures, however. In these instances, consultation with the hospital's infection control nurse should be considered to initiate transmission-based precautions properly.

The working environment should be assessed before an exposure control plan is written. In the catheterization laboratory, procedure-specific hazards exist. Some methods of protection are listed in Table 1.11.

Eye, Nose, Mouth, and Skin Protection

The eyes and nose should be protected from potential splashing of blood and contaminated fluids. Personnel at most risk are the operator and assistant, the circulating personnel, and the person removing the catheter and sheath and holding arterial puncture site pressure. Personnel performing these high-risk tasks should wear glasses or goggles, a facemask, or a facemask with an incorporated plastic eye shield if glasses or goggles are not worn (Fig. 1.9A).

Table 1.11

Methods of Protection.

Area Protected	Method
Eyes	Glasses with side shields or goggles
Nose, mouth	Masks
Skin	Gloves, fluid-resistant gowns
Parenteral	Proper methods of sharp instruments storage and disposal; do not recap or resheath needles

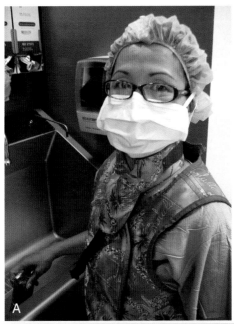

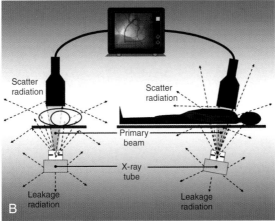

Fig. 1.9 **(A)** Nurse and technicians wear protective glasses, gloves, gowns, and face masks satisfying Occupational Safety and Health Administration (OSHA) standards. Thyroid shields should be worn by all personnel inside the catheterization suite. **(B)** Diagram of radiation scatter in the catheterization laboratory. Most radiation scatter occurs through the patient's body and is increased with increasing angulations.

Continued

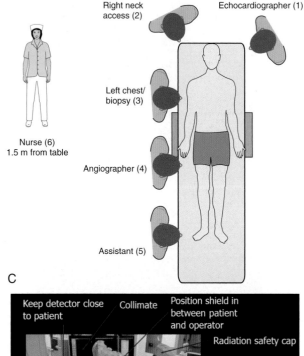

Right neck access (2)

Echocardiographer (1)

Left chest/biopsy (3)

Nurse (6)
1.5 m from table

Angiographer (4)

Assistant (5)

C

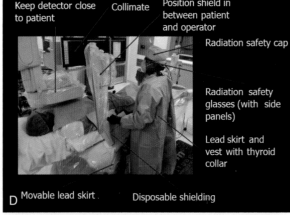

Keep detector close to patient   Collimate   Position shield in between patient and operator

Radiation safety cap

Radiation safety glasses (with side panels)

Lead skirt and vest with thyroid collar

D   Movable lead skirt   Disposable shielding

Fig. 1.9, cont'd (C) Diagram of locations that are exposed to radiation in the catheterization laboratory. Compared with the prestructural heart disease era, there are now personnel located closer to the x-ray tube for anesthesia and TEE operations. (Courtesy Dr. Robert Wilson) **(D)** Ways to reduce radiation injury in the catheterization laboratory. (Gautam Kumar, MD, FACC; Syed Tanveer Rab, MBBS, FACC Expert Analysis Radiation Safety for the Interventional Cardiologist—A Practical Approach to Protecting Ourselves From the Dangers of Ionizing Radiation. Jan 04, 2016. https://www.acc.org/latest-in-cardiology/articles/2015/12/31/10/12/radiation-safety-for-the-interventional-cardiologist)

Gloves should be worn whenever personnel are required to handle supplies or samples that are considered contaminated. Anyone involved in the sterile procedure should wear sterile gloves. Circulating personnel should wear gloves when accepting items being passed from the sterile field, such as used catheters or wires, syringes containing blood for blood gas and saturation analysis, and biopsy specimens. Gloves should be worn if a pressure transducer is being flushed with saline that has been contaminated with blood during the procedure. This point is of particular concern because the saline may not appear to be contaminated. However, it may have been aspirated through the same manifold through which blood has passed, producing an invisible contamination.

Glove integrity should be monitored. If personnel report holes or tears in gloves, double gloving or higher-quality gloves should be considered. Hand lotions containing petroleum products compromise latex glove material and should not be used.

Exposed skin should be covered when removing catheters and sheaths and holding puncture site pressure. An inexpensive disposable gown, such as an isolation gown or a disposable laboratory coat, should be donned first and the gloves pulled over the sleeves. This technique minimizes exposure to hands and arms. If the protective clothing becomes contaminated with blood or other body fluids, it should be removed immediately and the exposed skin should be washed with soap and water. Protective clothing worn during procedures should be removed before personnel leave the department or hospital building.

Equipment Considerations for Protection

As awareness of the hazards of blood-borne pathogens increases, a variety of protective equipment and instruments are being made available for use in the cardiac catheterization laboratory. Most companies that make angiographic manifolds offer closed drainage systems. This system incorporates a 1000-mL bag in the manifold system, which allows aspirated blood to be flushed directly into a sealed bag. This system reduces the potential exposure during the procedure and at the end of the procedure during cleanup.

Another product to reduce exposure improves on the conventional waste bowl often used on the sterile back table. The closed bowl design allows bloody, fluid-filled syringes to be emptied into the receptacle and prevents back splashing by incorporating a diaphragm slot in which the syringe can be inserted and emptied.

Employer Responsibility

Hepatitis B Virus Vaccination

The OSHA standard states that HBV vaccination must be made available as a prerequisite of employment to all employees with potential for occupational exposure. If the employee declines vaccination, it is mandatory that an HBV vaccine declination be signed.

Risk Category

The OSHA standard requires employers to inform employees of a job's risk category on employment. The three risk categories are:

Risk Category	Definition
I	Employment and procedures require exposure to blood and other body fluids.
II	Employment and procedures may require exposure to blood and other body fluids.
III	Employment and procedures usually do not require exposure to blood and other body fluids.

Most, if not all, catheterization laboratory staff fall into category I. The employer must provide proper training to employees regarding blood-borne pathogens and OSHA standards. Records must be kept documenting the dates, content, name of the person conducting the training, and names of persons attending the session. These records must be kept for at least 3 years.

Eliminating Careless Practices to Reduce Risks

In the cardiac catheterization laboratory, employees are often exposed as a result of carelessness and lack of attention to procedures. All incidents of employee exposure should be properly documented. A periodic review should be conducted to determine ways to eliminate future exposure. Careless practices that should be avoided in the catheterization laboratory include:

1. Vigorous squirting of blood in syringes into the back table waste bowl, resulting in splashing.
2. Throwing of bloody gauze across the table into trash receptacles.

3. Improper handling of guidewires and catheters, which may spring out of the saline bowl and cause splashing.
4. Failing to return needles properly to a needle counter or container on the back table.

Extra attention and care in such areas prevent unnecessary exposure of staff.

Radiation Safety

Radiation safety is everybody's business in the catheterization laboratory. While standard teaching about radiation safety is part of every team member's basic concepts and training, there have been very few major changes in our protective equipment over the years to reduce radiation exposure other than to employ the standard table-side and mobile shielding. Radiation dose is directly related to exposure time, determined by the operator's visualization needs (i.e., pedal time). The distance from radiation source is also a critical determinant of dose, the further the better. Methods to reduce exposure are summarized in Table 3.4 in Chapter 3. Significant radiation exposure has the potential to impact the health and well-being of interventional cardiologists and their teams.

The catheterization laboratory environment should be made as safe as possible for the staff and patient. Because radiation cannot be seen, felt, or heard, it is easy to become lackadaisical about proper protective measures. Standards for radiation protection (from the Society for Cardiac Angiography and Intervention) include four basic tenets and follow the ALARA principle (As Low As Reasonably Acceptable):

1. The less the exposure, the less chance there is of absorbed energy biologic interaction.
2. No known level of ionizing radiation is a permissible dose or absolutely safe.
3. Radiation exposure is cumulative. There is no washout phenomenon.
4. All participants in the cardiac catheterization laboratory have voluntarily accepted some degree of radiation exposure, but they are obliged to minimize and to reduce risks to other personnel and themselves.

The source of radiation is the primary x-ray beam emanating from the under table x-ray tube upward through the patient and onto the image intensifier. Scatter of this beam exposes all subjects to radiation in a dose geometrically inverse to the distance from the source. Radiation scatter is increased when the angle of the tube is set obliquely. A high degree of angulation increases the amount of radiation scatter (see Chapter 3). Acrylic shields and table-mounted lead aprons should be used to reduce the amount of scatter.

Fluoroscopy generates approximately one-fifth the x-ray exposure of cineangiography. The increased use of cineangiography for complex catheterization procedures has increased the total exposure and should be a consideration in procedures requiring extensive intracardiac manipulation, such as angioplasty, valvuloplasty, or electrophysiology studies. Figure 1.9B shows the radiation scatter distribution in the catheterization laboratory. Most radiation scatter occurs through the patient's body and is increased with increasing angulations. Figure 1.9C demonstrates locations that are at risk of higher exposure to radiation in the catheterization laboratory. Compared with the prestructural heart disease era, there are now personnel located closer to the x-ray tube for anesthesia and transesophageal echocardiogram (TEE) operations. Figure 1.9D demonstrates ways to reduce radiation injury in the catheterization laboratory. Figure 1.10 provides information on the positioning

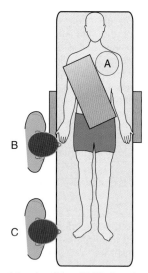

Fig. 1.10   Position of the absorbing shield, placed on the patient, between the image intensifier (A), the primary operator (B), and occasionally the secondary operator (C). From Wieneke Vlastra et al. Circ Cardiovasc Interv. 2017; 10:e006058.

of the absorbing shield, placed on the patient, between the image intensifier *(A)*, the primary operator *(B)*, and occasionally the secondary operator *(C)*.

Every cardiac catheterization laboratory should have a department-specific radiation safety policy. This policy should include:

1. Routine monitoring of personnel radiation exposure.
2. Continuing education programs on radiation safety for personnel.
3. Program to make personnel aware of the risks associated with radiation exposure.
4. Requirement for protective equipment be worn by all personnel.
5. Procedures to check safety of all equipment (x-ray dose output, integrity of lead aprons, and thyroid shields).

Lead Eyeglasses

A single x-ray exposure of 200 rad can result in cataract formation in humans. Eyeglasses made of 0.5- to 0.75-mm lead-equivalent glass should be worn by personnel exposed to radiation on a daily basis (see Fig. 1.9A). Glasses containing 0.5 mm of lead offer four times the protection of regular eyeglasses. Glasses with photochromic lenses offer two times the protection of regular eyeglasses. Plastic lenses offer no eye protection from radiation.

Radiation-protective glasses must contain a wraparound side shield. Glasses with proper-fitting side shields are not only effective for radiation protection but also provide protection from blood products splashing into the eyes.

Radiation Badges

All personnel should wear a radiation-monitoring badge when in the catheterization laboratory. To ensure accurate readings, a badge should always remain on the person to whom it is assigned. Badges should never be left lying on a counter or attached to a lead apron in an area where there is potential radiation exposure. When badges are not being used, they should be stored in an area away from any potential radiation exposure.

At the end of each month, exposed badges are collected and sent for analysis. A monthly exposure report indicates each staff member's exposure for that month. This information should be posted in the laboratory so that each staff member can monitor his or her individual exposure. The report should be reviewed each month by the laboratory medical director and the institution's radiation safety officer.

Radiation Dose Limitation

Although no known threshold for radiation exposure exists to define specific risks, the National Council on Radiation Protection and Measurements indicates that no dose greater than 3 roentgen equivalent man (rem) should be allowed over a 3-month period.

Definitions of Radiation Units

1. Roentgen (R) is the measure of ionization delivered to a specific point (exposure). One chest radiograph equals 3 to 5 mR.
2. Radiation absorbed dose (rad) is the amount of radiation energy deposited per unit mass of tissue. The amount of absorbed dose per given exposure depends on tissue type. For soft tissue, 1 R = 1 rad; for bone, 1 R = 4 rad (i.e., greater absorption).
3. Rem is used to express the biologic impact of a given exposure. For x-radiation, 1 rad = 1 rem.

Methods to Limit Exposure

1. Wear leaded aprons (preferably wraparound): 0.5 mm or more thickness provides 80% protection.
2. Limit the fluoroscopic or cineangiographic time (cineangiographic time produces much greater exposure than fluoroscopic time).
3. Use collimators.
4. Reduce the distance between the x-ray source and the patient.
5. Maximize the distance between the x-ray source and the operator and assistants.
6. Limit milliamperes per kilovolts as much as possible for an adequate image.
7. Use slower panning and provide good initial angiographic setup. Angled views almost double the radiation.
8. Keep the image magnification as low as possible.
9. Use extra shielding (leaded thyroid guards, lead glasses, and protective table shields).

Radiation Shielding

Radiation shielding provides only partial protection depending on location around the table, body heights, and imaging angles

(Fig. 1.9B). Personal Protection Equipment (PPE) alone has limits and is not sufficient to block all scatter radiation dose to the interventional catheterization laboratory staff. No current radiation protection strategy will protect the entire health care team in the interventional catheterization laboratory room (Fig. 1.9C). We need to account for additional staff locations around the table for TAVR, RightHeart procedures, biopsies and TEE, with operators at the head of the table and very close to radiation source. Although novel shield systems have been proposed over the last few years, none has been routinely used in most laboratories.

Radiation exposure is greater during angioplasty than during diagnostic catheterization. If the protective shields are used carefully, radiation exposure for single-vessel and double-vessel angioplasty may be comparable with diagnostic catheterization. Radiation exposures are generally higher for these procedures, however, especially when biplane angiography is performed.

Lead Aprons and Thyroid Shields

Lead aprons should contain 0.5-mm-thick lead lining. When properly cared for, an apron can provide years of service. However, the lead lining can crack or tear; this is usually caused by careless handling or improper storage. Aprons should be placed on an appropriate hanger or in a storage rack after use (Fig. 1.11A). Repeatedly throwing an apron over a chair or stretcher may damage the lead lining.

To assess the integrity of the lead, aprons should be examined under fluoroscopy at least once each year. There is an incorrect way to store lead aprons (Fig. 1.11B and C).

Documentation should be kept regarding the integrity of each apron. To do this, each apron should contain some sort of identification (e.g., number, color, or name).

Because of the nature of work in the catheterization laboratory, personnel are not always able to maintain a frontal position to the x-ray beam. Wraparound lead aprons should be considered. Aprons should be long enough to cover the long bones (femur) and should extend to the knee or just below the knee. Because proper fit is important, many companies take measurements to ensure a proper fit. A hanging rack for the lead aprons should be used to prevent cracking resulting from excessive folding of aprons left lying over chairs or benches.

Because the thyroid gland is particularly sensitive to ionizing radiation, a lead thyroid shield should be worn in the presence of ionizing radiation. Similar to aprons, thyroid shields

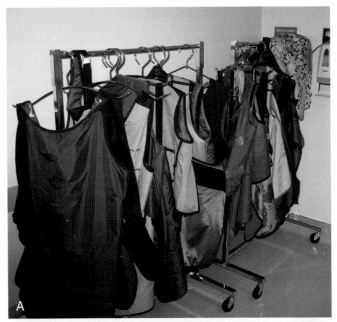

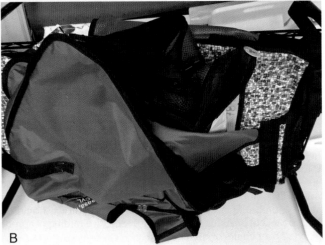

Fig. 1.11 **(A)** One correct storage method to prevent lead aprons from developing cracks, thereby reducing radiation protection. All aprons should be hung when not in use. **(B)** Incorrect way to store lead aprons.

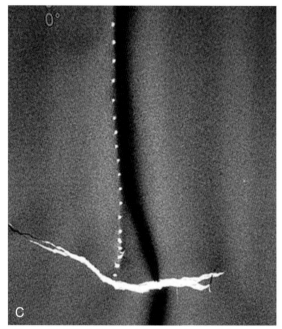

Fig. 1.11, cont'd (C) Folded and improperly cared for aprons show cracks defeating their role of radiation protection.

should be stored properly and the lead periodically checked radiographically.

Physician Training Requirements in Cardiac Catheterization

Diagnostic Catheterization in Adults

Training in Diagnostic and Interventional Cardiac Catheterization published by the American College of Cardiology (ACC) and endorsed by the Society for Cardiovascular Angiography and Interventions (COCATS Training Recommendations) provides guidance to the trainee's overall professional goals and further determines the requisite knowledge and skill set to be acquired in the training fellowship program. In general, trainees may be divided into three broad groups with differing training requirements:

· Level 1: Trainees who will practice noninvasive cardiology and whose invasive activities will be confined to critical care unit procedures. However, this level also provides cognitive training in the indications, risks, and outcomes for the procedures and in the accurate interpretation of data obtained in the catheterization laboratory.

- Level 2: Trainees who will practice diagnostic but not interventional cardiac catheterization.
- Level 3: Trainees who will practice diagnostic and interventional cardiac catheterization.

Each level has specific goals for training that build on one another and they are described in the following text. All cardiologists should have Level 1 knowledge and skills. Jacobs et al. (2008) in the Task Force 3 recommendations outline requisites for program accreditation, goals, structure, activity level and patient mix, training program curriculum, and the need for conferences.

The following are the proposed physician requirements for certification in the performance of cardiac catheterization. The physician should spend a minimum of 12 months in the cardiac catheterization laboratory. The trainee acquires a clear understanding of the indications, limitations, complications, and medical and surgical implications of the findings of cardiac catheterization and angiography. This background includes an understanding of the pathophysiology and the ability to interpret a wide variety of hemodynamic and angiographic data in adults. (Pediatric catheterization requires a special training track.) All trainees receive basic instruction in radiation safety, use of fluoroscopy, and radiologic anatomy.

The trainee learns to perform catheterization of the right and left sides of the heart by the various percutaneous routes. Routine ventriculography and coronary angiography are taught. Temporary RV pacing, endomyocardial biopsy, and pericardiocentesis are part of the training experience, if available. A working knowledge of catheterization laboratory equipment, including physiologic recorders, pressure transducers, blood gas analyzers, image intensifiers, and other x-ray equipment, and angiographic image management is emphasized for trainees seeking advanced catheterization laboratory experience.

Trainees should be exposed to adult patients with valvular, congenital, cardiomyopathic, ischemic heart disease and peripheral vascular and structural heart disease. Studies of acutely ill patients (cardiogenic shock, acute myocardial infarction, or unstable angina) are currently a routine part of invasive cardiology. At the end of the cardiac catheterization training period, for Level 2 training, a trainee should have performed at least 300 catheterization procedures; in 150 of them, the trainee should have been

Table 1.12

| | | | | Cumulative | Minimal |
| Task | | | Minimal Number of | Duration of Training | Cumulative Number of |
Force	Area	Level	Procedures	(Months)	Cases
3	Diagnostic	1	100	4	100
	catheterization	2	200	8	300
	Interventional	3	250	20	550
	catheterization				

Summary of Training Requirements in Diagnostic and Interventional Cardiac Catheterization.

From Jacobs AK, Babb JD, Hirshfeld JW, et al: Task Force 3: training in diagnostic and interventional cardiac catheterization. Endorsed by the Society for Cardiovascular Angiography and Interventions. *Cathet. Cardiovasc. Intervent.*, 2008;71:447–453.

the primary operator. The number of cases required to meet the training levels are shown in Table 1.12.

Because the potential for harm is greater with interventional techniques, only highly skilled physicians thoroughly trained in the fundamentals of diagnostic catheterization should undertake the additional year of training that is needed for competency in interventional cardiology (percutaneous coronary and peripheral vascular interventions, and interventions for structural heart disease [e.g., TAVR, mitral clip, balloon valvuloplasty, septal defect closures, left atrial appendage closure; see Chapter 6]).

Recommendations from the SCAI Best Practices in the Catheterization Laboratory, 2016 (see Naidu SS et al. Suggested Readings)

Institutional and operator qualifications:

The provider and institutional competency documentation sections suggest three features to make this action operational:

1. Physicians should participate in quarterly QI, peer review, and/ or morbidity/mortality (M and M) meetings for privileging and assessment of procedural appropriateness evaluation.

2. Operators should perform >50 PCI/year, averaged over two years, and >11 primary PCIs for STEMI. The Institution should perform >200 PCIs/year and >36 primary PCIs for STEMI per year. (These metrics are unchanged from 2012).

3. For those institutions without onsite cardiac surgery, an overview is paramount to ensure quality of procedures. Should the hospital's operators have insufficient volumes (as noted above), the institution should consider recruiting more experienced operators.

Catheterization Laboratory Governance

1. All cardiac catheterization laboratories (CCL) have a physician director and nonphysician manager.
2. The CCL director should work with the manager of QI, physician/ hospital administration, nurse and heart team training, to have an overview of debriefing of adverse events and the delegation of authority to facilitate education and mentorship to all team members.

Naidu and colleagues provide a comprehensive list of recommendations on the responsibilities of the cardiac catheterization laboratory physician director, such as the catheterization laboratory director should co-chair CCL administrative meetings, resolve personnel problems with the cardiac catheterization laboratory manager, attend cardiac catheterization laboratory staff meeting, act as a liaison between staff and physicians, resolve scheduling issues among physicians, coordinate catheterization laboratory call schedule, and assist catheterization laboratory manager with other problems.

Integrity in the Catheterization Laboratory

Admiral Sizemore describes principles of Operational Excellence in Navy Aviation, and after reading his article I immediately noticed parallels with our work in the catheterization laboratory from his experience with naval aviation and how it related to the practice of medicine. How does experience in naval aviation apply to the catheterization laboratory, and how do the lessons from training and experience help naval aviators support their missions? Table 1.13 shows that the training and experience of the catheterization laboratory team reflects the critical principles that support our mission.

The Navy provides safety and protection for all of us in our great country. It is a never-ending mission. Although of considerably smaller scope than that of the US Navy, the mission is the same for the catheterization laboratory. Patients who come into the catheterization laboratory expect safety and protection that we endeavor to achieve with excellence as they undergo their procedures. A high level of task performance by naval aviators is required to maintain readiness within the extraordinarily stressful environment of working on aircraft carriers patrolling the oceans. In a similar manner, working in the catheterization laboratory, at times a stressful environment, also requires flexibility and rapid

Table 1.13

Principles of Operational Excellence in Navy Aviation[a] (and the Catheterization Laboratory).	
Principle	**Metric**
1. Integrity	Do the right thing; adhere to the high standards at all times.
2. Procedural knowledge	Know your job and procedures; never stop learning.
3. Procedural compliance	By the book procedure; no short cuts; fight complacency.
4. Formal communications	Use clearly stated and standardized language that minimizes misunderstanding.
5. Question attitudes	Speak up, ask, and investigative when you are unsure of when you sense or know something is not right.
6. Forceful backups	Speak up, ask, and act when you know something is wrong.
7. Risk management	Identify, understand, mitigate, and manage risks.

[a]From Sizemore WG 2nd. U.S. Naval air training and operational excellence. *Tex Heart Inst J.* 2013;40(5):562–563.

responses. Admiral Sizemore notes that "aviation is extraordinarily complex and requires enormous commitment both in materials and in the individuals" with highly specialized training backgrounds. One could easily substitute "medicine" for "aviation" in the preceding sentence without changing the meaning.

Just as in naval aviation, the requirements to maintain proficiency in the catheterization laboratory should be a part of everyday life. In the catheterization laboratory with the near-continuous introduction of new devices and procedures, becoming proficient and maintaining proficiency is necessary to ensure safety and quality. Hopefully the materials in this book will help our catheterization laboratories succeed in their mission to our patients.

References

1. Kern M. Cath lab safety. *Cath Lab Digest.* 2014;22:6-8.
2. Weaver J. The latest ASA mandate: CO_2 monitoring for moderate and deep sedation. *Anesth Prog.* 2011;58:111-112.
3. Annala AP, Karjalainen PP, Porela P, Nyman K, Ylitalo A, Airaksinen KE. Safety of diagnostic coronary angiography during uninterrupted therapeutic warfarin treatment. *Am J Cardiol.* 2008;102:386-390.

Suggested Readings

Bashore TM, Balter S, Barac A, et al. 2012 American College of Cardiology Foundation/Society for Cardiovascular Angiography and Interventions expert consensus document on cardiac catheterization laboratory standards update: a report of the American College of Cardiology Foundation Task Force on Expert Consensus documents developed in collaboration with the Society of Thoracic Surgeons and Society for Vascular Medicine. *J Am Coll Cardiol.* 2012;59:2221-2305.

Blankenship JC, Gigliotti OS, Feldman DN, et al. Ad hoc percutaneous coronary intervention: a consensus statement from the Society for Cardiovascular Angiography and Interventions. *Catheter Cardiovasc Interv.* 2013;81:748-758.

Dehmer GJ, Weaver D, Roe MT, et al. A contemporary view of diagnostic cardiac catheterization and percutaneous coronary intervention in the United States: a report from the CathPCI Registry of the National Cardiovascular Data Registry, 2010 through June 2011. *J Am Coll Cardiol.* 2012;60:2017-2031.

Fornell, D. New Technologies to reduce staff dose in the Cath Lab. Radiation dose management. *Diagn Interv Cardiol Mag.* August 9, 2016.

Harold JG, Bass TA, Bashore TM, et al. ACCF/AHA/SCAI 2013 update of the clinical competence statement on coronary artery interventional procedures: a report of the American College of Cardiology Foundation/American Heart Association/American College of Physicians Task Force on Clinical Competence and Training (writing committee to revise the 2007 clinical competence statement on cardiac interventional procedures). *J Am Coll Cardiol.* 2013;62(4):357-396.

Kern MJ. Reducing Complications in the Very High 'BMI' Patient. October 2012. http://www.cathlabdigest.com/articles/Reducing-Complications-Very-High-%E2%80%98BMI%E2%80%99-Patient.

Kern MJ, ed. *Hemodynamic Rounds: Interpretation of Cardiac Pathophysiology From Pressure Waveform Analysis.* 3rd ed. Wiley-Liss, New York, 2017.

Kern MJ. Notes From the Editor's Corner of Cath Lab Digest: A Compilation. *Interventional Cardiology Education;* 2010:175.

Kern MJ, ed. *The Cardiac Catheterization Handbook.* 5th ed. Philadephia, PA: Elsevier; 2011:456.

Kern MJ, ed. *The Interventional Cardiac Catheterization Handbook.* 3rd ed. Philadelphia, PA: Saunders/Elsevier; 2013:450.

Kern MJ. Conversations in cardiology: the end of the end-hole LV gram. *Cath Lab Digest.* 2013.

Kern MJ. Cath Lab Safety. April 2014. http://www.cathlabdigest.com/articles/Cath-Lab-Safety. April 2014.

Kern MJ. How Should a "Code Blue" be Managed in the Cath Lab? February 2014. http://www.cathlabdigest.com/articles/How-Should-%E2%80%9CCode-Blue%E2%80%9D-be-Managed-Cath-Lab.

Kern MJ, King SB. Cardiac catheterization, cardiac angiography, and coronary blood flow and pressure measurements. In: Fuster V, Alexander RW, O'Rourke RA, eds. *Hurst's the Heart.* 13th ed. New York, NY: McGraw-Hill; 2014:490-538.

Klein LW, Ho KKL, Singh M, et al. Quality assessment and improvement in interventional cardiology: a position statement of the Society of Cardiovascular Angiography and Interventions, part II: public reporting and risk adjustment. *Catheter Cardiovasc Interv.* 2011;78:493-502.

Klein LW, Uretsky BF, Chambers C, et al. Quality assessment and improvement in interventional cardiology: a position statement of the Society of Cardiovascular Angiography and Interventions, part 1: standards for quality assessment and improvement in interventional cardiology. *Catheter Cardiovasc Interv.* 2011;77:927-935.

Madder RD, LaCombe A, VanOosterhout S, et al. Radiation exposure among scrub technologists and nurse circulators during cardiac catheterization: the impact of accessory lead shields. *JACC Cardiovasc Interv.* 2018;11:206-212.

Moscucci M. *Grossman & Baim's Cardiac Catheterization, Angiography, and Intervention.* 8th ed. Philadelphia, PA: Wolters/Kluwer/Lippincott Williams & Wilkins; 2014.

Naidu SS, Aronow HD, Box LC, et al. SCAI expert consensus statement: 2016 best practices in the cardiac catheterization laboratory: (Endorsed by the cardiological society of India, and sociedad Latino Americana de Cardiologia intervencionista; Affirmation of value by the Canadian Association of interventional cardiology-Association canadienne de cardiologie d'intervention). *Catheter Cardiovasc Interv*. 2016;88:407-423

Rao SV, Tremmel JA, Gilchrist IC, et al. Best practices for transradial angiography and intervention: a consensus statement from the Society for Cardiovascular Angiography and Intervention's Transradial Working Group. *Catheter Cardiovasc Interv*. 2014;83:228-236.

Sanborn TA, Tcheng JE, Anderson HV, et al. Structured Reporting in the Cardiac Catheterization Laboratory ACC/AHA/SCAI 2014 health policy statement on structured reporting for the cardiac catheterization laboratory. A report of the American College of Cardiology Clinical Quality Committee Developed in Collaboration With the American Association for Critical-Care Nurses, Asian Pacific Society of Cardiology, Canadian Cardiovascular Society, Health Level Seven International, Inter-American Society of Cardiology, Integrating the Healthcare Enterprise, Society of Thoracic Surgeons, and Society for Vascular Surgery. *J Am Coll Cardiol*. 2014;129:2578–2609.

Sizemore WG II. U.S. Naval air training and operational excellence. *Tex Heart Inst J*. 2013;40:562-563.

U.S. Public Health Service. Updated U.S. Public Health Service guidelines for the management of occupational exposures to HBV, HCV, and HIV and recommendations for postexposure prophylaxis. *MMWR Recomm Rep*. 2001;50(RR-11):1-52.

Vlastra W, Delewi R, Sjauw KD, et al. Efficacy of the RADPAD protection drape in reducing operators' radiation exposure in the catheterization laboratory: a sham-controlled randomized trial. *Circ Cardiovasc Interv*. 2017;10:e006058.

To view Video 1.1, please activate your
book on www.ExpertConsult.Inkling.com
using the pin code on the inside front cover.

Arterial and Venous Access

ADNAN K. CHHATRIWALLA • MICHAEL LIM •
PAUL SORAJJA

Vascular Access

A critical part of any catheterization procedure is attaining proper vascular access. Arterial access can be obtained in the femoral, brachial, or radial arteries. Preprocedure planning, careful detail to technique, proper equipment, and operator skill are all highly important. Some of the critical points of vascular access may not seem important to the uninitiated, but they are crucial to the safety and success of the procedure. The site of access is determined by planned investigation and the anticipated anatomic and pathologic conditions of the patient, in addition to anticipated bleeding risk. If possible, previous procedures and any difficulties encountered therein should be reviewed from old reports. Preprocedural assessment of the quality of all peripheral pulses is mandatory.

For patient comfort, adequate premedication and generous local anesthesia should be administered using a gentle approach. Pain during entry into the vessel may cause a vagal reaction or arterial spasm, potentially prolonging the procedure and causing significant complications.

Arterial Access Site Selection

For arterial access, femoral and radial approaches are most commonly used. Historically, brachial access was employed, but observed complication rates were relatively greater. A comparison of femoral versus radial artery catheterization is provided in Table 2.1. The greatest advantage of the radial approach is a reduction in bleeding and vascular complications, which has also been associated with a mortality benefit in high-risk patients. Because of this advantage, use of radial access in the United States has risen dramatically in the past few years. In 2007, 1.3% of all percutaneous coronary interventions (PCIs) were performed via the radial artery, but radial PCI had increased to >35% by 2017 (Fig. 2.1).

Table 2.1

Comparison of Femoral and Radial Access for Cardiac Catheterization.

Feature	Femoral	Radial
Access site bleeding	3%–4%	0%–0.6%
Artery complications	Pseudoaneurysm, retroperitoneal bleed, AV fistula, hematoma	Rare local irritation, pulse loss 3%–9%
Patient comfort	Acceptable	Excellent
Ambulation	1–4 hours	Immediate
Extra costs	Closure device (optional)	Hemostasis Band
Procedure time	Perceived shorter	Perceived longer
Estimated radiation exposure	Perceived lower	Perceived higher
Access to LIMA	Typically straightforward	Difficult from right radial artery
Use of artery for CABG surgery	N/A	Unknown
Learning curve	Short	Longer
>8-F guide catheters	Typically not a problem	Maximum 7 F (in men)
PVD, obese	Possibly problematic	Less problematic

Modified from Kern MJ, ed. Editor's corner: radial artery catheterization: the way to go, *Cath Lab Digest.* 2009;17:4–5.

AV, Arteriovenous; *CABG,* coronary artery bypass graft; *F,* French; *LIMA,* left internal mammary artery; *N/A,* not applicable; *PVD,* peripheral vascular disease.

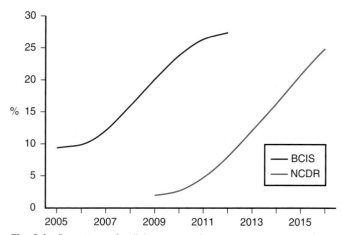

Fig. 2.1   Percentage of radial access use in percutaneous coronary intervention (PCI) cases over time. *BCIS: British Cardiovascular Intervention Society (Database)* and *NCDR: National Cardiovascular Data Registry.*

Femoral Artery Access

Percutaneous femoral arterial catheterization is still the most widely used technique in the United States. However, in patients with a history of claudication, signs of chronic arterial insufficiency, diminished or absent pulses, or bruits over the iliofemoral area, an alternate entry site may be considered to avoid the risk of further impairment of the arterial circulation in the legs (Box 2.1). The presence of arterial conduit grafts or previous balloon angioplasty of the iliofemoral system is not an absolute contraindication to femoral artery access. Prosthetic graft puncture has been shown to be safe if small-diameter sheaths are used and careful management for hemostasis is followed at the end of the procedure. Nonetheless, an alternative route should be considered.

Artery Location

Femoral artery access is usually obtained using the patient's right femoral artery with the operator standing at the right side of the patient. The common femoral artery is defined as that portion of the femoral artery below the lowest margin of the inferior epigastric artery and above the bifurcation of the superficial and profunda branches of the femoral artery. The goal is to access the common femoral artery over the mid portion of the femoral head so that there is a hard surface against which to compress the femoral artery when achieving hemostasis (Fig. 2.2). The mid portion of the femoral head is located approximately 2 cm below the inguinal ligament. The inguinal ligament is located by palpating the anterior superior iliac spine and the pubis and drawing an imaginary line between them. Then, using the middle and index fingers placed parallel to the long axis of the femoral artery,

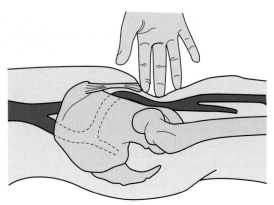

Fig. 2.2   Manual compression over the femoral head.

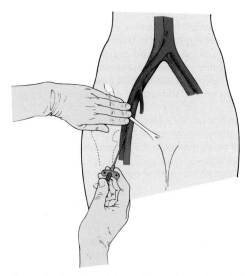

Fig. 2.3   Femoral artery (or vein) puncture with needle entering ~2 cm below the inguinal ligament and aiming medially toward the umbilicus. (From Tilkian AG, Daily EK. *Cardiovascular Procedures: Diagnostic Techniques and Therapeutic Procedures.* St Louis; Mosby: 1986.)

find the arterial pulse ~2 cm below this imaginary line (Fig. 2.3). A metal clamp can also be placed over the proposed entry site and the site can be confirmed by fluoroscopy (Fig. 2.4). Some operators place the tip of the clamp at the lower border of the femoral head to indicate where they will numb the patient and

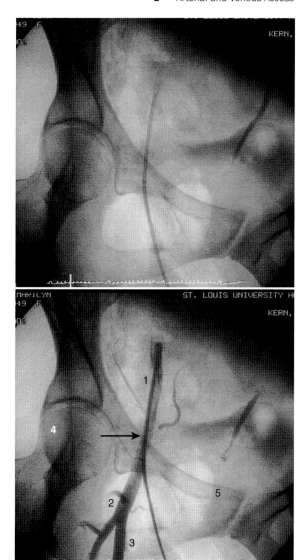

Fig. 2.4 Femoral artery landmarks. *Top:* Angiogram of sheath in the femoral artery in the anteroposterior projection. *Bottom:* Correct positioning is seen relative to angiographic landmarks. *1,* External iliac artery; *2,* bifurcation of profunda; *3,* superficial femoral artery; *4,* midpoint of femoral head; *5,* iliac-symphysis pubis ridge (inguinal ligament line). Upper limit of common femoral artery is lower margin of the inferior epigastric artery *(black arrow).*

then angle their needle such that they access the artery approximately 1 cm above this skin entry location. Identification of the femoral artery based on the skin crease as an anatomic landmark is no longer advocated because of its variability, particularly in obese patients.

Local Anesthesia

With a 25-gauge needle, the skin is infiltrated superficially with 1% lidocaine ~1 cm below (caudal to) the desired arterial entry site. This point is the skin entry site. In obese patients with thick subcutaneous tissue, the entry site should be slightly lower to ensure a needle entry angle of 45 degrees or less. Because large amounts of lidocaine may obscure the pulse, inject small amounts repeatedly instead of administering a large bolus. Next, with a 21-gauge needle, introduce 1% lidocaine into the deep tissue planes on each side of the artery. During lidocaine infiltration, palpate the arterial pulse with the middle and index fingers to avoid accidental puncture of the artery and ensure infiltration of tissue above and around the artery.

Gentle aspiration before the injection of lidocaine is essential to ensure that the needle tip is not in a blood vessel. Inserting the needle first to the deepest level desired and then continuing infiltration at several more shallow layers may decrease the patient's discomfort. Local anesthesia should cover the whole depth of the expected skin-to-artery path. Give sufficient lidocaine (~15 to 20 mL of a 1% solution) over 2 to 3 minutes for the full anesthetic effect to take place. Hint: Give lidocaine early and while the anesthetic is taking effect, other preparations such as connecting tubing and flushing catheters can be completed. During access, listen to the heart rate monitor or watch the electrocardiogram (ECG) for slowing of the rate as an early warning of a vagal reaction. Alternatives to lidocaine are listed in Box 2.2.

Skin Entry and Access Channel Preparation

Some operators perform a small skin incision before inserting a Seldinger needle. Other operators prefer to nick the skin over the entry needle or guidewire after the puncture. The latter approach usually results in only one nick if the operator does not obtain access on the first attempt. With the fingers placed over the artery as described previously, the operator can make a skin incision of 2 to 3 mm with a scalpel blade. For large-diameter sheaths, a subcutaneous tunnel can be made with blunt dissection using forceps.

Box 2.2   Anesthetic Alternatives to Lidocaine.

Group I
   Procaine (ester prototype)
   Benoxinate (Dorsacaine), benzocaine, butacaine (Butyn), butethamine
      (Monocaine), butylaminobenzoate (Butesin), chloroprocaine
      (Nesacaine), procaine (Novocain), tetracaine (Pontocaine)
Group II
   Lidocaine (amide prototype)
   Amydricaine (Alypin), bupivacaine (Marcaine), cyclomethycaine (Surfa-
      caine), dibucaine (Nupercaine), dimethisoquin (Quotane), diperodon
      (Diothane), dyclonine (Dyclone), etidocaine (Duranest), hexylcaine
      (Cyclaine), mepivacaine (Carbocaine), oxethazaine (Oxaine), phenacaine
      (Holocaine), piperocaine (Metycaine)
   Pramoxine (Tronothane), prilocaine (Citanest), proparacaine
      (Ophthaine), pyrrocaine (Endocaine)

From Tilkian AG, Daily EK. *Cardiovascular Procedures: Diagnostic Techniques and Therapeutic Procedures.* St Louis: Mosby;1986.

This channel makes the catheter and sheath entry easier and permits blood to drain outside the leg if the puncture site bleeds after the catheters have been removed. It is important to avoid extensive disruption of skin and subcutaneous tissue while creating the channel because these are the natural barriers to infection.

Arterial Puncture

The single anterior arterial wall entry (modified Seldinger) technique is preferred for femoral artery access (Fig. 2.5). This is especially important in patients treated with anticoagulants, antiplatelet agents, or thrombolytic agents. Access can be performed with a micropuncture kit or 18-gauge multipurpose needle. Ultrasound may be used to examine vessel size and the presence of untoward plaque and to identify the common femoral artery, thus avoiding puncture of bifurcations. Furthermore, ultrasound-guided access has been shown to facilitate anterior wall entry.

    The original Seldinger double-wall puncture technique is not explained here. The single-wall technique begins with the operator's fingers positioned over the femoral artery as described earlier. Hold the arterial needle (without an obturator) with the tip of the bevel directed upward. Introduce the needle through the skin and advance slowly toward the artery at a 30- to 45-degree angle to the horizontal plane. An entry into the artery that is too vertical creates problems in advancing the guidewire and promotes sheath and catheter kinking. A pulsation may be felt when the needle contacts the arterial wall. A slight resistance to the needle can be felt as it

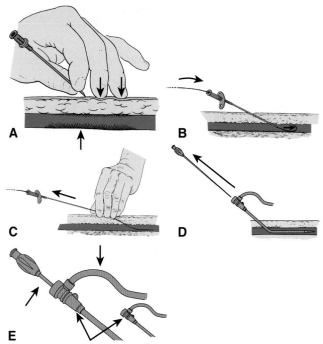

Fig. 2.5 **(A)** Femoral artery has been entered by a large-bore needle with backflow of blood. Note the operator's finger positions. As soon as the needle passes into the vessel through the anterior wall, brisk pulsatile flow occurs. This technique, called the front wall stick, prevents occult bleeding through the posterior wall. **(B)** The flexible tip of the guidewire is passed through the needle into the vessel. **(C)** A valve sheath is introduced into the artery. The needle is withdrawn, the artery is compressed, and the wire is pinched and fixed. **(D)** The valve sheath is advanced over a guidewire, and the dilator and guidewire are removed. **(E)** Position of sewing rings to attach valve to skin (*arrows*), should prolonged insertion be required. (A, B, C, and E: from Uretsky B, ed. *Cardiac Catheterization: Concepts, Techniques, and Applications.* Walden, MA: Blackwell Science; 1997.)

passes through the arterial wall. At this point, blood return from the needle hub confirms arterial puncture. Maintain the intraarterial needle position by holding the needle hub in a stable position. Resting the wrist on the patient's thigh may be helpful to stabilize needle position.

If the artery is not accessed, completely withdraw the needle, flush it of clot or fat, and advance in a different direction. Because of the sharp edge of the needle used for single-wall entry, the direction of the needle should not be changed when the needle tip is in the subcutaneous tissue.

Guidewire Insertion

Advance the guidewire gently into the artery. A soft J-tipped guidewire is the safest. Although straight-tipped guidewires have been used, they may increase the potential for subintimal dissection or vessel perforation. The wire should advance freely, without resistance. If resistance is encountered, the wire may be pulled back and advanced under fluoroscopic guidance, or the wire may be pulled back completely to confirm needle position via pulsatile blood return. Repositioning the needle may be necessary if the wire cannot be advanced freely. Sometimes the needle tip partially penetrates the posterior wall. In this case, there is good blood return, but the wire cannot be advanced because it is directed into the posterior wall of the artery rather than the arterial lumen. Withdrawing the needle 1 to 2 mm usually solves this problem. Lowering the needle hub several millimeters, or moving it medially or laterally, may improve alignment of the needle tip with the artery and permit easier guidewire passage. However, to avoid arterial injury, it is important not to move the needle hub excessively in any direction. The operator should attempt to puncture the artery close to the midline of the anterior vessel wall. Puncturing the lateral arterial wall may create a problem in advancing the guidewire or, worse, in controlling bleeding after the procedure.

   If it is not possible to advance the wire or if the needle comes out of the artery, withdraw the needle from the skin and apply pressure over the puncture site for at least 2 minutes to ensure hemostasis. Repeat the procedure using a slightly different angle or direction.

Micropuncture Access

The use of a 21-gauge micropuncture needle to obtain femoral artery access is appealing, because less bleeding may occur and hemostasis may be more easily achieved following needle removal compared with the use of larger gauge needles. This technique involves placement of a small micropuncture sheath into the femoral artery over a micropuncture guidewire once access has been obtained. The dilator of the micropuncture sheath can then be removed and the micropuncture sheath can be exchanged for a larger sheath over a 0.035-inch guidewire. However, micropuncture technique has not been proven to be superior to standard technique in preventing bleeding complications.

Ultrasound Imaging

If the artery cannot be located by palpation, ultrasound imaging can be used to localize and enter the artery (Fig. 2.6). A Doppler-tipped needle (Smart Needle), which differentiates between high-pitched (arterial) or low-pitched (venous) flow velocity sounds, can also be used.

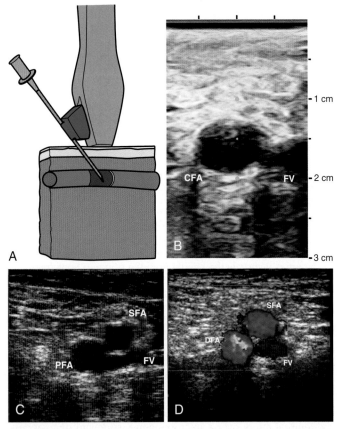

Fig. 2.6 Ultrasound visualization for femoral arterial access. **(A)** Hand-held sterile covered transducer with needle guide for arterial access. **(B)** Ultrasound image of common femoral artery (CFA) and femoral vein (FV). **(C)** Ultrasound image of profunda femoral artery (PFA), superficial femoral artery (SFA), and FV. **(D)** Doppler color flow images of deep femoral artery (DFA) and SFA (blue) and vein flow (red).

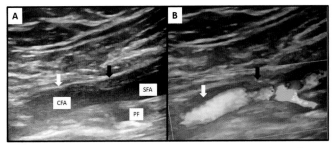

Fig. 2.7 **(A)** Ultrasound image demonstrating the common femoral artery *(CFA)* and its bifurcation into the superficial femoral artery *(SFA)* and profunda femoris *(PF)*. The artery appears normal proximally *(white arrow)* but atherosclerosis and resultant stenosis is apparent distally *(black arrow)*. **(B)** Color Doppler imaging of the same vessel demonstrating the normal vessel proximally *(white arrow)* and the extent of disease distally *(black arrow)*.

Routine ultrasound imaging may be useful in visualizing the femoral artery bifurcation and ensuring that access is obtained above the bifurcation in the common femoral artery. In addition, ultrasound imaging can be used to identify (and avoid) areas of atherosclerosis and/or vessel calcification (Fig. 2.7). Routine ultrasound imaging has been shown in large trials to increase the success of the first access attempt (83% vs. 46%, $P<0.001$) and thereby reduce the number of attempts needed to gain access and the time to arterial access. Furthermore, complications such as inadvertent venipuncture and access site hematoma are reduced with routine ultrasound imaging. The depth penetration should be adjusted to visualize the femoral artery and vein, and the centerline guide should be turned on. The femoral artery is imaged in the axial plane by holding the probe perpendicular to the course of the artery. The artery pulsates with gentle compression. Align the artery with the centerline guide on the display and insert the needle directly underneath the center marking of the probe, as close to the probe as possible. Using short in-and-out movements to visualize the needle course, move the needle toward the artery until it eventually compresses the artery and then punctures through.

From Guidewire to Catheter Insertion

If no resistance is encountered, advance the guidewire several centimeters at first and then into the abdominal aorta using fluoroscopy. Fluoroscopy of the guidewire moving through the iliac artery identifies large arterial plaques and excessive tortuosity, which complicates later catheter manipulation. As noted earlier, use of a J-tipped soft-spring guidewire is recommended because a straight wire may pass under a plaque, resulting in dissection. After the guidewire is correctly positioned above the iliac artery, remove the arterial needle. Apply firm pressure over the puncture site (to control bleeding) with the fingers while removing the needle from the skin and maintain puncture site pressure. The guidewire should be held firmly to avoid accidental wire removal as the needle is taken off the guidewire from the artery.

Advancement of the Sheath

After guidewire insertion into the artery, advance the sheath-dilator assembly over the wire while holding the guidewire straight. Introduce the sheath-dilator assembly into the artery by firmly holding it close to the tip, making clockwise and counterclockwise half-rotations (to reduce forward friction), and applying firm forward pressure. The sheath should not be advanced if significant resistance is encountered, as in the case of scar tissue. If significant resistance is encountered, serial dilatation of the tissue tract with increasingly larger dilators can be performed before the final sheath is inserted. The guidewire should be held straight and taut because it may otherwise kink. After the sheath is inserted completely, hold the sheath hub firmly in place and remove the dilator and guidewire together. Aspirate 2 to 3 mL of blood from the side arm of the sheath and flush the sheath with heparinized saline solution. The arterial pressure can be checked immediately by connecting a pressure manifold to the side arm of the sheath.

Patient Awareness

For both radial and femoral access, three steps may be associated with pain and vagal reaction: (1) initial administration of lidocaine, (2) arterial needle insertion, and (3) sheath assembly advancement. The operator should monitor the heart rate and feel the strength of the arterial pulse to detect early vagal responses. A vasovagal reaction of hypotension can occur with no change in heart rate, most commonly in elderly patients.

Sheath Removal and Manual Pressure Hemostasis

After catheterization has been completed, the patient's blood pressure is monitored and the catheter is removed. The sheath is aspirated and flushed to clear any thrombi. If heparin has been given during the procedure, an activated clotting time (ACT) should be obtained. Protocols vary, but the sheath is generally not removed until the ACT falls below 200 s. To remove the sheath, the operator places his or her fingers over the femoral artery. Because the actual puncture site is more cranial (toward the patient's head) than the skin incision, the operator's fingers should be placed over the femoral artery above the skin puncture site. The operator applies gentle pressure and removes the sheath from the leg, taking care not to crush the sheath and strip clot into the distal artery. When a small spurt of blood purges the arterial site of retained thrombi, the operator should apply firm downward pressure. Firm three-finger pressure should be adequate to achieve hemostasis in most cases. A rolled gauze pack may be placed over the artery to the groin and pressure applied with the palm of the hand. Standing on a short stool at bedside permits the operator's upper body weight to be used for pressure application.

Manual pressure is held firmly for approximately 3–5 minutes per sheath size, i.e., 15 to 25 minutes for a 5-F sheath and 18 to 30 minutes for a 6-F sheath. In patients treated with antiplatelet therapy, longer puncture site compression may be necessary. Compression time should be divided into four periods: full pressure, three-quarters pressure, half pressure, and one-quarter pressure, over the prescribed duration. During pressure application, pedal pulses should be intermittently evaluated and the entire leg should be uncovered to identify duskiness of the extremity. A diminished pulse is acceptable during brief full-pressure application, but distal pulses should not be obliterated completely at any time during manual compression. If the pedal pulse is absent during compression, the pressure over the artery should be decreased slightly periodically to allow distal circulation. Complete artery occlusion prevents clotting factors and platelets from being deposited at the arterial wall puncture site and in extreme cases can lead to vessel thrombosis, particularly in lower extremity bypass grafts. In patients with low cardiac output and a narrow pulse pressure, the femoral artery can easily be obliterated. In these patients, distal pulses should be checked more often and less pressure should be applied to the groin.

Hematoma Monitoring and Groin Dressings

After an appropriate time for manual pressure, the operator's hand is removed slowly and the area is inspected for hematoma or bleeding. Hemostasis may be difficult to secure in obese, hypertensive, or elderly female patients. Likewise, hemostasis may take longer to achieve in patients with a coagulopathy or who are receiving anticoagulant or antiplatelet agents. In all such patients, an extended monitoring period is prudent. In larger patients, greater than 500 mL of blood can be lost in a thigh or pannus before the problem is identified.

After hemostasis is obtained, clean the puncture area with an antiseptic solution and apply a small clear sterile dressing (e.g., Opsite, Tegaderm). This permits visualization of the entry site and surrounding tissues. One should not use gauze under the plastic dressing because this forms a culture medium if left in place after discharge. Likewise, large pressure dressings or sandbags should not be used, because they are ineffective in preventing bleeding and obscure the puncture site so that early hematoma formation may be missed.

If the femoral artery and vein are used in the procedure, arterial hemostasis should first be ensured and then the venous sheath should be removed to decrease the risk of AV fistula formation. In addition, preservation of venous access for the first 15 minutes of arterial compression may provide a useful access to treat hypotension resulting from blood loss or a vagal reaction should the peripheral IV line be inadequate for large volume resuscitation.

Mechanical Compression and Vascular Closure Devices

FemoStop Pressure System

The FemoStop (Fig. 2.8) is an air-filled clear plastic compression bubble that molds to skin contours. It is held in place by straps passing around the hips. The amount of applied pressure is controlled with a sphygmomanometer gauge. The clear plastic dome allows the operator to see the puncture site. The FemoStop is used most often for patients in whom prolonged compression is anticipated or whose bleeding persists despite prolonged manual compression. The duration of FemoStop compression and time until removal of the device vary depending on the patient and staff protocols. In some hospitals, the time from application to removal may be less than 30 minutes. In other patients in whom hemostasis is required, the device may be left at lower pressures for a longer duration. During the entire time of placement, direct visualization and monitoring should be performed by a trained individual. Caution should be used not to apply too much pressure to the groin, particularly for long durations, which may increase the risk of arterial or deep venous thrombosis.

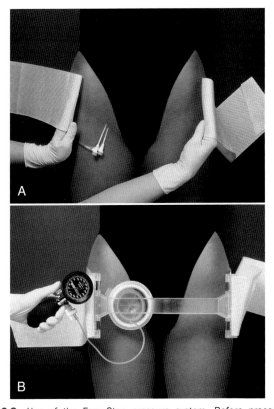

Fig. 2.8 Use of the FemoStop pressure system. Before proceeding, (1) examine the puncture site carefully, (2) note and mark edges of any hematoma, and (3) record patient's current blood pressure. **(A)** and **(B)** Step 1: position belt. The belt should be aligned with the puncture site equally across both hips. Step 2: center the dome and adjust the belt. The dome should be centered over the arterial puncture site above and slightly toward the midline of the skin incision. The sheath valve should be below the rim of the pressure dome. Attach the belt to ensure a snug fit. The center arch bar should be perpendicular to the body. Step 3: connect the dome pressure pump. Step 4: for a venous sheath, inflate dome to 20 or 30 mm Hg and remove the sheath. To minimize formation of arteriovenous fistula, obtain arterial hemostasis before the venous sheath is removed. Step 5: for the arterial sheath, pressurize the dome to 60 to 80 mm Hg, remove the sheath, and increase the pressure in the dome to 10 to 20 mm Hg above systolic arterial pressure. Step 6: maintain full compression for 3 minutes. Then, reduce pressure in the dome by 10 to 20 mm Hg every few minutes until 0 mm Hg is reached. Check arterial pulse. Observe for bleeding. After hemostasis is obtained, remove FemoStop and dress wound. (Courtesy Abbott Vascular, Santa Clara CA)

Vascular Closure Devices

Several different types of vascular closure devices (VCDs) are currently available. All VCDs have demonstrated rapid hemostasis and a decreased time to ambulation when compared with manual compression, but none has been shown to decrease vascular complications in randomized controlled trials. These devices may be especially helpful in patients who have back pain or cannot lie flat. Active closure methods include suture type (Perclose Proglide, Abbott Vascular, Santa Clara, CA), extravascular plug (Angio-Seal, St. Jude Medical, Santa Clara, CA; Mynx, Abbott Vascular, Santa Clara, CA), and surgical staple/clip technology (Abbott Vascular, Santa Clara, CA, Cardinal Health, Dublin OH; EVS-Angiolink, Medtronic, Inc., Minneapolis, MN). Theoretically, Angio-Seal has a higher risk of thromboembolic events because of the intravascular collagen anchor. The suture-mediated devices use primary healing (end-to-end anastomosis at the arteriotomy site) but have the highest rate of device and operator failure because of the learning curve associated with their use. Because VCDs do not ensure freedom from bleeding or vascular complications, diligent monitoring is still essential. The advantages and disadvantages of the various arterial closure devices are summarized in Table 2.2.

All VCDs should be used with caution in patients with peripheral vascular disease or with a high (above upper third of the femoral head) or low (at or below the femoral bifurcation) arterial puncture. Suture-mediated devices should not be used in small arteries (<4 mm). Caution is also needed in patients with scar tissue at the site of prior femoral artery procedures. Femoral angiography with an ipsilateral oblique angle (i.e., right anterior oblique [RAO] for right femoral artery, left anterior oblique [LAO] for left femoral artery) lays out the bifurcation, although the sheath entry site is often obscured. On the other hand, the contralateral oblique angle nicely demonstrates the sheath entry site but obscures the bifurcation (Fig. 2.9). The ipsilateral oblique angle is generally preferred and then the sheath is gently pulled medially to determine its entry point. For patient comfort, and to minimize contrast administration, femoral angiograms can be performed with a 50/50 contrast mixture.

Postcatheterization Patient Instructions and Discharge

Depending on the catheter and sheath size and whether or not a VCD was used, bed rest is recommended for 1 to 4 hours after femoral artery puncture. In the recovery area, the patient is

Table 2.2

Vascular Closure Devices.

Device	Mechanism	Advantages	Disadvantages	Sheath Sizes (F)	Ipsilateral Access <90 Days
Angio-Seal (Abbott Vascular, Santa Clara, CA)	Collagen and suture mediated	Secure closure	Intraarterial component, possible thromboembolic complications, infection related to wick	6 and 8	1 cm higher
Perclose (Abbott Vascular, Santa Clara, CA)	Suture mediated	Secure closure, ability to preclose for large-bore access	Intraarterial component, steep learning curve, device failure may require surgical repair	5 to 8	No restrictions

Continued on following page

Table 2.2

Vascular Closure Devices (Continued)					
Device	**Mechanism**	**Advantages**	**Disadvantages**	**Sheath Sizes (F)**	**Ipsilateral Access <90 Days**
StarClose (Abbott Vascular, Santa Clara, CA)	Nitinol clip	No intraarterial component	Adequate skin tract needed to prevent device failure	5 and 6	Not fully established
Mynx (Cardinal Health, Dublin OH)	PEG hydrogel plug	No intraarterial component, potential use in PVD	Possible intraarterial injection of sealant	5 to 7	No restrictions

PEG, Polyethylene glycol; *PVD,* peripheral vascular disease.

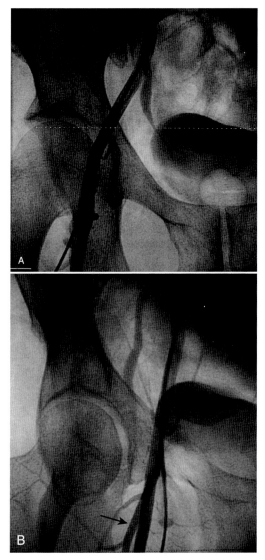

Fig. 2.9 Femoral angiograms. **(A)** Anteroposterior projection. The femoral bifurcation is obscured, although the insertion of the sheath can be visualized. **(B)** Right anterior oblique projection. The bifurcation of the femoral artery is now visible *(arrow)*. The sheath insertion site is made visible by gently pulling the sheath medially during the angiogram.

instructed (1) to stay in bed, (2) to keep the head down, (3) to hold the groin site when coughing, (4) to keep the punctured leg straight, and (5) to call a nurse for assistance if there is any bleeding, leg numbness, or leg pain. Following bed rest, the patient can sit up in bed for 30 minutes and can then walk with nursing assistance. At this point, the groin is rechecked and if there is no sign of hematoma or bleeding, the discharge process can continue.

Radial Artery Access

The radial artery is easily accessible in most patients and is not located near significant veins or nerves (Fig. 2.10A). The superficial location of the radial artery enables easy access and control of bleeding. No significant clinical sequelae after radial artery occlusion occur in patients with a normal Allen or Barbeau test because of the dual blood supply to the hand through the ulnar artery (see Fig. 2.10B). Lastly, patient comfort is enhanced by the ability to sit up and walk immediately after the procedure.

Use of the Allen or Barbeau Test

Performance of the Allen or Barbeau test is recommended to assess ulnar flow into the palmar arch prior to consideration of radial artery access. The Allen test is performed as follows: The patient makes a fist. The radial and ulnar arteries are occluded simultaneously. When the hand is opened, it appears to be blanched. Release of the ulnar artery should result in return of pink hand color within 8 to 10 seconds.

The Barbeau test uses pulse oximetry and plethysmography and is felt to be more sensitive, excluding only 1.5% of patients (Fig. 2.11). Using a pulse oximeter on the thumb, the pulse wave is displayed with both arteries open. The radial artery is then compressed and the pulse wave of ulnar flow can be observed. If the pulse wave does not change, it is classified as a Barbeau type A. If the pulse wave temporarily decreases in amplitude but then returns to the original amplitude, it is a Barbeau type B. If the pulse wave disappears but then returns at a decreased amplitude, it is a Barbeau type C. Finally, if the pulse wave disappears and there is no return of the pulse wave after 2 minutes, it is a Barbeau type D. Radial artery cannulation can proceed with types A, B, or C but is not recommended for type D. Similarly, a reverse Allen or Barbeau test can also be performed to check for radial artery patency by occluding the ulnar artery, which can be useful for patients with a history of prior radial artery access. It is important to emphasize that the Barbeau test can provide false reassurance if the pulse

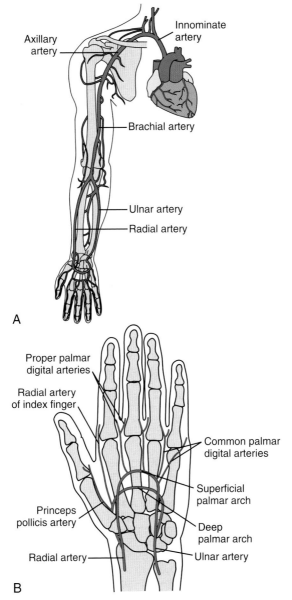

Fig. 2.10 Arterial anatomy of the upper extremity **(A)** and hand **(B)**.

Type   Precompression   Ulnar artery compression

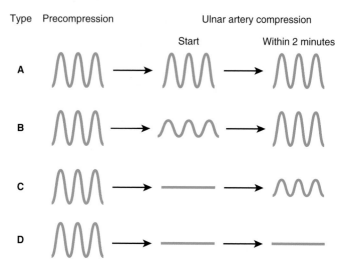

Fig. 2.11 The Barbeau test. (Courtesy James Bonnett. Adapted from Barbeau GR, Arsenault F, Dugas L, et al. Evaluation of the ulnopalmar arterial arches with pulse oximetry and plethysmography: comparison with the Allen's test in 1010 patients. *Am Heart J.* 2004;147:489–493.)

oximeter is placed on the index or other fingers as opposed to the thumb, because pulse oximetry in patients with an incomplete palmar arch may remain normal in the other fingers of the hand despite impairment of blood flow to the thumb with radial artery occlusion.

Patient Selection

Age need not be a factor in patient selection for radial artery access, because numerous series have reported high rates of success in patients older than 80 years. Although the risk of spasm and unsuccessful arterial access may be higher in smaller and older females, this group has the highest risk of bleeding and the most to gain from this approach. Similarly, patients with acute coronary syndromes, particularly ST-segment elevation myocardial infarction (STEMI), have higher bleeding risks and may benefit from the radial approach. However, the operator must be very comfortable with radial procedures before attempting the radial approach in these patients, for whom time is of the essence.

Patient Preparation

The patient should be comfortably positioned. Several positioning techniques have been suggested. Arm abduction at a 70-degree angle on an arm board or placement immediately next to the femoral access site has been used for sheath insertion. A movable arm board allows the arm to be positioned at the patient's hip next to the femoral artery during the procedure, and placement next to the leg allows decreased operator radiation exposure and removes the need for specialized drapes. A roll of sterile towels or a wrist splint is used to support and flex the wrist in a hyperextended position (Fig. 2.12). A topical anesthetic cream placed over the planned puncture site early in the patient preparation area for highly sensitive or anxious patients may help to decrease the amount of local lidocaine infiltration over the radial pulse, and small amounts of nitroglycerin added to lidocaine for topical infiltration may also reduce spasm. Large amounts of injected lidocaine may obscure the pulse and make cannulation more difficult. Pain management is important to minimize the risk of spasm during and after access.

Placement of intravenous (IV) lines must be considered preprocedurally. There should be no IVs near the hand or wrist that will get in the way of obtaining access or achieving hemostasis. IVs that will be used for infusions are preferably placed in the contralateral arm. With radial access occurring in the ipsilateral arm and infusion IVs being placed in the contralateral arm, blood pressure cuffs need to be placed on the patient's leg.

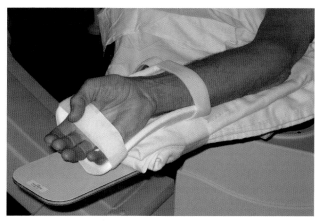

Fig. 2.12   Hyperextension of the wrist for radial access.

Right Versus Left Radial Approach

A right radial approach is often used because it is the side at which most operators are used to working. However, the left radial approach has been shown to have a shorter learning curve and reduced radiation exposure, and it may be easier in patients who are short (<165 cm) or elderly (age >75 years), because these patients develop more tortuosity in their innominate artery. This is also the preferred side for patients who have a left internal mammary artery (LIMA) graft that must be cannulated. Once access is obtained on the left side, the left arm should be brought over the abdomen so that the operator can work from his or her usual position on the right side of the patient. If the patient has mammary artery bypass grafts, the operator may choose to use the ipsilateral radial artery or the femoral artery because cannulating the contralateral mammary artery from the wrist can be challenging. Likewise, if the patient has a known arteria lusoria (an aberrant right subclavian artery arising from the descending aorta posterior to the esophagus, producing dysphagia) or other anatomic variation that will make the ipsilateral radial approach excessively difficult, the contralateral radial artery or femoral artery may be preferable. Lastly, consideration may be given as to whether the radial artery might subsequently be used as a bypass conduit, in which case the contralateral radial (or femoral) artery may be accessed instead.

Equipment Selection

There are two techniques for arterial puncture: the use of a micropuncture needle or the use of an angiocatheter needle. The choice is based on personal preference, although some data suggest that the angiocatheter needle technique is easier to learn and decreases the time and number of attempts used to gain access. Using the micropuncture technique, the operator punctures only the front wall of the radial artery, whereas with the angiocatheter technique, a through-and-through puncture must be used, whereby the needle is sent through the posterior wall of the radial artery. This is done to ensure access to the lumen and does not increase vascular complications as it might if the same approach were used for the femoral artery. Ultrasound imaging (see later) can also facilitate radial artery access.

Several radial artery sheath systems (10 to 36 cm) with a graduated dilator system are available, although there are no data demonstrating an advantage to using a longer sheath (Fig. 2.13). Sheathless systems have also been developed, but these are not available in the United States. Instead, a homemade system must be made if this approach is to be used. Several variations have

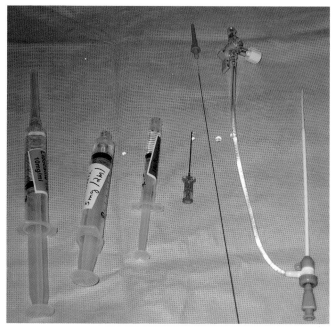

Fig. 2.13 Equipment used for radial artery access.

been proposed, and each involves the creation of a distal transition so that the guide can be passed smoothly through the skin and into the artery. An example is the insertion of a 5 F × 125-cm ShuttleSelect (Flexor) sheath inside a 6-F guide catheter.

A final important aspect of any sheath used is that it must be hydrophilic. This minimizes spasm, patient discomfort, and trauma to the vessel wall. Careful catheter selection for the radial approach is also important and is discussed in Chapter 3. Minimizing catheter exchanges has been shown to decrease the incidence of spasm, and all catheter exchanges should be done over a wire to maintain access in the ascending aorta and to avoid trauma to the great vessels.

Radial Artery Access and Sheath Introduction

Once the arm is draped, the radial pulse is palpated (Fig. 2.14). The point of puncture should be 1 to 2 cm proximal to the bony

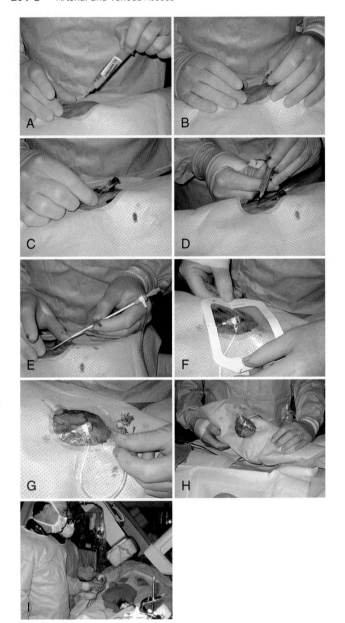

Fig. 2.14 Radial artery access and sheath introduction. Once draped, the radial pulse is palpated. The point of puncture should be 1 to 2 cm cranial to the bony prominence of the distal radius. **(A)** Administer a small amount of lidocaine into the skin. **(B)** Use the needle (micropuncture needle shown here) at a 30- to 45-degree angulation. Slowly advance until blood pulsates out of needle. It is not a strong pulsation because of the small bore of the needle. **(C)** Fix the needle position and carefully introduce 0.018-inch guidewire with a twirling motion. There should be little or no resistance to wire introduction. Remove the needle. **(D)** Make a small incision over the wire in preparation to introduce sheath (this step is optional). **(E)** Advance the sheath over the wire into the artery. If sheath moves easily, advance to hub. If resistance is felt with the sheath halfway in artery, remove the wire and administer the vasodilator cocktail. Reinsert the wire and continue to advance sheath. **(F)** and **(G)** After the sheath is positioned and flushed, secure the sheath with clear plastic dressing or suture (also optional). **(H)** and **(I)** The arm can now be moved to the patient's side for catheter introduction.

---

prominence of the distal radius. Inject a small (≤1 cc) amount of 1% lidocaine into the superficial skin. Hold the needle at a 30- to 45-degree angulation and slowly advance until blood pulsates out of the needle (in the case of a micropuncture technique) or advance until blood stops filling the reservoir in the angiocatheter needle. With the micropuncture needle, there is not a strong pulsation because of the small bore of the needle. With the angiocatheter needle, there is generally no blood return after withdrawal of the needle. Instead, blood pulsations are obtained once the small catheter is pulled back into the lumen. Once in the lumen, carefully introduce the guidewire; there should be little or no resistance to the wire introduction. Investigate any resistance with fluoroscopy. Care must be taken if a hydrophilic-coated guidewire is used, because these wires can easily perforate small branch vessels and lead to hematoma. Remove the needle and, if necessary, make a small skin incision over the wire (or prior to needle insertion) in preparation to introducing the sheath, although this is generally not necessary with hydrophilic sheaths unless a patient's skin is particularly tough. Advance the sheath over the wire into the artery. If the sheath moves in easily, advance it to the hub. If resistance is felt with the sheath halfway in the artery, remove the wire, administer the vasodilator cocktail, and consider performing a small injection of a 50/50 contrast mixture under fluoroscopic guidance. Reinsert the wire and dilator and continue to advance the sheath under fluoroscopic guidance. After the sheath is positioned and flushed (and an antispasm cocktail is given, if not already given), one can secure the sheath with clear plastic dressing or a suture. The arm may then be moved to the patient's side for catheter introduction.

Ultrasound Imaging

Ultrasound can be used to facilitate radial artery access, and studies have demonstrated improved first-pass rates, reduced number of attempts, and lower times to achieve success when using ultrasound compared with palpation alone. The ultrasound probe can be set up prior to access in order not to prolong the procedure. The ultrasound should be set at a minimum of depth penetration (i.e., 2 cm) and high gain, and the centerline guide should be turned on. The radial artery is imaged in the axial plane by holding the probe perpendicular to the course of the artery. The artery pulsates with gentle compression. Align the artery with the centerline guide on the display and insert the radial needle directly underneath the center marking of the probe, as close to the probe as possible. Using short in-and-out movements in order to visualize the needle course, move the needle toward the artery until it eventually compresses the artery and then punctures through. This technique may take some practice but ultimately can save time, particularly for difficult access cases.

The Radial "Cocktail"

After inserting the arterial sheath, infuse a radial "cocktail" for arterial spasm prevention through the side arm. Numerous cocktails are used, but they generally include verapamil, nitroglycerin, or a combination of both (Box 2.3). Diltiazem, papaverine, or nitroprusside may also be used. Verapamil in doses of 2.5 or 5 mg has been given

---

Box 2.3   Medical Regimen for Radial Catheterization.[a]

1. Before the procedure:
    Topical anesthetic cream over the radial artery (optional)
2. Through the sheath (before catheter insertion):
    Heparin 5000 U or 50 U/kg (better intravenously), verapamil 2.5 mg, and/or nitroglycerin 100 to 200 mcg
    1% lidocaine 1 to 2 mL (optional)
3. After the procedure and before sheath removal:
    Verapamil 2.5 mg, and/or nitroglycerin 100 to 200 mcg (optional)

[a]Other vasodilator cocktails can be used according to laboratory routines.

alone or in a cocktail without unwanted side effects, such as hypotension or bradycardia. Nitroglycerin and nitroprusside must be given cautiously in patients with severe aortic stenosis or any LV outflow obstruction; many operators forgo these drugs altogether. Lidocaine added to the cocktail may improve patient comfort during catheter manipulation. Heparin is typically given to prevent radial artery occlusion at a dose of 5000 U or 50 U/kg IV. Heparin may be given intraarterially (IA) as part of the cocktail, but if doing so, it should be mixed with plenty of blood to reduce burning. Alternatively, heparin can be given via IV to reduce local irritation and pain. Comparative studies have shown similarly efficacy for prevention of occlusion with heparin administered IV or IA. Bivalirudin is also an acceptable alternative to heparin and should be standardly dosed in a weight-based bolus and infusion.

Repeat injections of antispasm medications are not necessary with catheter exchanges or prior to sheath removal unless the patient is developing spasm. If the operator notes the development of spasm (the catheter becomes harder to manipulate and the patient reports pain), another round of spasmolytic cocktail can be given. Spasm occurs more commonly in women and with excessive catheter manipulation, multiple catheter exchanges, and less operator experience.

Navigating Up the Arm

Once the sheath is in place, advance the catheter up the arm, around the shoulder, and to the aortic root over a 0.035-inch guidewire. Generally, a standard J-wire with a very small J curve is sufficient, although operators often use other preferred wires, such as a short-tipped J-wire, a Wholey (Covidien ev3, Plymouth, MN) or a Bentson (Cook Medical, Bloomington, IN). If any resistance is encountered, use fluoroscopy. If the J-wire will not advance, a hydrophilic wire may be useful. However, hydrophilic wires should be used with caution, because they can enter (and potentially perforate) small branches without the tactile feedback from a standard J-wire. On rare occasions, an angiogram of the arm will be necessary. If there is tortuosity or looping in the innominate artery, having the patient take a deep breath can help straighten the anatomy and ease catheter motion.

For small caliber vessels, tortuosity/loops, or resistance as a result of spasm/atherosclerosis, a technique called *balloon-assisted tracking* (BAT) can be helpful. This involves dilating a coronary balloon at the distal end of the catheter (generally, a balloon 15 to 20 mm in length is used, with 7 to 10 mm protruding distal to the catheter tip) to create a nontraumatic tip that is more flexible or pushable. For more flexibility, the balloon can be dilated to 3 atm, whereas for more pushability, it can be dilated to 6 atm. A 1.5-mm diameter balloon can be used in a 5-F catheter/guide, and a 2-mm diameter balloon can be used in a 6-F catheter/guide. Then, advance the catheter/guide up the arm over a 0.014-inch coronary wire.

Sheath Removal and Postprocedure Care

A number of devices have been designed to provide hemostasis, from a simple plastic hemodialysis band compressing a gauze bullet over the radial arterial puncture to specifically designed compression bands, such as the Radistop (St. Jude Medical, St. Paul, MN) or TR Band (Terumo Medical Corp., Somerset, NJ; Abbott Vascular, Santa Clara, CA). Regardless of the chosen device, there are a few critical steps in this process.

Position the device snugly around the wrist before sheath removal; the compression portion of the device should be positioned to cover both the skin nick and arteriotomy site (Fig. 2.15). Gauze can be placed under the device as a wick to collect any blood leakage and then removed once hemostasis is achieved. The sheath should be removed slowly and smoothly while slowly tightening the device. One common mistake is tightening the device too aggressively before the sheath is removed, leading to patient discomfort. For both patient comfort and adequate hemostasis, the removal of the sheath and the tightening of the device should be done simultaneously. The device should be tight enough to ensure hemostasis but not too tight to occlude the flow through either the radial or ulnar arteries. This is called *patent hemostasis*, and it is an essential technique for reducing radial artery occlusion. Once the device is in place and hemostasis is achieved, a reverse Barbeau test can be performed to ensure patent hemostasis. Patent hemostasis of the radial artery will be confirmed by a Barbeau type A, B, or C while the ulnar artery is being compressed. If there is a Barbeau type D, try loosening the device. If the device cannot be loosened any further without blood leakage, send the patient to recovery and try again after 15 minutes. Generally, further loosening can be performed after a short period of time to obtain patent hemostasis. Recovery room nurses should be adept at performing the Barbeau test and maintaining patent hemostasis.

Numerous protocols have been used for removal of the hemostatic device. One protocol commonly used is to ensure (or achieve) patent hemostasis upon arrival to the recovery room for 1 hour and then to start loosening the device after 90 minutes. The device is loosened further at 105 minutes and then removed at 120 minutes, as long as there is no active bleeding. If there is still bleeding, minimally tighten the device to achieve hemostasis

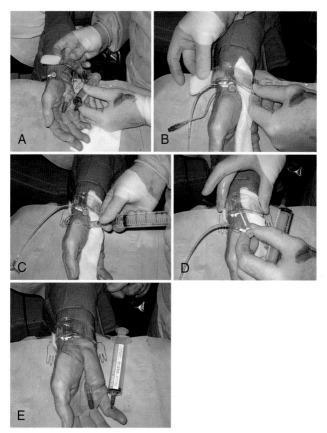

Fig. 2.15 **(A)** Radial sheath removal with Terumo band, which has an inflatable compression pad for hemostasis. **(B)** TR band is applied around the wrist with green dot over the arterial (not skin) puncture. A thin gauze wick is placed beneath the band to absorb blood when pressure is released to assess proper compression pressure in pad. **(C)** Compression pad is inflated. **(D)** Sheath is removed. **(E)** Final result.

for an additional 15 minutes and then make another attempt to remove the device. Repeat this until successful. If late bleeding occurs, give the patient instructions about using the fingers to compress the puncture site. In addition, instruct the patient to limit lifting any item weighing more than 10 pounds for 3 days following the procedure.

Complications: Radial Artery Spasm

Some spasm during sheath withdrawal is common. It is wise to tell patients that removal of the sheath may be associated with discomfort. Take the sheath out quickly (but gently); usually the duration of discomfort (if any) is short. Do not allow the patient to experience significant pain; analgesics and sedation should be administered. If spasm is severe and the sheath (or catheter) is stuck, the following actions can be undertaken:

1. Administer nifedipine 10 mg orally or nitroglycerin 400 mcg sublingually.
2. Administer more analgesia and sedation.
3. Place warm compresses over the forearm to relax the spastic artery.
4. Administer nitroglycerin 200 mcg IA; repeat if necessary.
5. Give verapamil 2.5 mg intra-arterial (diltiazem can also be used). This should be mixed with blood prior to injection via the side-arm of the sheath because direct injection will cause significant discomfort.

If these do not work, wait for an hour and try again. During this time, maintain proper anticoagulation (heparin), sedation, and analgesia. If nothing helps, an axillary block, propofol, or general anesthesia might be required to relax the radial artery. One should never apply excessive force. This might result in rupture or avulsion of the radial artery.

Bleeding and Vascular Complications

Early recognition of vascular complications is vital, because an unrecognized hematoma can develop even under the watchful eyes of a provider. These can be subtler than those seen from the femoral approach and without overt bleeding. Patients complaining of pain or paresthesias (numbness) warrant a close evaluation. Developing hematomas can be averted with gentle manual pressure followed by a careful arm-wrapping technique. While maintaining the wristband in place, wrap the arm loosely with gauze and secondarily with elastic tape or an ACE bandage, providing compression to the forearm. After several minutes, remove the tape and recheck the forearm; it should be softer. If not, rewrap with slightly higher tension. An unnoticed and untreated hematoma can produce a forearm compartment syndrome, threatening the viability of the forearm and hand. Figure 2.16 gives a schema for

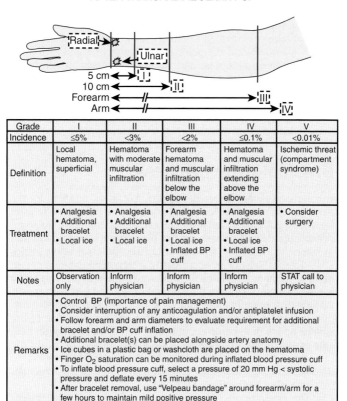

EASY HEMATOMA CLASSIFICATION
AFTER TRANSRADIAL/ULNAR PCI

Grade	I	II	III	IV	V
Incidence	≤5%	<3%	<2%	≤0.1%	<0.01%
Definition	Local hematoma, superficial	Hematoma with moderate muscular infiltration	Forearm hematoma and muscular infiltration below the elbow	Hematoma and muscular infiltration extending above the elbow	Ischemic threat (compartment syndrome)
Treatment	• Analgesia • Additional bracelet • Local ice	• Analgesia • Additional bracelet • Local ice	• Analgesia • Additional bracelet • Local ice • Inflated BP cuff	• Analgesia • Additional bracelet • Local ice • Inflated BP cuff	• Consider surgery
Notes	Observation only	Inform physician	Inform physician	Inform physician	STAT call to physician
Remarks	• Control BP (importance of pain management) • Consider interruption of any anticoagulation and/or antiplatelet infusion • Follow forearm and arm diameters to evaluate requirement for additional bracelet and/or BP cuff inflation • Additional bracelet(s) can be placed alongside artery anatomy • Ice cubes in a plastic bag or washcloth are placed on the hematoma • Finger O$_2$ saturation can be monitored during inflated blood pressure cuff • To inflate blood pressure cuff, select a pressure of 20 mm Hg < systolic pressure and deflate every 15 minutes • After bracelet removal, use "Velpeau bandage" around forearm/arm for a few hours to maintain mild positive pressure				

Fig. 2.16 Schema for easy recognition and management of arm hematoma after radial artery catheterization. *BP,* Blood pressure; *PCI,* percutaneous coronary intervention; *STAT,* statium (immediately). (Courtesy Dr. Oliver Bertrand, Laval Hospital, Quebec, Canada.)

easy recognition and treatment of arm bleeding after radial artery catheterization and PCI.

Dissection or perforation of the radial or brachial artery can occur from wires or catheters. In this situation, the initial reaction is often to abort the procedure, but in fact, if the procedure can be continued safely, it is best to do so. The catheter will serve to tamponade the vessel, and the dissection/perforation will typically resolve by the end of the procedure. This can be confirmed by arteriography at the end of the case.

Postprocedure radial arterial occlusion has been reported to occur at rates of <1% to 10% and is usually asymptomatic. If ulnar flow is adequate and the palmar arch is patent, supportive treatment with acetaminophen and warm compresses are all that is necessary. With the preventive measures discussed earlier, including use of heparin, a small sheath, and patent hemostasis, radial artery occlusion rates can be minimized. Brachial arterial thrombosis is a rare complication that should be treated by thrombectomy followed by an evaluation for a hypercoagulable state.

Brachial Artery Access

Percutaneous brachial arterial access should be reserved for patients in whom neither the radial nor femoral artery can be used for access. Although similar to femoral arterial puncture, there are several important differences. The brachial artery is smaller (3 to 5 mm in diameter) than the femoral artery. The brachial artery varies considerably. Spasm can occur easily with considerable decrease in pulse amplitude, making the puncture more difficult. The artery is also more mobile than the femoral artery and prone to spasm, making the puncture more difficult. Care should be taken to puncture the artery successfully on the first attempt. Because of the smaller space in the arm, uncontrolled hematoma formation here can readily cause compartment syndrome with ischemia of the forearm and hand. The median nerve lies immediately medial to the artery, and unintentional contact with it may cause a peculiar electrical shock sensation in the hand.

The operator should check the brachial and radial pulses before attempting brachial arterial puncture. In patients in whom femoral access is not possible because of severe atherosclerosis, vascular surgery, or the presence of an IABP or LV support device, the same type of atherosclerotic disease may exist in the subclavian arterial system.

Anesthesia Administration

The maximum point of brachial arterial pulse is located approximately 1 cm above the elbow crease. With a 25-gauge needle, infiltrate the skin and subcutaneous tissue with 2 to 3 mL of 1% lidocaine. Injection of excessive amounts of local anesthetic may make palpation of the artery difficult or obscure the pulse completely.

Puncture of the Artery and Introduction of the Guidewire

Similar to the radial artery entry technique, a micropuncture needle with a 0.018-inch guidewire is used to enter the brachial artery. The through-and-through puncture with an angiocatheter needle is not recommended in this location. To facilitate the arterial puncture, the operator can stabilize the artery with the index and middle fingers placed below and above the puncture point. Upon blood return from the needle, the guidewire is advanced into the artery, and the sheath is placed as with radial artery cannulation. Additional lidocaine can be applied to the deeper tissue planes. Heparin (40 to 50 U/kg) is given via IV. The brachial artery can accommodate up to size 8-F sheaths in large men. In most patients, especially smaller men and women, smaller sheaths (e.g., 6-F) are preferred.

Hemostasis after Brachial Artery Catheterization

A board is placed behind the patient's elbow to facilitate pressure application. Check the radial pulse before removing the sheath. If the pulse is weak or absent, 200–400 mcg of nitroglycerin can be delivered into the artery through the sheath and then the pulse should be rechecked. Remove the sheath while applying firm finger pressure over the puncture site. A small amount of bleeding is allowed to purge possible clots. The operator should not strip the sheath, pushing thrombus into the artery. Continuously palpate the radial pulse either with manual palpation or plethysmography and adjust the amount of pressure applied over the artery to stop bleeding without completely obliterating the radial pulse. After 15 to 20 minutes, slowly release the pressure. Check and record the patient's radial pulse. The arm circumference at the site of puncture can be measured to facilitate the detection of hematoma formation. Instruct the patient to keep the arm in a relaxed but straight position for 2 to 4 hours. Sitting up in bed is permitted, but ambulation is restricted until after the hemostasis period of 2 to 4 hours.

Femoral Vein Access

The femoral arterial pulse is the landmark for the femoral vein. The femoral vein is located approximately 1 cm medial to the femoral artery, but sometimes it is located partially behind the artery. The procedure for femoral vein percutaneous entry involves the following steps: (1) The femoral arterial pulse is located as described previously. If arterial and venous puncture are planned, the area infiltrated by lidocaine must be wide enough to provide adequate anesthesia to both puncture sites. (2) The skin is entered 0.5 to 1 cm medial and 0.5 to 1 cm caudal (toward the foot) to the arterial entry site. (3) Because venous pressure is low, a syringe is attached to the Seldinger needle and gently aspirated during needle advancement. The operator inserts the needle medially through the skin at a 30- to 45-degree angle to the horizontal plane while palpating the femoral arterial pulse (remember: *N-A-V = nerve, artery, vein*, from outside in; i.e., lateral to medial). Be sure not to press so hard on the artery that the vein is occluded. If arterial pulsations are felt at the tip of the needle, withdraw and redirect the needle at a slightly more medial angle.

If the vein has been entered, venous (nonpulsatile) dark blood fills the syringe. Blood should come easily into the syringe on the needle without application of much negative pressure. If the vein has not been entered, flush and reintroduce the needle in a slightly more lateral or medial direction. If the artery is entered and not used, the needle is removed and firm manual pressure is applied over the artery for several minutes. Another attempt to enter the vein can be made after the bleeding has stopped. Sometimes it may be necessary to direct the needle close to the artery because the vein may be located partially under the artery. Ultrasound imaging guidance can reduce the number of venous puncture attempts.

A vein that has been entered mistakenly during a femoral artery puncture attempt should be used only if the needle tip did not puncture both walls of the artery and go into the vein behind it. Placing a sheath through the artery into the vein may create an AV fistula or cause uncontrolled bleeding from a large hole in the posterior wall of the femoral artery. The remainder of the venous sheath placement is completed in the same way as described for the femoral arterial sheath insertion.

After the catheterization is completed, finger pressure is applied over the vein as described for femoral artery sheath removal, although much less pressure is needed. After femoral vein access with a 5-F or 6-F sheath, 5 to 10 minutes of compression is usually enough time to obtain adequate hemostasis.

Note for Accessing Both Femoral Artery and Vein

For cases in which femoral artery and vein access is planned, the method of vascular access can be modified from the standard approach described previously. In some laboratories, venous access is performed first, but instead of proceeding to insert a sheath after the wire is introduced, the wire remains in the vein until the artery has been punctured and the artery guidewire is in place. The insertion of sheaths then follows after skin nicks are made. The sheaths are inserted over each wire sequentially, usually vein, then artery. The advantage of this minor change is the elimination of puncturing the venous sheath while searching with the needle for the nearby artery.

Internal Jugular Vein Access

The internal jugular vein is lateral to the carotid artery, medial to the external jugular vein, and usually just lateral to the outer edge of the medial head of the sternocleidomastoid muscle. To identify landmarks, the operator instructs the patient to lie supine without a pillow and, in the case of the right internal jugular, with the head turned 30 degrees to the left. Patients with low venous pressures may be placed in the Trendelenburg (head lower than feet) position. Ultrasound imaging is recommended to facilitate access.

Several approaches to internal jugular vein access exist. A high anterior approach from the top of the triangle formed by the two heads of the sternocleidomastoid muscle and clavicle is recommended. This location moves the puncture site away from the upper lung tip. In obese patients, the triangle can be difficult to localize correctly, but it is helpful to put a finger in the suprasternal recess and move the finger to the right (for right internal jugular access). The first elevation palpated is the medial head of the sternocleidomastoid muscle. Move the finger over the medial head and follow the edge superiorly until the top of the triangle is palpated.

After infiltrating the skin with lidocaine, insert the needle through the skin, pointing slightly toward the ipsilateral nipple. When blood is aspirated, the guidewire is inserted, followed by the sheath, using a standard Seldinger technique.

Brachial Vein Access

Right heart catheterization may be performed via the brachial vein. Access can be obtained from the arm by placing a 20-gauge IV in the ipsilateral antecubital vein. All superficial veins lead to the deep veins, although a medial antecubital vein is preferable over a lateral antecubital vein, which courses through the cephalic venous system over the deltoid muscles, making catheter advancement difficult through the relatively sharp turns in the shoulder area. This IV is then prepped and draped in the usual manner. An

0.018-inch guidewire is advanced through the IV and up the arm. The IV is removed and a sheath is placed over the wire. A small amount of 1% lidocaine to the area prior to sheath insertion will reduce discomfort. Next, a hydrophilic sheath can be advanced through the skin with no nick needed. The veins will generally accommodate up to a 7-F sheath, but a 5-F sheath is preferable, if a 5-F balloon-tipped PA catheter is available. Advancing the catheter over the wire is often easier than simply advancing it through the vein without a wire, because the veins can be small and valves can get in the way. Continuous injection of saline through the catheter during advancement can help negotiate venous valves as a liquid guidewire. The balloon should not be expanded until the catheter approaches the superior vena cava. If IV placement was not done prior to the intervention, or was unsuccessful, the operator can gain antecubital venous access using a micropuncture needle with ultrasound guidance. Application of a tourniquet several centimeters above the elbow may facilitate the identification of a suitable vein.

Vascular Access Through Synthetic Graft Conduits

If possible, avoid access through synthetic peripheral vascular grafts. Limited experience indicates that complications are less than 2% if 5-F to 9-F sheaths are used for diagnostic (not interventional) procedures in grafts greater than 6 months old. If it is necessary to use grafts for access, diligent care must be taken during hemostasis not to occlude the graft completely, which can lead to graft thrombosis.

Large-Bore Access

Many mechanical circulatory support systems, structural procedures (e.g., aortic valvuloplasty, transcatheter aortic valve replacement) and peripheral therapies (e.g., endovascular graft) require large-bore access. The use of these large-bore sheaths necessitates careful attention to procedural planning and postprocedural hemostasis.

Ultrasound-guided access is essential for proper large bore access. Alternatively, some operators will also initially access the contralateral artery (to visualize the side to be used for the femoral artery) and cross over to the ipsilateral femoral with a guidewire and exchange for a pigtail catheter. After injecting contrast through the pigtail catheter and assuring absence of vascular disease and proper access site and vessel size, access is obtained for the large-bore sheath, often using the center of the pigtail catheter as the needle target.

The most commonly used device for hemostasis in this setting is the Perclose ProGlide system using a pre-close technique. The preclose technique utilizes two devices placed after initial arterial access is achieved. The first device is oriented slightly off the vertical at the 10 o'clock position. Use standard placement technique, but the suture knots are not tightened down on the arteriotomy but rather clamped and placed under a sterile towel to be closed at the end of the procedure. The second device is oriented at the 2 o'clock position relative to vertical. After the second device is placed in a similar way to the first device, the sutures are set aside to be used later. At this point, reintroduce a guidewire through the port of the VCD and exchange it for the large-bore sheath to proceed with the main procedure (Fig. 2.17).

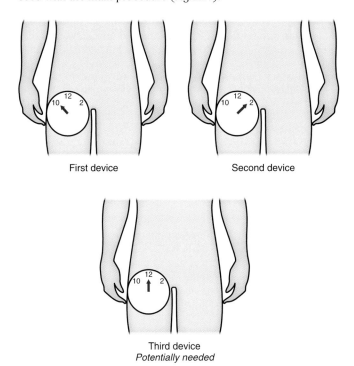

First device

Second device

Third device
Potentially needed

Fig. 2.17 Preclose technique signifies that the Perclose ProGlide suture is placed around the arteriotomy at the beginning of the procedure and knot advancement is placed on hold until the procedure is complete. The preclose technique using at least two devices must be used when closing sheath sizes from 8.5 F to 21 F. See the text for more information. (Redrawn with permission of Abbott Vascular, copyright 2013)

After completing the main procedure, place a guidewire through the large-bore sheath. If desired, a contralateral balloon catheter can be placed in the ipsilateral iliac artery and inflated to obstruct antegrade blood flow. Aspirate, flush, and slowly remove the sheath and advance the first suture knot with the guidewire position maintained, but do not yet lock the sutures on the arteriotomy site. Reinsertion of the sheath introducer prior to sheath removal may allow for an easier transition as the sheath is removed and the suture knot is advanced, resulting in less bleeding. The second set of pre-closed sutures is then similarly tightened on the arteriotomy site. The site is now assessed for relative hemostasis (if an iliac balloon inflation was performed, it should be deflated to assess hemostasis). There may be some slight bleeding, but it should not be pulsatile. If significant bleeding is identified, a third VCD can be inserted at 12 o'clock (Figs. 2.17 and 2.18). Once bleeding is controlled, the guidewire can be removed, and the first and then subsequent sutures locked on the arteriotomy. Finally, the sutures should be held taut and cut in the order in which they were made (Fig. 2.19). If full hemostasis is achieved, a final angiogram can be performed to assess vascular integrity. Having an iliac balloon in place during the deployment of the Perclose devices provides an additional measure of safety should the closure not hold and additional procedures become necessary to provide hemostasis.

Tips and Tricks: Options to Achieve Success

Vessel Tortuosity

The most commonly encountered difficulty in advancing guidewires or catheters into the aorta is iliac or subclavian vessel tortuosity, a problem often found in elderly patients. A wire with a flexible and atraumatic steerable tip (e.g., 0.035-inch Wholey or hydrophilic Glidewire) may be useful in these circumstances. In cases of extreme tortuosity, it might be necessary to advance a catheter close to (within several centimeters of) the guidewire tip in order to increase the torque control of the guidewire. A Judkins right (JR) or a multipurpose (MP) coronary catheter can also be used to change the direction of the guidewire tip.

In patients with tortuous iliac vessels, a long (>20 cm) sheath may be used, recognizing the tradeoff of multiple friction points for some straightening of the vessel. Catheter exchanges over a long (300 cm) exchange guidewire may be required to avoid undue prolongation of the procedure by repeated attempts to advance catheters across tortuous atherosclerotic segments.

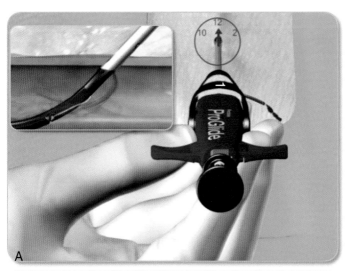

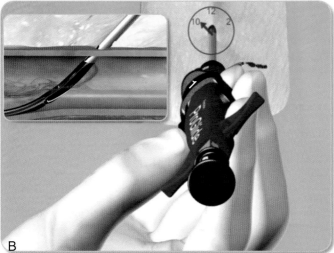

Fig. 2.18 **(A)** With the device lever (marked #1) and the logo facing the ceiling (12 o'clock), advance the device into artery until brisk pulsatile flow is observed exiting the marker lumen. **(B)** Rotate the device approximately 30 degrees toward the patient's right side (~10 o'clock). (Used with permission from Abbot Vascular, copyright 2013)

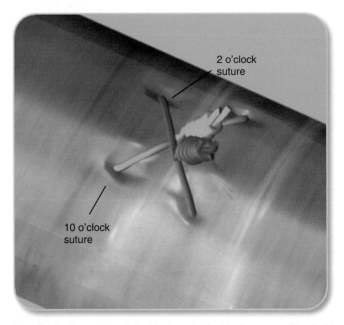

Fig. 2.19 Illustration of 2 o'clock and 10 o'clock sutures. (Used with permission from Abbott Vascular, copyright 2013)

In some cases, a stiff guidewire can straighten tortuous vessels, but vessel folding and kinking at the curves may cause pain. In the upper extremities, trauma with extra-stiff guidewires is also a concern. A deep breath, as already mentioned, can dramatically ease difficulties of catheter passage to the central aorta when the catheter is advancing from the radial artery.

Remember: Wire contact with blood forms thrombi despite anticoagulation. Limit wire-loaded catheter manipulations to 2 to 3 minutes, maintain adequate ACT, and use meticulous wire wipe and sheath flush techniques.

Complications of Arterial Access

The most common complication of femoral artery access is local hematoma formation. Other common complications (in order of decreasing frequency) include retroperitoneal hematoma, pseudoaneurysm, AV fistula formation, and arterial thrombosis secondary to intimal dissection. The frequency of these complications is increased in women, the elderly, patients with renal failure or

peripheral arterial disease, patients undergoing high-risk procedures, and patients receiving anticoagulation, antiplatelet, or fibri-
nolytic therapies. In addition, although there is an increased risk in
patients with morbid obesity, patients with a low body mass index
(BMI) are actually at the highest risk.

A retroperitoneal hematoma is the first diagnosis to consider
in patients with hypotension, tachycardia, pallor, a rapidly falling
postcatheterization hematocrit, lower abdominal or back pain, or
neurologic changes in the leg in which the puncture was made.
Small women, particularly those with a high puncture (above the
upper third of the femoral head) are at greatest risk of retroperitoneal hematoma.

Pseudoaneurysm presents as a painful palpable mass and is
associated with a low puncture (usually below the femoral head).
In the past, all femoral pseudoaneurysms were routinely repaired
by the vascular surgeon to avoid further neurovascular complication or rupture. With ultrasound imaging techniques, these false
channels can be easily identified and nonsurgical closure pursued.
Manual compression of the expansile growing mass guided by
Doppler ultrasound with or without thrombin or collagen injection
is an acceptable therapy for femoral pseudoaneurysm (Fig. 2.20).

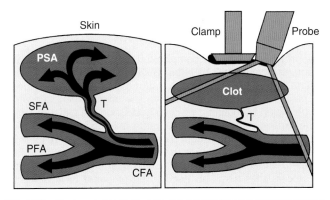

Fig. 2.20 Noninvasive technique for closure of a femoral artery pseudoaneurysm *(PSA)* by external compression. *Arrows:* Course and direction of blood
flow. *Left:* Blood is shown flowing from the common femoral artery *(CFA)* into
a large PSA through a large tract *(T)*. *Right:* External application of pressure
using a vascular clamp guided by Doppler ultrasound color flow probe results
in obliteration of the tract and clot formation in the pseudoaneurysm. *PFA,*
Profunda femoris artery; *SFA,* superficial femoral artery. (Redrawn from
Agrawal SK, Pinheiro L, Roubin GS, et al. Nonsurgical closure of femoral
pseudoaneurysms complicating cardiac catheterization and percutaneous
transluminal coronary angioplasty. *J Am Coll Cardiol.* 1992;20:610–615.)

AV fistula formation is also associated with a low puncture. Most go undetected, but if the formation is large enough, patients can experience pain and swelling in the lower extremity. Very large AV fistulae can lead to high-output heart failure. In such cases, repair may be indicated.

Infections are more common in patients who undergo repeat ipsilateral (same site) femoral punctures or prolonged femoral sheath maintenance (within 1 to 5 days).

Compared with the femoral approach, the brachial (but not radial) approach has a higher risk of bleeding and vascular complications. On the other hand, such complications are less frequent when the transradial approach is used.

Access and Hemostasis: Nurse-Technician Viewpoint

The nursing and technical staff play an integral role in obtaining safe and successful arterial and venous access and hemostasis. Their knowledge of anatomy, patient positioning, and equipment is essential to providing optimal patient care and support during all phases of the cardiac catheterization procedure.

Precatheterization Assessment

Any procedure may be complicated by the inherent vascular trauma associated with bleeding. Therefore, planning ahead is important. Before the procedure, a staff member should describe to the patient the sensations that he or she might experience while the physician is obtaining vascular access. On the patient's arrival at the cardiac catheterization laboratory, the nursing and technical staff must position the patient properly on the procedure table for the femoral or radial approach and prepare the access site in a manner that facilitates vascular access by the physician. Alternative access sites may also need to be prepared in advance for unanticipated entry problems. Pertinent pulses should be palpated or, when necessary, Doppler assessment should be performed. Information concerning the presence and stability of the pulse must be conveyed to the physician. Even the uninvolved extremities may lose pulse from a central embolus or dissection.

Baseline Vascular Assessment

The patient's preprocedure peripheral vascular status (i.e., pulse quality) should be assessed and documented on the catheterization chart before the start of the procedure. In some laboratories, assessment is the responsibility of the nurse, whereas in other laboratories, all personnel share this duty. It is a good idea for the person responsible for postcatheterization care to perform the initial assessment so that any changes in vascular status can be easily recognized. Many laboratories are set up so that the same staff members manage patient entry and preparation and recovery areas. This setup is ideal because the staff member responsible for precatheterization assessment and postcatheterization care can easily assess any change in the patient's baseline status.

If the femoral approach is used, the femoral artery, dorsalis pedis artery (top of the foot), and posterior tibial artery (inside behind the ankle) pulses should be assessed, graded, and recorded on a scale of 0 to 4+ (4 being maximal or a bounding pulse). It is helpful to use a marking pen to indicate the location and grade of the pulse on the patient's foot to facilitate postcatheterization assessment. If the radial arterial approach is used, a precatheterization assessment of the radial and ulnar pulses should be performed. Mark the location and document the grade on the chart.

Patient Positioning

Femoral Approach

Proper positioning of the patient on the catheterization table by laboratory personnel is important to facilitate arterial and venous access. For the femoral approach, the patient should be in the supine position. In some laboratories, the patient's arms are placed behind the head, ensuring that the hands and arms are away from the sterile field and will not be in the way of the C-arm of the x-ray unit. However, the problem with placement of the arms above the head is that the patient will likely become uncomfortable (and fatigued) during a long procedure. Positioning the arms at the patient's side is the most common method. Instruct patients to keep their arms as close to the body as possible and under the sterile drape at all times. Instructing patients to tuck their hands under their hips may help remind them to keep their arms at their sides and aid in maintaining a comfortable position during the procedure. Positioning of the patient's arms at their sides causes the arms to appear in the x-ray field and compromises angiography performed in severe oblique (angled) projections. For a lateral projection, arms should be raised and placed behind the head.

Position patients with their legs spread slightly so that their knees are 8 to 12 inches apart. This position facilitates access to the groin by pulling the skin folds apart at the inguinal crease and creates a space on the catheterization table to hold equipment, syringes, gauze, and so forth.

Position the patient as far toward the head of the catheterization table as possible. This positioning allows travel of the C-arm to cover the inguinal area and fluoroscopic landmarks (e.g., the femoral head). If access is difficult because of vessel obstruction or tortuosity, it may be necessary to perform fluoroscopy at the access site. If the patient is positioned too far toward the foot of the x-ray table, fluoroscopic visualization of this area may be hindered.

The Obese Patient for the Femoral Approach. Obese patients present a challenge to the staff in terms of positioning and site preparation. The first problem usually encountered is that most catheterization tables are narrow, which leaves no room for comfortable positioning of the patient's arms. An arm retainer gives some support and helps keep the patient's arms at his or her sides. Positioning the arms above the head for short procedures is recommended for obese patients.

The second challenge is that of groin preparation. The protruding abdomen and panniculus of obese patients usually extend and rest over the groin area, presenting an obstacle to access and preparation. The abdomen wall can be retracted toward the chest and retained in this position by using 3- to 4-inch-wide tape. The tape can be crisscrossed over the retracted abdomen and secured to the sides of the catheterization table. When the abdominal folds are retracted, the groin can be prepared in the usual fashion. Because excessive skin folds in the obese patient may result in higher than normal amounts of skin bacteria, extra care should be taken when cleaning the skin and applying antiseptic solutions.

Radial Artery Approach

For the radial artery approach, the arm can be positioned on an arm board to stabilize the position of the wrist, or the arm may be placed next to the body on a pillow in an arm cradle. Most x-ray tables have accessory arm boards that mount on the side of the x-ray table. Proper orientation of the radial artery occurs if the arm is placed with the hand secured in the palm-up position and the wrist is hyperextended with a small pad underneath it. Place the drape so that it exposes only the area targeted for access. Because the radial artery will be accessed ~2 cm proximal to the bony prominence of the distal radius, the distal edge of the drape hole can start there, leaving more of the forearm exposed and available for access (Fig. 2.21). After obtaining vascular access, bring the arm to the patient's side near the femoral artery if an arm board is used, and catheter insertion and manipulation can proceed as with femoral access.

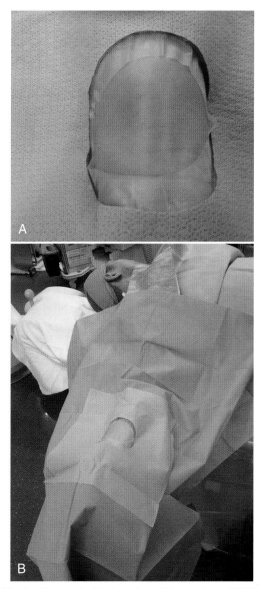

Fig. 2.21 Positioning of wrist drape for radial procedures. **(A)** The hole is placed so that the most distal end is at the bony prominence of the distal radius. **(B)** A full sterile radial drape is placed prior to the arm being moved to the right hip for catheter insertion.

Equipment Used for Access

A variety of needles, guidewires, vessel dilators, and introducer sheaths are available for use in obtaining vascular access. Because the components necessary for access come in many different sizes, staff members must be knowledgeable regarding compatibility of the different components. Certain needles accept only certain sized guidewires. The same is true for compatibility among wires, catheters, and introducer sheaths. Component package inserts contain information regarding size and component compatibility. The catheterization team members should understand the anatomy of the vascular system for access and catheter placement depending on the clinical presentation when the patient needs a right-sided, left-sided, or combined right- and left-sided heart catheterization procedure (see Chapter 4).

Postprocedure Assessment

Prior to arriving in recovery, it is important that the nurse accepting the patient understands what transpired during the procedure. They should know what procedure was performed, access site(s) used, and drugs given, and whether there were any complications during the procedure. In addition, knowing the patient's mental status and vital signs during the procedure will help in determining whether anything has changed once in recovery.

If femoral access was used, the patient may arrive in recovery with a sheath in place, or with the sheath removed, and hemostasis achieved through manual compression or with a VCD. If the sheath remains in place, clear communication is needed regarding sheath management and the timing of sheath removal. Regardless of whether the sheath remains in place, initial assessment in the recovery area should include careful inspection of the access site for hematoma and a pulse assessment in the ipsilateral leg, so that any changes in status can be easily discerned.

If radial access was used, the patient should arrive in recovery with a hemostatic wristband in place. One of the first important steps, after establishing that the patient is hemodynamically stable, is assessing for patent hemostasis. With the device on the wrist and the pulse oximetry with plethysmography on the ipsilateral thumb, the nurse occludes the ulnar artery to determine the Barbeau type. If it is a Barbeau D, the nurse attempts to let some air out while maintaining hemostasis. If unsuccessful, another attempt should be made in 15 minutes and every 15 minutes thereafter until a Barbeau A, B, or C pattern is present, indicating that patent hemostasis has been achieved. Once patent hemostasis is achieved, it should be confirmed once every hour. If the nurse is unsuccessful in achieving patent hemostasis by the time the device is to be removed, the physician should be notified.

Protocols vary, but patients who have had a femoral procedure may be prescribed bed rest for a duration of 1 to 4 hours but should still ambulate as soon as safely possible after their procedure. Patients who have had a radial procedure can be immediately ambulatory as long as they are safe to do so from a hemodynamic and neurologic (sedation) perspective. Early ambulation increases patient satisfaction, expedites recovery, and promotes early discharge, which has been shown to reduce medical costs.

Safe and effective vascular access and hemostasis are key components to an overall successful cardiac catheterization procedure. Key steps must be followed throughout the entire process, from preprocedure to recovery, requiring a cooperative effort of the whole team. In addition, as new techniques continue to be introduced, such as radial and large-bore access, the entire catheterization laboratory must have a method of quickly educating the staff and seamlessly adapting to change.

Suggested Readings

Amin AP, Patterson M, House JA, et al. Costs associated with access site and same-day discharge among medicare beneficiaries undergoing percutaneous coronary intervention: an evaluation of the current percutaneous coronary intervention care pathways in the United States. *JACC Cardiovasc Interv.* 2017;10:342-351.

Annala AP, Karjalainen PP, Porela P, Nyman K, Ylitalo A, Airaksinen KE. Safety of diagnostic coronary angiography during uninterrupted therapeutic warfarin treatment. *Am J Cardiol.* 2008;102:389-390.

Bertrand OF, De Larochellière R, Rodés-Cabau J, et al. A randomized study comparing same-day home discharge and abciximab bolus only to overnight hospitalization and abciximab bolus and infusion after transradial coronary stent implantation. *Circulation.* 2006;114:2636-2643.

Bertrand OF, Bélisle P, Joyal D, et al. Comparison of transradial and femoral approaches for percutaneous coronary interventions: a systematic review and hierarchical Bayesian meta-analysis. *Am Heart J.* 2012;163:632-648.

Brueck M, Bandorski D, Kramer W, Wieczorek M, Höltgen R, Tillmanns H. A randomized comparison of transradial versus transfemoral approach for coronary angiography and angioplasty. *JACC Cardiovasc Interv.* 2009;2:1047-1054.

Campeau L. Percutaneous radial artery approach for coronary angiography. *Cathet Cardiovasc Diagn.* 1989;16:3-7.

Carey D, Martin JR, Moore CA, Valentine MC, Nygaard TW. Complications of femoral artery closure devices. *Catheter Cardiovasc Interv.* 2001;52:3-7.

Dauerman HL, Applegate RJ, Cohen DJ. Vascular closure devices: the second decade. *J Am Coll Cardiol.* 2007;50:1617-1626.

Deftereos S, Giannopoulos G, Raisakis K, et al. Moderate procedural sedation and opioid analgesia during transradial coronary interventions to prevent spasm: a prospective randomized study. *JACC Cardiovasc Interv.* 2013;6:267-273.

Dehghani P, Mohammad A, Bajaj R, et al. Mechanism and predictors of failed transradial approach for percutaneous coronary interventions. *JACC Cardiovasc Interv.* 2009;2:1057-1064.

Chhatriwalla AK, Amin AP, Kennedy KF, et al. Association between bleeding events and in-hospital mortality following percutaneous coronary intervention. *JAMA.* 2013; 309:1022-1029.

Farouque HM, Tremmel JA, Raissi Shabari F, et al. Risk factors for the development of retroperitoneal hematoma after percutaneous coronary intervention in the era of glycoprotein IIb/IIIa inhibitors and vascular closure devices. *J Am Coll Cardiol.* 2005;45:363-368.

Feldman DN, Swaminathan RV, Kaltenbach LA, et al. Adoption of radial access and comparison of outcomes to femoral access in percutaneous coronary intervention: an updated report from the national cardiovascular data registry (2007-2012). *Circulation.* 2013;127:2295-2306.

From AM, Bell MR, Rihal CS, Gulati R. Minimally invasive transradial intervention using sheathless standard guiding catheters. Catheter Cardiovasc Interv. 2011;78:866-871.

Hildick-Smith D. Use of the Allen's test and transradial catheterization. *J Am Coll Cardiol.* 2006;48:1287.

Jolly SS, Amlani S, Hamon M, Yusuf S, Mehta SR. Radial versus femoral access for coronary angiography or intervention and the impact on major bleeding and ischemic events: a systematic review and meta-analysis of randomized trials. *Am Heart J.* 2009;157:132-140.

Jolly SS, Yusuf S, Cairns J. Radial versus femoral access for coronary angiography and intervention in patients with acute coronary syndromes (RIVAL): a randomized, parallel group, multicenter trial. *Lancet.* 2011;377:1409-1420.

Karrowni W, Vyas A, Giacomino B, et al. Radial versus femoral access for primary percutaneous interventions in ST-segment elevation myocardial infarction patients. JACC *Cardiovasc Interv.* 2013;6:814-823.

Kern MJ. Cardiac catheterization on the road less traveled: navigating the radial versus femoral debate. *J Am Coll Cardiol Interv.* 2009;2:1055-1056.

Kiemeneij F, Laarman GJ, Odekerken D, et al. A randomized comparison of percutaneous transluminal coronary angioplasty by the radial, brachial and femoral approaches: the access study. *J Am Coll Cardiol.* 1997;29:1269-1275.

Kim D, Orron DE, Skillman JJ, et al. Role of superficial femoral artery puncture in the development of pseudoaneurysm and arteriovenous fistula complicating percutaneous transfemoral cardiac catheterization. *Cathet Cardiovasc Diagn.* 1992;25:91-97.

Lesnefsky EJ, Carrea FP, Groves BM. Safety of cardiac catheterization via peripheral vascular grafts. *Cathet Cardiovasc Diagn.* 1993;29:113-116.

MacDonald LA, Meyers S, Bennett CL, et al. Post-cardiac catheterization access site complications and low-molecular weight heparin following cardiac catheterization. *J Invasive Cardiol.* 2003;15:60-62.

Nguyen N, Hasan S, Caufield L, Ling FS, Narins CR. Randomized controlled trial of topical hemostasis pad use for achieving vascular hemostasis following percutaneous coronary intervention. *Catheter Cardiovasc Interv.* 2007;69:801-807.

Pancholy S, Coppola J, Patel T, Roke-Thomas M. Prevention of radial artery occlusion-patent hemostasis evaluation trial (PROPHET study): a randomized comparison of traditional versus patency documented hemostasis after transradial catheterization. *Catheter Cardiovasc Interv.* 2008;72:335-340.

Pancholy SB, Patel TM. Effect of duration of hemostatic compression on radial artery occlusion after transradial access. *Catheter Cardiovasc Interv.* 2012;79:78-81.

Pancholy SB, Sanghvi KA, Patel TM. Radial artery access technique evaluation trial: randomized comparison of Seldinger versus modified Seldinger technique for arterial access for transradial catheterization. *Catheter Cardiovasc Interv.* 2012;80: 288-291.

Patel T, Shah S, Pancholy S, Rao S, Bertrand OF, Kwan T. Balloon-assisted tracking: a must-know technique to overcome difficult anatomy during transradial approach. *Catheter Cardiovasc Interv.* 2014;83:211-220.

Seto AH, Roberts JS, Abu-Fadel MS, et al. Real-time ultrasound guidance facilitates transradial access: RAUST (Radial Artery access with Ultrasound Trial). *JACC Cardiovasc Interv.* 2015;8:283-291.

Sandoval Y, Burke MN, Lobo AS, et al. Contemporary Arterial Access in the Cardiac Catheterization Laboratory. *JACC Cardiovasc Interv.* 2017;10:2233-2241.

Seto AH, Abu-Fadel MS, Sparling JM, et al. Real-time ultrasound guidance facilitates femoral arterial access and reduces vascular complications: FAUST (Femoral Arterial Access With Ultrasound Trial). *JACC Cardiovasc Interv.* 2010;3:751-758.

Sharieff W, Chisholm RJ, Kutryk MJ, et al. Mechanism and predictors of failed transradial approach for percutaneous coronary interventions. *JACC Cardiovasc Interv.* 2009;2:1057-1064.

Uretsky B, ed. Cardiac Catheterization: Concepts, Techniques, and Applications. Walden, MA: Blackwell Science; 1997.

Wang HJ, Lee KW, Hsieh DJ. Brachial loop: transradial technique to overcome this rare anatomic variation. *Catheter Cardiovasc Interv.* 2006;68:260-262.

To view Videos 2.1, 2.2, and 2.3, please
activate your book on www.ExpertConsult.
Inkling.com using the pin code on the inside front cover.

Coronary Angiography and Ventriculography

MORTON J. KERN • ANDREW J. KLEIN •
PRANAV M. PATEL

Catheter-based coronary angiography is the gold standard for the diagnosis of coronary artery disease (CAD). From preprocedure assessment to the acquisition of images to the postprocedural follow-up, care must be taken at each step to maximize high-quality data collection with minimal patient risk and discomfort. Optimal angiographic imaging is the result of a series of linked steps. Failure of any link breaks the imaging chain and may cause loss of all or part of the data. The chain begins with positioning the patient on the table, followed by vascular access, catheter placement, correct imaging views, contrast injection during acquisition of the images, display of the images for review, and finally the analysis and archiving of the digital images. The major causes of poor angiograms include factors specific to the patient (size, medical devices/hardware that interfere with imaging), angiographic technique, equipment-related problems, and optical and digital imaging system issues (Box 3.1).

Indications

Coronary angiography is widely used to evaluate patients with known or suspected CAD. Angiography may be combined with the measurement of left ventricular (LV) pressures (left heart catheterization) and/or the evaluation of LV systolic function and wall motion (left ventriculography). The decision to perform a left heart catheterization and left ventriculography is left to the discretion of the operator and the patient's primary physician.

All catheterization laboratory personnel should recognize the importance of preprocedure assessment and be aware of the indications why the patient is having the procedure performed. As a measure of quality within the laboratory, appropriate documentation should describe the indications for the procedure and, ideally,

Box 3.1 Causes of Poor Angiograms.

Patient Factors

- Size
- Movement
- Hardware (pacemaker, Harrison rods, multiple surgery with clips, silicone prosthesis)
- Anatomic conditions (scoliosis, scarred lungs, large heart [fluid])

Angiographer Factors

- Poor catheter seating (wrong catheter shape or size, anomalous origin, subselective cannulation)
- Poor contrast opacification (weak injection, volume too small, diluted contrast material)

Equipment Factors

- X-ray generator problems (high heat, quantum mottle, too high kilovoltage, too short or too long pulse width)
- X-ray tube problems (anode pitting, wrong focal spot, beam geometry, proximity to image intensifier, poor collimation)
- Digital imaging program malfunction

Biologic Factors

- Variation in contrast medium concentration, which is reduced during diastole due to increased blood flow, can cause subtle vessel border defining issues due to incomplete contrast mixture encountered with large diameter native vessel or bypass grafts.
- Hyperviscosity and hyperosmolality of contrast can shift tissue water into capillaries and affect imaging quality. Nonionic, Isosmotic can improve this diagnostic accuracy.
- Motion blurring can result from the movements of coronary arteries during the cardiac can affect imaging especially in distal vessels.

should reference the indication category from the American College of Cardiology/Society for Cardiovascular Angiography and Interventions (ACC/SCAI) appropriate use criteria (AUC) document. Using the AUC, patient indications that fall in the uncertain (U) or inappropriate (I) categories can be addressed before the procedure occurs because the AUC categories do not address all individual patient level decision-making. AUCs are intended as guiding documents. The AUC will aid in justifying the final clinical decision and indication for a procedure after discussion about treatment and patient goals. Furthermore, the SCAI has developed a smart phone application (available through the SCAI website, www.scai.org). After answering a few short questions, the app can display the indication category for any individual patient.

Patient Preparation for Coronary Angiography

Before proceeding with cardiac catheterization, informed consent must be obtained from all patients and/or family. It is critical to confirm this documentation prior to the procedure and the administration of conscious sedation to ensure the procedure is performed in concordance with the patient's wishes and hospital policies.

Medications that are part of a catheterization laboratory routine for CAD evaluations and other patient's clinical conditions are continued unless they might interfere with the technique of the procedure (i.e., continuation of novel/direct oral anticoagulants or warfarin). The administration of other antiplatelet medications including clopidogrel, prasugrel, or ticagrelor before the ascertainment of coronary anatomy is to be guided by individual laboratory protocols and any anticipated need for surgery.

Coronary Angiography

The goal of coronary angiography is to visualize the coronary arteries, branches, collaterals, and anomalies with enough detail to make a precise diagnosis and plan for the treatment of CAD. With percutaneous coronary interventions (PCIs; e.g., stents), the coronary angiographer must demonstrate the precise location of disease relative to major and minor side branches and any associated vascular anomalies, such as thrombi, calcifications, or aneurysms. For the performance of PCI, visualization of vessel bifurcations, vessel tortuosity, origin of side branches, the portion of the vessel proximal to a significant lesion, and specific lesion characteristics (e.g., length, eccentricity and calcium) is crucial. The routine coronary angiographic views should visualize the origin and course of the three major vessels and their branches in at least two different planes. Because coronary anatomy varies widely, appropriate angiographic projections must be modified for each patient. In the case of a total vessel occlusion (also called *chronic total occlusion* [CTO]), the distal vessel should be visualized as clearly as possible by opacifying the contralateral coronary artery and collateral vessel pathways. CTO angiograms require extended cineangiographic imaging runs that are long enough to visualize late collateral vessel filling with appropriate panning across the heart. The features of the proximal segment, the distal cap (point of occlusion), and length of the occluded segment help determine the suitability for CTO revascularization strategy. CTO PCI starts with a careful review of the coronary angiogram that, in nearly all cases, should be performed using dual injection. Procedural plans are then made based on the lesion angiographic characteristics.

Angiographic Catheters

The initial choice of catheters for coronary angiography depends on the approach (radial or femoral access) and physician preferences. Regardless of approach, the angiographic catheter is advanced over a J-wire (or other angled tip or soft/floppy tipped wire) to the aortic root under fluoroscopic guidance. Engagement of the left main coronary artery (LMCA) can be performed in anterior-posterior (AP) or left anterior oblique (LAO), whereas engagement of the right coronary artery (RCA) is performed in LAO. Regardless of the catheter or the artery, coaxial alignment of the catheter with the artery should be obtained by subtle movement of the catheter while carefully observing the catheter tip pressure waveform on the hemodynamic monitor. Before contrast injection through the catheter, operators must pay careful attention to the catheter tip pressure waveform, which can indicate obstruction or malpositioning of the catheter. A waveform that shows dampening or ventricularization (Fig. 3.1) suggests that the catheter may be placed into a small side branch (e.g., conus) or up against a plaque or is touching left main (LM) roof where injection might lead to ventricular fibrillation and/or dissection. Care also must be taken to notice deep seating of the catheter, which may lead an operator to miss an ostial lesion beyond which the catheter has moved. During contrast injection into the coronary tree, the operator should note an adequate contrast reflux back into the aorta to see whether an ostial lesion is present. Many laboratories routinely administer intracoronary nitroglycerin to prevent or to resolve catheter-induced spasm that can mimic stenosis. Catheter-induced spasm is typically more common in the RCA than the LCA.

X-ray Imaging

For all catheterization laboratories, the x-ray source is under the table, and the image intensifier (II) is directly above the patient. The source and *flat-panel detector* in fully digital laboratories

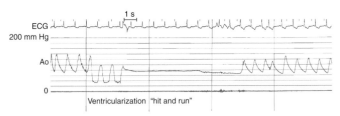

Fig. 3.1 Damping of aortic (*Ao*) pressure in the left main coronary artery with ventricularization in which immediate angiography was performed with removal of the catheter in a hit-and-run maneuver, rapidly restoring flow and perfusion after contrast media injection.

(*II In older labs*) move in opposite directions in an imaginary circle around the patient who is positioned in the center. The body surface of the patient facing the observer determines the specific view. This relationship holds true regardless of whether the patient is supine, standing, or rotated (Fig. 3.2).

Angiographic Nomenclature

AP position: The detector is directly over the patient with the beam traveling perpendicularly back to front (i.e., from posterior to anterior) to the patient lying flat on the x-ray table.

RAO position: The detector is on the right side of the patient. *A,* Anterior; *O,* oblique.

LAO position: The detector is on the left side of the patient.

Note: Think of the oblique view as turning the left or right shoulder forward (anterior) to the camera (II).

Cranial: The detector is tilted toward the head of the patient.

Caudal: The detector is tilted toward the feet of the patient.

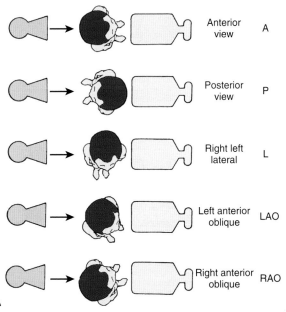

Anterior view	A
Posterior view	P
Right left lateral	L
Left anterior oblique	LAO
Right anterior oblique	RAO

A

Fig. 3.2 Nomenclature for radiographic projections. *Small black arrows:* Directions of the x-ray beam. **(A)** Anterior, posterior, lateral, and oblique.

Continued

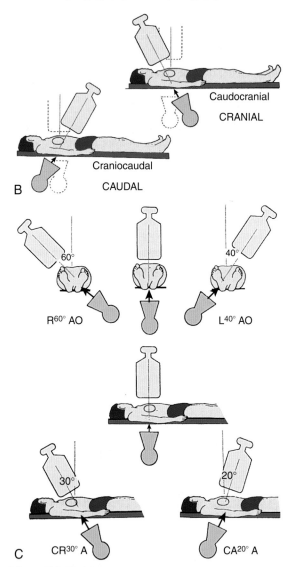

Fig. 3.2, cont'd (B) If the intensifier is tilted toward the feet of the patient, a caudal view is produced. If the intensifier is tilted toward the head of the patient, a cranial view is produced. **(C)** Cranial *(CR)* and caudal *(CA)* oblique views. (Redrawn from Paulin S. Terminology for radiographic projections in cardiac angiography. *Cathet Cardiovasc Diagn.* 1981;7:341-344.)

Angiographic Projections Made Simple: An Easy Way to Understand Oblique Views

Trainees in the catheterization laboratory need to understand coronary angiograms and how the arteries change position with specific angulations. The following section illustrates how the heart and the coronary arteries move in the different projections. The changing positions can be easily remembered by using the left hand as a representation of the coronary tree as it sits over the heart and changes position with different angulations while the right or left shoulder is rotated toward the detector to duplicate LAO and RAO views.

The Cardiac Silhouette in Left Anterior Oblique and Right Anterior Oblique

The heart is the size of a fist (Fig. 3.3) and is shaped like an ice cream cone, with the tip toward the sternum. The open hand is positioned as it would be seen in an AP projection. When the left shoulder is moved forward (LAO projection), the hand is seen more on end; that is, the heart is made shorter and rounder in the LAO (Fig. 3.4A). When the right shoulder is moved forward (RAO projection), the hand is seen in profile; that is, the heart is made longer with the tip extending to the left chest wall. These two movements of the hand in the LAO and RAO remind you how the heart should look in each projection, whether seen on a plain chest x-ray or on fluoroscopy or ventriculography during cardiac catheterization (see Fig. 3.4B).

The Left Coronary Arteries: Left Anterior Oblique Views

By placing the left-hand fingers over the clenched right fist, the index finger becomes the left anterior descending (LAD) artery and runs over the knuckles, which represent the anterior interventricular groove (Fig. 3.5). The middle finger is spread lying on the finger joints and represents the circumflex (CFX) artery. The thumb runs horizontal to the wrist joint and represents the initial course of the RCA arising from the right sinus of Valsalva.

Left Coronary Artery With Left Anterior Oblique Cranial and Caudal Angulations

In cranial angulation, the detector moves toward the head of the patient and produces a downward tilt of the LAO view, exaggerating

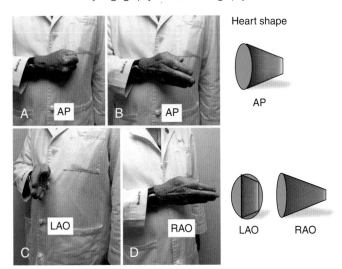

Heart shape

Fig. 3.3 **(A)** Anterior-posterior (AP) view of the heart (closed fist) in the chest. **(B)** AP view of the left ventricle (LV) shape (open hand) in the chest. *Right diagrams,* The approximate shapes as might be seen on x-ray. **(C)** Left anterior oblique *(LAO)*: The left shoulder forward rotation causes foreshortening of the LV with the apex toward the viewer and rounding of the cardiac silhouette *(right diagram, LAO)*. **(D)** Right anterior oblique *(RAO)*: The right shoulder forward causes the heart to elongate as it rotates with the tip of the heart to the left side. *Right diagram*: The LV image as it might appear on x-ray. (Reprinted with permission from Kern M. *Cath Lab Digest.* 2011;19(8), copyright HMP Communications.)

the LM segment but keeping the relationship between LAD and CFX almost the same (Fig. 3.6A).

In caudal angulation, the detector moves toward the foot of the patient. This position views the coronary arteries from underneath, tipping the LAO view upward to produce a branching appearance that some refer to as the spider view. Figure 3.6B and similar images provide a computed tomography angiography (CTA) reconstruction of the coronary arteries, with the lower panels showing a subtracted image duplicating what would be seen on traditional coronary angiography in the catheterization laboratory. The lower right panel of Figure 3.6B shows the LAO-caudal angulation and is called the spider view for obvious reasons.

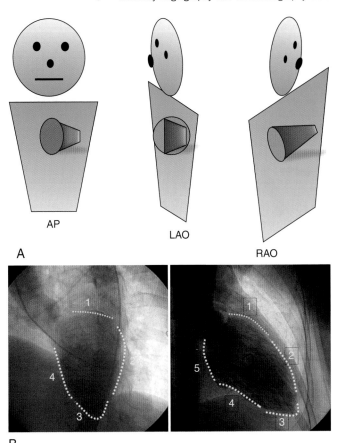

Fig. 3.4 **(A)** Left ventricle (LV) diagrams in patients as the LV shape changes from anterior-posterior *(AP)* to left anterior oblique *(LAO)* and right anterior oblique *(RAO)*. **(B)** Cineangiographic frames of left ventriculograms in the LAO *(left)* and RAO *(right)*. LAO segments: *1,* Basal; *2,* lateral; *3,* apical; and *4,* septal. RAO segments: *1,* Anterior basal; *2,* anterior; *3,* apical; *4,* inferior; *5,* inferior basal. (Reprinted with permission from Kern M. *Cath Lab Digest.* 2011;19(8), copyright HMP Communications.)

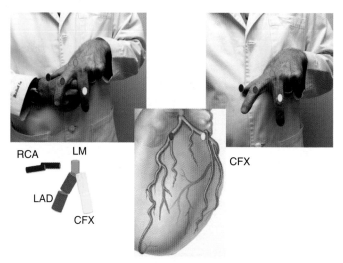

Fig. 3.5 *Top left,* Fingers of the left hand represent the coronary arteries. The colored bars depict the coronary arteries of the drawing in the center. When placed over the heart *(fist),* the left anterior descending *(LAD) (orange, index finger)* runs down the anterior interventricular groove. The circumflex *(CFX)* artery *(yellow, middle finger)* runs over the left side of the fist. The proximal portion of the right coronary artery *(RCA) (blue, thumb)* starts at the top of the fist, runs to the wrist, and then runs down the atrio-ventricular (AV) groove *(wrist joint).* The posterior descending artery (PDA) is shown in the heart illustration. *Top right,* Coronary arteries *(fingers)* are shown with the heart *(fist)* removed in the anterior-posterior (AP) projection. *Green block,* The left main *(LM)* artery segment position. Note that the colored dots *(orange* for LAD, *yellow* for CFX, *green* for LM, and *blue* for RCA) correspond to the same color codes used in Figures 3.6 to 3.8. (Reprinted with permission from Kern M. *Cath Lab Digest.* 2011;19(8), copyright HMP Communications.)

The Left Coronary Arteries: Right Anterior Oblique Projections

In the LAO projection (see Fig. 3.6), the LAD (index finger) is on the right side and the CFX (middle finger) is on the left side. When rotated over to RAO, the position of the fingers (LAD/CFX) changes the orientation such that the LAD is now on the left and the CFX is in the middle or more rightward than in the LAO view (Fig. 3.7A).

The RAO with caudal angulation (see Fig. 3.7A, *top left*) tips the CFX downward, separating it further from the LAD. For the RAO with cranial angulation (see Fig. 3.7A, *top right*), the CFX is tipped upward, foreshortened, and overlapped with the LAD. Cranial views are best used to see the LAD and diagonals, whereas caudal views are best to see the CFX and LM segments. Figure 3.7B shows the angiograms of the RAO-caudal and RAO-cranial angulations.

The Right Coronary Artery and Posterior Descending Artery: Left Anterior Oblique and Right Anterior Oblique

Using the left hand over the fist, the thumb represents the proximal part of the RCA. The RCA continues down the wrist (atrioventricular [AV] groove) to the posterior descending artery (PDA) portion

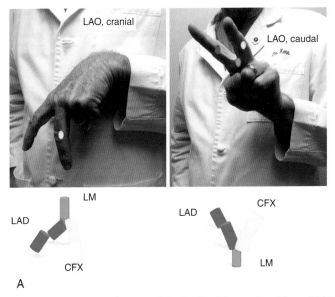

A

Fig. 3.6 **(A)** Coronary finger models showing left anterior oblique *(LAO)* with cranial *(left)* and caudal *(right)* angulations. The coronary arteries *(fingers)* are tipped downward as the image intensifier (II) moves toward the head (cranially). The arteries are tipped upward *(right)* as the II moves toward the feet (caudally). *Green bloc:* The left main *(LM)* artery segment position. *(Orange blocks:* Left anterior descending *[LAD]* artery; *yellow blocks:* circumflex *[CFX]* artery.)*

Continued

LAO, cranial   LAO, caudal

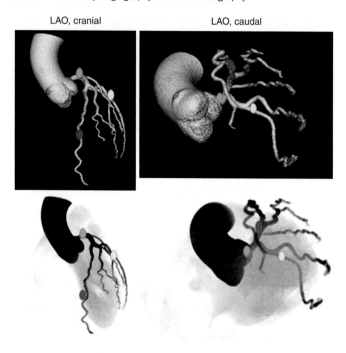

B

Fig. 3.6, cont'd (B) Computed tomography angiography (CTA) reconstruction of left coronary arteries in LAO-cranial *(left)* and LAO-caudal *(right)* angulations. *Bottom:* Simulations of images seen on contrast angiography. *Lower right:* The left coronary artery (LCA) in the LAO-caudal view is called the spider view for obvious similarities to the arachnid. Color codes are the same as shown in Figures 3.5 to 3.8. (Reprinted with permission from Kern M. *Cath Lab Digest.* 2011;19(8), copyright HMP Communications.)

of the RCA, which runs along the inferior interventricular groove. The PDA along the bottom of the heart can be represented by the index finger (Fig. 3.8A). In the LAO cranial angulation, the PDA runs along the bottom of the heart and is tipped downward to visualize better the length without foreshortening (Fig. 3.8A). In the RAO without cranial or caudal angulation, the PDA is seen lengthwise running from the base to the apex of the heart (Fig. 3.8A, *right panels*). Figure 3.8B shows the CTA and contrast-filled angiograms of the RCA in the LAO-cranial and RAO projections.

Using this model, it should be easy to visualize and to remember the coronary and ventriculographic images in the different oblique views with and without cranial and caudal angulations.

Left Coronary Artery Imaging

1. The AP-caudal or shallow RAO view displays the LMCA in its entire perpendicular length (Fig. 3.9). In this view, the proximal segments of the LAD and left CFX arteries are displayed, but the branches are overlapped. After the LM segment, slight RAO or LAO angulation may be necessary to clear the density of the vertebrae and the catheter shaft in the thoracic descending aorta from covering the artery.

2. The LAO-cranial view also shows the LMCA (slightly foreshortened) and the LAD and its diagonal branches. Septal (coursing

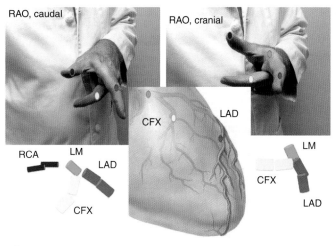

A

Fig. 3.7 (A) *Top left:* The coronary arteries in the right anterior oblique *(RAO)* with caudal angulation. As the right shoulder moves anteriorly, the position of the left anterior descending *(LAD)* artery *(red)* moves from the left side to the right side of the cardiac silhouette. The circumflex *(CFX)* artery *(yellow)* moves toward the left side or center of the heart. *Top right:* RAO with cranial angulation showing the turning upward with foreshortening of the CFX artery. In most left coronary artery (LCA) images with RAO cranial, there is overlapping of the proximal LAD and CFX (see Fig. 3.3B).

Continued

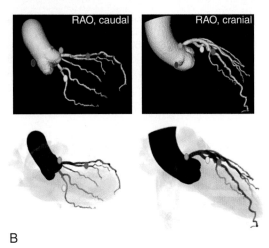

B

Fig. 3.7, cont'd (B) Computed tomography angiography (CTA) reconstruction of LCAs in the RAO-caudal *(left)* and RAO-cranial *(right)* angulations. *Bottom:* Simulations of the images seen on contrast angiography. Note the overlapping of the proximal LAD and CFX. Color codes are the same as shown in Figures 3.4 to 3.7. *LM,* Left main; *RCA,* right coronary artery. (Reprinted with permission from Kern M. *Cath Lab Digest.* 2011;19(8), copyright HMP Communications.)

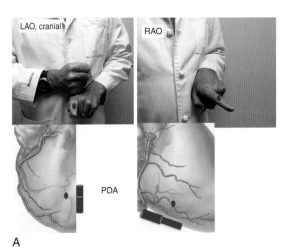

A

Fig. 3.8 (A) The posterior descending artery *(PDA)* portion of the right coronary artery (RCA) runs along the inferior interventricular groove. *Top left:* In the left anterior oblique *(LAO)*-cranial angulation, the PDA runs along the bottom of the heart and is tipped downward to visualize better the length without foreshortening. *Top right:* In the right anterior oblique *(RAO)* without cranial or caudal angulation, the PDA is seen lengthwise running from the base to the apex of the heart.

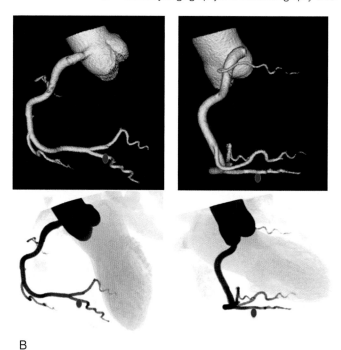

B

Fig. 3.8, cont'd (B) Computed tomography angiography (CTA) reconstruction of the RCA in the LAO-cranial *(left)* and RAO (no cranial or caudal) *(right)* angulations. *Bottom:* Simulations of the images that are seen on contrast angiography. Color codes are the same as shown in Figures 3.4 to 3.6. (Reprinted with permission from Kern M. *Cath Lab Digest.* 2011;19(8), copyright HMP Communications.)

to the left) and diagonal (to the right) branches are separated clearly. The CFX artery and marginal branches are foreshortened and overlapped, although the posterolateral and posterior descending branches of left-dominant circulation are displayed clearly. Deep inspiration, which moves the density of the diaphragm down and out of the field, is helpful. The LAO angle (>45 degrees) should be set so that the LAD artery course is parallel to the spine and stays in the "lucent wedge" bordered by the spine on the medial edge and the curve of the diaphragm. Imaging over the spine degrades the quality of the angiogram and moving more LAO will bring the LAD off the spine for optimal opacification. Cranial angulation tilts the LMCA down and

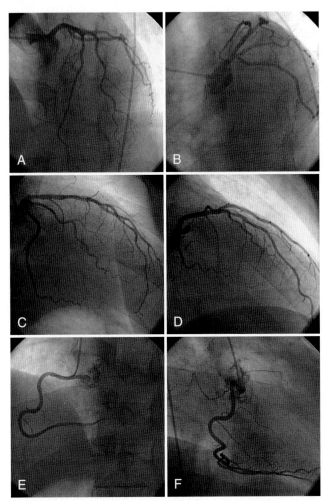

Fig. 3.9 Frames from coronary angiograms in several standard views. **(A)** Left coronary artery (LCA) left anterior oblique (LAO)-cranial projection; **(B)** LAO-caudal projection; **(C)** right anterior oblique (RAO)-caudal projection; **(D)** RAO-cranial projection; **(E)** right coronary artery (RCA) in LAO-cranial projection; **(F)** RCA in RAO-straight projection.

permits a view of the LAD/CFX bifurcation. LAO-cranial angulation that is too steep or inspiration that is too shallow produces considerable overlapping with the diaphragm and liver, degrading the image.

3. The RAO-caudal view shows LMCA bifurcation, perpendicular to that of the LAO-cranial angle. The origin and course of the CFX/obtuse marginal branches, ramus intermedius branch, and proximal LAD segment are seen clearly. This view is one of the two best for visualization of the CFX artery. Overlapped diagonals obscure the LAD artery beyond the proximal segment; however, the apical segment of the LAD artery is displayed clearly.

4. The RAO-cranial view is used to see the origins of the diagonals along the mid and distal LAD artery. Diagonal branch bifurcations are well visualized. The diagonal branches are projected upward. The proximal LAD and CFX usually are overlapped. Marginal branches may overlap, and the CFX artery is foreshortened, but distal circumflex and left-sided posterolateral branches are well visualized in this projection.

5. The LAO-caudal view ("spider" view) shows the LMCA (foreshortened) and bifurcation of the LMCA into the CFX and LAD arteries. Proximal and mid portions of the CFX artery are usually seen clearly with the origins of obtuse marginal branches. Poor image quality may be caused by an overlapping of the diaphragm and spine. Good separation of the vessel is more difficult in vertically displaced hearts, such as those in patients with chronic obstructive pulmonary disease, and more angulation is required to obtain an unobstructed view. The LAD artery is considerably foreshortened in this view.

6. A lateral view (detector rotated 90 degrees, parallel with the floor) is the best view to show the mid and distal LAD arteries. The LAD and CFX arteries are well separated. Diagonals are usually overlapped. The ramus intermedius branch course is well visualized. This view best shows insertions of bypass grafts (usually LIMA) into the mid LAD artery. Occasionally, slight caudal or cranial angulation is needed to visualize the segment of interest.

Right Coronary Imaging

In contrast to left coronary angiography, selective engagement of the RCA requires torqueing of the catheter anteriorly and to the right (Fig. 3.9E,F). The catheter must be advanced to the right coronary cusp and then pulled back slowly while applying clockwise torque. A push-pull motion while torqueing the catheter will help transmit the twisting down to the catheter tip. As with cannulation of the LM, the operator should observe the pressure waveform. Damping signals engagement of the conus branch. Injection of this vessel can lead to ventricular fibrillation. Once selective coronary engagement is accomplished, intracoronary nitroglycerin is often given to prevent or to alleviate catheter-induced spasm. If spasm occurs or if an ostial lesion is suspected, a smaller-diameter catheter might be used. If selective engagement of the RCA using standard catheters is not successful, consider using special catheters, such as 3DR or no-torque RCA catheters. Anomalous positions of the RCA should be considered when one cannot find the RCA in the usual location in the right sinus of Valsalva. A high anterior takeoff of the RCA might be present. If the RCA cannot be found, a review of left coronary angiography should be examined for unsuspected collateral flow or the RCA potentially coming off the left coronary cusp.

1. The LAO-cranial view shows the origin of the RCA, the entire length of the mid RCA, and the PDA bifurcation (crux) (see Figs. 3.4 and 3.5). Cranial angulation tilts the PDA down to see vessel contour and to reduce foreshortening. Deep inspiration is necessary to clear the diaphragm. The PDA and posterolateral branches are slightly foreshortened in this view.

2. The RAO view (no cranial or caudal angulation is generally necessary) shows the mid RCA and the length of the PDA and posterolateral branches. Septal branches coursing upward from the PDA, supplying occluded LAD artery via collaterals, may be clearly identified. The posterolateral branches are overlapped and may need the addition of a cranial view.

3. The AP-cranial view shows the origin of the RCA. The mid segment is foreshortened. However, this is the best view to display the posterior descending and posterolateral branches of a dominant RCA system as well as the size of a collateralized LAD artery.

4. The lateral view also shows the RCA origin (especially in patients with more anteriorly oriented orifices) and mid RCA. The PDA and posterolateral branches are foreshortened.

Technical note: Because of individual variations in anatomy, small (1 to 2 mL) test injections during patient inspiration help the operator obtain the appropriate oblique and axial (cranial/caudal) angulations and setup for panning.

Bypass Graft Angiography

In patients who have undergone coronary artery bypass graft (CABG) surgery, review of the operative report is important. The number and type of grafts should be noted, particularly if there are arterial grafts and they are in situ (right internal mammary artery [RIMA] or left internal mammary artery [LIMA]) or harvested (often radial artery). The proper technique to engage these grafts depends on the type of graft.

Left Internal Mammary Angiography

Selective injection of the LIMA is required for any patient who had this graft used for CABG (typically to the LAD). The LIMA is a branch of the left subclavian artery and is most easily accessed using the left radial approach. From the femoral approach, selective intubation of the left subclavian in an LAO projection (Fig. 3.10) using an internal mammary (IM) catheter can be performed after passing the catheter into the subclavian artery over a J-wire. Marked tortuosity of the proximal subclavian artery may require a soft-tipped atraumatic wire (Wholey, Versacore or Terumo Glidewire) to permit passage of the IM catheter into the subclavian artery. There is also an IM catheter that often permits easier cannulation of the LIMA. Any pressure gradient between aortic and subclavian arteries should be noted because a subclavian artery stenosis with an LIMA can lead to anterior wall ischemia (coronary-subclavian steal syndrome). Subclavian stenosis can be stented with high success and low procedural complication rates. Selective LIMA engagement can be performed in AP, RAO, or LAO (usually easiest in RAO). Turning the patient's head to the right or left can sometimes assist in LIMA intubation. When selective angiography of the LIMA is not possible because of extreme tortuosity, nonselective injection of the left subclavian artery can be obtained with the brachial artery occluded with a blood pressure cuff inflated to suprasystolic pressure.

The best views for imaging the LIMA-LAD graft are the same as those used for evaluation of the LAD (i.e., RAO- and LAO-cranial projections). The lateral view is especially useful to visualize LIMA-LAD anastomosis and may help determine whether scar tissue has formed tacking the LIMA to the sternum, a finding important to surgeons planning a reoperation with a second sternotomy.

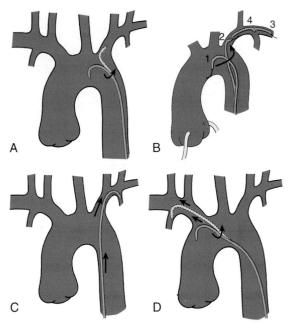

Fig. 3.10 **(A)** Catheterization of the internal mammary (IM) arteries. **(B)** *1:* To catheterize the left internal mammary artery (LIMA), the catheter is located in the aortic arch in a neutral position, with its tip pointing downward. (Arrows depict catheter motion and direction of movement) The catheter is rotated counterclockwise until it falls into the left subclavian artery. *2:* The catheter is advanced with a slight anterior rotation until it engages the origin of the LIMA. *3:* The right internal mammary artery (RIMA) is entered by counterclockwise rotation of the catheter at the origin of the right innominate artery and advanced until the origin of the RIMA is engaged. *4:* A guidewire is inserted in the IM graft catheter until it is passed into the left subclavian artery. **(C)** The catheter is advanced over the guidewire and then removed, withdrawing the catheter into the IM artery (IMA). **(D)** Positioning the IMA catheter to engage the RIMA. (B: from Tilkian AG, Daily EK. *Cardiovascular Procedures: Diagnostic Techniques and Therapeutic Procedures.* St Louis; Mosby: 1986. D: from King SB, Douglas JS, Jr. *Coronary Arteriography and Angioplasty.* New York: McGraw-Hill; 1985)

Right Internal Mammary Coronary Angiography

The RIMA is a branch of the right subclavian artery that arises from the innominate artery. Selective angiography of the RIMA is required when this vessel has been used as an arterial bypass graft (typically to the RCA). Use of the right radial approach permits easiest canalization of the RIMA, whereas the femoral approach can be challenging, especially in an older patient with an elongated aorta (type III aortic arch). From the femoral approach, the innominate must be engaged using an IM catheter in the LAO projection followed by advancing a J-wire into the subclavian artery (Fig. 3.10D). Care must be taken not to wire the right common carotid, which is the other major branch of the innominate. Engagement of the RIMA can be performed in AP projection or LAO. Head positioning or caudal arm movement sometimes assists in selective RIMA intubation.

Saphenous Graft Angiography

Locating saphenous vein graft (SVG) ostia can be challenging and blind movement up and down an atheromatous arch can be risky, which underscores the need to know preprocedurally how many aortotomies where made. Sometimes, surgeons place graft markers (clips or rings) near the SVG ostium, permitting easier future angiography although these markers may not be exactly at the graft opening. Classically, the orientation of SVGs from lowest (caudal) to highest (cranial) has been RCA, LAD, diagonals, and then obtuse marginals.

Coronary artery SVGs are visualized in at least two views (LAO and RAO). It is important to show the aortic anastomosis, body of the graft, distal anastomosis (Fig. 3.11), distal runoff, and collateral channels. The optimal view of graft-vessel anastomosis is usually seen in the view that depicts the native vessel best. Stumps of occluded SVGs should be recorded for future reference.

General Strategy for Coronary Artery Bypass Graft Angiography

Following native LCA and RCA angiography and visualization of missing or reciprocally filled vessel segments, the operator proceeds to SVG angiography using key views for specific coronary artery segments and taking into account the subsequent need to determine contingency views or addition of special views.

1. **SVG to RCA** (lowest): This graft is best engaged in an LAO projection and travels downward, paralleling the RCA. It can be easily cannulated with a multipurpose (MP) catheter or Judkins right (JR) catheter. Other catheters useful for this type of graft include a right coronary bypass (RCB) graft catheter or an

Amplatz right modified (AR mod) catheter. The best views for these grafts are LAO cranial, RAO, and AP cranial.

2. **SVG to LAD** (second lowest, above RCA): The LAD SVG graft typically originates from the anatomic leftward aspect of the anterior aorta and is best engaged in RAO using a JR4 (Judkins right, 4 cm), left coronary bypass (LCB), or Amplatz left (AL) catheter. The best views for a LAD graft are lateral, RAO cranial, LAO cranial, and AP (the lateral view is especially useful to visualize the anastomosis to the LAD).

3. **SVG to diagonal:** Diagonal SVGs are also best visualized in the RAO projection and using the same catheters as those used for SVG to LAD. Often, a slight clockwise rotation from an inferior graft permits the JR4 to engage this graft. The best views for SVGs to diagonal are LAO cranial and RAO cranial.

4. **SVG to obtuse marginal** (highest SVG on the aorta): SVG marginal grafts are best engaged in RAO projections using a JR4,

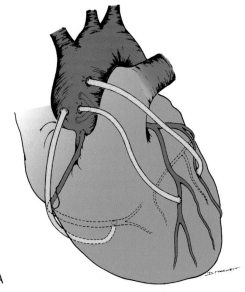

A

Fig. 3.11 **(A)** Usual insertion sites of vein grafts to coronary arteries. The proximal (aortic) anastomosis site of the graft to the right coronary artery (RCA) is most anterior and usually the lowest. Grafts to the branches of the left coronary artery (LCA) are usually inserted in a progressively higher and more posterolateral position. Variations frequently occur.

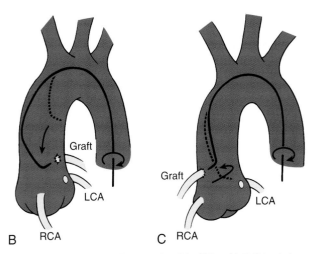

Fig. 3.11, cont'd (B) Use of the Judkins right (JR) and left (JL) vein bypass catheters. For RCA grafts, the catheter is rotated clockwise in the left anterior oblique (LAO) projection until the tip is superior to the graft orifice. It is then advanced down the aortic wall to the orifice of the graft. **(C)** For LCA grafts, clockwise rotation is applied in the left or right anterior oblique (RAO) projection. (From Tilkian AG, Daily EK. *Cardiovascular Procedures: Diagnostic Techniques and Therapeutic Procedures*. St Louis: Mosby; 1986.)

LCB, or AL catheter. The best views for an SVG to obtuse marginal are caudal (LAO to RAO).

Right Gastroepiploic Artery

Because of the strong patency of arterial grafts, some surgeons graft the RCA or PDA using the right gastroepiploic artery (GEA). The right GEA, a branch of the gastroduodenal artery, originates from the common hepatic artery, which is one of the three main branches from the celiac trunk. If the operative report is not available, use of this graft should be considered if median sternotomy extends inferiorly into the abdominal cavity or numerous surgical clips extend up from the abdominal cavity to the inferior wall of the heart. Selective angiography of these grafts requires special technique. It is recommended that only operators familiar with peripheral anatomy and angiography perform GEA angiography because it requires knowledge of the vessel anatomy and selective canalization of the GEA. First, the celiac trunk (located anterior and inferiorly directed) must be engaged using specialized peripheral catheters, such as the Cobra (Cook Medical, Bloomington, IN) or Simmons Sidewinder. Anticoagulation with heparin or bivalirudin is recommended, given the need for subbranch vessel wiring. Once the celiac trunk is engaged, an angioplasty style wire (typically, 0.018 or 0.014 inches) should be passed through the common hepatic to the gastroduodenal and then to the GEA using roadmap imaging. Over this wire, a smaller 4-F or 5-F catheter (Terumo straight glide catheter) or transit catheter (0.035-inch Quickcross [Spectranetics]) can be advanced to perform selective GEA graft angiography. Care must be exerted not to cause vessel dissection. The prophylactic administration of nitroglycerin should prevent vessel spasm.

Contrast Media Injection Techniques: Power Versus Hand Injection

Contrast medium, a viscous, iodinated solution used to opacify the coronary arteries, can be injected either by hand through a multivalve manifold or by a variable rate power injector. For hand injections, flow rates are usually 2 to 4 mL/s with volumes of 2 to 6 mL in the RCA and 7 to 10 mL in the LCA. Operators should keep the tip of the syringe pointed down (handle raised up) so that any small bubbles float up and are not injected into the circulatory system (Fig. 3.12). The use of disposable manifolds, syringes, and tubing is cost effective and safe.

Power injection of contrast media is as safe as hand injections, with operator-controlled rate and volume injections producing excellent opacification. Coronary power injectors use sterile hand controls, permitting precise operator touch-sensitive variable volume injectors (ACIST Medical Systems; Bracco Research USA; Medrad, Inc.), and a computer touch screen allows precise contrast delivery settings (Fig. 3.13). The system is especially helpful for small-diameter catheters (<5 F). In addition, it is also highly cost effective with the large contrast reservoir. Typical settings for power injections are as follows:

· RCA: 6 mL at 3 mL/s; maximal 450 psi
· LCA: 10 mL at 4 mL/s; maximal 450 psi

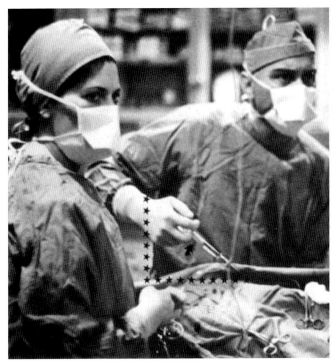

Fig. 3.12 Pioneer Dr. Goffredo Gensini performing coronary angiography. Note the raised angle (30 degrees) of the injection syringe to keep out air bubbles. (From Gensini GG. *Coronary Angiography.* Mount Kisco, NY: Futura; 1975.)

Cineangiographic Frame Rates

Images may be acquired at different frame rates but a frame rate of 15 frames/s is most commonly used. In some pediatric cases or if the heart rate is greater than 95 beats/min, the rate of 60 frames/s may be used. In many adult laboratories, 7.5 to 15 frames/s is standard and reduces radiation dosage to patient and staff.

Panning Techniques

Most laboratories use x-ray image screen sizes (e.g., 8 inches in diameter or less) that may preclude having the entire coronary artery course visualized without panning over the heart to include

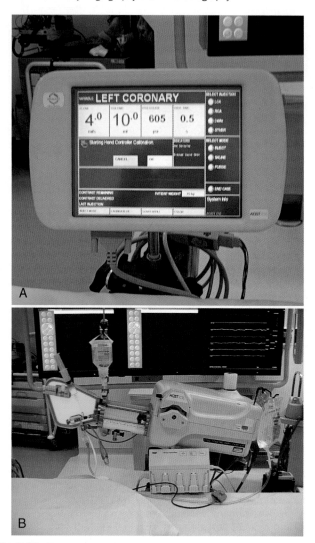

Fig. 3.13 Power injector (Bracco Research USA, Princeton, NJ). **(A)** Operator touch screen selects injection of coronary arteries or ventriculography. **(B)** Mounted on the injector, a large contrast bottle permits multiple patient studies because only the hand control and patient injection tubing are sterile and changed for each patient. The injection syringe with piston has several valves and bubble detectors used to prevent contamination and inadvertent air injection.

the late filling portions of the arterial segments and any collateral filling. In addition, in most views, some degree of panning is necessary to identify regions that are not seen from the initial setup position. Some branches may unexpectedly appear later from collateral filling or other unusual arterial input sources. Imaging runs should be long enough to see contrast in the cardiac veins, which is generally long enough to pan to see late-filling collateralized coronary vessels.

Angiographic View Setup Keys

Panning motion that is too fast or overshoots the image targets causes information to be lost. The key to accurate, optimal coronary cineangiography (that is, obtaining the most information for the least amount of movement) is the initial setup of the catheter on the fluoroscope screen. Figure 3.14 shows the catheter–LM artery setup keys for LAO views in the straight AP, cranial, and caudally angled projections. When the patient is positioned correctly and the setup key followed, only minimal panning is necessary to obtain the information. In the LAO view, the operator pans down the LAD artery then rightward to identify collaterals going to the RCA. If the CFX is occluded, then leftward panning will include collaterals going to the distal CFX artery. For the RCA, in the LAO position, the operator pans downward and to the left toward the LAD artery. This visualizes late-filling collaterals from the right coronary system to the LAD artery. These motions are shown in Figure 3.14.

In RAO projections for the LCA and RCA, the operator pans downward to the apex to identify late-filling, left-to-left, or right-to-left collaterals. The initial setup keys for catheter tip position on the fluoroscope, summarized in Table 3.1, help the operator include all crucial information for coronary angiography.

Collateral Circulation

The opacification of a totally or subtotally (99%) occluded vessel from antegrade or retrograde filling is defined as collateral filling. The collateral circulation is graded angiographically in Table 3.2.

It is useful but difficult to establish the exact size of the recipient vessel. The operator determines whether the collateral circulation is ipsilateral (e.g., same-side filling, proximal RCA to distal RCA collateral supply) or contralateral (e.g., opposite-side filling, LAD artery to distal RCA collateral supply) and identifies exactly which region is affected by collateral supply and stenoses in the artery feeding the collateral artery. He or she notes whether the opacification is forward (anterograde) or backward (retrograde).

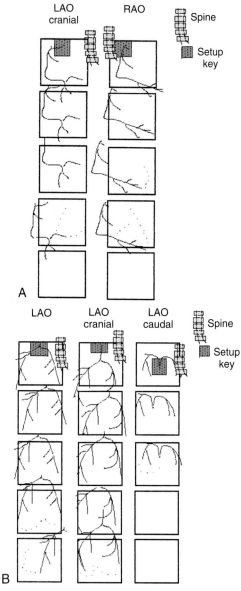

Fig. 3.14 Setup keys for panning during coronary angiography. **(A)** Right coronary artery *(RCA)*. **(B)** Left coronary artery *(LCA)*.

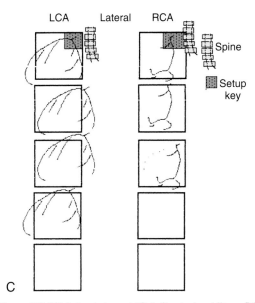

C

Fig. 3.14, cont'd **(C)** Lateral views. *LAO,* Left anterior oblique; *RAO,* right anterior oblique.

This evaluation is important for making decisions regarding which vessels might be protected or lost during coronary angioplasty.

Usefulness of Biplane Coronary Angiography

Simultaneous biplane cineangiography, although uncommonly used, provides accurate images from two different simultaneous points of view and is advantageous in performing complete coronary or ventriculography with reduced contrast volumes and radiation exposure. Biplane angiography is most useful for the pediatric population and those patients with need for reduced contrast load (e.g., patients with renal failure).

The value of biplane information must be balanced against the difficulty of use. The traditional biplane coronary angiography setup required the patient's heart to be in the exact center of the two planes (the isocenter) and then the AP and lateral planes were rotated from vertical or horizontal to *orthogonal projections* (i.e., perpendicular imaging planes, LAO cranial, and RAO caudal; Fig. 3.15). This setup often resulted in more difficulties than it solved, in that panning in one plane moved the heart out of the field of the other plane. Alternatively, setting up the biplane using

Table 3.1

Setup Key Locations for Angiographic Views.			
Artery	View	Setup Region on Angulation Grid (below)[a] (No.)	Comment
LAD	LAO cranial	2	Setup on screen
	LAO caudal	5	Top, midline
	RAO cranial	1	Top, left upper coronary
	RAO caudal	4	Middle, left side
RCA	LAO cranial/caudal	1, 2	Left upper coronary
	RAO cranial/caudal	1, 4	Left upper coronary
LAD/RCA AP	Cranial	2	

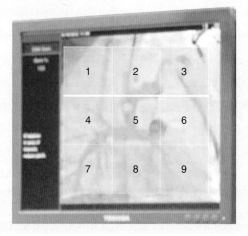

For either LAD or RCA (LAD/RCA) in AP, cranial angulation, use position 2.

AP, Anterior-posterior; *LAD,* left anterior descending; *LAO,* left anterior oblique; *RAO,* right anterior oblique; *RCA,* right coronary artery.

[a]Fluroscreen grid.

The rectangle of the TV monitor showing the position of the catheter tip can be divided into a grid of nine boxes. The position on the screen shown by the number below can be used to position the beginning point of the imaging run.

concordant imaging views (i.e., with both C-arms in the same direction), such as using cranially angled LAO and RAO projections and then moving both C-arms to caudally angled LAO and RAO projections (see Fig. 3.15), makes biplane angiography simple, quick, and effective. In this way, angiographic information is not lost when panning because the heart moves in a similar direction, albeit

Table 3.2

Collateral Angiographic Grade Scale.	
Grade	Collateral Appearance
0	No collateral circulation
1	Very weak (ghost-like) reopacification
2	Reopacified segment, less dense than the feeding vessel, and filling slowly
3	Reopacified segment as dense as the feeding vessel and filling rapidly

from the opposite side (but not cranial vs. caudal). With the concordant biplane setup, contrast use is halved, radiation dose reduced, and procedure time shortened. Although biplane coronary angiography is not generally considered critical for routine studies, if the laboratory has biplane capability, this form of angiography can improve procedure times, contrast use, and information quality.

Rotational Coronary Angiography

To avoid radiation exposure and reduce consumption of contrast dye, some institutions use rotation of the C-arm during coronary angiography. Rotational coronary angiography has been established for noncoronary angiographic procedures, particularly in the diagnosis and treatment of cerebrovascular disease. Rotational angiography, like biplane, is dependent upon the placement of the patient in an isocenter position. Various vendors have distinct programs that permit the attainment of images across a cranial or caudal plane while injecting contrast or in the case of dual-axis rotational angiography, complete assessment of the left coronary system with a single injection. Rotational angiography has been shown to reduce radiation, contrast, and procedural time. The critical aspects of rotational angiography are proper patient positioning because panning is not possible and proper coronary injection. The use of power injectors is recommended in order to maintain a consistent injection to provide adequate opacification.

Coronary Angiographic Catheters

The femoral arterial catheterization technique initially performed by Dr. Melvin Judkins continues to bear his name and has been highly successful because of its simplicity and ease of use with preshaped catheters (Fig. 3.16). As discussed earlier, operators using the radial artery for access can use a different array of specially designed catheters. Regardless of the vascular access, all catheters are inserted with a J-tipped guidewire. This J-wire is advanced into the ascending thoracic aorta under fluoroscopic guidance. The catheter follows the guidewire to the central position. When the catheter tip has reached the desired location in the aorta,

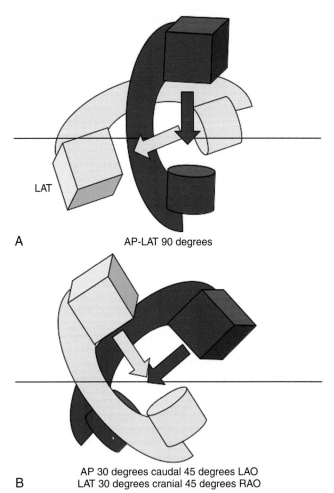

Fig. 3.15 Diagrams of biplane angiographic C-arm orientations. **(A)** Biplane C-arms in perpendicular anterior-posterior *(AP)* and lateral starting configuration. **(B)** Biplane C-arms rotated in opposing cranial/caudal, left anterior oblique/right anterior oblique *(LAO/RAO)* angulations. Panning in one plane moves the heart out of the other plane.

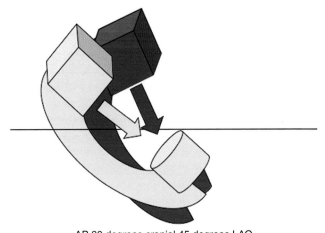

AP 30 degrees cranial 45 degrees LAO
C LAT 30 degrees cranial 45 degrees RAO

Fig. 3.15, cont'd (C) Biplane C-arms rotated in a concordant cranial orientation. Panning keeps images visible on both screens. *LAT,* Lateral.

the guidewire is removed and the catheter is aspirated (2 to 3 mL of blood), flushed, and connected to the pressure manifold. The guidewire or catheter tip should always be visible on the fluoroscopy screen when the catheter or guidewire is manipulated.

Judkins-Type Coronary Catheters

Judkins catheters have preshaped curves and tapered end-hole tips. The Judkins left (JL) coronary catheter has a double curve. The length of the segment between the primary and secondary curve determines the size of the catheter (i.e., 3.5, 4, 5, or 6 cm). The proper size of the JL catheter is selected depending on the length and width of the ascending aorta and the approach. A JL3.5 is best from the right radial while a JL4 is best from the left radial, which mirrors the femoral approach with respect to catheter selection. In a small person with a small aorta, a 3.5-cm catheter is appropriate, whereas in a large person or in an individual with an enlarged or dilated ascending aorta (e.g., as a result of aortic stenosis, regurgitation, or Marfan syndrome), a 5-cm or 6-cm catheter may be required (Fig. 3.17).

The ingenious design of the JL catheter permits cannulation of the LCA without any major catheter manipulation. The catheter

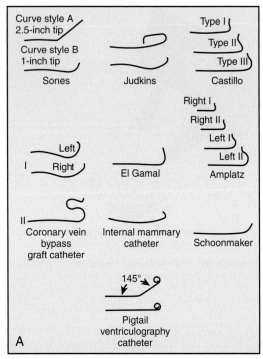

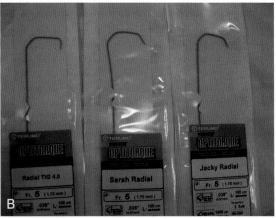

Fig. 3.16 **(A)** Coronary angiographic catheter shapes. **(B)** Preformed catheters for radial approach: Radial TIG 4.0, Sarah Radial, Jacky Radial.

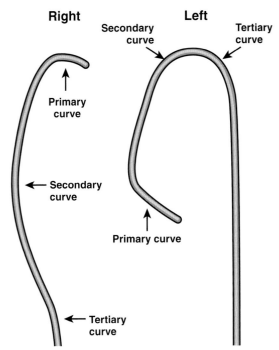

Fig. 3.17 Judkins right (JR) and Judkins left (JL) coronary catheters, identifying primary, secondary, and tertiary curves of each catheter. These curves are designed to facilitate entry into the ostia of each coronary artery.

tip follows the ascending aortic border and falls into the LM coronary ostium, often with an abrupt jump. In the words of its inventor, from the femoral approach "the [Judkins] catheter knows where to go if not thwarted by the operator." Because of the ease of seating in most patients, the slow advance of the catheter under fluoroscopic control will prevent rapid engagement into an unexpected LM narrowing.

A JL4 catheter fits most adults with the catheter tip aligned parallel with the long axis of the LM coronary trunk. A smaller (3.5 cm) catheter in the same patient angles upward and a larger (5 cm) catheter angles downward into the coronary cusp. When the coronary ostium cannot be seated correctly or placed in a stable position, the catheter should be replaced with a better-fitting catheter rather than aggressively manipulated into the coronary artery (Fig. 3.18). A slight rotation of the catheter may be necessary to improve alignment of the catheter tip with the LM coronary trunk.

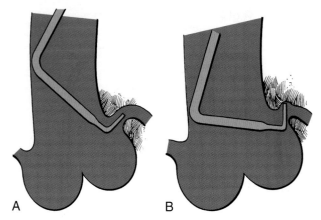

Fig. 3.18 Judkins left (JL) coronary catheter position. **(A)** Correct alignment. **(B)** Incorrect position and overinsertion. (From King SB, Douglas JS Jr. *Coronary Arteriography and Angioplasty.* New York: McGraw-Hill; 1985.)

The JR coronary catheter is sized by the length of the secondary curve and is available in 3.5-cm, 4-cm, and 5-cm sizes. In most cases, the 4-cm catheter is adequate. The JR catheter is advanced into the ascending aorta (usually with LAO projection) with the tip directed caudally (Fig. 3.19).

The RCA can be entered in most cases by one of two maneuvers:

1. Advance the catheter into the right coronary cusp and rotate the catheter 45 to 90 degrees clockwise as the tip is pulled back 2 to 3 cm. As the right coronary orifice is engaged, the fluoroscope shows rotation of the tip toward the right coronary cusp and downward motion of the catheter.

2. Advance the catheter tip to 2 to 4 cm above the valve. When the catheter is rotated clockwise for 45 to 90 degrees, the tip rotates toward the right cusp and descends approximately 1 to 2 cm, engaging the right coronary ostium from above.

If the coronary ostium is not engaged, the maneuvers are repeated, starting at a slightly different level each time. A brief contrast media injection into the right coronary cusp may help the operator direct the catheter. A slight but firm push-pull motion on the catheter is necessary to translate rotational motion at the hub down to the tip.

If stored rotational energy is not released by a small counter rotation after seating, the catheter may spring out of the right

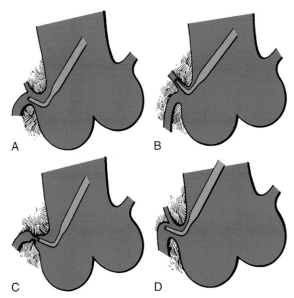

Fig. 3.19 Judkins right (JR) coronary catheter position. **(A)** Correct alignment. **(B)** Tip subselectively in conus artery. **(C)** Tip wedged in proximal stenosis. **(D)** Tip impinging on lateral vessel wall. (From King SB, Douglas JS Jr. *Coronary Arteriography and Angioplasty*. New York: McGraw-Hill; 1985.)

coronary ostium when the patient takes a deep breath. After seating, the operator checks for pressure damping associated with ostial stenosis or conus branch cannulation.

Amplatz-Type Catheters

The left Amplatz-type catheter is a preshaped half-circle with the tapered tip extending perpendicular to the curve (Fig. 3.20). Amplatz catheter sizes (left 1, 2, and 3 and right 1 and 2) indicate the diameter of the tip curve. In most normal-sized adults, no. 2 left and no. 1 right (modified) Amplatz catheters give satisfactory results. In the LAO projection, the tip is advanced into the left aortic cusp. Further advancement of the catheter causes the tip to move upward into the LM aortic trunk. It may be necessary to push Amplatz catheters down to move the tip up and out of the ostium to disengage the catheter from the LM ostium. If the catheter is pulled instead of being advanced, the tip moves downward and into the LM or CFX artery. Unwanted deep cannulation of the CFX artery might tear this

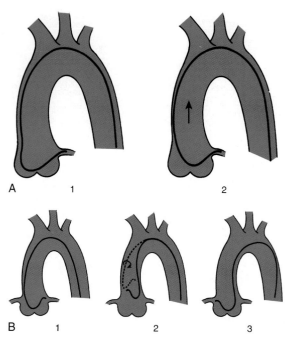

Fig. 3.20 Catheterization of the coronary arteries (Amplatz technique, left anterior oblique [LAO] projection). **(A)** Catheterization of the left coronary artery (LCA). (Arrows depict catheter movement and direction) *1:* The left coronary catheter is advanced until the secondary curve rests in the noncoronary posterior aortic cusp and its tip points to the left coronary ostium. *2:* The catheter is gently advanced and retracted until the left coronary ostium is engaged. **(B)** Catheterization of the right coronary artery (RCA). *1:* The right coronary catheter may initially point to the left coronary sinus. *2:* It is withdrawn slightly and rotated clockwise until the tip points toward the RCA and the secondary curve rests against the left aortic cusp. *3:* The RCA is engaged as the catheter is advanced and withdrawn. (From Tilkian AG, Daily EK. *Cardiovascular Procedures: Diagnostic Techniques and Therapeutic Procedures.* St Louis: Mosby; 1986.)

branch or the LM aortic trunk. The incidence of coronary dissection is higher with Amplatz catheters than with Judkins-type catheters.

The AR mod catheter has a smaller but similar hook-shaped curve. The catheter is advanced into the right coronary cusp. As with JR catheters, the catheter is rotated clockwise by 45 to 90 degrees. The same maneuver is repeated at different levels until the RCA is entered. After coronary injections, the catheter may be pulled, advanced, or rotated out of the coronary artery.

Multipurpose Catheters

MP catheters are those that are primarily straight or slightly angled with an end hole and two side holes placed close to the tapered tip. An MP catheter can be used for left and right coronary injections. Extra care is required if this catheter is used for ventriculography.

Special-Purpose Femoral Angiography Catheters

The right coronary vein graft catheter is similar to a JR catheter but has a wider, more open primary curve that allows cannulation of a vertically oriented coronary artery vein graft. The left coronary vein graft catheter is similar to the JR catheter but has a smaller and sharper secondary curve that allows easy cannulation of LAD and left CFX vein grafts, which are usually placed higher and more anterior than right coronary grafts with a relatively horizontal and upward takeoff from the aorta.

The internal mammary artery (IMA) graft catheter has a peculiar hook-shaped tip configuration that facilitates the engagement of IMA grafts, especially in patients with a vertical origin of the IMA.

Preformed Coronary Catheters from the Radial Artery Approach

Coronary Catheters from the Radial Artery Approach

Cannulation of the LCA using a preformed catheter is easier than cannulation using an MP catheter. JL and JR coronary catheters can be used through the left or right arm with satisfactory results. Compared with the femoral technique, a JL3.5 catheter may be necessary with the right radial technique.

An Amplatz catheter can be used effectively from either the right or the left arm. This catheter is manipulated in a fashion similar to that described for the femoral approach. The coronary catheters can be removed without a guidewire, but the pigtail ventriculography catheter should be removed over a guidewire to straighten the pigtail loop and prevent it from kinking or lodging in the subclavian or axillary artery. Torturous subclavian arteries may make catheter manipulation very difficult when trying to engage the coronary arteries. In these instances, substitution with stiffer (5 F) guiding catheters may provide more success.

A special consideration from the arm approach is negotiating a sharp caudal turn near the origin of the right carotid artery. To facilitate passage into the central aorta, the patient should be instructed to take a deep breath to pull down the great vessels and heart while the operator advances the guidewire and catheter. The manipulations to seat the preformed radial catheter are similar to those for the Amplatz and MP techniques (see Fig. 3.20C).

Radial Universal Catheters

Catheters used for coronary angiography from the radial approach are generically called universal catheters because they can engage both the left and right coronary ostia. Among the most common is the Jacky catheter (see Fig. 3.16B). This catheter is positioned in a similar way to the Amplatz maneuver catheters. The advantages of the Jacky and other universal catheters are reduced catheter exchanges with reduced potential for radial/brachial artery spasm, radiation exposure, and procedure time. The Jacky has a less acute terminal curve than the Tiger (TIG) catheter and has a tendency to sit more coaxially with the LMCA and engage the RCA with fewer movements.

Although some operators perform ventriculography through universal catheters because there are side holes near the catheter tip, a technique that is not recommended (see end of the end-hole left ventricle [LV] gram, page 172 and Fig. 3.21). We do not recommend it because a hand injection for ventriculography may be inadequate and the Jacky catheter tip frequently points directly toward the anterior wall of the LV, causing ventricular ectopy and possible perforation.

Saphenous Vein Graft and Internal Mammary Artery Angiography Catheters

The RCB graft catheter is similar to a JR catheter but has a wider, more open primary curve that allows cannulation of a vertically oriented coronary artery vein graft. The LCB graft catheter is similar to the JR catheter but has a smaller and sharper secondary curve that allows easy cannulation of LAD and left CFX vein grafts, which are usually placed higher and more anterior than right coronary grafts with a relatively horizontal and upward takeoff from the aorta. The IMA graft catheter has a peculiar hook-shaped tip configuration that facilitates the engagement of IMA grafts, especially in patients with a vertical origin of the IMA.

Ventriculography Catheters (Pigtail, Halo, Multipurpose)

The pigtail catheter is the safest choice for ventriculography and is the most commonly used ventriculography catheter, with a pre-shaped tip making nearly a full circle ~1 cm in diameter. There are 6 to 12 side holes on the straight portion of the catheter above the curve. To enter the LV, the pigtail catheter is advanced to the aortic

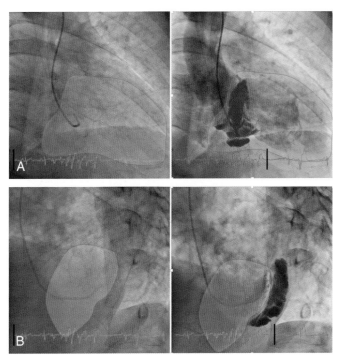

Fig. 3.21 **A.** Left to right, A 5F Jacky catheter positioned in the RAO projection followed by power contrast injection with the ACIST medical injector, 13ml/sec to maximal volume of 45cc (less was injected when staining was noted). Right side shows significant myocardial staining. **B.** Left to right, Simultaneous RAO LV gram with the 5F Jacky catheter recorded during the power contrast injection as in figure above. Right side shows significant myocardial staining. There is little reason to use end hole catheters for ventriculography.

valve. The loop is positioned to the left in the RAO projection (resembling a 6), and the catheter is pushed against the valve to make a U shape that facilitates entry into the ventricle during deep inspiration. Inside the ventricle, the catheter can be placed in front of the mitral valve with the loop directed toward the apex, away from the valve (in the RAO position). A slight rotation, advancement, or withdrawal may be necessary to find a quiet position (one that does not cause frequent premature ventricular contractions) (Fig. 3.22). An angled (145 degrees) pigtail catheter may be helpful for this purpose, especially for horizontally oriented hearts.

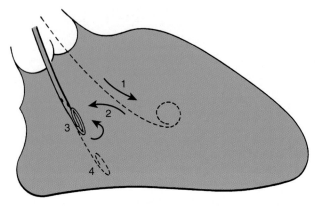

Fig. 3.22 Method of left ventricle (LV) catheterization. *1:* Having crossed the aortic valve, the pigtail catheter is in position. *2:* The catheter is withdrawn 2 to 3 cm and rotated 70 to 90 degrees counterclockwise. *3:* The coiled loop is in the inflow tract of the mitral valve. *4:* If the catheter moves excessively in this position, it should be advanced until it is stable. (From Judkins MP, Judkins E. Coronary arteriography and left ventriculography: Judkins technique. In: King SB, Douglas JS Jr, eds. *Coronary Arteriography and Angioplasty.* New York: McGraw-Hill; 1985.)

A Halo catheter is a novel 5-F catheter with a perpendicular helical tip with an inwardly and upwardly directed tip. The side holes are located on the helix and produce equivalent left ventriculograms with minimal ectopy because the contrast jets are directed inward and not to the myocardium (Fig. 3.23). It is excellent for measuring distal LV chamber pressure in hypertrophic cardiomyopathy because, in contrast to a pigtail catheter, there are no holes along the shaft to create a falsely low distal intraventricular pressure gradient.

In the past, the MP and other end-hole-type catheters have been used for ventriculography. This and other end-hole catheters are no longer recommended for ventriculographic studies because the high-pressure contrast jet may produce ventricular tachycardia (VT), contrast injection in the myocardial tissue (contrast staining), or ventricular perforation (Fig. 3.21).

Common Problems in Accessing and Cannulating Coronary Arteries and Grafts

Left Coronary Artery

Short Left Main, Separate Ostia for Left Anterior Descending and Circumflex Arteries. In patients with a short LM artery segment or separate ostia, it may be necessary to cannulate the

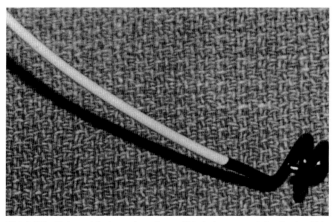

Fig. 3.23 Halo ventriculography catheter. Side holes are contained only within the spiral, which is directed inward to reduce premature ventricular contractions.

LAD and CFX arteries separately. Using a smaller JL catheter (i.e., JL3.5, not JL4) often permits selective cannulation of the LAD artery. Slight withdrawal and clockwise rotation or use of a larger JL5 catheter also favors cannulation of the CFX artery. An Amplatz-type catheter is especially useful to cannulate the CFX artery separately but must be used with care to avoid artery dissections.

High Left Coronary Artery Takeoff. An unusually high origin of the LMCA from the aorta can usually be cannulated with use of an MP catheter or an Amplatz-type catheter (e.g., AL 2). A long, tapered-tip MP catheter may be used to cannulate the high-origin LM trunk through the radial approach.

Wide Aortic Root. In patients with a relatively horizontal or wide aortic root with upward takeoff of the LMCA, a large-curve JL5 or JL6, AL coronary, or MP catheter may be required.

Right Coronary Artery

The origin of the RCA shows more variation than that of the LCA. When encountering difficulty in locating the ostium, a contrast injection low into the right coronary cusp helps direct the catheter. If the RCA is not seen with this flush injection, it may be totally occluded or may originate anteriorly on the aorta or from the left sinus of Valsalva. In this case, the orifice is usually located above the sinotubular ridge. An AL catheter or a left bypass graft catheter can be used successfully to engage the RCA orifice located anteriorly or in the left cusp. Minimal anterior displacement of the RCA from the right coronary sinus is more common. In this case, the JR catheter tip may not be directed toward the right but looks foreshortened in the familiar LAO view. Directing the catheter tip to the right in the usual fashion using the lateral view permits easy cannulation of the anteriorly directed right coronary orifice. Rarely, an aortogram is necessary to ascertain the location of the RCA.

Wide Aortic Root. In a patient with a horizontal and wide aortic root, cannulation of the right coronary orifice and right coronary cusp may require an Amplatz or MP catheter.

High Right Coronary Artery Takeoff. A relatively high origin of the RCA may require an AL or AR mod catheter. The most common coronary anomaly (see section Angiography of Common Coronary Anomalies) is the CFX artery originating from the RCA or right coronary cusp and coursing posteriorly and downward. This location may be cannulated easily with use of an AR catheter or multipurpose catheter.

Assessment of Coronary Stenoses

The degree of an angiographic narrowing is estimated as the percentage lumen reduction of the most severely narrowed segment compared with the adjacent angiographically normal vessel segment, seen in the worst x-ray projection. Because the operator uses visual estimations, an exact evaluation is impossible; in general, there can be a ±20% variation between readings of two or more experienced angiographers. Stenosis severity alone should not always be assumed to be associated with abnormal physiology (blood flow) and ischemia. Moreover, CAD is a diffuse process, and thus, minimal luminal irregularities on angiography may represent significant albeit nonobstructive CAD at the time of angiography. The stenotic segment lumen is compared with a nearby lumen that does not appear to be obstructed but that may have diffuse atherosclerotic disease (Fig. 3.24). This explains why postmortem examinations and intravascular ultrasound (IVUS) imaging reveal much more plaque than is seen on angiography. The percent diameter is estimated from the angiographically normally appearing adjacent segment. Because coronary arteries normally taper as they travel to the apex, proximal segments are always larger than distal segments, often explaining the large disparity among several observers' estimates of stenosis severity.

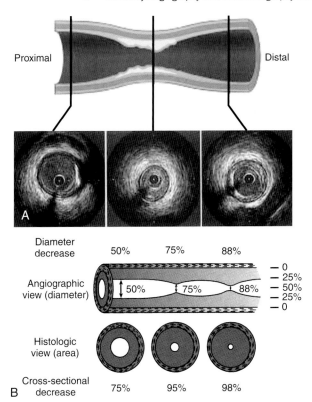

Fig. 3.24 **(A)** Diagram of coronary artery with stenosis *(top)* and corresponding intravascular ultrasound (IVUS) images demonstrating diffuse nature of coronary artery disease (CAD). **(B)** The percent narrowing is compared only with the angiographic lumen that appear normal but might not be normal at all.

Percent diameter is the common measurement reported to convey stenosis severity. Recall that area of stenosis is greater than diameter stenosis. Estimates of narrowing assume that the lumen is circular, but the lumen is more often eccentric. Although the practice has been to report exact measurements (even when using only the naked eye), realistically and for practical purposes, there are only four categories of lesion severity:

1. Minimal or mild CAD, narrowings <40%
2. Moderate, stenosis between 40% and 70%

3. Severe, stenosis between 70% and 95%

4. Total occlusion (100%)

Technical note: Stenosis anatomy should not be confused with abnormal physiology (flow) and ischemia, especially for lesions 40% to 70% narrowed. For nonquantitative reports, the length of a stenosis is simply mentioned (e.g., LAD proximal segment stenosis diameter 25%, long or short). Other features of the coronary lesion may not be appreciated by angiography and may require IVUS or optical coherence tomography (OCT) (Fig. 3.25).

Several different angiographic pathologies commonly seen during coronary or peripheral vascular angiography include thrombus, dissection, aneurysms, and coronary fistulae.

A thrombus is defined as a lucency within a vessel or chamber surrounded by at least three sides of contrast in an appropriate clinical setting (e.g., acute coronary syndromes). In the coronary vessels, a thrombotic occlusion may totally block the flow of contrast and have a meniscus appearance (Fig. 3.26A).

A dissection is defined as a linear lucency in a vessel that may or may not be associated with slow angiographic flow (Fig. 3.26B).

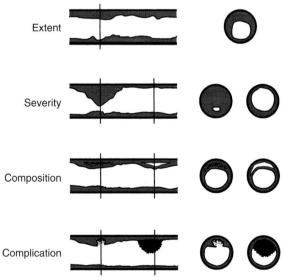

Fig. 3.25 Angiographic features that may not be appreciated on cineangiographic imaging and can be evaluated by intravascular ultrasound (IVUS).

An aneurysm in a coronary artery is typically associated with a bulbous segment of the vessel often with slow flow (Fig. 3.26C). The aneurysms may be diffuse or isolated and are usually associated with atherosclerotic arterial disease.

A coronary artery fistula connects the artery to the pulmonary circuit and other regions of the heart directly into the LV cavity or the right-sided structures (Fig. 3.26D).

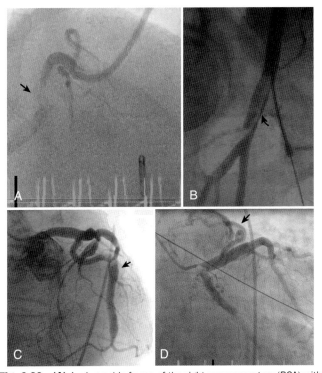

Fig. 3.26 **(A)** Angiographic frame of the right coronary artery (RCA) with thrombus showing faint opacification around the thrombotic material after the proximal segment. **(B)** Image of femoral artery dissection with linear lucency extending below the puncture site, down the common femoral artery toward the bifurcation of the profunda and superficial artery. **(C)** Cineangiographic frame showing large ectatic and aneurysmal coronary arteries. This one involves both the circumflex (CFX) and left anterior descending (LAD) coronary artery. **(D)** Cineangiographic frame of patient who has fistula from the proximal LAD moving upward over the anterior surface of the pulmonary artery. This fistula might or might not be the cause of symptoms.

Continued

CORONARY IMAGING DEVICES IN THE CATHETER LAB

	Angio	IVUS	NIRS	Angioscopy	OCT
Resolution (μm)	100 – 200	80 – 120	=	<200	10 – 15
Probe size (m)	N/A	700	1000	800	140
Contact	No	Yes	Yes	Yes	Yes
Ionizing radiation	Yes	No	No	No	No
Other	Lumen only	N/A	N/A	Surface only	Plaque character

Fig. 3.26, cont'd Coronary imaging devices used in the catheterization laboratory. *Angio,* angiography *IVUS,* Intravascular ultrasound; *NIRS,* near-infrared spectroscopy; *OCT,* optical coherence tomography.

Non-angiographic Lesion Assessment Tools (Fractional Flow Reserve, Intravascular Ultrasound, and Optical Coherence Tomography).

Because the angiographic image is a two-dimensional (2D) projection of a three-dimensional (3D) structure, it does not accurately reflect the physiologic consequences of a stenosis alone, especially for narrowings in the intermediate ranges (40% to 80%). The use of nonangiographic lesion assessment tools overcomes this limitation. There are various commonly used nonangiographic lesion assessment tools: a pressure sensor guidewire measurement for *fractional flow reserve* (FFR) or nonhyperemic pressure ratios (NHPR, e.g. instantaneous wave-free ratio [iFR], diastolic pressure ratio [dPR], and Pd/Pa); and two intravascular imaging methods, one using ultrasound (IVUS) and the other using laser light (OCT), to create intraluminal images of the vessel. FFR (distal/aortic pressure at hyperemia) is used to determine the functional significance of a coronary stenosis, that is, whether the lesion is responsible for ischemia. iFR is a nonhyperemic pressure-based index of stenosis severity using the distal pressure value obtained during the wave-free period of diastole. Both FFR and NHPRs are used to determine whether a lesion is causing significant ischemia.

IVUS and OCT provide visualization of intraluminal and transmural coronary anatomy but cross-sectional areas should not be used to replace FFR/NHPRs. OCT has higher resolution than IVUS and further improves visualization of various plaque components and vessel structures. These adjunctive diagnostic procedures, summarized in Figure 3.26E, influence the decision for coronary revascularization, guide the performance of PCIs and optimize procedural outcomes.

Classification of Angiographic Blood Flow (TIMI Grades)

Angiographic blood flow has been qualitatively assessed by observing the distal runoff and is classified into four grades (also known as *TIMI flow grades*). The TIMI grade was developed from the Thrombolysis in Myocardial Infarction Studies during the late 1980s.

The four grades of flow are described as follows:

- TIMI 3: Flow rate equal to that in noninfarct arteries
- TIMI 2: Distal flow in the artery less than that in noninfarct arteries
- TIMI 1: Some contrast filling beyond the culprit lesion but no significant antegrade flow
- TIMI 0: No flow beyond the total occlusion

To quantitate TIMI flow rates, the number of angiographic frames required for contrast media to traverse the coronary artery was reported by Gibson et al. It was originally calculated as the number of frames from the initial appearance of the dye in the coronary artery to a distal predetermined landmark. Gibson et al. proposed a correction of this frame count called the *corrected TIMI frame count*, which uses the distal targets in the LAD artery as the distal bifurcation, the distal target in the CFX artery as the distal bifurcation of the terminal segments at the longest distance, and the RCA as the first branch of the posterolateral artery. Today, TIMI frame counts are used almost exclusively in research.

Coronary Angiography: Common Problems and Solutions

Coronary Spasm

Spontaneous or catheter-induced coronary artery spasm may appear as a fixed stenotic lesion. Catheter spasm has been observed in right and left coronary arteries (including the LMCA) and must be considered and excluded (by the administration of intracoronary nitroglycerin) before the narrowing is considered to be an organic lesion. Catheter-induced spasm may occur not only at the tip of the catheter touching the artery but also more distally. Repositioning of the catheter and administration of nitroglycerin (100 to 200 µg through the catheter) determines whether the presumed lesion is structural or spastic. A change to a smaller-diameter (4 F or 5 F) catheter or to catheters that do not seat deeply may also help.

Vessel Overlap

The purpose of coronary angiography is to visualize adequately each segment of the coronary tree in at least two orthogonal imaging planes. Given the individual variations of the coronary tree, multiple angles are often required to reveal locations of lesions. Depending on lesion location, steeper angles or even AP-cranial or AP-caudal views are often helpful to minimize vessel overlap. For lesions whose significance remains uncertain, IVUS or physiologic measurements (FFR and coronary flow reserve [CFR]) should be considered.

Inadequate Vessel Opacification

Poor contrast opacification of the vessel may lead to a false impression of an angiographically significant lesion or lucency that could be considered a clot. Inadequate mixing of contrast material and blood (streaming) could be seen as a luminal irregularity. A satisfactory bolus injection of contrast material must be delivered if adequate opacification is to be achieved and the angiogram interpreted correctly. Contrast delivery can be enhanced by use of a larger catheter, injection during Valsalva maneuver phase III, or use of a power injector. For patients who have elevated cardiac outputs (liver failure patients) or who have large coronary arteries, use of a guiding catheter that has a larger luminal diameter can be considered to preclude this common problem.

Total Coronary Occlusion

Total occlusion of a vessel may be erroneously suspected if the catheter injection site is subselective or an anomalous origin or course of a vessel is not recognized. A short LMCA may lead to selective opacification of only the LAD artery and a presumption of a CFX occlusion or anomalous origin of the CFX. To address this, an aortic cusp flush of contrast may reveal the second vessel. When target vessels are not clearly seen, the operator should consider anomalous origins of the coronary artery and review the aortogram and left ventriculogram (see page 184, Angiography of common coronary anomalies).

Dominance Determination

Which vessel supplies the PDA determines the dominance of the coronary circulation and the majority of people are right-dominant (85%). Left dominance is present in 7% of the population, and the PDA is best visualized in the LAO-cranial injection during left coronary angiography, laying in the interventricular groove and feeding the inferior septum. In these left-dominant individuals, the RCA is often small and only supplies a few RV arteries marginally. These nondominant RCAs are often small and may be prone to catheter-induced spasm. The remaining 7% to 8% of people are codominant and the inferior septum is supplied by parallel left and right PDAs.

Special Clinical Situations and Problems

Left Main Coronary Artery Stenosis

A commonly encountered and potentially critical problem is coronary angiography of patients who have LMCA stenosis (Fig. 3.27), which is one of the few situations wherein the routine performance of angiography may be life threatening. An LM stenosis may occur at the ostium, mid body, or distal bifurcation of LAD or CFX arteries, and the correct diagnosis of lesion severity is critical for CABG and PCI decisions.

LMCA stenosis is commonly associated with two clinical presentations:

1. Patients who show evidence of significant low workload ischemia or hypotension during exercise treadmill testing. Unstable angina may be caused by LMCA stenosis in ~10% of patients.
2. Patients with atypical angina. The clinical history and resting or stress electrocardiogram (ECG) may not be helpful and patients with resting or atypical chest pain syndromes often do not have previous exercise test data.

Technical notes for angiography of LMCA stenosis:

1. Either femoral or radial vascular access approach may be used safely. Access should be based on the operator's best working method.
2. Coronary angiography before left ventriculography is recommended to obtain the most important information first, should a complication (e.g., arrhythmia, pulmonary edema) occur.

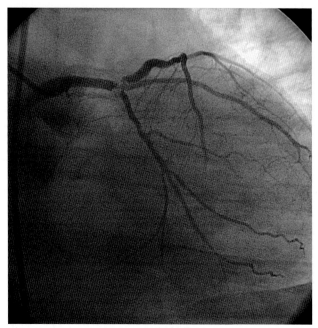

Fig. 3.27 Cineangiographic frame showing distal left main (LM) coronary stenosis at the trifurcation branch of the left anterior descending (LAD), ramus intermedius, and circumflex (CFX) arteries. In critical LM stenoses, only one or two views may be necessary. In this case, only one view was obtained before recommending urgent coronary artery bypass graft (CABG) surgery.

3. Careful slow advancement and seating of the left coronary catheter prevents the Judkins preshaped catheter from jumping into the left coronary ostia. This maneuver is important for an aorta-ostial narrowing. Continuous observation of the arterial pressure for damping is key for safe engagement. Most universal shaped radial catheters have end and side holes at the tip and may not demonstrate damping.

4. For patients in whom there is high suspicion of LMCA stenosis, the catheter can be positioned beneath the ostia, and a cusp flush of contrast material in the aortic sinus in an AP or shallow LAO or RAO projection may identify an ostial LM stenosis.

5. After catheter engagement, the operator should look for aortic pressure wave deformation (damping). If pressure damping occurs, a limited contrast flush (1 to 2 mL) and rapid catheter

withdrawal (hit and run) during cineangiography should be performed to obtain a first look (Fig. 3.1). Rarely, aortic pressure damping occurs without LMCA narrowing because the coronary catheter is seated deeply subselectively into the LAD artery or positioned against the vessel wall. Gradual withdrawal and repositioning of the catheter may eliminate pressure damping. The absence of reflux of contrast media into the aortic root on coronary injection is also associated with an ostial LMCA stenosis. Some operators have advocated the use of a 6-inch collimated initial view of the LM performed in shallow LAO (LAO 5 to 20 degrees) to obtain the best visualization of the LM ostia for all coronary angiography.

6. Limit the number of coronary injections. Distal coronary artery anatomy suitable for bypass grafting is assessed from the few views (usually two or three) that are available. Additional injections should be kept to a minimum. Two projections, an LAO with cranial angulation and a steeper RAO with caudal angulation, are usually sufficient. An LAO-caudal projection for an ostial narrowing is sometimes better. Occasionally, one image may be sufficient. Frequent catheter engagement of the LMCA segment and contrast jet stimulation of the lesion may precipitate coronary spasm or occlusion. In less critical LMCA stenosis with 40% to 60% narrowing, FFR or IVUS may be critically important for an accurate diagnosis.

7. After the left coronary views are completed, right coronary angiography is performed. In symptomatic patients with RCA occlusion and a critical LMCA stenosis, abdominal aortography and insertion of an intraaortic counterpulsation balloon or percutaneous LV support device, intensive-care-unit admission, and early CABG surgery should be strongly considered.

Important points for postcatheterization care of the patient with LMCA stenosis:

1. Prevention of hypotension is paramount. If we assume an LMCA stenosis pressure gradient of 40 mm Hg, aortic diastolic blood pressure of 80 mm Hg, and LV end-diastolic pressure of 10 mm Hg, the coronary perfusion pressure can be approximated to be $80 - (40 + 10) = 30$ mm Hg. If diastolic blood pressure decreases to 60 mm Hg, the perfusion pressure can decrease to 10 mm Hg, exacerbating myocardial ischemia and hypotension, leading to a downward spiral of LV dysfunction and death.

2. Treat the hypotension of vasovagal reactions immediately. Vagal reactions can occur during painful sheath removal. Consider a vascular closure device (VCD), preferably starting with the radial approach.

3. Administer adequate volumes of intravenous (IV) fluids (at least 1000 mL of normal saline in 4 hours) and monitor the patient's blood pressure and urine output.

4. Any signs of ischemia in the postcatheterization period require immediate evaluation and urgent revascularization. LV support with an IABP, TandemHeart, or Impella pump should be strongly considered.

5. Change the patient's admission status and monitor patient in an intensive care unit.

6. Urgent consultation with a cardiothoracic surgeon to determine the best timing for CABG surgery is important to achieve an optimal result. If a problem should develop, immediate communication between the cardiologist and surgeon makes a crucial difference in timing for urgent intervention.

7. Under urgent conditions or complicating comorbidities that preclude urgent surgery, LM stenting may be lifesaving and is recommended.

Angiography of Common Coronary Anomalies

Coronary artery anomalies should be considered when on a routine angiography there appears to be a missing coronary artery or a large area of myocardium that is not perfused by visible vasculature. It is an error to assume that a vessel is occluded when it has not been visualized because of an anomalous origin. Because the natural history of a patient with an anomalous origin of a coronary artery may depend on the initial course of the anomalous vessel, it is the angiographer's responsibility to define accurately the origin and course of the vessel. Historically, the simple 'dot and eye' method for determining the proximal course of an anomalous artery was performed using RAO ventriculography and/or aortography. During the injection, the location of the dot and eye in relation (anterior or posterior) to the aorta aids in determination of the vessel course. Placement of right-sided catheters or injection of contrast material into the PA is unnecessary and often misleading. Among all coronary anomalies, the highest potential for adverse sequelae is with an anomalous vessel that runs an interarterial course. These malignant variants can manifest in young individuals as sudden cardiac death, angina, syncope, angina, myocardial infarction, acute pulmonary edema, dyspnea, and palpitations. The mechanism causing myocardial ischemia appears to be the slit-like opening in the aortic wall that narrows further during activity with dynamic compression of the obliquely arising LMCA ostium as it courses between the aortic root and the root of the pulmonary trunk. The performance of coronary CTA should be considered when angiography is unclear in confirming the diagnosis of specific anomalies of the coronary vasculature.

Absent Left Main Trunk (Separate Ostia of Left Anterior Descending and LCX)

Likely to be the most common coronary anomaly (incidence ~0.47%), separate ostia of the two major branches of the LCA is often referred to as a double-barrel LM. Subselective cannulation of only one branch may mistakenly lead to the belief that there is an occlusion of the other. If the LAD is subselectively cannulated, the catheter should be pulled back into the aorta and clockwise torque administered to gain access into the CFX. If this is unsuccessful, a longer catheter such as a JL5 may be preferable. The converse is true for subselective cannulation of the left CFX: a smaller catheter (JL3.5) can be used to engage the LAD.

Anomalous Origin of the Circumflex Coronary Artery

The next most common coronary anomaly (0.45%) is the origin of the left CFX from the right coronary cusp or from the RCA ostia. This feature is often suggested during left coronary angiography when the operator sees a long LMCA segment (Fig. 3.28) with a presumed small or trivial CFX branch (sometimes thought to be occluded). When this occurs, a visual reflex should suggest the following mantra to the operator: 'That LM seems very long… I wonder if there is an anomalous CFX?' When the CFX coronary artery arises from the right coronary cusp or the proximal RCA, it invariably follows a retroaortic course and passes posteriorly around the aortic root to its normal position. During RAO ventriculography, aortography, or coronary angiography, the CFX artery is seen on end, appearing as a radiopaque dot posterior to the aorta. The missing CFX coronary artery is often found arising from the right coronary cusp or the proximal RCA and invariably follows a posterior path, moving behind and around the aortic root ultimately supplying the lateral wall of the LV. The retroaortic course can be easily seen in the RAO projection as the CFX moves leftward and behind the aorta (Fig. 3.29).

For all artery pathways that travel behind the aorta, the RAO projection during left ventriculography, aortography, or coronary angiography will visualize the artery on end and appear as a radiopaque dot posterior to the aorta. The anomalous CFX from the RCA is a benign variant of no clinical significance unless a significant stenosis is also present.

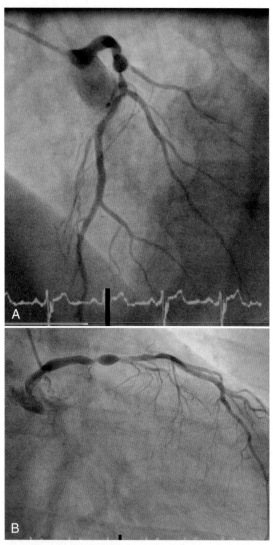

Fig. 3.28 **(A)** Left anterior oblique (LAO) projection of left main (LM) and left anterior descending (LAD) with 70% stenosis. The circumflex (CFX) is not visible. **(B)** Long LM artery segment with stenosis. Note that the CFX is not evident. (Reprinted with permission from the *Cath Lab Digest,* copyright HMP Communications.)

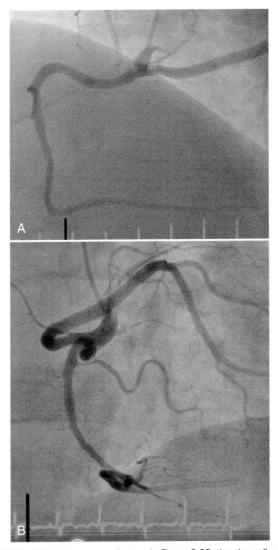

Fig. 3.29 **(A)** In the same patient as in Figure 3.28, the circumflex (CFX) artery can be seen originating in the proximal ostial part of the right coronary artery (RCA) in the left anterior oblique (LAO) projection. **(B)** Right anterior oblique (RAO) projection of RCA with anomalous CFX traveling behind the aorta, looping around to the lateral aspect of the heart. (Reprinted with permission from the *Cath Lab Digest,* copyright HMP Communications.)

Anomalous Origin of the Left Main Coronary Artery from the Right Sinus of Valsalva

This very rare anomaly (0.02%) can be malignant, depending on its course. Although most variants are benign, it is imperative to exclude the interatrial course of this anomaly. When the LMCA arises from the right sinus of Valsalva or the proximal RCA, it may follow one of four pathways (Table 3.3):

1. Septal course (benign):The LMCA runs an intramuscular course through the septum along the floor of the RV outflow tract (RVOT) (Fig. 3.30). It then surfaces in the mid septum, at which point it branches into the LAD artery and left CFX artery. Because the artery divides in the mid septum, the initial portion of the CFX artery courses toward the aorta (the normal position of the proximal LAD), and the LAD artery is relatively short (i.e., only the mid and distal LAD are present). During RAO ventriculography, aortography, or coronary angiography, the LMCA and the CFX coronary artery form an ellipse (similar to the shape of an eye) to the left of the aorta. The LMCA forms the inferior portion and the CFX artery forms the superior portion. Septal perforating arteries are evident branching from the LMCA.

2. Anterior free wall course (benign): The LMCA crosses the anterior free wall of the right ventricle and then divides at the mid septum into the LAD and CFX arteries (Fig. 3.31). Because the artery divides at the mid septum, the initial portion of the CFX artery courses toward the aorta (the normal position of the proximal

Table 3.3

Radiographic Appearance of Anomalous Origin of the Left Main Coronary Artery From the Right Sinus of Valsalva.				
	Right Anterior Oblique Aortography or Ventriculography			
Course of LMCA	**Dot**	**Eye**	**LAD Length**	**Septal Branches Arising from LMCA**
Septal	−	+ (Upper CFX) (lower LMCA)	Short	Yes
Anterior	−	+ (Upper LMCA) (lower CFX)	Short	No
Retroaortic	+ (Posterior)	−	Normal	No
Interarterial	+ (Anterior)	−	Normal	No

+, Present; −, absent. *Posterior* and *anterior* are in reference to the aorta root. *CFX,* Circumflex coronary artery; *LAD,* left anterior descending coronary artery; *LMCA,* left main coronary artery.

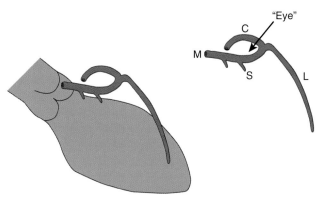

Fig. 3.30 Diagram of septal course of anomalous left coronary artery (LCA). *C*, Circumflex; *L*, left anterior descending artery; *M*, left main; *S*, septals.

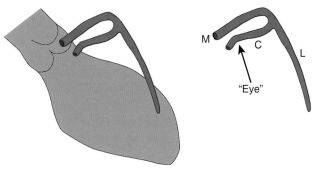

Fig. 3.31 Diagram of anterior course of anomalous left coronary artery (LCA). *C*, Circumflex; *L*, left anterior descending artery; *M*, left main.

LAD), and the LAD artery is relatively short (i.e., only the mid and distal LAD are present). During RAO ventriculography, aortography, or coronary angiography, the LMCA and the CFX artery form an ellipse (eye) to the *left of the aorta*, with the LMCA forming the superior portion and the CFX forming the inferior portion.

3. Retroaortic course (benign): The LMCA passes posteriorly around the aortic root to its normal position on the anterior surface of the heart (Fig. 3.32). It divides into LAD and CFX arteries at the normal point and gives rise to LAD and CFX coronary arteries of normal length and course. During RAO ventriculography, aortography, or coronary angiography, the LMCA is seen on end, *posterior to the aorta*, and appears as a

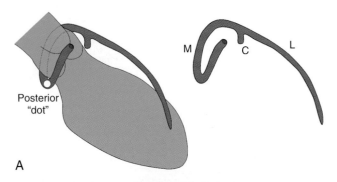

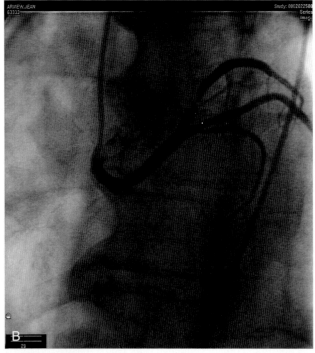

Fig. 3.32 **(A)** Diagram of retroaortic course of anomalous left coronary artery (LCA). **(B)** Intraseptal course of left main coronary artery (LMCA) from right sinus. The LMCA, when it originates within the right sinus of Valsalva or from the proximal right coronary artery (RCA), may take an inferior and intraseptal course, a superior course anterior to the pulmonary artery, or a serpentine course between the great arteries (which carries a risk of sudden death). *C*, Circumflex; *L*, left anterior descending artery; *M*, left main.

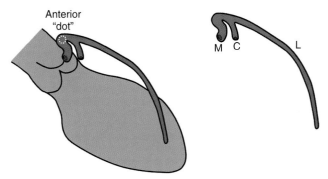

Fig. 3.33 Intraarterial course of left main coronary artery (LMCA) from right sinus. *C,* Circumflex; *L,* left anterior descending artery; *M,* left main.

radiopaque dot, which signifies a posteriorly coursing anomalous vessel. (It is also seen with anomalous origin of CFX from the right sinus.)

Note: This variant is considered benign, and evidence of myocardial ischemia has been reported in only a few individuals.

4. Interarterial course (malignant): The LMCA courses between the aorta and PA to its normal position on the anterior surface of the heart (Fig. 3.33, top part). It divides into LAD and CFX arteries at the normal point and gives rise to LAD and CFX coronary arteries of normal length and course. During RAO ventriculography, aortography, or coronary angiography, the LMCA is seen on end, *anterior to the aorta,* and appears as a radiopaque *dot to the left* of the aortic root. This variant is considered malignant and coronary revascularization with translocation is indicated in patients with myocardial ischemia. The need for revascularization in older patients with this anomaly is less clear. A decision for revascularization should be based on the severity of concomitant obstructive coronary disease and inducible myocardial ischemia.

Anomalous Origin of the Right Coronary Artery From the Left Sinus of Valsalva (Malignant)

When the RCA arises from the left coronary cusp or the proximal LMCA, it generally follows only one path, although other courses are theoretically possible and have been reported. The RCA generally courses between the aorta and PA to its normal position. During RAO ventriculography (Fig. 3.34), the anomalous RCA (ARCA) is seen on end, anterior to the aorta, and appears as a radiopaque

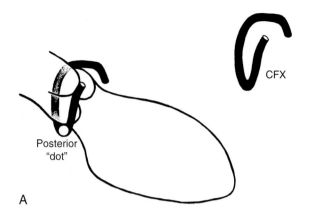

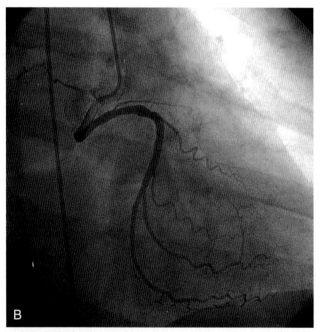

Fig. 3.34 **(A)** Diagram of retroaortic course of circumflex *(CFX)* from the left coronary cusp. **(B)** The anomalous CFX artery usually originates from the right sinus of Valsalva with a separate ostium or from the proximal right coronary artery (RCA). The typical course of this benign anomaly is retroaortic as it travels to the lateral surface of the left ventricle (LV). The right anterior oblique (RAO) view shows a dot of the anomalous retroaortic course of the CFX.

dot. This coronary anomaly has been associated with symptoms of myocardial ischemia, particularly when the RCA is dominant. Coronary revascularization should be considered when this anomaly is associated with symptoms of myocardial ischemia. When the ARCA arises from an anterior location or high above the sinus of Valsalva, an aortic root injection will help locate the ostium for subselective catheter engagement using AL2 or MP catheters.

Anomalous Right Coronary Artery Above the Sinus of Valsalva or From the Anterior Aortic Wall (Benign)

The RCA may arise from an anterior location or high above the sinus of Valsalva. Aortic root flush injection helps locate the ostium for proper, subselective catheter selection (using AL2 or MP catheters, for example).

Anomalous Origin of the Left Anterior Descending Coronary Artery From the Right Sinus of Valsalva (Benign)

When the LAD artery arises from the right aortic cusp or the proximal RCA, it generally follows one of two pathways, although other courses are possible.

1. Anterior free wall course: The LAD coronary artery crosses the anterior free wall of the right ventricle and then at the mid septum turns toward the apex. During RAO ventriculography, aortography, or coronary angiography, the LAD artery is seen passing to the left and upward before turning toward the apex. This coronary anomaly is benign.
2. Septal course: The LAD coronary artery runs an intramuscular course through the septum, along the floor of the RVOT. It then surfaces in the mid septum and turns toward the apex. During RAO ventriculography, aortography, or coronary angiography, the LAD artery is seen passing to the left and downward before turning toward the apex. This anomaly is benign.

Ventriculography

The left ventriculogram is an integral part of every coronary arteriographic study and provides information about LV wall motion and overall function of the heart. Figure 3.35 shows the LV in systole and diastole in RAO and LAO projections. In the RAO view,

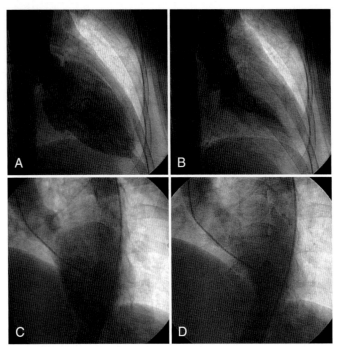

Fig. 3.35 **(A)** Left ventriculographic frame 30-degree right anterior oblique (RAO) projection in diastole and **(B)** in systole. In the LAO projection **(C** and **D). (B)** In systole. **(C** and **D)** Left ventriculographic frame in diastole and systole, respectively.

from the 1 o'clock position, LV segments are the anterior base, anterior, apical, inferior, and inferior base. The lateral wall cannot be seen in the RAO projection. In the LAO view, the LV segments, moving clockwise from 12 o'clock, are the high lateral, lateral, apical, septal, and base (see Fig. 3.4).

Abnormal wall motion indicates the presence of coronary ischemia, infarction, aneurysm, or hypertrophy. Left ventriculography also provides quantitative information, such as the ventricular volumes during systole and diastole, ejection fraction (EF), rate of ejection, quality of contractility, presence of hyperdynamic hypertrophic contraction, and valvular regurgitation. Ventricular function in general and EF in particular predict the long-term outcome of patients with CAD. Ventriculography may be performed before or after coronary angiography. Coronary angiography is routinely performed first because ventricular function can be obtained through noninvasive methods in case of complications that

---

Box 3.2   Indications and Complications of Left Ventriculography.

Indications

1. Identification of LV function for patients with CAD, myopathy, or valvular heart disease
2. Identification of VSD
3. Quantitation of the degree of mitral regurgitation
4. Quantitation of the mass of myocardium for regression of hypertrophy or other similar research studies

Indications for Right Ventriculography

1. Documentation of tricuspid regurgitation
2. Assessment of RV dysplasia for arrhythmias
3. Assessment of pulmonary stenosis
4. Assessment of abnormalities of pulmonary outflow tract
5. Assessment of right-to-left ventricular shunts

Complications

1. Cardiac arrhythmias, especially nonsustained brief VT, do not require treatment; sustained VT and ventricular fibrillation require immediate cardioversion. (Note: Arrhythmias and staining are more common with the use of end-hole catheters than with any other pigtail catheters.)
2. Intramyocardial contrast media staining during power injection (generally transient and of no clinical importance unless it is deep or perforating producing tamponade).
3. Embolism (thrombi or air)
4. Contrast-related complications
5. Transient hypotension (<15 to 30 seconds) was common with ionic high-osmolar contrast media.

CAD, Coronary artery disease; *LV,* left ventricular; *RV,* right ventricular; *VSD,* ventricular septal defect; *VT,* ventricular tachycardia.

---

terminate the study prematurely. The indications, contraindications, and complications for ventriculography are shown in Box 3.2.

Technical Notes for Ventriculography

Catheter Selection: End of the End-Hole Left Ventricle Catheter

Left ventriculography, once an integral part of every cardiac angiographic procedure, has been reconsidered as often unnecessary in light of high-quality echocardiography for LV functional assessment. The practice of end-hole ventriculography often performed through a JR catheter with a hand injection for operator convenience has come under scrutiny as an inappropriate catheterization laboratory technique that should be abandoned. End-hole LV catheter angiography can cause serious harm with poor catheter positioning. An operator can cause LV perforation with an end-hole catheter (e.g., an MP catheter) when the tip is against the LV wall and contrast is injected directly into or through the myocardium, followed by tamponade and cardiac arrest.

Another practice to be discouraged is the use of hand injection for left ventriculography. Hand delivery of a large contrast bolus to opacify adequately the LV results more often than not in an inadequate and nondiagnostic study. Although some operators perform hand injections to reduce contrast use (e.g., in patients with chronic kidney disease at risk of contrast nephropathy), these images are nearly always suboptimal and may be misleading because too little contrast might not identify hypokinetic LV segments. Quantitative left ventricular ejection fraction (LVEF) and wall motion assessment are optimal, but they have been reserved generally for research studies. The visual estimate of the LVEF is acceptable with qualitative grading by 10% variance (i.e., <20%, 20% to 30%, 30% to 40%, etc.)

Some operators prefer to omit left ventriculography from both routine and emergency catheterizations. Cited reasons include (1) preference for echo assessment, (2) concern for extra contrast load, (3) fear of hypotension or complications of ventriculography, and (4) extra time needed to perform the left ventriculogram. These fears arise from a dated experience wherein the left ventriculogram, performed with ionic, hyperosmolar contrast media, was associated with worsening congestive heart failure (CHF), hypotension, arrhythmias, and death. These events do not occur with modern low-osmolar or nonionic low-osmolar contrast media (LOCM). A left ventriculogram at the time of catheterization provides an accurate prediction of the patient's outcome relative to his or her coronary status. A low-volume left ventriculogram (20 to 25 mL) has a very remote chance of complication and will be immediately available for review in the catheterization laboratory at the time of surgical consultation for a one-stop visit with full disclosure. Hence, in most patients the benefits of ventriculography outweigh the risks.

Left ventriculography should be omitted in compromised patients not responding to conventional medical treatment for heart failure (i.e., with LV end-diastolic pressure >35 mm Hg) as well as in patients with chronic kidney disease or those at higher risk for contrast-induced nephropathy (diabetics, patients with proteinuria, or dehydrated/hypotensive patients) to limit contrast exposure.

Operator Technique

During contrast injection, the physician performing the ventriculogram should be holding the catheter with the right hand at the connection to the high pressure tubing and the sheath with the left, preparing to withdraw the catheter if necessary, observing the physiologic monitor, and looking for problems, such as myocardial contrast staining, VT, or sudden hypotension. Rapid catheter withdrawal may be required in the event of a perforation or other complication. A pull-back distance of 10 to 15 cm from the femoral approach or 5 to 10 cm from the arm is needed to take out the slack before the end of the catheter moves out of the ventricle. Small-diameter (e.g., 4 F to 5 F) catheters require high injection pressures and do not allow flow rates >13 mL/s. Injector connections to the manifold or direct connection to the catheter must be secured so that inadvertent catheter-injector tubing separation does not spray the operator, patient, and laboratory with contrast media. Patients should be forewarned about the sudden warm sensation they will feel during ventriculography. This will last for 30 to 60 seconds and usually passes without incident.

Ventriculography Views

Standard left ventriculographic views are (1) a 30-degree RAO that visualizes the high lateral, anterior, apical, and inferior LV walls and (2) a 45- to 60-degree LAO, 20-degree cranial angulation that best identifies the lateral and septal LV walls. The LAO with cranial angulation provides a view of the interventricular septum, projected on edge and tilted downward to give the best view of ventricular septal defects and septal wall motion. Biplane ventriculography provides simultaneous RAO and LAO ventriculography with more radiation but less contrast. If no biplane system is available, patients with coronary disease affecting the lateral wall should have a second left ventriculogram in an LAO projection 40- to 60-degree LAO, 20-degree cranial view.

Historically, cineangiographic frame rates have been 30 to 60 frames/s depending on heart rate (30 frames/s for rates of <95 beats/min). Recent information suggests that 7.5 frames/s will produce satisfactory images with markedly reduced radiation. A 10-inch image field is routine, and collimating should be used to limit radiation scatter. Recommended views for valvular regurgitation are shown in Table 3.4. The angiographic quantitation of valvular regurgitation is shown in Table 3.5.

Regional Left Ventricle Wall Motion

The normal pattern of LV contraction has been defined as a uniform, concentric, inward motion of all points along the ventricular

Table 3.4

Recommended Sites of Injection and Angiographic Projections in the Evaluation of Valvular Regurgitation and Shunts.		
	Filming Projections	Site of Injection
Type of Valvular Regurgitation		
Aortic	LAO, RAO	Aortic root
Mitral	RAO cranial, LAO (lateral)	LV
Tricuspid	RAO (shallow, lateral)	RV
Pulmonic	RAO, LAO, AP	Main PA
Type of Cardiac Shunt		
ASD	LAO cranial	PA
VSD	LAO cranial	LV
PDA	AP cranial	Aorta

AP, Anterior-posterior; *ASD,* atrial septal defect; *LAO,* left anterior oblique; *LV,* left ventricle; *PA,* pulmonary artery; *PDA,* patent ductus arteriosus; *RAO,* right anterior oblique; *RV,* right ventricle; *VSD,* ventricular septal defect.

Table 3.5

Angiographic Quantitation of Valvular Regurgitation.	
Mitral Regurgitation	**Aortic Regurgitation**
+ Mild LA opacification; clears rapidly; often jetlike	+ Small regurgitant jet only; LV ejects contrast each systole
++ Moderate LA opacification < LV	++ Regurgitant jet faintly opacifies LV cavity; not cleared each systole
+++ Diffuse contrast regurgitant; LA opacification = LV; LA significantly enlarged[a]	+++ Persistent LV opacification = aortic root density; LV enlargement[a]
++++ LA opacification > LV, persistent; systolic pulmonary vein opacification may occur; often marked LV enlargement[a]	++++ Persistent LV opacification > aortic root concentration; often marked LV enlargement[a]

+, 1; ++, 2+; +++, 3+; ++++, 4+; *LA,* left atrium; *LV,* left ventricle.
[a]Chronic regurgitation.

inner surface during systole. Uniform wall motion depends on the cooperative and sequential contraction of the heart muscle, producing maximal effective work at minimal energy costs. This coordinated contraction is called *synchrony.* Uncoordinated contractions of LV wall motion are given names according to the severity of asynergy. Abnormal LV wall motion is particularly obvious in patients with severe CAD or cardiomyopathy. Several methods exist to analyze LV wall motion (Fig. 3.36). In general, individual

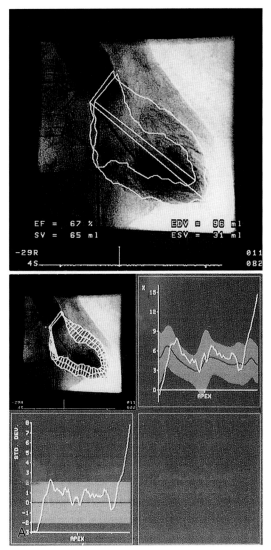

Fig. 3.36 Left ventriculographic wall motion analysis. **(A)** Normal left ventricle (LV) wall motion shows concentric inward motion of all LV wall segments. *Bottom panel:* Chords and deviation from midline.

Continued

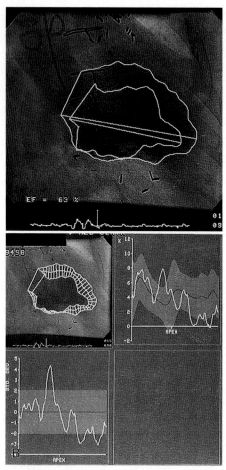

Fig. 3.36, cont'd (B) Inferior wall motion abnormality on left ventriculo-gram. Note failure of the LV to move inward on inferior wall. *Bottom panel:* Abnormal chords above mean values. The centerline method of regional wall motion analysis uses end-diastolic and end-systolic LV endocardial contours. Lower panels show how a centerline is constructed by the computer midway between the two contours. Motion is measured along 100 chords constructed perpendicular to the centerline. Motion at each chord is normalized by the end-diastolic perimeter to yield a shortening fraction. Motion along each chord is plotted for the patient *(dark out line, thin is inner line).* The mean motion in the normal ventriculogram group *(thin line)* and 1 standard deviation (SD) above and below the mean *(dotted line)* are shown for comparison. Wall motion also is plotted as the difference in units of SDs from the normal mean *(right panel). Horizontal zero line:* Normal ventriculogram group mean.

segments are evaluated and reported to have normal contraction, hypokinesis (sluggish or slowed contraction), akinesis (lack of contraction), or dyskinesis (movement of the segment outward during systole and suggestive of a ventricular aneurysm).

Setup of Contrast Medial Power (High-Pressure) Injectors

Because contrast media is viscous and great force is necessary to inject contrast rapidly through small catheters, power injectors are always used to deliver a preset contrast volume over a brief period. Three steps are critical for safe ventriculography: (1) contrast loading, (2) air bubble clearing from the injection syringe and high-pressure connecting tubing, and (3) correct injector settings.

The most important step of the setup is to clear all air and bubbles from the transparent pressure injection syringe and tubing before any injection. This is an obligation for all physicians and nurses in the laboratory. There is no excuse for injection of air during contrast ventriculography.

Typical injection pressure settings for ventriculography are:

- flow rate (10 to 15 mL/s)
- total volume (20 to 50 mL)
- pressure limit (900 to 1200 psi)
- rise time (0.2 to 0.5 s)

Catheter Position

The optimal catheter position for left ventriculography is one that avoids contact with the papillary muscles and is not positioned too close to the mitral valve, so that mitral regurgitation is not produced artificially. For most catheters, a mid-cavity position seems best because contrast material fills most of the LV chamber and apex, and the catheter during injection does not interfere with mitral valve function. In this position, pigtail catheter side holes are well below the aortic valve, which improves chamber opacification. Angled (45 degrees) pigtail catheters and helical tip designs (Halo catheter; see Fig. 3.6) may provide better quality ventriculography with less induced ectopy and mitral regurgitation.

The pigtail loop of the catheter may be coiled upward or downward in front of the mitral valve in the RAO plane as long as it does not interfere with mitral valve apparatus and produce ectopy. Twisting and opening of the pigtail loop with each beat indicates interference with the mitral valve apparatus. When the position of the catheter is in question, a test injection of 5 to 8 mL of contrast material confirms proper catheter position (i.e., catheter is not entrapped in the valve structures or trabeculae).

For right ventriculography, a 7-F Berman balloon-tipped catheter (with no end hole and side holes proximal to balloon) produces excellent opacification. The angiographic projection of right ventriculography is not standardized. An AP-cranial or AP-lateral projection is commonly used to visualize the septum and RVOT. Injection rates range from 8 to 10 mL/s for volumes of 20 to 30 mL.

Contrast Volumes

Adequate visualization and opacification of the ventricular chambers are accomplished by delivery of a large bolus (20 to 50 mL) of x-ray contrast medium over a short period (1 to 3 seconds). For best quality, a powered injection technique should be used. Typical power injector settings for an average adult are total volume 20 to 50 mL at 10 to 15 mL/s. The rate of rise to maximal pressure is also a variable that can be set for smoother contrast delivery, typically a 0.5-second rise time. With the catheter in the far apical position, a lower rate and volume can be used (e.g., 10 mL/s for 20 to 25 mL).

Ventricular Ectopy

Ventricular ectopy during powerful contrast material injection is common and generally does not require antiarrhythmic medications. A stable rhythm should be maintained before contrast material injection by careful catheter positioning between the papillary muscles and the inferior LV wall. Ventricular ectopy is commonly produced by use of end-hole (e.g., MP) catheters. A pigtail shape is safer. A Halo catheter is an out-of-plane pigtail loop with all holes directed into the center of the loop and produces LV grams with nearly no ectopy.

Measurements of Left Ventricle Contractility

The most common measures of LV function are the EF and stroke volume (SV). The EF (%) is calculated as:

$$EF = \frac{EDV - ESV}{EDV} \times 100$$

$$SV = EDV - ESV$$

where EDV is end-diastolic volume and ESV is end-systolic volume. Most EF calculations are estimated by visual examination at the time of ventriculography. SV requires a quantitative assessment with a calibration marker of true volume. This technique is not used for clinical practice.

Assessment of Mitral Regurgitation

The severity of mitral regurgitation is semi quantitative on the basis of the degree of contrast opacification of the left atrium during left ventriculography (Figs. 3.37 and 3.38). Although an angiographically derived regurgitant fraction can be calculated, the use of echocardiography has supplanted the angiogram as the gold standard to assess mitral regurgitation. Methods other than subjective grading are rarely performed in today's catheterization laboratory.

Ascending Aortography

Ascending aortography may be necessary to determine the position and/or patency of bypass grafts and degree of aortic

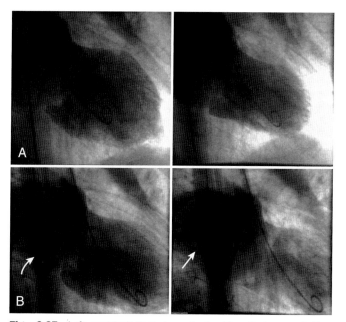

Fig. 3.37 Left ventriculogram in patient with mitral regurgitation. **(A)** Early opacification of the left atrium (LA) *(arrow)*. **(B)** *Left:* Denser opacification of LA. *Right:* LA is more densely opacified than left ventricle (LV) after several beats. This is severe (4+) mitral regurgitation (MR).

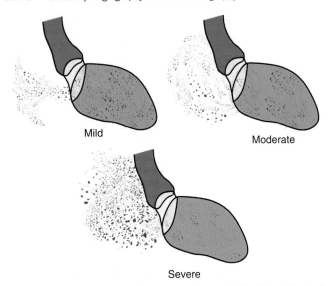

Mild

Moderate

Severe

Fig. 3.38 Angiographic evaluation of mitral regurgitation. (From Pujadas G. *Coronary Angiography in the Medical and Surgical Treatment of Ischemic Heart Disease.* New York; McGraw-Hill: 1980.)

insufficiency or to exclude aortic dissection (Box 3.3). Aortography should be performed using side hole catheters (e.g., pigtail) to reduce the risk of extending or inducing a dissection during contrast medium injection. The catheter should be positioned just above the aortic valve, but not close enough to interfere with valve opening or closing. For descending aortic dissection, the catheter is positioned above the suspected proximal tear. Catheter position should be checked with a contrast test before full-volume injection. Aortic regurgitation is estimated semiquantitatively as +1, +2, +3, or +4, depending on the opacification of the ventricle after the third cycle following contrast injection (Figs. 3.39 and 3.40). Care should be taken to avoid entrapping the catheter in a false lumen of a suspected aortic dissection by careful manipulation of the catheter and J-tipped guidewire.

Aortography can be performed by use of a minimum flow rate of 15 to 20 mL/s for total volumes of 40 to 60 mL. High-flow (≥5 F) catheters are required with standard power injectors. Cineangiographic frame rates of 15 frames/s are satisfactory. Aortography can be performed in LAO or lateral projection and RAO projection (Figs. 3.40 and 3.41).

Box 3.3 Indications and Contraindications for Thoracic Aortography.[a]

Indications

1. Aortic aneurysm or aortic dissection
2. Aortic insufficiency
3. Nonselective visualization of coronary bypass grafts
4. Supravalvular aortic stenosis
5. Brachiocephalic or arch vessel disease
6. Coarctation of the aorta
7. Aortic-to-PA or aortic-to-right-side heart (e.g., sinus of Valsalva fistula) communication
8. Aortic or periaortic neoplastic disease
9. Arterial thromboembolic disease
10. Arterial inflammatory disease

Contraindications

1. Contrast media reaction
2. Injection into false lumen of aortic dissection
3. End-hole catheter malposition
4. Inability of the patient to tolerate additional radiographic contrast media

PA, Pulmonary artery.
[a]Note: In modern cardiac catheterization laboratories, cineangiography is acceptable for patients with suspected dissection of the aorta.

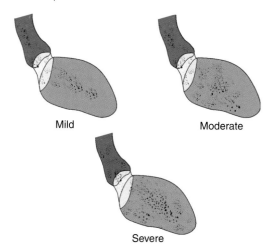

Mild   Moderate

Severe

Fig. 3.39 Angiographic evaluation of aortic regurgitation, right anterior oblique (RAO) view. When the left anterior oblique (LAO) view is used, over-estimation of aortic regurgitation occurs. (From Pujadas G. *Coronary Angiography in the Medical and Surgical Treatment of Ischemic Heart Disease.* New York: McGraw-Hill; 1980.)

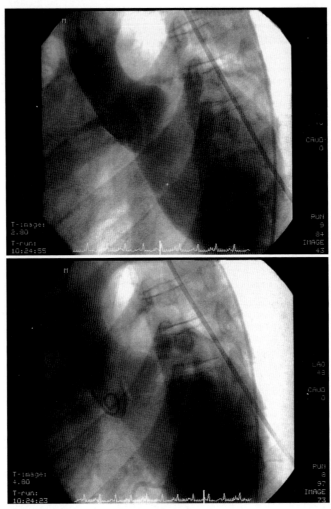

Fig. 3.40 *Top:* Cineframe showing aortic regurgitation from left anterior descending (LAD) aortogram. Note equal opacification of left ventricle (LV) and aorta. *Bottom:* LV is still opacified after several beats. This is severe aortic regurgitation.

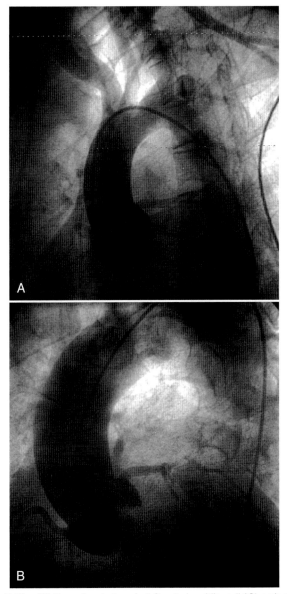

Fig. 3.41 **(A)** Normal aortogram in left anterior oblique (LAO) projection. **(B)** Dilated ascending aorta.

Left Anterior Oblique or Lateral Projection

The LAO view (LAO 40 degrees) is excellent for identifying dissection of the ascending aorta extending up to the neck vessels; optimally delineating the aortic arch; and opening the aortic curvature and providing clear views of the innominate, common carotid, and left subclavian arteries. The coronary arteries at the root of the aorta are displayed in a semilateral projection.

Right Anterior Oblique Projection

The descending thoracic aorta and the ascending aorta may be superimposed across the arch in the AP or LAO projection. The RAO view is more helpful in delineating the effect of dissection on the lower thoracic aorta and intercostal arteries, the origin of bypass grafts to the left coronary system, or assessing aortic insufficiency. There are no advantages to cranial or caudal tilts for viewing the aorta. In nonselective coronary angiography in which aortic root angiography may help identify a vein graft takeoff, cranial and caudal angulation may provide some increased detail.

Basics of X-Ray Generation and Radiation Safety

Cardiac angiography uses a complex interaction of radiographic x-ray elements to transform energy into a visual image. The x-ray image generation chain can be simplified into three major components: (1) x-ray generator, (2) x-ray tube, and (3) II or detector. The details of x-ray equipment should be familiar to all personnel working in the catheterization laboratory. Figure 3.42 shows the x-ray system in a cardiac catheterization laboratory (Fig. 3.43).

X-Ray Generator

The x-ray generator provides the power source necessary to accelerate the electrons through the x-ray tube. The duration of x-ray exposure is similar to the shutter speed on a regular camera. During the cardiac imaging examination, exposure is usually set at a fast enough speed to stop blurring caused by heart movement. During selective coronary angiography, the shorter the exposure time, the better the image. Exposure times of 3 to 6 ms reduce movement blur. Most modern generators are capable of delivering adequate power and providing precise and automatically adjusted exposure timing. They are equipped with either multiphase (alternating on and off) or short and long pulse widths that are adjusted automatically for correct exposure. Manual settings, which the operator can select, are limited to cineangiographic frame rates (e.g., 15 to 60 frames/s).

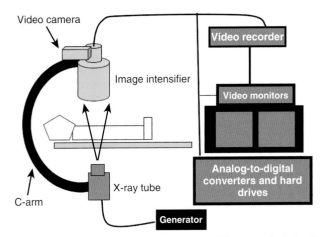

Fig. 3.42 Schematic diagram of an x-ray system. The x-ray tube below the table radiates upward through the patient table to the image intensifier. The video camera transmits the signal to video recorder, monitors, and signal processors.

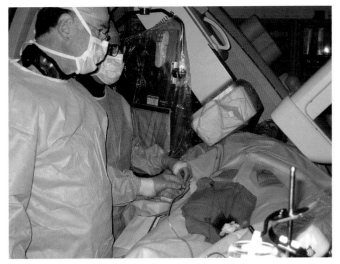

Fig. 3.43 Cardiac catheterization laboratory with C-arms over patient. Operators are observing images on fluoroscopic monitors.

X-Ray Tubes

The function of the x-ray tube is to convert electrical energy, provided from the generator, to an x-ray beam. Electrons emitted from a heated filament (cathode) are accelerated toward a rapidly rotating disk (anode) and at contact undergo conversion to x-radiation (Fig. 3.44). This process generates extreme heat. The heat capacity of the tube is a major limiting factor in the design of x-ray tubes. Only 0.2% to 0.6% of the electrical energy provided to the tube is eventually converted to x-rays.

In addition to the exposure times (controlled by the generator system) and the size of the imaging field (controlled by the x-ray tube), two other factors determine the quality of x-ray for proper imaging:

1. Electrical current (mA): The number of photons (electrical particles) generated per unit of time. The greater the electrical current, the greater the number of photons. More photons result in improved image resolution. If the photon volume is marginal,

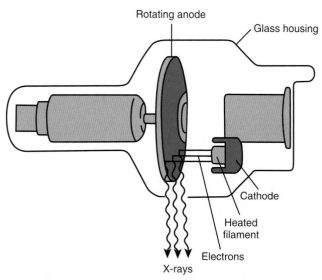

Fig. 3.44 Schematic of x-ray tube and x-ray production. A tungsten rotating anode is the target of high-energy electrons from the cathode and heating elements. The electrons striking the target release x-rays at a 90-degree angle. (Redrawn from Baim DS, Grossman W. *Grossman's Cardiac Catheterization, Angioplasty, and Intervention.* 6th ed. Philadelphia: Lippincott, Williams, and Wilkins; 2000.)

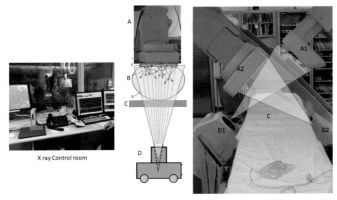

Fig. 3.45 Left Panel. X-ray control room. Middle Panel. **A,** Image intensifier flat panel collector. **B.** Patient with arrows showing scatter. **C.** Patient table. D. X-ray source. Right Panel. D1, D2 sources for biplane system, A1, A2 image flat panels for biplane system.

the resulting image may be mottled or have a spotty appearance. Increasing the milliamperage improves this result, but the level of milliamperage is limited by the heat capacity of the x-ray tubes. In addition, increasing the number of milliamperes markedly increases radiation exposure and scatter to the patient and catheterization laboratory personnel.

2. Level of kilovoltage (kV): The energy spectrum (wavelengths) of the x-ray beam. The higher the level of kilovoltage, the shorter the wavelength of radiation and the greater the ability of x-rays to penetrate target tissue. Increased kilovoltage is especially important in obese patients. To obtain better images through more tissue, a higher kilovolt level is required. However, a high-kilovolt level also produces lower resolution because of wide scatter and results in a greater radiation exposure to patients and laboratory personnel. An automatic exposure control system sets exposure times to incorporate changes in voltage and amperage to provide the desired images at the best exposures possible (Fig. 3.45).

Image Intensifier and Detector

After the x-rays have penetrated the body (Figs. 3.45 and 3.46), the partially absorbed beams are cast as shadows on the input screen of the II or flat-panel detector. The II/detector converts the invisible x-ray image into a visual image. Each x-ray photon hits the

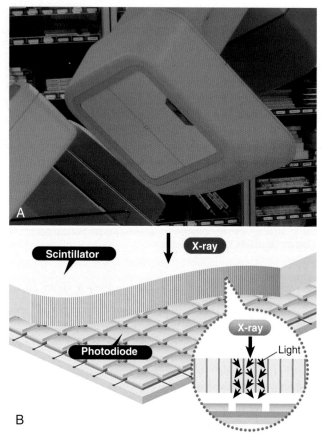

Fig. 3.46 (A) Flat-panel image intensifier (II). **(B)** Screen of flat panel showing how x-rays trigger the photodiode to produce digital signals that are transmitted and reconverted into an x-ray image.

phosphorus-covered plate of the intensifier resulting in a light particle, whose position and intensity are noted. The sum of all events produces an image for video. The development of the flat-panel image detector offers efficient (low-dose) x-ray image acquisition and better image clarity and provide ability to change field size without a great loss of resolution. Image size (5- to 7-inch) screens are better suited for coronary angiography. In contrast, for large area examinations (i.e., left ventriculography, aortography, or peripheral angiography), field diameters of 9 to 11 inches are used with the known tradeoff of loss of resolution for small structures.

Image Distortion

Magnification

The x-ray image casts an x-ray shadow onto the image intensifier. The distance of the object from the panel determines the image sharpness or resolution. Figure 3.47 displays the effect of the object–screen distance on image quality. When an object is held close to the surface on which the shadow falls, the image is sharp. The farther the object is moved away from this surface, the larger and more indistinct the image. When the II/detector is closest to the chest wall and the heart, the image is sharp. When the heart is far away from the II/detector and closer to the x-ray source, the image is magnified but poorly defined. Increasing the distance of

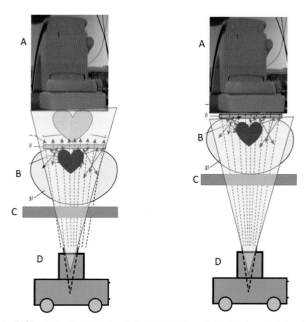

Fig. 3.47 Left, The heart will appear larger when the image intensive **(A,B)** is further from the object. Right, the heart is closer to actual size when the image intensifier is close to the chest. **A** is image intensifier, **B** is patient, **C** is table, **D** is x-ray tube.

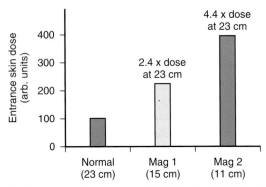

Fig. 3.48 The effect of electronic magnification on entry skin dose. The radiation dose increases by the square of the ratio of image intensifier (II) diameter. *arb,* Arbitrary; *Mag,* magnification.

the heart to the II/detector also requires more kilovoltage to produce the image and further reduces image quality. Increased magnification increases the radiation exposure required to produce the magnified image. Figure 3.48 shows the effects of increasing image size on radiation dosing. The closer the patient is to the source without moving the II/detector, the greater the spread of the beam and higher the radiation exposure. Keep the II/detector close to the patient whenever possible. Minimizing the angulation of the C-arm also reduces x-ray exposure (Fig. 3.49).

Foreshortening

Distortion of the object's perspective is called *foreshortening.* Figure 3.50 displays the effects of the shadow cast by an object, such as a pencil, that has a concentric narrowing (similar to an artery stenosis) in the middle portion. Because of foreshortening, an angiographic narrowing that may appear severe in one projection may not appear at all or may seem significantly less severe in other projections. For this reason, multiple projections are used to characterize the severity of lesions within the coronary tree.

The best practices to maximize image quality and to reduce radiation exposure are:

1. The II/flat-plate detector should be as close to the patient's chest as possible. This position optimizes the image detail and decreases scatter radiation (see tube height and radiation exposure).

2. All ECG electrodes, lead wires, metal snaps on the patient's gown, and jewelry should be out of the field of view before the

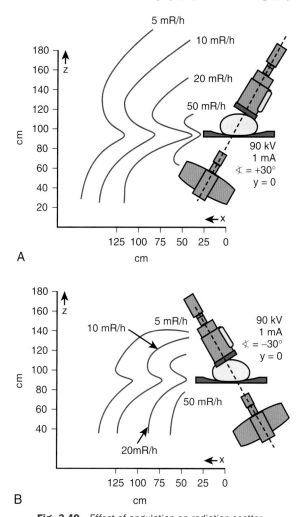

Fig. 3.49 Effect of angulation on radiation scatter.

start of the procedure. Stopping the IV lines and wires from hanging down under the table prevents the x-ray tube from pulling out a lead or IV tube when rotating around the patient.
3. Use of the collimators (shutters) is mandatory. The operator should focus on the exact area of interest to be imaged and

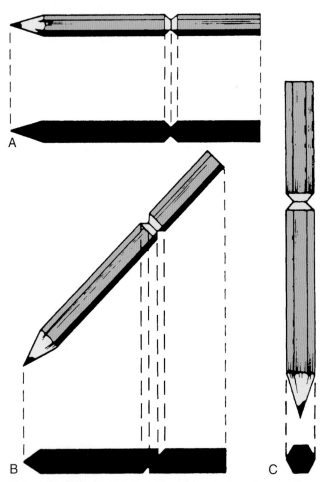

Fig. 3.50 **(A to C)** Foreshortening of the shadow of an object occurs when it is not parallel with the filming plane.

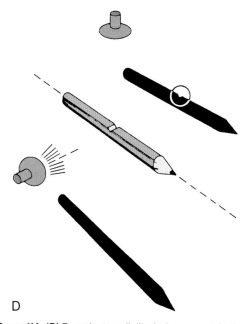

D

Fig. 3.50, cont'd (D) To evaluate a slit-like lesion accurately, the operator must use a view perpendicular to the longitudinal axis of the vessel but parallel to the longest diameter of the lesion. The foreshortening (change of true length) of the pencil causes the image to change depending on the axis in relation to the beam of the x-ray. When the pencil's long axis is perpendicular to the image plane (parallel to the x-ray beam), all contour details are lost, and the shadow is seen as a dot. When the longitudinal axis is seen at an oblique angle, the length shadow is foreshortened, and when the axis is perpendicular to the x-ray beam (parallel to the image plane), a full and true image of the length and contour details can be seen. (From Pujadas G. *Coronary Angiography in the Medical and Surgical Treatment of Ischemic Heart Disease.* New York; McGraw-Hill: 1980.)

eliminate unwanted lung field brightness. This helps optimize settings for the automatic brightness control system.

4. Minimize the number of cineangiograms obtained to only those that are necessary. Maximize use of newer features of angiographic systems, such as fluoro save, that save images obtained during fluoroscopic imaging without having to use higher-radiation cineangiography.

5. Use the ceiling mounted screen and table-side skirt to block scatter radiation from above and below the table.

Digital Angiography Archives

The x-ray image is converted into a quantitative digital format for storage and display on a computer. Archival storage uses magnetic tapes, disks, or other electronic media and permits compact storage, image enhancement, and retrieval for quantitative image analysis.

Radiation Safety

Radiation safety is also addressed in Chapter 1. Personal radiation protection equipment must be available for all personnel in every cardiac catheterization laboratory. Standards for radiation protection have been published by the Society of Cardiac Angiography and Interventions, ACC, and American Heart Association (AHA). Four principles of radiation safety should be self-evident:

1. The lower the exposure, the smaller the chance of absorbed energy biologic interaction.

2. No known level of ionizing radiation is a permissible dose or absolutely safe.

3. Radiation exposure is cumulative and occurs over a lifetime. No washout phenomenon occurs.

4. All participants in the cardiac catheterization laboratory have voluntarily accepted some degree of radiation exposure but are obligated to minimize and to reduce risks to other personnel and themselves.

The source of radiation in the cardiac catheterization laboratory is the primary x-ray beam that emanates from the under the table tube, upward and outward toward the II/detector. Scatter of this beam (mostly because of transit through the patient) exposes all subjects to radiation in a dose geometrically inverse to the distance from the source. Radiation scatter is increased when the angle of the tube is set obliquely. A high degree of angulation with large obliquities increases the amount of radiation scatter. Acrylic lead shields and table-mounted lead aprons should be used to reduce the amount of scatter.

Fluoroscopy generates x-ray exposure approximately one-fifth that of cineangiography. The increased use of cineangiography for complex catheterization procedures increases the total radiation exposure in the laboratory and should be a consideration in procedures requiring extensive intracardiac manipulation, such as PCI, electrophysiologic (EP) studies, or valvuloplasty.

Personal Radiation Protection

Radiation protection for laboratory personnel should include eye, neck, and body shielding. Room-installed radiation shields should protect physicians performing cardiac angiography. Exposure with a shield resulting from performing 25 examinations per week on a continuous basis should be within the recommendations of the National Commission on Radiologic Protection and Units.

Radiation exposure is greater during PCI than during diagnostic catheterization. If protective shields are used carefully, radiation exposure may be comparable for single- and double-vessel angioplasty procedures and for diagnostic catheterization procedures. Radiation exposure is higher for diagnostic and angioplasty procedures using biplane imaging.

During angiographic studies, 90% of the x-ray energy entering the body is absorbed. It has been shown that a single exposure of 200 R can produce cataract formation in humans. Thyroid cancers and other carcinomas are associated with x-rays. Techniques often used to improve image quality (e.g., increased amperage, voltage, LAO views) have resulted in increased exposure. A summary of radiation safety for the cardiac catheterization laboratory is provided in Box 3.4 (also discussed in Chapter 1).

Box 3.4   Radiation Safety Considerations During Cardiac Catheterization.

Radiation to Patient

1. Originates from the primary x-ray beam and then scatters on passing through the body.
2. Affects thyroid, eyes, gonads, bone marrow, or gastrointestinal tract.
3. Highest exposure of any diagnostic test.
4. Deterministic radiation effects, such as skin injury, and stochastic effects such as malignancy and congenital abnormalities.

Radiation to Staff

1. Long-term low dose from scatter and tube leakage
2. Affects thyroid and eyes
3. Accepted occupational exposure

Means of Limiting Dose

1. Maintain equipment safeguards
2. Optimize milliamperage and kilovoltage
3. Minimize exposure time
4. Minimize scatter with shielding and techniques
5. For staff, maximize distance from source
6. Use all protective measures
7. Use of fluorography ("store fluro") compared to cineangiography may be effective in decreasing the radiation exposure for selected patients

Angiographic Equipment

Injectors and Contrast Materials

The angiographic power injector allows the angiographer to administer a precise volume (bolus) of contrast material at a rapid, preset flow rate. Power injectors are necessary for performing ventricular and great vessel angiography. The injector uses a large syringe for radiographic contrast media. Power injector settings are selected and, on receiving an electronic signal, a calibrated motor discharges the exact amount of contrast material at the predetermined rate through a connecting tube and catheter to the patient. The quantity and type of contrast material (concentration or dilution) and rate of injection are selected by the operator or physician. The signal to the injector to inject the contrast media is transmitted from a hand- or foot-operated switch.

Power Contrast Injector: Responsibilities of the Nurse or Technician

1. For an off-table freestanding injector, the nurse or technician loads the syringe with contrast media.
2. The nurse or technician sets the volume, flow rate, and rate of pressure rise parameters as instructed by the physician.
3. The nurse or technician presses the inject button that triggers the injection. Releasing the button stops the injection.

The staff members and physicians must be aware of the following points regarding safe power injection. Some injector systems (e.g., ACIST) have physician-operated touch-sensitive injection controls on the table.

Be sure to clear air bubbles. All air must be expelled from the contrast-filled syringe before making the injector available to the physician for the catheter connection. Under no circumstances should the head of the power injector be tilted toward the catheterization table or made available to the physician if air is in the syringe. Several techniques are used to establish a bubble-free system when connecting the catheter to the syringe. A running connection (fluid-to-fluid interface) is a technique in which a small amount of contrast material is squirted out of the syringe while the catheter is being connected to the syringe. Merging the fluid streams of blood from the catheter and the forward flow of contrast material from the syringe prevents any large air bubbles from entering the system on connection. After connection, the injector operator always aspirates more fluid (usually contrast material in the connector tube) into the syringe to ensure that no air bubbles are present. If air is present, it is expelled, and the clearing procedure is repeated. Variable rate automatic injectors operated from the sterile table have air bubble detectors that prohibit injection if air is detected anywhere in the injection pathway. The operator must be careful when aspirating blood into the contrast syringe for two reasons: (1) A large blood volume in the syringe dilutes the contrast material, and (2) more important, but rarely, after some time the blood may clot in the injector syringe.

Test Injection in Ventricle

When the system is free of air, the injector operator and physician should be sure that the catheter is cleared of blood. The injector operator squirts a small amount of contrast material out of the tip of the catheter under x-ray visualization. This small test injection of contrast material also helps the physician ascertain proper catheter position for ventriculography.

Confirming Injector Settings

The physician should orally confirm the power injector settings for the contrast volume and delivery rate desired. The injector operator should repeat the injection parameters back to the physician to eliminate any chance of error in injector setup. Before injecting, the staff member must ensure that the catheter being used can accept the flow rate that has entered the injector.

Safety Features

When the physician has initiated a cineangiographic run, the injector operator must listen for the physician's command to start the injection. The nurse or technician should be prepared to stop the injection (by hitting or releasing the trigger button) at any time as directed by the physician or at their own discretion (e.g., when the catheter is pulled back or a contrast stain in the heart muscle is seen).

Note: All personnel should be watching the power injection setup and injections for small bubbles or other problems. Six (or more) eyes are better than four for seeing catheterization laboratory problems. Power injectors have many safety features that must be understood by the cardiac catheterization laboratory staff. To ensure patient safety during angiography, staff members must understand all aspects of the operation of the power injector and built-in safeguards.

Contrast Media

During angiography, the catheterization laboratory staff provides technical support with regard to contrast media in the following areas:

1. Contrast agents should be warmed to body temperature before administration. Commercial warmers are available from companies that manufacture contrast media.

2. The nurse or technician preparing the patient for angiography should ask the patient whether he or she is aware of any known contrast allergy. Iodine gives contrast material its radiopaque qualities and is a known allergen. Although some believe that a history of seafood allergy (iodine is found in certain seafood, especially shellfish) is significant, this does not appear to be the case. The physician may wish to give corticosteroids or antihistamines to these patients before performing angiography (see Chapter 1).

3. Before the administration of contrast agents, the patient should be told about the sensations associated with contrast administration. Rarely, patients have nausea and vomiting, so patients should not have ingested food or water before angiography. If vomiting occurs, staff members should be quick to respond; the patient's head should be turned to the side (away from the sterile field) to prevent aspiration. This is particularly important when patients have been heavily sedated for the procedure.

4. Patients should be told that they may feel a hot flushing sensation (caused by artery vasodilation) during the LV injections of contrast media. Direct injection of contrast material into peripheral vessels may produce a painful burning and cramping sensation. These reactions are uncommon with the nonionic low-osmolar agents that are used today.

During angiography, it is important for the nurse to document the type and amount of contrast material delivered and any signs of allergy, such as hives, flushed skin, bronchospasm, or laryngeal edema (hoarseness). Appropriate medications for treatment of anaphylaxis, such as epinephrine, and an airway should always be easily accessible during the procedure.

Although uncommon with nonionic LOCM, hypotension, bradycardia, and arrhythmias have been reported during injections. Therefore, the ECG and arterial pressure should be monitored continuously and postinjection the pressure manifold needs to be turned back to pressure. Atropine, vasopressors, and antiarrhythmic agents should be available for prompt administration. Transient bradycardia or hypotension can be overcome with a brief forceful cough. Use of nonionic LOCM has greatly reduced the incidence of bradycardia, arrhythmias, hypotension, and the need for coughing during coronary angiography.

Selection of Radiographic Contrast Media

The contrast material is selected for the specific examination to be conducted. All contrast agents contain iodine, an effective absorber of x-rays, which makes iodine-filled structures x-ray dense when compared with other body structures. Those tissues without iodinated material are more x-ray lucent and absorb x-rays to provide different gray shades in x-ray images. The quantity and concentration of contrast materials used are specific medical decisions. Factors included in these decisions are the patient's age, size, general health, allergies, and cardiac condition.

Although all agents are derivatives of benzoic acid, the number of iodine molecules and ionic and osmolar composition vary (Table 3.6). Osmolality, viscosity, sodium content, and other additives and properties are different among these agents. Table 3.7 summarizes commonly used contrast agents for coronary and LV angiographic studies. Selection of a contrast agent for the particular laboratory is, to a large extent, a matter of personal preference. Major differences between ionic and nonionic contrast agents include cost, effect of hemodynamics, and LV and renal function.

Table 3.6

Classification and Distinguishing Properties of Various Contrast Agents.

Quality	High	Low	Low	Iso-osmolar
Osmolality	>1500	600	600–1000	280
Ionicity	Ionic	Ionic	Nonionic	Nonionic
Number of benzene rings	Monomer	Dimer	Monomer	Dimer
Name	Diatrizoate Iothalamate	Ioxaglate Iopamidol Ioversol Iopromide Iomeprol	Iohexol	Iodixanol
Viscosity	Low	Low	Intermediate	High
Ratio (iodine/ osmotically active particles	1.5	3	3	6

From Klein L, Sheldon MW, Brinker J, et al. The use of radiographic contrast media during PCI: a focused review: a position statement of the Society of Cardiovascular Angiography and Interventions. *Catheter Cardiovasc Intervent.* 2009;74:728-746.

Table 3.7

Contrast Agents in the Catheterization Laboratory.			
Contrast Type	**Chemical Name**	**Trade Name**	**Manufacturer**
High-osmolar ionic	Diatrizoate	Renografin	Bracco
	Diatrozoate	Hypaque	GE Health Care
	Iothalamate	Conray	Mallinckrodt
	Metrizoate	Isopaque	Sanofi
Low-osmolar nonionic	Iopamidol	Isovue	Bracco
	Iohexol	Omnipaque	Amersham
	Ioversol	Optiray	Mallinckrodt
	Ioxilan	Oxilan	Guerbet
Low-osmolar ionic dimer	Ioxaglate	Hexabrix	Mallinckrodt
Iso-osmolar nonionic dimer	Iodixanol	Visipaque	Amersham

From Klein L, Sheldon MW, Brinker J, et al. The use of radiographic contrast media during PCI: a focused review: a position statement of the Society of Cardiovascular Angiography and Interventions. *Catheter Cardiovasc Intervent.* 2009;74:728-746.

Historically, ionic contrast media produced hypotension by peripheral arterial vasodilation, transient myocardial dysfunction, and decrease in circulating volume and blood pressure after osmotic diuresis (initially contrast media increase circulating fluid volume by osmotically shifting fluid into the vascular space).

Nonionic LOCM have been shown to be safer than ionic, high-osmolar agents. LOCM are routinely used in all catheterization laboratories around the world and produce satisfactory diagnostic imaging quality, especially for high-risk patients. Despite numerous studies and meta-analyses, there is no consensus on which of the LOCM is superior with regard to contrast-induced renal injury or nephropathy.

Contrast-Induced Renal Injury or Nephropathy

For the vast majority of patients, exposure to contrast media has no sequelae; however, in a small percentage, it can result in contrast-induced nephropathy (CIN). CIN is one of the leading causes of in-hospital renal dysfunction. It is associated with a significant increase in morbidity and mortality as well as an increased length of hospital stay and costs. CIN is related to underlying renal function. Hypoxia, vasoconstriction, and cytotoxic effects of the contrast media themselves all play a significant role in CIN. Risk factors for CIN are summarized in Table 3.8. Serum creatinine level is a crude

Table 3.8

Risk Factors for Contrast-Induced Nephropathy.[a]		
Patient Related	**Extrinsic**	**Possible**
PRI	Volume of contrast	Metabolic syndrome
CHF	High-osmolar contrast	Diabetes
Diabetes mellitus with PRI	Intraaortic balloon	Prediabetes
Age >70 years	Nephrotoxic drugs	Hyperuricemia
Volume depletion	MCA within 72 hours	ACE-I/ARB
Hypotension	Urgent/emergent PCI	Female gender
Anemia	Multiple myeloma	
Hypertension	Cirrhosis	
PVD	Intraarterial contrast	

Modified from Best PJ, Berger PB, Davis BR, et al. Impact of mild or moderate chronic kidney disease on the frequency of restenosis: Results from the PRESTO trial. *J Am Coll Cardiol.* 2004;44:1786-1791; Parfrey P. The clinical epidemiology of contrast-induced nephropathy. *Cardiovasc Intervent Radiol.* 2005;28(suppl 2):S3-S11; McCullough PA, Adam A, Becker CR, et al. Epidemiology and prognostic implications of contrast-induced nephropathy. *Am J Cardiol.* 2006;98(suppl):5K-13K; and Weinrauch LA, Healy RW, Leland OS, et al. Coronary angiography and acute renal failure in diabetic azotemic nephropathy. *Ann Intern Med.* 1977;86:56-59.

ACE-I, Angiotensin-converting enzyme inhibitor; *ARB,* angiotensin II receptor blocker; *CHF,* congestive heart failure; *GFR,* glomerular filtration rate; *MCA,* multiple contrast administration; *PCI,* percutaneous coronary intervention; *PRI,* preexistent renal insufficiency; *PVD,* peripheral vascular disease.

[a]Factors in bold contribute to risk scores of Mehran et al. and/or Bartholomew et al. (Mehran R, Aymong ED, Nikolsky E, et al. A simple risk score for prediction of contrast-induced nephropathy after percutaneous coronary intervention: Development and initial validation. *J Am Coll Cardiol.* 2004;44:1393-1399; Bartholomew BA, Harjai KJ, Dukkipati S et al. Impact of nephropathy after percutaneous coronary intervention and a method for risk stratification. *Am J Cardiol.* 2004;93:1515-1519).

indicator of true glomerular filtration rate (GFR), whereas creatinine clearance (CrCl), calculated using the Cockcroft-Gault formula, has repeatedly been shown to be a more reliable indicator of GFR.

Recommendations to Prevent Contrast-Induced Nephropathy Based on Glomerular Filtration Rate

1. GFR or CrCl greater than 60 mL/min
   a. Hold Metformin until 48 hours post-procedure. Metformin, an oral antihyperglycemic medication, is excreted predominantly by the kidneys. If patients who receive metformin become azotemic, increased tissue levels of metformin may induce life-threatening lactic acidosis.

2. GFR or CrCl 30 to 60 mL/min
   a. Hydrate the night before the procedure with at least four to six glasses of water up to 4 hours preprocedure.
   b. Hold angiotensin-converting enzyme (ACE) inhibitors, angiotensin receptor blockers, diuretics, diuretics, nonsteroidal antiinflammatory drugs (NSAIDs), and cyclooxygenase-2 (COX-2) inhibitors 24 hours preprocedure. The aforementioned medications may be resumed at 24 hours postprocedure.
   c. Hold Metformin until 48 hours postprocedure or until creatinine is stable.
   d. Minimize contrast use (biplane imaging in the catheterization laboratory, if possible).
   e. Consider using a nonionic, iso-osmolar contrast.
   f. Check serum creatinine at 48 to 72 hours postprocedure.
3. GFR or CrCl less than 30 mL/min
   a. IV hydration recommendations
   b. For inpatient cases[a]:
      i. Preprocedure: 1 mL/kg/h × 12 h[b]
      ii. Postprocedure: 1 mL/kg/h × 12 h[b]
   c. For same-day cases[a]:
      i. Preprocedure: 3 mL/kg/h × 1 h (maximum rate = 330 mL/h)
      ii. Postprocedure: 1–2 mL/kg/h × 6 h
   d. Hold ACE inhibitors, angiotensin receptor blockers, diuretics, NSAIDs, and COX-2 inhibitors and diuretics 24 hours before the procedure. The aforementioned medications may be resumed at 24 to 72 hours postprocedure.
   e. Hold Metformin until 48 hours postprocedure or until creatinine is stable.
   f. Minimize contrast use (biplane imaging in the catheterization laboratory, if possible).
   g. Use a nonionic, iso-osmolar contrast.
   h. Check serum creatinine at 48 hours postprocedure.
   i. For same-day cases[a]:
      i. Preprocedure: 3 mL/kg/h × 1 h (maximum rate = 330 mL/h)
      ii. Postprocedure: 1 to 2 mL/kg/h × 6 h
   j. Hold ACE inhibitors, angiotensin receptor blockers, diuretics, NSAIDs, and COX-2 inhibitors and diuretics 24 hours before the procedure. The aforementioned medications may be resumed at 24 to 72 hours postprocedure.

k. Hold Metformin until 48 hours postprocedure or until creatinine is stable.

l. Minimize contrast use (biplane imaging in the catheterization laboratory, if possible).

m. Use a nonionic, iso-osmolar contrast.

n. Check serum creatinine at 48 hours postprocedure.

Allergy to Iodinated Contrast Media

The development of nonionic low-osmolar iodinated contrast media has greatly reduced the incidence of adverse reactions to contrast media. The majority of reactions are self-limited and present as dermatological manifestations. Premedication with steroids is only recommended for individuals identified as high risk of an adverse reaction. Life-threatening reactions occur in up to 0.2% of individuals. There is no evidence that allergy to shellfish alters the risk of reaction to intravenous contrast more than any other allergy.

LVEDP Guidance for Fluids

An alternative approach to IVF administration is to use an upfront fluid bolus with 3 mL/kg/h × 1 h (maximum rate = 330 mL/h) and then to assess the LVEDP immediately upon access and prior to coronary angiography.

1. Preprocedure: 3 mL/kg/h × 12 h[b]

2. Intraprocedurally fluid administration varied by LVEDP

   LVEDP <13: 5 mL/kg/h

   LVEDP 13–18: 3 mL/kg/h

   LVEDP >18: 1.5 mL/kg/h

This LVEDP-guided approach has been shown to be valid in the reduction of CIN and should be considered. ([b]IV hydration for 6 to 12 hours preprocedure and/or for 6 to 12 hours postprocedure can be considered.)

Cautionary Note

1. Patients who are at risk of developing fluid overload should be given less IV hydration and observed carefully for development of heart failure.

2. Avoid repeat contrast exposure. Delay angiography until serum creatinine level has peaked and stabilized.

   a. In patients with diabetes and renal disease, delay angiography >72 hours.

   b. In patients with no risk factors, delay angiography >48 hours.

Suggested Readings

Best PJ, Skelding KA, Mehran R, et al: SCAI consensus document on occupational radiation exposure to the pregnant cardiologist and technical personnel. *Catheter Cardiovasc Interv.* 2011;77:232-2411.

Chambers CE, Fetterly KA, Holzer R, et al. Radiation safety program for the cardiac catheterization laboratory. *Catheter Cardiovasc Interv.* 2011;77:546-556

Christopoulos G, Makke L, Christakopoulos G, et al. optimizing radiation safety in the cardiac catheterization laboratory: a practical approach. *Catheter Cardiovasc Interv.* 2016;87:291-301.

Klein LW, Miller DL, Balter S, et al. Occupational health hazards in the interventional laboratory: time for a safer environment. *Radiology.* 2009;250:538-544.

*To view Videos 3.1, 3.2, and 3.3, please activate
your book on www.ExpertConsult.Inkling.com
using the pin code on the inside front cover.*

Invasive Hemodynamics

NAVIN K. KAPUR • PAUL SORAJJA

Pressure Waves in the Heart

Blood within the heart and vessels exerts pressure. A pressure wave is created by cardiac muscular contraction and is transmitted from the heart chambers through the vessels. This wave can be measured by a catheter, which enables a closed fluid-filled column to be connected to a pressure transducer. The transducer in turn converts mechanical pressure to an electrical signal that is displayed on a video monitor.

Cardiac pressure waveforms are cyclical, with the pressure rising and falling from the onset of one cardiac contraction (systole) to the onset of the next contraction. The complete description of cardiac physiology can be found elsewhere, but an examination of the cardiac cycle, electrocardiogram (ECG), and corresponding pressures (Figs. 4.1 and 4.2) provides a starting point to understand basic hemodynamics in the cardiac catheterization laboratory.

Collection of hemodynamic data is an integral part of every catheterization protocol. Even complex hemodynamic data recording can be accomplished accurately and rapidly if an efficient method is consistently used in the laboratory. A measurement sequence used in our laboratory is shown in Boxes 4.1, 4.2, and 4.3. This sequence facilitates simultaneous pressure measurements across the heart. As with most brief techniques, it is not all-inclusive; different hemodynamic measurements for specific clinical situations are necessary. Specific examples are illustrated later.

The collection of routine hemodynamic data obtained from the right and left sides of the heart, with appropriate sampling of blood for oxygen saturations and CO measurements, can be accomplished in less than 30 minutes. Although the Fick CO method is considered to be more accurate, CO by the thermodilution (TD) technique is the routine. Depending on the clinical scenario, both methods of CO determination have their advantages and limitations. Arterial, vena caval, right atrial (RA), and pulmonary artery

(PA) blood for oxygen saturation measurements are collected to screen for and, if identified, quantitation of intracardiac shunts.

Right- and Left-Sided Heart Catheterization

The protocol used during right-sided heart catheterization is summarized in Box 4.1. Right-sided heart catheterization is performed for specific indications, most commonly in patients with a history of dyspnea, valvular heart disease, or intracardiac shunts (Box 4.4). Patients with a history of pulmonary edema that occurred on a previous hospital admission often have only dyspnea with no objective evidence (e.g., after chest film, echocardiography) of left ventricular (LV) dysfunction. Dyspnea caused by lung disease cannot be differentiated from that caused by pulmonary hypertension or LV dysfunction. Right-heart catheterization (RHC) is most commonly performed with a pulmonary artery catheter (PAC),

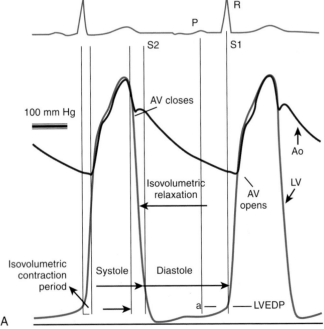

Fig. 4.1 **(A)** Normal left ventricular *(LV)* and aortic *(Ao)* pressure with electrocardiogram (ECG). Scale mark indicates 100 mm Hg.

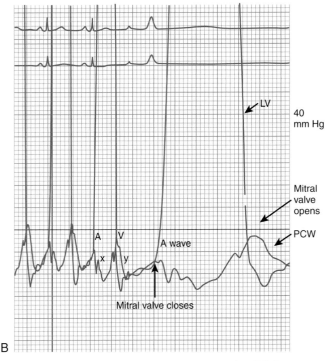

Fig. 4.1, cont'd (B) LV and pulmonary capillary wedge *(PCW)* pressures on a 0- to 40-mm Hg scale. *A,* a wave; *AV,* atrioventricular; *LVEDP,* left ventricular end-diastolic pressure; *P,* P wave; *R,* R wave; *S1 and S2,* first and second heart sounds; *V,* v wave corresponding to mitral valve opening and closing; *x,* x descent; *y,* y descent.

although larger-bore end-hole catheters may be used and provide high-fidelity tracings. First designed in the 1970s by Swan and Ganz, the PAC is available in sizes ranging from 5 F to 7 F and contains four ports: distal, proximal, thermistor, and balloon inflation. Additional ports for right ventricular (RV) pressure measurement, ventricular pacing, or drug infusion are available. The PAC may be inserted via femoral, subclavian, internal jugular, or basilic veins. Potential complications associated with RHC are shown in Box 4.5.

The most common complication of right-sided heart catheterization is arrhythmia resulting from mechanical catheter stimulation of the right ventricular outflow tract (RVOT), which can lead to ventricular tachycardia (VT), atrioventricular (AV) block or, rarely, right bundle-branch block. Significant but transient ventricular

NORMAL PRESSURES AND O₂ SATURATIONS

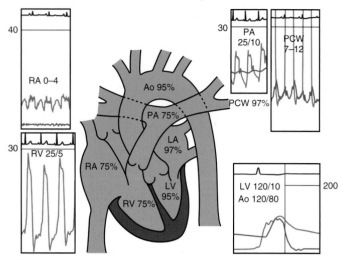

Fig. 4.2 Normal oxygen saturation, oxygen volume percentage, and pressure ranges (mm Hg) in heart chambers and great vessels with pressure tracings in relation to an electrocardiogram (ECG). *Ao,* Aortic; *LV,* left ventricle; *PA,* pulmonary artery; *PCW,* pulmonary capillary wedge; *RA,* right atrium; *RV,* right ventricle.

Box 4.1   Right-Sided-Heart Catheterization Protocol.

Right Atrium

1. Advance catheter to inferior vena cava (IVC).
2. Obtain oxygen saturation sample (1-mL heparinized syringe).[a]
3. Advance catheter to superior vena cava (SVC).
4. Obtain oxygen saturation sample (1-mL heparinized syringe).[a]
5. Advance catheter to right atrium (RA).
6. Record phasic and mean pressure (0- to 40-mm Hg scale, 25-mm/s sweep speed).

Right Ventricle

1. Advance catheter to right ventricle (RV).
2. Record phasic pressure (0- to 40-mm Hg scale, 25-mm/s sweep speed).

Pulmonary Artery and Pulmonary Capillary Wedge

1. Advance catheter to pulmonary artery.
2. Record phasic/mean/phasic pressure (25/10/25-mm/s sweep speed).

Box 4.1   Right-Sided-Heart Catheterization Protocol
(Continued)

3. Obtain oxygen saturation sample (1-mL heparinized syringe).[a]
   Flush catheter and advance to pulmonary capillary wedge (PCW).
   Obtain oxygen saturation sample to confirm wedge position.
4. Record phasic/mean/phasic pressure (25/10/25-mm/s sweep speed).
5. Obtain oxygen saturation samples for arterial.
   Perform Thermodilution Cardiac Output

[a]Only one to two drops of heparin should be aspirated and flushed out of 1- to 3-mL heparinized syringes.

Box 4.2   Left-Sided Heart Catheterization Protocol.[a]

Aortic Valve Assessment

1. Match peripheral to central aortic (Ao) pressure. If using pigtail catheter inserted through arterial sheath (sheath should be 1 F larger than catheter). If using double lumen catheter, match two Ao pressures before crossing valve.
2. Administer heparin (40 U/kg per laboratory routine).
3. Advance wire and catheter across Ao valve.
4. Obtain zero left ventricular (LV) pressure.
5. Obtain zero sheath/Ao pressure.
6. Record sheath/Ao pressure and LV pressure simultaneously (0- to 200-mm Hg scale).

[*]Right-sided heart hemodynamic studies often precede left-sided heart studies. Simultaneous pressures of the left and right sides of the heart provide the most precise and accurate information.

Box 4.3   Combined Left- and Right-Heart Hemodynamic Protocol.

1. Perform right-sided-heart catheterization and position catheter in pulmonary capillary wedge (PCW).
2. Advance left-heart catheter to left ventricle (LV).
3. Aortic (Ao) valve assessment: Follow left-sided heart protocol (see Table 4.2).
4. Mitral valve assessment:
   Obtain zero PCW and femoral arterial (FA) and LV pressures.
   Record LV vs. PCW (50-mm/s speed, 0- to 40-mm Hg scale).
   Let down balloon or pull back PCW to pulmonary artery (PA) (40-mm Hg scale).
   Note: If mitral valve gradient is present, 100-mm/s sweep.
   Measure cardiac output (CO): Thermodilution (TD) outputs × 3.
   Obtain arterial oxygen and pulmonary arterial oxygen (PAO$_2$) saturation samples.

Continued on following page

Box 4.3   Combined Left- and Right-Heart Hemodynamic Protocol (Continued)

5. Right-sided heart pull back:
   Record PCW to PA (40-mm Hg scale).
   Record PA to right ventricular (RV) pressure.
   To assess constrictive/restrictive physiology, record RV and LV simultaneously (capture both 0-40 mm Hg and 0-200 mm Hg to observe dynamic RV/LV respiratory changes).
   Record RV to RA (0- to 40-mm Hg scale).
   Left ventriculography usually performed at this point.
6. Postventriculography hemodynamics:
   Record postventriculography left ventricular end-diastolic pressure (LVEDP) (0- to 40-mm Hg scale).
   Perform LV pull back to aorta with sheath/Ao pressures displayed (0- to 200-mm Hg scale).

Box 4.4   Indications and Contraindications for Right-Sided Heart Catheterization.

Indications

Differentiation of shock (cardiogenic, distributive, hypovolemic, or obstructive)

Complications associated with acute myocardial infarction (i.e., hypotension, pulmonary edema, mitral regurgitation, ventricular septal defect, right ventricular (RV) ischemia, or tamponade)

Heart failure with reduced or preserved ejection fraction (diagnosis and management)

Primary and secondary pulmonary hypertension (diagnosis and management)

Valvular heart disease

Cardiac tamponade

Intracardiac shunts

Candidacy evaluation for orthotopic heart transplantation (OHTx)

Left ventricular (LV) assist device dysfunction

Acute pulmonary embolism

Assessing volume status in renal or hepatic failure

Postoperative monitoring after cardiac surgery

Primary lung disease

Contraindications (relative)

Prosthetic tricuspid or pulmonic valve

Coagulopathy

Severe thrombocytopenia

Endocardial pacemaker

Ventricular arrhythmias

Left bundle-branch block

Box 4.5 Potential Complications of Right-Sided Heart Catheterization.

Arrhythmias (atrial or ventricular)
Cardiac perforation
Pulmonary infarction
Pulmonary artery (PA) rupture
Air embolism
Endocarditis
Venous thrombosis
Arterial puncture
Pneumothorax

---

arrhythmias occur in 30% to 60% of RHC procedures and are self-limited (not requiring treatment). The arrhythmia is terminated when the catheter is readjusted. Sustained ventricular arrhythmias have been reported, especially in unstable patients or those with electrolyte imbalance, acidosis, or concurrent myocardial ischemia. In patients with left bundle-branch block, a temporary pacemaker may be necessary if right bundle-branch block occurs.

Proper catheter positioning is essential for proper waveform interpretation. Upon catheter insertion to 20 to 25 cm, a normal RA pressure tracing includes five components: (1) a wave of atrial contraction, (2) x descent illustrating atrial diastole, (3) c wave of tricuspid valve closure, (4) v wave of ventricular systole and passive atrial filling, and (5) y descent of passive atrial emptying (remember as a/x, c, v/y).

Advancing the PAC to 30 to 35 cm yields a RV waveform that can be identified by an abrupt increase in systolic pressure and a diastolic pressure that normally approximates the RA pressure. Rotation of the catheter through the RVOT and advancing across the pulmonic valve at 45 to 55 cm results in a PA waveform identified by three hallmark findings: (1) abrupt increase in diastolic pressure from RV to PA, (2) development of a small dicrotic notch in the PA tracing, and (3) alignment of the peak PA systolic pressure within the electrocardiographic T wave. Further advancement of the PAC results in occlusion of a secondary or tertiary branch of a PA and generates the pulmonary capillary wedge pressure (PCWP) waveform, characterized by a and v waves of reflected left atrial (LA) and LV contraction, respectively.

Use of Pulmonary Balloon Occlusion (Wedge) Pressure

The PCWP closely approximates the LA pressure, reflecting the filling pressure of the LV in the in most patients. PCWP is not a reliable surrogate for LA pressure in patients with absence of mitral stenosis, cor triatriatum, or pulmonary veno-occlusive disease (e.g., pulmonary vein [PV] stenosis after atrial fibrillation [AF] ablation) (Fig. 4.3A). Reported discrepancies between LA pressure and PCWP may be caused in part by different types of catheters: Balloon-tipped flotation catheters are soft with small lumens, and transseptal pressure catheters (e.g., Brockenbrough or Mullins-type sheath) are stiff with large lumens. Transseptal LA catheterization should be considered when there is concern for these discrepancies.

Rules for obtaining an accurate PCWP that agrees with LA pressure are:

1. Position the catheters correctly and verify position through waveform, oximetry (oxygen saturation >95%), and fluoroscopy. The wedged position of the catheter is confirmed by an oxygen saturation sample >95%. Note: Obtaining this saturation uncontaminated by low-saturation PA blood can be challenging because of the volume of low-saturation blood that must be discarded before wedge blood is collected. Use of a large-bore

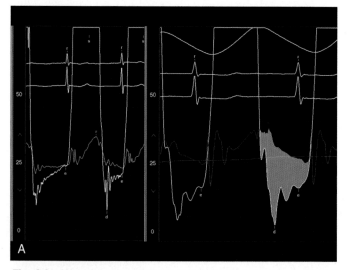

Fig. 4.3 **(A)** *Left panel:* Left atrium (LA) (by transseptal access, *orange*) with left ventricular (LV) pressure *(yellow)*. *Right panel:* pulmonary capillary wedge pressure (PCWP) by pulmonary artery catheter (PAC) with LV pressure showing the higher pulmonary capillary wedge (PCW)-LV gradient of 16 mm Hg compared with direct LA-LV gradient of 4 mm Hg. For best accuracy in assessing mitral valve gradients, use the transseptal approach.

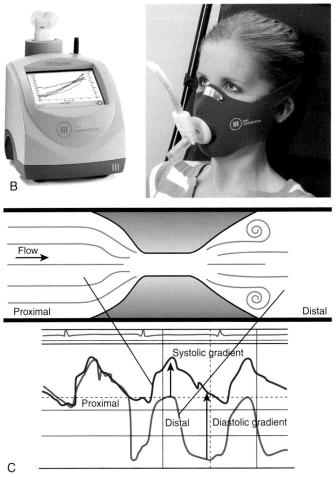

Fig. 4.3, cont'd (B) MCG Diagnostics oximetric mask. **(C)** Diagram of pressure gradient across a stenosis or narrowing. The pressure gradient is the difference between proximal and distal pressure. Pressure distal to the narrowing shows a systolic and diastolic pressure gradient. (B: courtesy MCG Diagnostics.)

catheter and saline flushing during antegrade movement into the pulmonary capillary wedge (PCW) position can help with obtaining accurate oxygen saturation measurements.

2. Confirm that PCWP is not a damped PA pressure by using a precise a and v waveform timed against the ECG or LV pressure.

Use a stiff, large-bore, end-hole catheter and connect it to the pressure manifold with stiff, short pressure tubing. The system should be thoroughly flushed and bubble free.

Fick Principle for Measurement of Cardiac Output

The Fick principle states that uptake or release of a substance by any organ is the product of the arteriovenous concentration difference of the substance and blood flow to that organ. Pulmonary blood flow (which is equal to systemic blood flow in the absence of an intracardiac shunt) is determined by measuring the arteriovenous difference of oxygen across the lungs and the uptake of oxygen from room air by the lungs. CO is calculated as oxygen consumption divided by the arteriovenous oxygen (AVO_2) concentration difference. The AVO_2 consumption difference is calculated (in milliliters of oxygen) as the difference in left ventricular oxygen (LVO_2) content ($1.36 \times$ hemoglobin $\times LVO_2$ saturation $\times 10$) minus the pulmonary arterial (mixed venous) oxygen (PAO_2) content ($1.36 \times$ hemoglobin $\times PAO_2$ saturation $\times 10$).

With accurately measured oxygen consumption, the Fick technique is the most accurate method of assessing CO, particularly in patients with low CO. Supplemental oxygen is often administered to a patient during diagnostic cardiac catheterization. Mixing the supplemental oxygen with room air makes determination of the oxygen content of the inspired air difficult (if not impossible) to calculate. Supplemental oxygen therapy should be discontinued at least 10 to 15 minutes before determination of CO by the Fick technique.

There are several formulae used to compute assumed oxygen consumption (VO_2). Studies have shown that measured VO_2 differed significantly using values derived from formulae of Dehmer, LaFarge, and Bergstra (Box 4.6) with median absolute differences of 28, 38, and 32 mL/min, respectively ($P < 0.0001$ for each). The measured and estimated values differed by $>25\%$ in 17% to 25% of patients, depending on the formula used. Median absolute differences were greater in severely obese patients (body mass index >40 kg/m^2) but were not affected by sex or age.

Compared with measured oxygen consumption, the assumed Fick at 3 mL O_2/kg correlated poorly. This assumption using the LaFarge equation is based on pediatric measurements and is specifically *not* recommended for use in adults, despite the fact that it is common practice. The most accurate method is direct measurement of VO_2 at the time of PA and arterial blood sampling and can be facilitated by metabolic carts (e.g., MCG Diagnostics) (see Fig. 4.3B). These direct measurements of VO_2 also enable cardiac function assessment with cardiopulmonary exercise testing.

Box 4.6   Formula for Assumed Oxygen Consumption.

1. Dehmer formula: $\dot{V}O_2$ (mL/min) = 125 × BSA
2. LaFarge formula: $\dot{V}O_2$ (mL/min) = 138.1 − (11.49 × log age) + (0.378 × HR) × BSA (male); $\dot{V}O_2$ (mL/min) = 138.1 − (17.04 × log age) + (0.378 × HR) × BSA (female)
3. Bergstra formula: $\dot{V}O_2$ (mL/min) = 157.3 × BSA + 10 − (10.5 × log age) + 4.8 (male); $\dot{V}O_2$ (mL/min) = 157.3 × BSA − (10.5 × log age) + 4.8 (female)

BSA, Body surface area; *HR*, heart rate; *$\dot{V}O_2$*, assumed oxygen consumption.

Box 4.7   Clinical Scenarios Favoring Invasive Hemodynamic Assessment.

1. Aortic Stenosis and/or Regurgitation
   a. Poor Doppler signature by echocardiography
   b. Discrepancy between symptoms and noninvasive testing
   c. Severe anemia
   d. Concomitant subvalvular/supravalvular stenosis
   e. Low-output/low-gradient AS with angiographic assessment for concomitant coronary disease before dobutamine challenge
   f. Low-output/low-gradient AS with preserved left ventricular (LV) ejection fraction; vasodilator challenge if high peripheral vascular resistance
2. Mitral stenosis and/or regurgitation
   a. Discrepancy between symptoms and transmitral gradient or pulmonary pressures by noninvasive testing
3. Pulmonary hypertension (primary and secondary)
4. Heart failure with preserved ejection fraction (HFpEF) without valvulopathy
5. Candidacy evaluation for LV assist device or orthotopic heart transplantation (OHTx)
6. Right ventricular (RV) failure
7. Hypertrophic cardiomyopathy (HCM)
8. Constrictive and/or restrictive cardiomyopathy

Estimates of resting VO_2 derived from conventional formulae are inaccurate, especially in severely obese individuals. When accurate hemodynamic assessment is important for clinical decision-making (Box 4.7), VO_2 should be directly measured.

Indicator Dilution Cardiac Output Principle

The indicator dilution technique is based on the principle that a single injection of a known amount of an indicator (e.g., cold saline for the TD technique) injected into the central circulation mixes completely with blood and changes concentration as it flows to a more distal location. The change in the indicator concentration (or temperature) is plotted over time; the area under the curve is used to calculate CO.

Thermodilution Indicator Method

The TD indicator method requires a PA balloon flotation catheter (Swan-Ganz) with a thermistor at the tip. The TD Swan-Ganz catheter is a triple lumen design. The proximal port, located 30 cm from the tip, is used for RA pressure measurement and rapid infusion of the saline indicator during CO determination, the distal end-hole is used for pressure measurement, and the lumen is used to inflate the balloon. A thermistor at the distal tip measures blood temperature.

The balloon serves two purposes: (1) a positioning aid and (2) facilitation of PCWP. The inflated balloon helps to direct the catheter into the PA by "floating" with the flow of blood through the right-heart chambers. When positioned in the PA, the catheter can be advanced to the distal pulmonary vasculature, "wedging" in a small branch. The balloon forms a seal that isolates the tip from PA flow to measure LA pressure. The thermistor at the end of the catheter is positioned in the PA when the proximal port is in the RA.

Measuring Cardiac Output

CO is determined by rapid-injection 10 mL of iced (4°C) or room temperature (20°C) saline injected as the indicator through the proximal port of the PAC. An external thermistor measures the temperature of the saline injectate. Complete mixing of the injectate with blood causes a decrease in blood temperature, detected by the distal thermistor. The CO computer calculates the change in indicator concentration (temperature over time) to determine CO in liters per minute. To obtain consistent, reliable results, the physician and technical staff must use appropriate technique. The following steps contribute to TD CO accuracy.

1. Position the catheter properly in the PA. Excessive coiling of the catheter in the RA or RV can result in poor positioning of the dual thermistor in relation to the injectate port. This problem is sometimes encountered with a large, dilated right side of the heart. In these instances, a 0.025-inch guidewire can be used to give additional stiffness to the catheter. A wedged catheter does not register the appropriate temperature change.

2. Most TD systems require input of a specific computation constant (in the output computer) depending on the system used. Some computers provide a table that gives a constant corresponding to the injectate volume and temperature and size and type of catheter used.

3. Deliver the precise amount of injectate, which is relatively cool in temperature relative to the patient. In adults, 10 mL is the commonly used volume, and 5 mL is typical in children. In adults for whom fluid restriction is important, a smaller bolus of injectate may be desired. If so, remember to change the computation constant on the output computer to reflect the change in injectate volume.

4. Coordinate the start button and bolus injection. Press the start button on the computer followed within a few seconds by the bolus injection. Injection before the release of the start button is a common error. When this happens, the computer does not recognize the full bolus of injectate delivered.

5. Deliver the bolus rapidly at a constant flow rate. Use two hands to inject.

6. Securely connect the catheter to the computer. The interface cable from the CO computer is nonsterile so care should be taken not to contaminate the catheterization table.

7. If room temperature saline is used, there should be at least a 10°C difference between the injectate and body temperature. Most computers have built-in sensors that enable the technician to check these parameters before the start of the procedure.

8. Obtain three to five CO values. Erroneous values are ignored in the final averaging of results.

9. Keep in mind that TD technique is inaccurate with tricuspid regurgitation or low CO or significant arrhythmia, which may occur from ectopy caused by placement of the catheter. Both conditions interfere with the normal flow of injectate past the sensing thermistor. Intracardiac shunts further reduce the accuracy of TD.

Left-Sided Heart Catheterization

The protocol for left-sided heart catheterization is summarized in Box 4.2 and indications for left-sided heart catheterization are summarized in Chapter 1. A combined right-side and left-side heart protocol is a precise and complete method for addressing the most common hemodynamic problems in the catheterization laboratory (see Box 4.3).

Computations for Hemodynamic Measurements

When hemodynamic data have been obtained, specific computations quantify cardiac function. In this section, some of the most common computations and standard formulae are provided for measurement of cardiac work, flow resistance, valve areas, and shunts. Complete derivations and applications of these formulae can be found elsewhere.

CO using the Fick principle and O_2 consumption is:

$$CO = \frac{O_2 \text{ consumption (mL/min)}}{A \, \mathrm{V}O_2 \text{ difference (mL } O_2/100 \text{ mL blood)} \times 10}$$

Oxygen consumption is best measured from a metabolic "hood." (This device is widely used except in a pulmonary function laboratory.) It is more commonly estimated as 3 mL O_2/kg or 125 mL/min/m^2. The true O_2 consumption for an adult based on the preceding estimate has been strongly questioned. A VO_2 difference is calculated from arterial–mixed venous (PA) O_2 content, where O_2 content is saturation $\times$ 1.36 $\times$ hemoglobin.

For example, if arterial saturation is 95%, O_2 content 0.95 $\times$ 1.36 $\times$ 13.0 g = 16.7 mL, PA saturation 65%, O_2 consumption 210 mL/min (70 kg $\times$ 3 mL/kg) or measured value, CO is determined as follows:

$$\frac{210}{(0.95 - 0.65) \times 1.36 \times 13.0 \times 10} = \frac{210}{53} = 3.96 \text{ L/min}$$

1. Cardiac index (CI; L/min/m^2) is

$$CI = \frac{CO \text{ (mL/beat)}}{BSA \text{ (}m^2\text{)}}$$

where CO is cardiac output; BSA is body surface area.

2. Stroke volume (SV; mL/beat) is

$$SV = \frac{CO \text{ (mL/min)}}{HR \text{ (bpm)}}$$

where HR is heart rate.

3. Stroke index (SI; mL/beat/m^2) is

$$SI = \frac{SV \text{ (mL/beat)}}{BSA \text{ (}m^2\text{)}}$$

4. Stroke work (SW; g · m) is

SW = (mean LV systolic pressure − mean LV diastolic pressure)
  × SV × 0.0144

5. Pulmonary arteriolar resistance (PAR; Wood units) is

$$PAR = \frac{mean\ pulmonary - mean\ LA\ pressure\ (or\ mean\ PCW)}{CO}$$

6. Total pulmonary resistance (TPR; Wood units) is

$$TPR = \frac{mean\ pulmonary\ arterial\ pressure}{CO}$$

7. Transpulmonary gradient (TPG; mm Hg) is

TPG = mean pulmonary artery pressure (mPAP) − mean RA
  pressure

8. PA capacitance (PAC: mL/mm Hg) is

PAC = stroke volume/PA pulse pressure

9. Systemic vascular resistance (SVR; Wood units) is

$$SVR = \frac{mean\ systemic - mean\ right\ arterial\ pressure}{CO}$$

Resistance calculations follow the form of Ohm's law, where

$$R = \Delta p / \bar{Q}$$

  where R is resistance; Δp is mean pressure differential across the vascular bed, and $\bar{Q}$ is blood flow. Resistance units (mm Hg/L/min) are also called *hybrid resistance units* or *Wood units*. To convert Wood units to metric resistance (dynes × s × cm^{-5}), multiply by 80.

Computations of Valve Areas From Pressure Gradients and Cardiac Output

A pressure gradient is the pressure difference across a valvular or vascular obstruction, such as a stenosis or narrowed valve. Figure 4.3C is a diagram of a coronary stenosis with higher pressure proximal to the stenosis and lower pressure beyond the stenosis. The same principle applies to heart valves with higher pressure proximal to the stenotic valve and lower pressure distal

Box 4.8   Techniques to Measure Left Ventricular—Aortic Pressure Gradients (From Least to Most Accurate).

Single catheter left ventricular (LV)-aortic (Ao) pull back
LV and femoral sheath
LV and long Ao sheath
Bilateral femoral access
Double lumen pigtail catheter
Transseptal LV access with ascending Ao
Pressure guidewire with ascending Ao
Multitransducer micromanometer catheters

Box 4.9   Artifactual Variables Influencing Hemodynamic Accuracy.

Miscalibrated pressure transducers
Pressure leaks on catheter manifold or connecting tubing
Pressure tubing type, length, and connectors
Air in system
Catheter sizes (especially those with small diameters)
Fluid viscosity (viscous contrast material tends to damp pressure wave)
Position of catheter side holes moving across aortic (Ao) valve (see
    Fig. 4.16)

to the stenotic valve. Several methods are used to measure trans-valvular gradients.

Techniques to measure LV-aortic (Ao) pressure gradients are listed in Box 4.8.

All pressure gradients are affected by a number of physiologic, anatomic, and artifactual variables (Box 4.9). Physiologic variables include (1) rate of blood flow (e.g., CO, coronary blood flow), (2) resistance to flow, and (3) proximal chamber pressure and compliance. Anatomic variables include (1) shape and length of valve orifice; (2) tortuosities of the vessels (for arterial stenosis), folding of coronary artery by guidewire (i.e., pseudostenosis); and (3) multiple or serial lesions (for cardiac valves and arterial stenosis).

Valve Area Calculations

$$\text{Area (cm}^2) = \frac{\text{value flow (mL/s)}}{K \times C \times \sqrt{\text{MVG}}}$$

where MVG is mean valvular gradient (mm Hg), K (44.3) is a derived constant by Gorlin and Gorlin, C is an empirical constant that is 1 for semilunar valves and 0.85 for the mitral valve, and valve flow is measured in milliliters per second during the diastolic or systolic flow period.

For mitral valve flow,

$$\frac{CO\,(mL/min)}{(diastolic\ filling\ period)\,(HR)}$$

For Ao valve flow,

$$\frac{CO\,(mL/min)}{(systolic\ ejection\ period)\,(HR)}$$

where systolic ejection period (s/min) is systolic period (s/beat) × heart rate (HR).

Examples of Aortic and Mitral Valve Area Calculations

Most modern physiologic recording systems use computer-generated waveforms and gradient-producing valve areas automatically. When using femoral artery (FA) and LV pressure, time shifting the FA back to match upstroke of the LV will underestimate the true Ao valve gradient (Fig. 4.4). When calculating from the formula, convert CO to milliliters per minute, not liters per minute. When computing flow, convert the ejection period and filling period to fractions of the period in seconds.

Data obtained at catheterization for Ao stenosis (Fig. 4.5) are:

1. CO = 4 L/min = 4000 mL/min

2. HR = 60 beats/min

3. Pressure waves of LV-Ao pressures are displayed at 100-cm/s sweep speed. If FA pressure is used, greater accuracy is associated with *unshifted* Ao upstroke and LV pressure.

Step 1. Obtain the Ao-LV gradient area (if in AF, the average is 10 beats).

$$\text{Gradient area} = 12.20\ cm^2$$

Step 2. Measure systolic ejection period (SEP).

$$SEP = 4.1\ cm\ (next\ convert\ to\ time) = 4.1 \times 1\,s/10\ cm = 0.41\ s$$

Step 3: Compute mean systolic pressure gradient (Mean valve gradient (MVG) in systole).

$$MVG = 12.2\ cm^2 \times \frac{19.6\ mm\ Hg/1\ cm}{4.1\ cm} = \frac{239}{4.1} = 58\ mm\ Hg$$

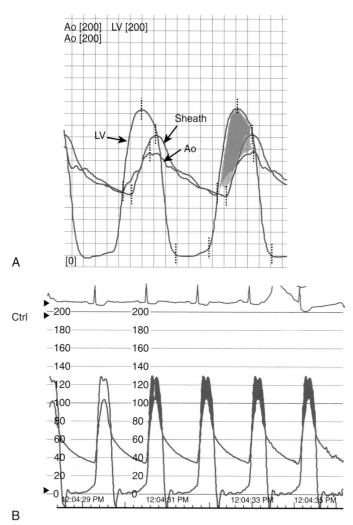

Fig. 4.4 **(A)** Aortic *(Ao)*-left ventricular *(LV)* pressure gradient for computing valve area by shifted and unshifted femoral artery (FA) pressure
compared with central Ao pressure. The unshifted additional gradient area
(orange) is bigger than the central area, overestimating the severity of
the valve area. The shifted area is smaller than the true central area, un-
derestimating valve area. **(B)** Computer-shifted LV-Ao pressure artificially
makes the gradient area smaller and hence overestimates the Ao valve
area.

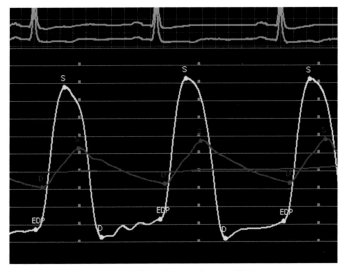

Fig. 4.5 Left ventricular (LV) and central aortic (Ao) pressure as measured by dual lumen pigtail catheter. Note immediate upstroke of Ao pressure measured just above Ao valve with no delay as seen with femoral artery pressure. (Scale 0 to 200 mm Hg.) *EDP*, End-diastolic pressure.

Step 4: Compute Ao valve flow.

$$\text{Flow} = \frac{\text{CO}}{\text{SEP} \times \text{HR}} = \frac{4000 \text{ mL/min}}{0.41 \text{ s/beat} \times 60 \text{ bpm}}$$

$$\frac{4000}{24.6} = 126.6 \text{ mL/min (Note: SEP now in s/beat.)}$$

Step 5: Compute aortic valve area (AVA).

$$\text{AVA} = \frac{\text{Ao value flow}}{1.0 \times 44.3\sqrt{\text{MVG}}} = \frac{162.6}{44.3 \times \sqrt{58}}$$

$$= \frac{162.6}{44.3 \times 7.6} = \frac{162.6}{336.6} = 0.48 \text{ cm}^2$$

Notes on the Aortic Valve Gradient

The mean pressure gradient (MPG) is the area of superimposed Ao and LV pressure tracings. Peak-to-peak pressure difference is easily measured and often used as an estimate of valve stenosis severity. Peak-to-peak pressure difference is not equivalent to the mean gradient for mild and moderate stenosis but is often close to the mean gradient for severe stenosis.

The delay in pressure transmission and pressure wave reflection from the proximal aorta to the FA artificially increases the mean gradient. If the pressure tracing is shifted to match the upstroke of the LV, femoral pressure overshoot (amplification) reduces the true gradient. In patients with low gradients (i.e., <35 mm Hg), more accurate valve areas were obtained with unshifted LV-Ao pressure tracings (see Fig. 4.4A). Consider changing the default option on the computer to shift Ao pressure automatically to correspond with LV pressure (see Fig. 4.4B). A dual lumen pigtail catheter will eliminate the delay in pressure transmission and femoral pressure amplification but the side arm must be meticulously flushed to avoid damping. Figure 4.5 shows LV-Ao pressure measurement from the central Ao catheter without delay in the upstroke of Ao pressure.

Simplified formulae provide quick in-laboratory determinations of AVA. AVA can be accurately estimated as CO divided by the square root of the LV-Ao peak-to-peak pressure difference.

$$\text{Peak-to-peak gradient} = 65 \text{ mm Hg}$$

$$CO = 5 \text{ L/min}$$

$$5 \text{ L/min}$$

$$\text{Quick valve area (Hakki formula)} = \frac{5 \text{ L/min}}{\sqrt{65}} = \frac{5 \text{ L/min}}{\sqrt{8}} = 0.63 \text{ cm}^2$$

Note: The quick formulae for valve area differ from the Gorlin formula by $18 \pm 13\%$ in patients with bradycardia (<65 beats/min) or tachycardia (>100 beats/min). The Gorlin equation at low-flow states overestimates the severity of valve stenosis.

Use of Valve Resistance for Aortic Stenosis

Although not commonly computed, valve resistance (a measure of valve obstruction) has been shown to have clinical value. Valve resistance has not been used because the units of dynes/s/cm^{-5} were not well related to clinical outcomes.

Valve resistance is calculated using the same variables for valve area measurement. In contrast to valve area, the MPG is considered to be a linear variable rather than taken as a square root term. The contribution of pressure gradient to the magnitude of valve resistance is greater. Resistance has also been shown to be more constant than valve area under conditions of changing CO. Figure 4.6 shows resistance and area calculated in a group of

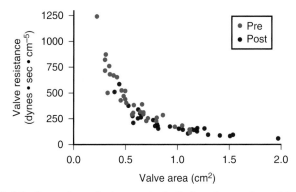

Fig. 4.6 Comparison of valve area by Gorlin formula vs. valve resistance before (pre) and after (post) aortic (Ao) valvuloplasty. Valve resistance <200 dynes/s/cm⁻⁵ is associated with minimal obstruction and >250 dynes/s/cm⁻⁵ with significant obstruction. This measure complements and refines valve area decision-making. (From Feldman T, Ford L, Chiu YC, et al. Changes in valvular resistance, power dissipation and myocardial reserve with aortic valvuloplasty. *J Heart Valve Dis*. 1992;1:55-64.)

patients before and after balloon Ao valve dilation. Resistance rises sharply above a valve area of 0.7 cm². The shoulder of this curve is 0.7 to 1.1 cm², which is the common area of indeterminate significance of Gorlin AVA. Some patients in this gray zone tend to have higher valve resistance than others. In this setting, it has been shown that patients with resistance >250 dynes/s/cm⁻⁵ are more likely to have significant obstruction than patients with resistance <200 dynes/s/cm⁻⁵. There is also a gray zone in using this index; some patients may have resistance <250 dynes/s/cm⁻⁵ despite a planar valve area of 0.7 to 0.8 cm². Resistance is a complementary index, not a replacement for valve area.

Catheter Selection for Aortic Stenosis

Initial catheter selection is a matter of operator choice and experience. In most cases, dual lumen pigtail ventriculography catheter is a good initial choice. Of note, the side port of the dual lumen catheter is prone to damping, should be flushed routinely, and must be carefully positioned to ensure its placement above the Ao valve in the central aorta. The Ao valve is usually crossed using a 0.038-inch straight-tipped guidewire loaded into a steerable catheter (e.g., AL-1 or Judkins right). Manipulation of the wire and catheter allows wire positioning in various directions to cross the valve. After wire crossing, advance the LV catheter over the wire and position correctly for ventriculography and hemodynamic studies. Only the pigtail catheter is suitable for LV angiography. It should not require more than several minutes to cross an Ao valve, even if severely stenosed. The wire should be removed every 3 minutes during an attempt to be wiped. If great difficulty is encountered with crossing, a transseptal approach should be considered.

Points to Remember When Crossing the Aortic Valve with Guidewires

1. Give adequate heparinization (a 40- to 50-U/kg bolus) anticipating 10 minutes of work. Perform frequent catheter flushing (approximately every 2 to 3 minutes) on removal of the guidewire.
2. To prevent guidewire clotting, a maximum of 3 minutes per crossing attempt is a good rule before wire withdrawal, wiping, and flushing of the catheter.
3. To prevent dissection of the coronary arteries, avoid positions of the catheter and guidewire that point to the coronary ostia. This is achieved most easily by using left anterior oblique views for crossing.
4. Practice gentle manipulation of the wire to avoid damaging the valve, lifting atheromas, or causing a perforation of the cusps or Ao root.
5. After valve crossing and during catheter exchanges, observe the distal guidewire position in the ventricle to avoid wire perforation. Once the catheter is in the ventricle, the tip of the exchange guidewire can be shaped in a curve to prevent perforation during further catheter exchanges.

When Do You Need to Cross the Aortic Valve for Hemodynamic Assessment?

An example of a class-I recommendation is when experts recommend a procedure for direct hemodynamic measurement in symptomatic aortic stenosis (AS) patients for whom noninvasive tests are inconclusive or in whom a discrepancy exists between the noninvasive test and clinical findings regarding the severity of Ao stenosis (level C).

It is a class III recommendation (experts agree procedure provides no benefit or may be harmful) *not* to cross the Ao valve during cardiac catheterization when noninvasive tests are adequate and concordant with clinical findings (level C), or for the assessment of severity of Ao stenosis in asymptomatic patients (level C).

If the echocardiogram can provide precise, accurate, reproducible, high-quality, and high-confidence information, crossing of the Ao valve is relatively superfluous. This would also apply to any routine catheterization, because LV function can readily be assessed by echocardiography. However, in the patient with Ao stenosis in whom there is a question about the adequacy of the noninvasive testing, retrograde cannulation with catheter-obtained hemodynamics of the Ao valve is certainly important in determining the true transvalvular gradient because aortic valve replacement is indicated when the stenosis is severe in symptomatic patients. Thus, the decision of whether to cross the valve or not remains patient-specific.

Data From the Catheterization Laboratory for Calculation of Mitral Valve Area

Figure 4.7 shows a hemodynamic tracing to calculate the MVA.

1. CO = 3.5 L/min = 3500 mL/min
2. HR = 80 beats/min
3. Scale factor = 1 cm = 3.9 mm Hg (40 mm Hg full scale)

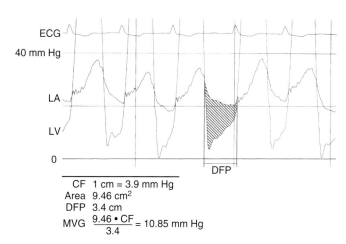

CF	1 cm = 3.9 mm Hg
Area	9.46 cm²
DFP	3.4 cm

$$MVG \quad \frac{9.46 \cdot CF}{3.4} = 10.85 \text{ mm Hg}$$

Fig. 4.7 Hemodynamic tracing used to calculate mitral valve area (MVA). *Shaded area*: Diastolic mean valvular gradient *(MVG)* surrounded by the diastolic filling period (DFP). *CF,* Correction factor or scale factor; *DFP,* diastolic filling period; *ECG,* electrocardiogram; *LA,* left atrial pressure; *LV,* left ventricular pressure (scale 0 to 40 mm Hg); *MVG,* mean valvular gradient.

4. Tracing of LV-PCW pressure at 100-mm/s paper speed = (10-cm/s paper speed) (align PCW v wave with downstroke of LV pressure)

Step 1. Planimeter five LV-PCW areas (10 if in AF).

$$\text{Area} = 9.46 \text{ cm}^2$$

Step 2. Measure diastolic filling period (DFP).

$$\text{DFP} = 3.4 \text{ cm (then convert to time)}$$

$$3.4 \text{ cm} \times 1 \text{ s}/10 \text{ cm} = 0.34 \text{ s}$$

Step 3. Convert planimetered area to mean diastolic pressure gradient.

$$\text{MVG} = 9.46 \text{ cm}^2 \times \frac{3.9 \text{ mm Hg}/1 \text{ cm}}{3.4 \text{ cm}} = 10.85 \text{ mm Hg}$$

Step 4. Compute mitral valve flow. For the mitral gradient (similar to AVAs), DFP is in centimeters at this point, owing to scale factor.

$$\text{Flow} = \frac{\text{CO}}{\text{DFP} \times \text{HR}} = \frac{3500 \text{ mL/min}}{0.34 \text{ s/beat} \times 80 \text{ bpm}} = \frac{3500}{0.34 \times 80}$$

$$= \frac{3500}{27.2} = 128.7 \text{ mL/min}$$

Step 5. Compute MVA.

$$\text{MVA} = \frac{\text{Mitral value flow}}{0.44 \times 44.3\sqrt{10.85}} = \frac{128.7}{0.85 \times 44.3 \times 3.3} = \frac{128.7}{124.3} = 1.0 \text{ cm}^2$$

Notes on Mitral Valve Gradient

Obtaining an accurate PCWP is crucial (see earlier discussion about PCW accuracy; see Fig. 4.3A). Use of direct LA pressure from transseptal measurement is the most accurate method. Transseptal catheterization will confirm pressure gradients, especially for suspected prosthetic mitral stenosis. However, if the PCWP-LV pressure tracings show no significant gradients, transseptal catheterization is unnecessary.

Simplified Mitral Valve Gradient Calculation by Cui et al.

Cui et al. (2007) simplified estimation of the mitral valve gradient and thus simplified the calculation of MVA from hemodynamic tracings. Because the mean mitral valve gradient is the pressure difference between the mean left atrium pressure (MLAP) and mean left ventricular pressure (MLVP) during diastole (i.e., MLVG = MLAP − MLVP), the computation of the mean mitral valve gradient depends on simply knowing the MLVP. The MLAP is easily obtained from the electronically meaned LA signal on the hemodynamic recorder. The area under the LV pressure during diastole is roughly a triangle with the three corners formed from the intersections of the DFP starting and ending points (mitral valve closure and opening) marking the vertical lines intersecting with the LV pressure line (rising diagonally across diastole; Fig. 4.8). This triangular area can be estimated from the rectangular area LVEDP × DFP divided by 2. Thus, the MLVP is equal to the LVEDP/2. From this key calculation, the mitral valve gradient is therefore simplified as

$$MVG = MLAP - LVEDP/2$$

There is strong correspondence between MVAs calculated by the Gorlin and Hakki formulae, both before and after mitral balloon valvuloplasty, with an error of estimates at 1.6 mm Hg. The Cui mitral valve gradient slightly overestimated the gradient before but not after mitral valvuloplasty. The Hakki formula significantly underestimated mitral valve gradients after mitral

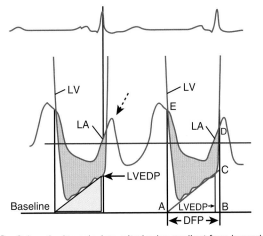

Fig. 4.8 Cui method to calculate mitral valve gradient from hemodynamic tracings. Left ventricular *(LV)* and left atrial *(LA)* pressures are superimposed. The LV-LA gradient is triangular in shape, representing half of the rectangle delineated by *A* and *B* diastolic filling period *(DFP)*; *C*, left ventricular end-diastolic pressure *(LVEDP)*; *D,* mitral value closing; and *E,* mitral value opening. (From Cui W, Dai W, Zhang G. A new simplified method for calculating mean mitral pressure gradient. *Catheter Cardiovasc Interv.* 2007;70:754-757.)

balloon valvuloplasty. Unlike Hakki, the Cui mitral valve gradient was not affected by mitral regurgitation, Ao insufficiency, AF, or HR.

Although simple, the Cui mitral valve gradient still has potential problems. HR changes will affect the shape of the triangular area under the LV pressure curve, and tachycardia may cause a potential overestimation of valve severity.

Tricuspid Valve Gradients

Because small gradients (5 mm Hg) across the tricuspid valve may lead to significant clinical symptoms, precise measurement of hemodynamics through two large-lumen catheters may be required. Match pressures through two catheters (or through the two lumens of a balloon-tipped catheter if correctly positioned) before placement in the RA and RV to avoid technical error. The Gorlin valve area formula has not been validated for the tricuspid or pulmonic valves.

Measurement of Cardiac Output

In the cardiac catheterization laboratory, CO is determined by one of two techniques: (1) Fick, with measurement of oxygen consumption (see earlier) or (2) indicator dilution (TD, using a PAC; see Chapter 1).

Intracardiac Shunts

A shunt is an abnormal communication between the left- and right-heart chambers. The direction of blood flowing through the shunt is left to right, right to left, or sometimes bidirectional. In the absence of shunting, the pulmonary blood flow (right side of the heart) is equal to the systemic blood flow. Table 4.1 lists intracardiac shunt locations. A left-to-right shunt increases the amount of blood to the right side of the heart and increases pulmonary blood flow, now the sum of the systemic blood flow plus shunt flow. With a right-to-left shunt, the amount of blood shunted from the right side of the heart to the left is added to that normally ejected into the systemic circulation, making systemic blood flow greater than pulmonary blood flow by the amount of blood flow in the shunt (Fig. 4.9). Intracardiac shunts have been evaluated by oximetry, radionuclide perfusion, and Doppler echo flow measurements. Oximetry is the most common method used in the catheterization laboratory.

Table 4.1

Cardiac Shunt Locations.	
Location	**Earliest Step-Up Location (for Left-to-Right Shunts)**
Atrial Septal Defects	
Primum (low)	RA, RV
Secundum (mid)	RA
Sinus venosus (high)	RA
Partial anomalous pulmonary venous return (pulmonary veins entering RA)	RA
Ventricular Septal Defects	
Membranous (high)	RV
Muscular (mid)	RV
Apical (low)	RV
Aorticopulmonary window (connection of aorta to PA)	PA
Patent ductus arteriosus (normally closed Ao-PA connection at birth)	PA

Ao, Aortic; *PA*, pulmonary artery; *RA*, right atrium; *RV*, right ventricle.

Oximetry Procedure: Diagnostic Saturation Run

A diagnostic "saturation run" uses 1- to 3-mL heparinized syringes to obtain blood from the superior vena cava (SVC), inferior vena cava (IVC), RA, RV, and PA in a rapid, organized manner. A standard balloon-tipped PA flotation catheter is satisfactory, but a large-bore end-hole or side-hole (multipurpose) catheter performs better rapid sampling. Heparinize saturation syringes with <0.5 mL. In addition, prepare the labels and list of sample sites in advance (Box 4.10).

The saturation run begins after diagnostic hemodynamic data and CO have been obtained and before right-sided heart pull back. With the catheter positioned in the right or left PA, measure oxygen consumption (Fick method). On catheter pull back, one operator manipulates the catheter under fluoroscopic and pressure control while an assistant aspirates the blood samples at each location along the run. Each new sample is obtained after several milliliters of blood have been withdrawn and discarded so that blood left from the previous catheter sampling location will not contaminate the new blood oxygen. The entire diagnostic run should take approximately 5 to 7 minutes.

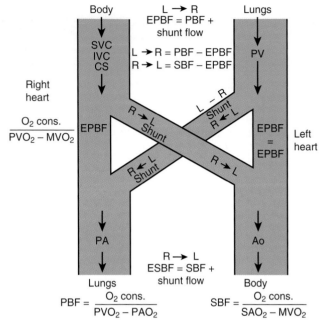

Fig. 4.9 Schematic diagram for right-to-left and left-to-right shunting across the heart. *Ao,* Aorta; *CS,* coronary sinus; *EPBF,* effective pulmonary blood flow; *ESBF,* effective systemic blood flow; *IVC,* inferior vena cava; *L,* left; *MVO₂,* mixed venous oxygen saturation or content; *O₂ cons.,* oxygen consumption; *PA,* pulmonary artery; *PAO₂,* pulmonary arterial oxygen saturation or content; *PBF,* pulmonary blood flow; *PVO₂,* pulmonary venous oxygen saturation or content; *PV,* pulmonary vein; *R,* right; *SAO₂,* systemic arterial oxygen saturation or content; *SBF,* systemic blood flow; *SVC,* superior vena cava.

Oxygen Step-Up: Evidence of a Shunt

A left-to-right shunt is suggested when an oxygen step-up or increase in oxygen content in that chamber or vessel exceeds that of a proximal compartment. A step-up in oxygen saturation at the PA by more than 7% above the RA saturation is indicative of a left-to-right shunt at the atrial level (Table 4.2). Similarly, the desaturation of arterialized blood samples from the left heart chambers and aorta suggests a right-to-left shunt. In determining the site of the right-to-left shunt, sequential sampling can be made from the LA, LV, and aorta.

Box 4.10 Sample Sites for Oxygen Saturations During Diagnostic Saturation Run.

Right Side of the Heart

Left PA
Right PA
Main PA
PA above pulmonary valve (PA_{pv})
RV below pulmonary valve (RV_{pv})
RV (mid)
RV (apex)
RV at tricuspid valve (RV_{TV})
RA at tricuspid valve (RA_{TV})
RA (mid)
SVC (high)
SVC (low)
RA (high)
RA (low)
IVC (high, just beneath heart, above hepatic vein)
IVC (low, above renal vein, but below hepatic vein)

Left Side of the Heart

Arterial saturation, Ao
If possible, cross ASD, pulmonary vein saturation
Patent foramen ovale or LA

Ao, Aortic; *ASD,* atrial septal defect; *IVC,* inferior vena cava; *LA,* left atrium; *PA,* pulmonary artery; *RA,* right atrium; *RV,* right ventricle; *SVC,* superior vena cava.

Table 4.2

Oxygen Saturation Values for Shunt Detection.

Level of Shunt	Significant Step-Up Difference[a] $O_2\%$ Saturation
Atrial (SVC/IVC to right aorta)	≥ 7
Ventricular	≥ 5
Great vessel	≥ 5

IVC, Inferior vena cava; *SVC,* superior vena cava.
$MVO_2 = (3\ SVC + 1\ IVC)/4$ and difference from PA should normally be $\leq 7\%$.
[a]Difference between distal and proximal chamber; for example, for atrial septal defect (ASD).

Mixed venous blood is assumed to be fully mixed PA blood. With a left-to-right shunt, measure mixed venous blood one chamber proximal to the step-up. In the case of an atrial septal defect (ASD), compute the mixed venous oxygen content from the weighted average of vena caval blood (i.e., as [$3 \times$ SVC + IVC]/4).

When pulmonary venous blood is not collected, assume that pulmonary venous oxygen (PVO_2) percentage saturation is 95%.

Shunt Calculation

The Fick or left-sided indicator dilution methods of CO determination are used to measure systemic flow (see Fig. 4.9). Using the Fick method, the following formulae apply:

1. Systemic flow

$$Q_s(L/min) = \frac{O_2 \text{ consumption (mL/min)}}{(\text{arterial} - \text{mixed venous}) \, O_2 \text{ content}}$$

2. Pulmonary flow, Q_P (L/min)

$$\frac{O_2 \text{ consumption (mL/min)}}{(\text{pulmonary venous} - \text{pulmonary arterial}) \, O_2 \text{ content}}$$

Thus, the effective pulmonary blood flow (EPBF) is

$$Q_{EPB} = \frac{O_2 \text{ consumption (mL/min)}}{(\text{pulmonary venous} - \text{mixed venous}) \, O_2 \text{ content}}$$

Normally, the EPBF is equal to the systemic blood flow. In a left-to-right shunt, EPBF is increased (by the amount of the shunt) as follows:

EPBF = systemic flow + shunt flow (left-to-right)

In a right-to-left shunt, EPBF is decreased (by the amount of the shunt):

EPBF = systemic flow − shunt flow (right-to-left)

Shunt volume is determined by use of equations 1 and 2 (later).

The shunt fraction is the ratio of pulmonary to systemic flow (called Qp/Qs, where Q is flow, P is pulmonary, and S is systemic) for a left-to-right shunt. Flow ratios (Q_p/Q_s) >1.5 often require closure.

Example for Left-to-Right Shunt Atrial Septal Defect Calculation

Data obtained at catheterization are:

Hemoglobin = 13 g

O_2 consumption = 210 mL/min

Location	Saturation (%)	Location	Saturation (%)
Arterial	92	PA	81
SVC	71	PV	98
Mid RA	85	IVC	70
Low RA	68		

1. Compute O_2 content.

$$\text{Arterial } O_2 \text{ content} = 0.98 \times 1.36 \text{ mL } O_2/g \times 14.1 \text{ g/dL} \times 10$$
$$= 188 \text{ mL } O_2/L$$

Mixed venous O_2 content (use estimate of mixed venous oxygen saturation):

$$\frac{3 \text{ SVC} + 1 \text{ IVC}}{4} \text{ for mixed venous oxygen saturation:}$$

$$\frac{(0.71 + 0.71 + 0.71 + 0.70)}{4} = 0.71$$

$$71 \times 1.36 \text{ mL } O_2/g \times 14.1 \text{ g/dL} \times 10 = 136 \text{ mL } O_2/L$$

$$\text{Pulmonary artery } O_2 \text{ content} = (0.81 \times 1.36 \text{ mL } O_2/g \times 14.1 \text{ g/dL} \times 10)$$
$$= 155 \text{ mL } O_2/L$$

$$\text{Pulmonary vein } O_2 \text{ content} = (0.98 \times 1.36 \text{ mL } O_2/g \times 14.1 \text{ g/dL} \times 10)$$
$$= 188 \text{ mL } O_2/L$$

2. Compute systemic flow (equation 1).

$$\frac{225 \text{ mL } O_2/\text{min}}{(188 - 136) \text{ mL } O_2/L} = \frac{225}{52} = Q_S = 4.3 \text{ L/min}$$

3. Compute pulmonary flow (equation 2).

$$\frac{225 \text{ mL } O_2/\text{min}}{(188 - 155) \text{ mL } O_2/L} = \frac{225}{33} = Q_P = 6.8$$

4. Compute.

$$\frac{Q_P}{Q_S} = \frac{6.8}{4.3} = 1.6$$

The L→R shunt is 6.8 L/min − 4.3 L/min or 2.5 L/min.

If absolute flows are not required, the Q_P/Q_S ratio can be determined using saturations only as follows:

$$\frac{Q_P}{Q_S} = \frac{SAO_2 - MVO_2}{PVO_2 - PAO_2}$$

where SAO_2 is systemic arterial oxygen saturation, PVO_2 is pulmonary venous oxygen saturation, MVO_2 is mixed venous oxygen saturation, and PAO_2 is pulmonary arterial oxygen saturation.

Using saturation data from the example of left-to-right shunt:

$$\frac{Q_P}{Q_S} = \frac{98 - 71}{98 - 81} = \frac{27}{17} = 1.6$$

Example for Right-to-Left Shunt

Data obtained at catheterization are:

$$\text{Hemoglobin} = 15 \text{ g}$$

$$O_2 \text{ consumption} = 195 \text{ mL/min}$$

Location	Saturation (%)	Location	Saturation (%)
Arterial	89	LA	88
SVC	81	PA	82
Mid RA	83	PV	96
Low RA	82	IVC	70

1. Compute O_2 content.

   Arterial = $(0.89 \times 15 \text{ g}/100 \text{ mL} \times 1.36 \text{ mL } O_2/\text{g} \times 10) = 182 \text{ mL } O_2/\text{L}$

   Mixed venous (estimated mixed venous) saturation = $(.81 + .81 + .81 + .70) \, 4 = 0.78$

   Mixed venous = $(0.78 \times 15 \text{ g/dL} \times 1.36 \text{ mL } O_2/\text{g} \times 10) = 159 \text{ mL } O_2/\text{L}$

   Pulmonary arterial = $(0.82 \times 15 \text{ g/dL} \times 1.36 \text{ mL } O_2/\text{g} \times 10) = 167 \text{ mL } O_2/\text{L}$

   Pulmonary venous = $(0.96 \times 15 \text{ g/dL} \times 1.36 \text{ mL } O_2/\text{g} \times 10) = 196 \text{ mL } O_2/\text{L}$

2. Compute systemic flow (equation 1).

   $$\frac{O_2 \text{ consumption}}{(\text{arterial} - \text{mixed venous}) \, O_2 \text{ content}} = \frac{195 \text{ ml } O_2/\text{min}}{(182 - 159) \text{ ml } O_2/\text{L}}$$

3. Compute pulmonary blood flow (equation 2).

   $$\frac{O_2 \text{ consumption}}{(\text{pulmonary venous} - \text{pulmonary arterial}) \, O_2 \text{ content}}$$

   $$= \frac{195 \text{ mL } O_2/\text{min}}{(196 - 167) \text{ mL } O_2/\text{L}} = 6.7 \text{ L/min}$$

4. Compute Q_{EPB}.

$$= \frac{O_2 \text{ consumption}}{(\text{pulmonary venous} - \text{mixed venous}) \, O_2 \text{ content}}$$

$$= \frac{195 \text{ ml } O_2/\text{min}}{(196 - 159) \text{ mL } O_2/\text{L}} = 5.3 \text{ L}$$

Shunt calculations:

$$\text{Left-right shunt} = Q_P - Q_{EPB} = 6.7 - 5.3 = 1.4 \text{ L/min}$$
$$\text{Right-to-left shunt} = Q_S - Q_{EPB} = 8.5 - 5.3 = 3.2 \text{ L/min}$$

Limitations of the Oximetric Technique

1. Because of its low sensitivity, oximetry may fail to detect small (<1) shunts.
2. The application of the Fick principle to calculate blood flow presumes a steady state during the diagnostic run and measurement of oxygen consumption (i.e., timely collection of saturation sample within a period during which oxygen consumption and CO are stable).
3. The oximetry method also assumes that complete mixing is achieved instantly and that blood samples obtained are representative of blood in the respective compartment.
4. The rate of systemic blood flow is important in detecting a shunt by oximetry. A high systemic flow tends to equalize the AVO_2 difference across a given vascular bed. In the presence of elevated systemic blood flow, the mixed venous oxygen saturation is higher than normal and intrachamber variability caused by streaming is reduced. In contrast, when systemic blood flow and mixed venous oxygen saturation are low, a larger step-up must be detected before a significant left-to-right shunt is diagnosed.

Angiography

Angiography is a qualitative method used to localize either left-to-right or right-to-left shunts. The shunt can be detected by injection of x-ray contrast medium into the closest proximal chamber. The left anterior oblique view with cranial angulation puts the interatrial and interventricular septae on face (i.e., on edge), which provides an ideal view for detection of contrast medium passage across the atrial and ventricular septal defects (see Chapter 3 for angiographic views to visualize an intracardiac shunt).

Equipment Used for Hemodynamic Study

Pressure Manifold and Setup

The optimal set of transducers, tubing, and manifolds for any laboratory is that which is cost effective, familiar, accurate, and simple to use. Several varieties of disposable manifolds exist (Fig. 4.10) that can be coupled to transducers positioned either on the manifold or at the side of the catheterization table. For research studies, special transducer-tipped micromanometer pressure catheters and pressure sensor guidewires are used to obtain high-fidelity pressure recordings. High-fidelity recordings are not necessary for routine clinical hemodynamic studies; accurate measurements can be obtained with fluid-filled systems if appropriate precautions in the setup are taken.

Some clear plastic manifolds have several ports: (1) pressure and zero line, (2) saline flush, (3) contrast media at the third, and (4) closed waste line (to minimize contamination of personnel and laboratory). A three-port manifold combines a saline flush and waste port with a one-way valve.

For best pressure waveforms, tubing should be short and stiff, with the transducer as close to the catheter as possible. Tubing

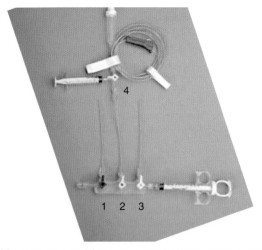

Fig. 4.10 Pressure manifold used for coronary angiography. At the end of the manifold the connection of the manifold to the catheter has a swivel connector. *1*, Stopcock to pressure; *2*, saline flush line; *3*, contrast line; *4*, waste line with a one-way valve.

length from the catheter to the transducer should also be mini-mized; longer tubing contributes to more resonating or "ringing" artifacts (Fig. 4.11).

The zero level is set at mid chest (i.e., the measured antero-posterior diameter of the patient divided by 2 and added to the position of the table). When the transducer is raised above zero level, pressure is artificially lower. When the transducer is lower than zero, pressure is artificially higher (Fig. 4.12). When abnor-mally low pressures are seen initially, recheck the zero for proper positioning (at mid chest) and check for air bubbles or loose con-nections.

Physiologic Recorder

The physiologic recorder system is now a digital system that pro-cesses the hemodynamic and electrocardiographic signals from the transducers and pacing electrode catheters used in electrophysio-logic studies. The typical physiologic monitor/recorder is a multi-channel unit that can process, display, and record ECG signals, pres-sure tracings, and direct current (DC) inputs from external sources (e.g., TD). The number of channels determines how many individual signals are displayed and recorded simultaneously. For routine cardiac catheterization, one ECG signal and two to three pressure channels are normally recorded. In certain complex cases, such as electrophysiology studies and cases with complex congenital or valvular heart disease, it is common to use four to 18 channels.

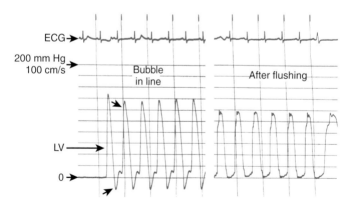

Fig. 4.11 Hemodynamic tracing showing the effect of an air bubble in a pressure line. Note the change in hemodynamic waveform after the bubble is flushed: The ringing artifact *(sharp points at arrows)* is eliminated and fine detail of precise pressure restored. *ECG,* Electrocardiogram; *LV,* left ventricle.

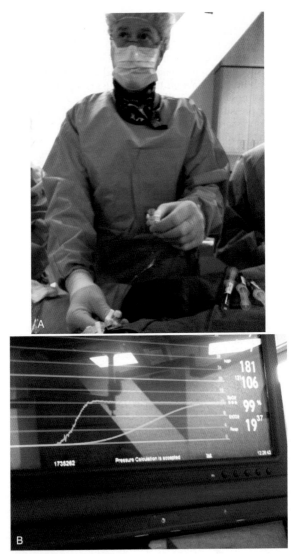

Fig. 4.12 **(A)** To demonstrate the effect of zero position, a transducer is connected to a fluid-filled tube and its stopcock is open to air. By lifting either the tubing (as shown in the left hand) or the transducer, the zero can be seen to move. **(B)** The effect of first raising the tubing shows how zero offset is affected by height on the table. The blue line goes up and then raising the transducer to the same level produces the same effect. Set the zero at bedside and keep the transducer fixed throughout the study.

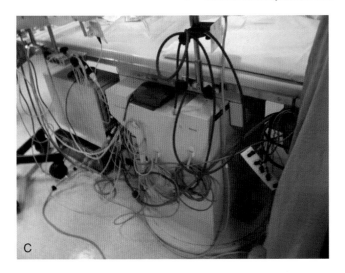

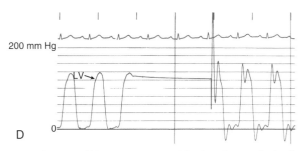

Fig. 4.12, cont'd (C) Picture shows cables hanging on the back of the catheterization table. Organization by color coding and coiling to protect cables against damage is very helpful to achieve optimal catheterization laboratory operation. **(D)** *Left:* Left ventricle *(LV)* pressure tracing showing normal damping with viscous contrast media in the fluid path. *Right:* After flushing with saline, the tracing is now seen as underdamped with an exaggerated ringing artifact. (A, B, and C: reproduced with permission from *Cath Lab Digest*, copyright HMP Communications.)

Most recorders have an electronic calibration that allows the operator to input an electronic pressure standard. This feature provides a convenient means for simulating pressure signals to calibrate the display. An external standard pressure reference can be input from a mercury manometer and the transducer calibrated to match the input pressure.

Display Settings for Hemodynamic Data

The laboratory has many choices when setting the display for hemodynamic waveforms. These settings include timing lines, signal display sweep speed, and pressure scale(s). The typical setting for a routine case is 1-second time lines (i.e., one line each second). Use a faster time line sequence for special studies or when a faster paper speed is used. For most procedures, the sweep speed of the monitor is 25 mm/s. Slower sweep speeds (10 and 5 mm/s) are used to examine changes in hemodynamics, such as respiratory variations in RV/LV pressure, over longer periods of time. Faster speeds can help in observing timing of diastolic and systolic pressures (e.g., LV and Ao; LA and LV).

For pressure scales, displaying more than one tracing may require setting each tracing's pressure scale on a different value. Right-heart scales range from 0 to 50 mm Hg, whereas typical left-heart pressure scales range from 0 to 200 mm Hg.

Hemodynamic Recording Techniques

Coordination between the recording technician and operators is required to obtain high-quality hemodynamic recordings. The following are some suggestions that aid in providing consistent, reliable data:

1. At the start of each procedure, enter the patient's identifiers, the date, and other key data. Calibrate the transducers and set at zero at the mid-chest level. Measure the mid-chest point with a ruler and mark for later reference.

2. Anticipate changes in the recording settings as the catheter is moved to new positions. Change pressure scales and sweep speeds as needed.

   Example: For monitoring RA pressure in a patient with pulmonary hypertension, a full-scale 0 to 50 mm Hg may be appropriate. As the catheter passes through the tricuspid valve, RV pressure may be >50 mm Hg. The technician should observe this, anticipate the change, and quickly change the scale (e.g., 0- to 100-mm Hg full scale) accordingly.

Hemodynamic Data Collection: Points of Confusion and Frustration

It is frustrating for nurses and technicians to enter a laboratory wherein all of the cabling connecting the transducers to the table and the table connectors to the hemodynamic recorder is un-plugged and lying all over the floor (see Fig. 4.12C). This may be a continuous battle if cleaning personnel between or after cases unplug the cables for better cleaning. Numbering or color-coding all cables and inputs for easy match-ups is one way to solve this problem. In addition to clear labeling, cable attachments to the table side with Velcro strips or tapes will help organization and eliminate confusion and wasted time.

Likewise, during a procedure on the catheterization table, it is worthwhile to color code the transducers or connecting tubing or to number them so that communication between the table and the recording technician can proceed smoothly. For example, "please zero transducer number 1, pressure is up on number 1" will clarify recording of FA pressure and not RA pressure.

Hemodynamic Examples and Artifacts

Artifacts of Hemodynamic Tracings

Pressure Fidelity: Underdamping and Overdamping

Normal pressure waveforms from fluid-filled systems are sharp without rounded contours. The correct frequency of the system permits some high-frequency oscillations to be visible at low pressures and maintain rapid upstrokes without overshoot or hyperoscillation at high pressure. If the transducer is too sensitive, a small pressure wave can cause a big deflection of the signal. Narrow spikes or exaggerated overshoot of the ventricular (right and left) pressure suggests underdamping. Conversely, if the transducer is not sensitive enough, the same pressure wave will not sufficiently deflect the signal, producing a dull or rounded waveform. This is called an *overdamped signal* and is usually produced by a problem in the fluid path to the transducer or a transducer that is not calibrated correctly.

Air Bubbles

An air bubble in a LV pressure line produces a tracing with exaggerated systolic and diastolic overshoot (see Fig. 4.11), demonstrating underdamping. After the line is flushed and the air bubble eliminated, the sharp, crisp upstroke of ventricular pressure shows a normal pressure rise. An accurate waveform for a properly flushed fluid-filled catheter system shows little overshoot during the high-frequency systolic period and at the same time shows mild vibratory waves during the low-frequency diastolic period. An underdamped tracing can be corrected by instilling diluted contrast media in the pressure line. Figure 4.12D shows a suitable LV pressure with normal (or only slightly rounded) waveform after flushing of the line (right side of tracing). Early diastolic and systolic portions of the pressure wave on the right show striking overshoot underdamping. Table 4.3 lists common problems and solutions for hemodynamic waveforms. Underdamping produces a "noisy" PCWP (Fig. 4.13). With instillation of contrast media into the catheter, underdamping is corrected, yielding a tracing with clearly interpretable waveforms. Figure 4.14 shows the effect of different timing signals of the transducers for pressure and ECG.

Table 4.3

Common Hemodynamic Recording Problems.

Problem	Possible Cause	Solution
Overdamping[a]	Bubble or clot in line or transducer	Reflush system
	Small lumen of tubing system	Increase internal diameter of tubing
	Soft or compliant tubing	Use stiffer tubing
	Loose catheter connection	Tighten catheter
	Kink in catheter	Unkink catheter
Underdamping[b]	System tubing too stiff	Use softer tubing
	System tubing too long	Shorten tubing
	Hyperdynamic state	Increase filter on amplifier; introduce small bubble or contrast media
	Catheter tip in turbulent jet	Reposition catheter
Loss of signal	Bad transducer	Change transducer
	Bad cable	Change cable
	Bad amplifier	Switch amplifier
	Catheter disconnected	Check connections
	Catheter obstructed/ kinked	Flush/change catheter
Pressures do not return to zero	Same causes as loss of signal as above	Readjust zero line
		Recalibrate
		Check zero at mid chest

Modified from Tilkian AG, Daily EK. *Cardiovascular Procedures: Diagnostic Techniques and Therapeutic Procedures*. St Louis: Mosby; 1986.
[a]Overdamping system is not sensitive enough and yields flat or rounded tracings.
[b]Underdamping system is too sensitive and produces too much ringing or overshoot of tracings.

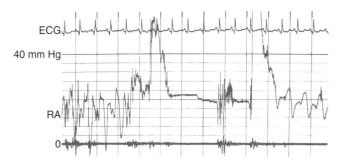

Fig. 4.13 Right atrial *(RA)* pressure tracing showing marked under-damped ringing artifact. Instillation of viscous contrast media damps the system, producing excellent waveforms. *ECG,* Electrocardiogram.

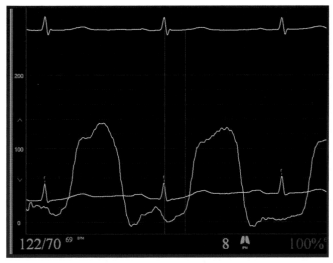

Fig. 4.14 Left ventricular (LV) pressure and electrocardiogram (ECG) show an artifact of amplifier miscalibration regarding timing between the two signals. Note that the ECG occurs in the middle of diastole rather than at the left ventricular end-diastolic pressure (LVEDP) *(second red line).* Reset the default time for each amplifier to rectify this problem. (Reproduced with permission from the *Cath Lab Digest*, copyright HMP Communications.)

Catheter Malposition or Movement

A false Ao valve stenosis gradient is shown in Figure 4.15. For measurement of LV and Ao pressures, all side holes of the pigtail catheter must be under the Ao valve. In Figure 4.15B, the pigtail catheter is partly out of the LV. LV pressure is partly contaminated by Ao pressure, which reduces the LV-Ao gradient. This artifact also is evidenced by the abnormal diastolic waveform, which shows a continued decline (downslope) in diastolic pressure (see Fig. 4.15C). LV diastolic pressure should be lowest in the first part of diastole, with a rising pressure across the mid and late diastolic period. Figure 4.15A shows the true gradient when the pigtail catheter is advanced slightly. This artifact is important and if unappreciated may lead to a false conclusion of only minimal Ao valve disease (Fig. 4.16).

Loose Tubing Connections

Loss of pressure may be due to loose connections among the tubing, catheter, manifold, or transducer (Fig. 4.17). An LV pressure lower than the Ao pressure is caused by this problem (unless the Ao pressure is increased by another source, such as heterotopic transplant or extra cardiac hemodynamic support).

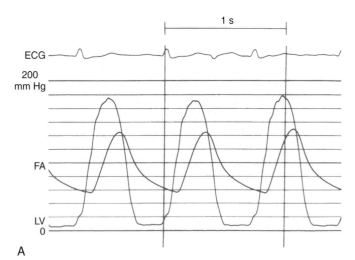

A

Fig. 4.15 (A) True gradient is seen when the pigtail catheter is advanced fully across the aortic (Ao) valve.

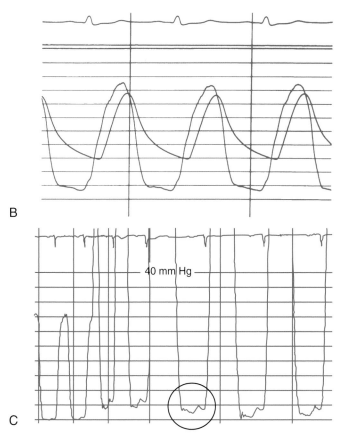

B

C

Fig. 4.15, cont'd (B) Falsely low aortic stenosis (AS) gradient caused by pigtail catheter side holes in the aorta. **(C)** Abnormal diastolic left ventricular *(LV)* pressure wave pattern showing relaxation failure of diastolic dysfunction. Note that the lowest diastolic pressure occurs in the middle of diastole, whereas normally the lowest diastolic pressure occurs at the very beginning of diastole. *ECG,* Electrocardiogram; *FA,* femoral artery pressure.

Normal Right Ventricular and Right Atrial Pressure Waves

The respiratory influences on RA pressure are shown in Figures 4.18 and 4.19. Simultaneous RV and RA pressures are shown in Figure 4.20. The atrial filling a wave and ventricular filling v wave correspond to the RV pressure tracing. Following the a wave is the

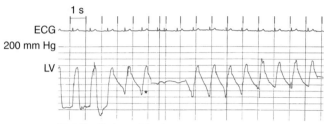

Pigtail catheter pull back

Fig. 4.16 A falsely wide aortic (Ao) pulse pressure *(*)* with the use of a pigtail catheter is caused by incomplete withdrawal of all side holes outside the left ventricle *(LV)*. On final catheter positioning *(far right)*, Ao pressure is normal. *ECG*, Electrocardiogram.

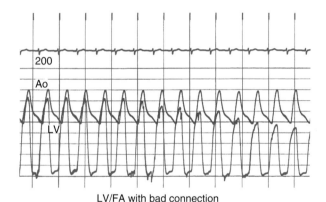

LV/FA with bad connection

Fig. 4.17 A loose connection on the left ventricle *(LV)* catheter to the pressure manifold causes loss of LV pressure *(right side)*. Few real conditions produce aortic *(Ao)* pressure higher than LV pressure. *FA*, Femoral artery.

x descent, and following the v wave is the normal y descent. These waveforms may be altered by specific heart disease or arrhythmias. The notch (Fig. 4.20, *left-facing arrow*) on the top of the RV tracing is the ringing artifact of an underdamped fluid-filled catheter. This ringing is also evident on the early diastolic part of the pressure wave (bottom of same beat, *right-facing arrow*).

Figure 4.21 shows the continuous pressure on pull back *(red arrow)* across the interatrial septum from the LA to the RA of a

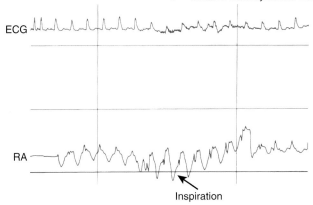

Fig. 4.18 Normal decrease in right atrial *(RA)* pressure during inspiration (scale 0 to 40 mm Hg). Note increase in y descent *(arrow)*. *ECG,* Electrocardiogram.

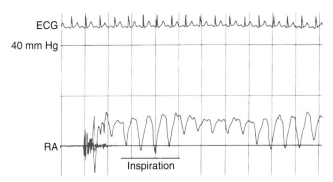

Fig. 4.19 Abnormal response of right atrial *(RA)* pressure to inspiration in a patient with constrictive physiology or heart failure. Although y descent is exaggerated, no corresponding fall in a or v wave height occurs. *ECG,* Electrocardiogram.

patient with Ao stenosis. It also shows the differences between LA and RA a and v waves. The v waves in the LA pressure wave are prominent with their corresponding x and y descents. In the RA, the a and v waves are less striking. In general, RA a waves are larger than v waves. In the LA, v waves are more prominent than a waves.

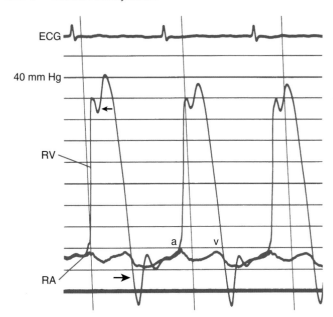

Fig. 4.20 Right atrial *(RA)* and right ventricular *(RV)* tracings in a normal patient. *Left-facing arrow:* notch of ringing or overshoot on RV pressure rise. *Right-facing arrow:* ringing and overshoot of decline in RV pressure at early diastole. *a,* Atrial wave; *v,* ventricular filling wave.

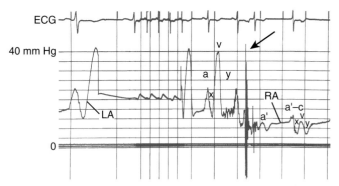

Fig. 4.21 Hemodynamic tracing of the left atrium *(LA)* with catheter pull back to the right atrium *(RA)* across the intraatrial septum. See text for details of waveform analysis. *ECG,* Electrocardiogram.

Right Atrial Pressure with Tricuspid Regurgitation

With tricuspid valvular regurgitation, blood is pushed backward into the RA during systole. In contrast to the normal pattern, RA pressure rises throughout RV systole. Figure 4.22 shows an example of a patient with tricuspid regurgitation. The RA pressure shows striking regurgitant v waves during systole without a gradient during diastole between RA and RV pressures, indicating no tricuspid stenosis. RV and RA pressure are elevated (RV systolic, 70 mm Hg; RA mean pressure, 17 mm Hg). A small gradient exists between the RA (higher tracing) and RV (lower tracing) during diastole because of mild tricuspid stenosis (a narrow and limited opening of the tricuspid valve).

Right Atrial Pressure in a Patient with Atrioventricular Dissociation

Normal a waves represent the pressure response to atrial contraction on ventricle pressure. During an AV block, the atria are not contracting at the proper time (just before ventricular contraction) (Fig. 4.23). Immediately after the QRS, the ventricles contract

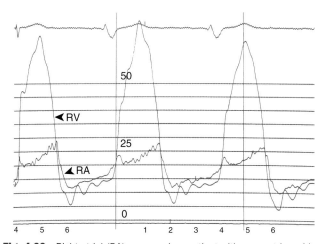

Fig. 4.22 Right atrial (RA) pressure in a patient with severe tricuspid regurgitation. When RA pressure is paired with simultaneous right ventricular (RV) pressure, tricuspid regurgitation can be seen associated with tricuspid stenosis as the separation (gradient) between the RA and RV pressures during diastole.

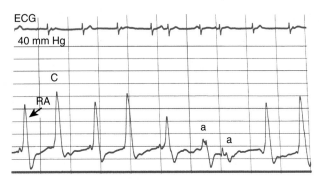

Fig. 4.23 Right atrial *(RA)* pressure during atrial-ventricular dissociation. *a,* Small a wave during synchrony of atrial and ventricular activity; *(C)* cannon wave; *ECG,* electrocardiogram. (See text for details.)

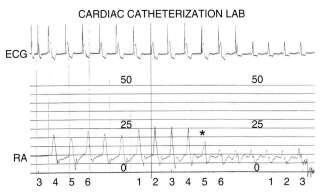

Fig. 4.24 Right atrial *(RA)* pressure during and after temporary right ventricular *(RV)* pacing. Electrocardiogram *(ECG)* shows large pacer spikes associated with giant a waves on RA pressure. Fusion beats begin at the asterisk, and the timing of an atrial contraction begins to precede ventricular activation, resulting in normal a waves.

and the tricuspid and mitral valves close. If the P wave (and atrial contraction) occurs after the tricuspid valve is closed, a giant a, or *cannon,* wave can be seen. With return of AV synchrony (normal sequence) on beats 6 and 7, a waves return, appropriate for the atrial contraction, emptying blood before ventricular systole (QRS). Similar findings may be seen when a pacemaker causes the dissociation; giant a waves occur during pacing (Fig. 4.24). The atrial contribution may be as much as 25% to 30% of CO and its effect on systemic pressure can be seen in Figure 4.25.

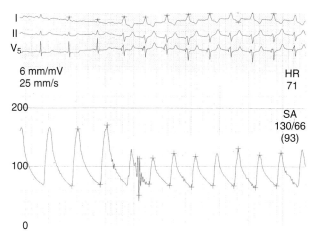

Fig. 4.25 Aortic (Ao) pressure changes occur when rhythm changes from sinus to junctional. *HR,* Heart rate.

Pulmonary Capillary Wedge Pressure and Left Atrial Pressure with Simultaneous Transseptal and Right-Sided Heart Catheterization

For every waveform, the LA pressure rise precedes that of PCWP by approximately 100 to 150 ms. Figure 4.26 shows simultaneous LA pressure and PCWP tracings. PCWP is measured through a 7-F fluid-filled, balloon-tipped catheter; LA pressure is measured through a Brockenbrough catheter. The correspondence of these two pressures is generally close and permits clinical use of PCWP for most standard hemodynamic cases.

Normal Femoral Arterial and Central Aortic Pressures

The femoral arterial (FA) and centrally measured Ao pressures have a fairly close correspondence. Normally, there is a slight overshoot of systemic pressures at the peripheral and FA locations. In the example in Figure 4.27, FA pressure measured through the side arm of the FA sheath (8 F) is matched against pressure in the pigtail catheter (7 F) positioned above the Ao valve. By observing the timing of the upstroke of the pressures, the operator can distinguish the central Ao pressure (first signal rising). The mean of the two pressures is identical. Figure 4.27 shows the high-fidelity

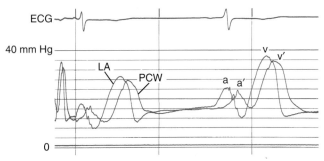

Fig. 4.26 Simultaneous left atrial *(LA)* and pulmonary capillary wedge *(PCW)* tracings. (The patient has aortic stenosis [AS] with high ventricular filling pressure.) *ECG*, Electrocardiogram.

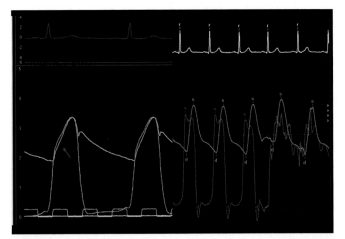

Fig. 4.27 *Left:* Simultaneous aortic (Ao) and left ventricular (LV) pressures recorded from a micromanometer high-fidelity dual transducer catheter. Note small impulse gradient of a normal left ventricular outflow tract (LVOT). *Right:* Simultaneous hemodynamic tracings of femoral arterial (FA) pressure, taken through the side arm of an 8-F sheath and central Ao pressures. Ao pressure is obtained through the 7-F pigtail catheter. Overshoot of FA pressure and the lag in the pressure upstroke are the normal characteristics of femoral tracings. (Reproduced with permission from the *Cath Lab Digest,* copyright HMP Communications.)

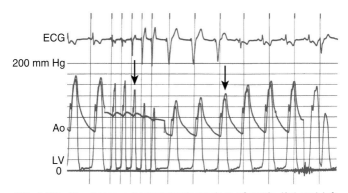

Fig. 4.28 Simultaneous hemodynamic tracings of aortic *(Ao)* and left ventricular *(LV)* pressures in a patient with a pacemaker. Loss of atrial contraction (paced beats between *arrows*) decreases ventricular filling with loss of systemic pressure. *Left arrow:* Initiation of ventricular pacing with loss of the atrial contribution to LV filling. *Right arrow:* return of atrial synchrony and normal sinus rhythm. Systemic pressures are increased markedly during normal sinus rhythm. *ECG,* Electrocardiogram.

pressure tracings of simultaneous LV and Ao pressures from a dual high-fidelity catheter.

The contribution of atrial filling to systemic pressure can be seen in Figure 4.28. The normal sinus beats (1 and 2) with simultaneous Ao (FA) and LV pressure tracings show a systolic pressure of 175 mm Hg and Ao diastolic pressure of 70 mm Hg. Atrial contribution is lost because of atrio-ventriular impulse dissociation (Fig. 4.28, *arrow*), and a pacemaker rhythm takes over. The systolic pressure falls dramatically to 118 mm Hg and gradually returns as atrial activity becomes more connected to the QRS.

Large v Waves on Pulmonary Capillary Wedge Tracing

LV and PCW pressures generally match well in diastole (Fig. 4.29). The PCW a wave (a′) follows the LV a wave by 150 ms (beat 1). The v wave is large. There is no important diastolic PCW-LV gradient. On beat 2, because of late atrial activity, loss of the LV a wave is shown by the different initial upstroke of the LV pressures. The PCW has large and late a and v waves. The v wave on a PCWP tracing may be associated with significant mitral regurgitation but is neither highly sensitive nor specific for mitral regurgitation. Large v waves may also be present with a ventricular septal defect or any condition in which the LA volume (e.g., ventricular septal defect) or LA pressure relationship (stiffness or compliance) is increased

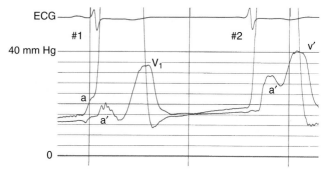

Fig. 4.29 Simultaneous pulmonary capillary wedge *(PCW)* and left ventricular *(LV)* pressures in a patient who has loss of atrial activity (beat 2). On beat 1, the a wave is evident on LV *(a)* and pulmonary capillary wedge pressure *(PCWP)* *(a′)*. The a wave is lost on beat 2, with no atrial activity. The a′ wave is considerably higher because of its contraction against the closed mitral valve. *ECG,* Electrocardiogram.

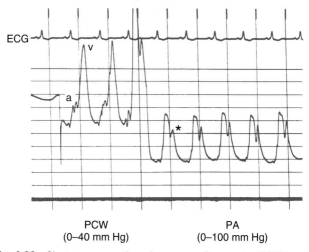

Fig. 4.30 Giant v waves on the pulmonary capillary wedge *(PCW)* tracing can be transmitted to pulmonary artery *(PA)* pressure, producing a notch *(*)* on the PA downslope. *ECG,* Electrocardiogram.

(e.g., rheumatic heart disease, postcardiac surgery, and infiltrative heart diseases). Mitral valve obstruction from any cause and congestive heart failure (CHF) in the absence of mitral regurgitation are also associated with large v waves. Giant v waves, also seen in Figure 4.30, may be large enough to be transmitted to the PA pressure, which causes a notch on the diastolic downslope.

Aortic Stenosis

The effect of increasing LV filling by a premature ventricular contraction (PVC) on simultaneous LV and Ao pressure tracings in a patient with minimal Ao stenosis can be seen with the higher LV pressure after an extrasystolic beat, called *postextrasystolic potentiation* (Fig. 4.31).

The atrial contraction is important in patients with Ao stenosis (Fig. 4.32). Simultaneous Ao and LV pressure (transseptal approach) shows that atrial activity is absent on the first beat, a junctional beat (Fig. 4.32, *asterisk*). Without the atrial contribution, Ao systolic pressure is 132 mm Hg, and LV systolic pressure is 190 mm Hg. On the following beat, number 3 atrial activity (P wave) precedes the QRS, and the Ao pressure increases to 160 mm Hg; LV pressure increases to 225 mm Hg, representing an approximately 25% increase in pressure augmentation. This effect is crucial in patients with poor LV function. Two additional features of this tracing are worthy of note. The a wave on the LV pressure tracing (see Fig. 4.31A and B, *arrow*) can be seen on LV beat 2, and Ao regurgitation may be present when a wide pulse pressure (Ao systolic-diastolic pressure) of >50 to 60 mm Hg is observed. The Ao pressure has decreased to <50 mm Hg at the end of diastole. Recall that the least accurate method to measure an LV-Ao gradient is with a single catheter pull back (see Fig. 4.31C)

Left Ventricular Gradient Below the Aortic Valve

Hypertrophic obstructive cardiomyopathy (HOCM) is a condition in which thick heart muscle contracts and may obstruct flow

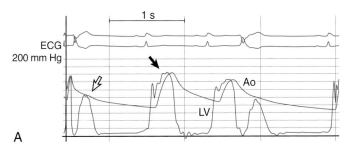

Fig. 4.31 **(A)** Postextrasystolic accentuation of left ventricular *(LV)* and aortic *(Ao)* pressures *(closed arrow)* after a premature ventricular contraction (PVC) *(open arrow)*. This patient does not have Ao stenosis. The PVC does not generate pressure sufficient to open the Ao valve and results in a dropped beat when the peripheral pulse rate is counted. *Continued*

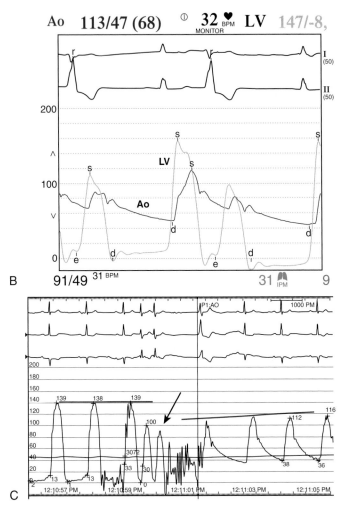

Fig. 4.31, cont'd (B) Postextrasystolic potentiation hemodynamics in a patient with mild aortic stenosis (AS). **(C)** LV to aorta pressure pull back with a single catheter, demonstrating difficulty in assessing a transvalvular gradient. (Fig. 4.31A From Kern MJ, Donohue T, Bach R, et al. Interpretation of cardiac pathophysiology from pressure waveform analysis: cardiac arrhythmias. *Cathet Cardiovasc Diagn.*1992;27:223–227.)

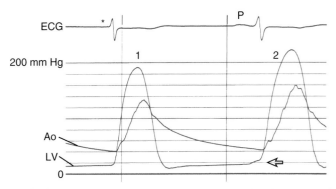

Fig. 4.32 Simultaneous left ventricular *(LV)* (obtained with transseptal technique) and aortic *(Ao)* pressures from fluid-filled catheter systems. Note the contribution of atrial contraction *(arrow)* to the change in LV and systemic pressures on beat 2. *, Absence of P wave on this tracing; *P,* P wave. The wide pulse pressure is also indicative of Ao insufficiency.

out of the ventricle, producing a pressure gradient inside the LV with a normal Ao valve. Figure 4.33 depicts simultaneous LV and Ao pressure showing a large Ao-LV gradient (LV pressure, 220 mm Hg; Ao pressure, 120 mm Hg). On pull back of the LV catheter (end-hole multipurpose) from the distal LV to a position just beneath the Ao valve, the Ao-LV gradient disappears (see the LV pressure matching with Ao pressure in Fig. 4.33, *far right.*)

A PVC in a patient with HOCM produces a longer LV filling period after the PVC beat, increases contractility, and may result in greater intraventricular muscular obstruction. Three characteristic changes in post-PVC pressure waveforms occur: (1) The LV-Ao gradient is greater, (2) Ao pulse pressure is narrower, and (3) Ao waveform if deformed shows a spike and dome pattern characteristic of early LV outflow obstruction. In addition, the Ao pressure upslope is very rapid and parallels the LV pressure upstroke. These post-PVC changes occur as a result of the increase in contractility, which outweighs the effects of the increase in preload and leads to worse outflow tract obstruction. Post-PVC findings in AS include a larger LV-Ao gradient but, unlike HOCM, they also include an increase in Ao pulse pressure, with preservation of the Ao waveform including the delayed Ao upstroke (Fig. 4.34). Table 4.4 lists provocative maneuvers to increase an outflow tract gradient in patients with hypertrophic cardiomyopathy (HCM).

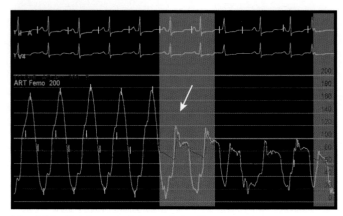

Fig. 4.33 Simultaneous left ventricular (LV) and aortic (Ao) pressures in a patient with hypertrophic obstructive cardiomyopathy (HOCM) during pull back of the catheter from the distal portion of the LV. The pressure gradient between the aorta and LV is lost. LV systolic pressure matches Ao pressure during catheter pull back before the catheter is pulled out of the LV. There is no true Ao valve gradient. This LV-Ao gradient is located in the mid-LV wall beneath the Ao valve. Matching Ao and LV systolic pressures in the proximal chamber (*arrow* indicates transition from distal LV to proximal LV under the aortic valve). (See text for details.)

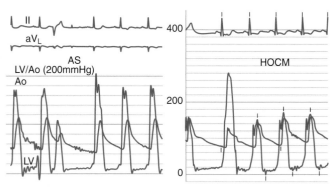

Fig. 4.34 Comparison of postpremature ventricular contraction (PVC) hemodynamics in patients with aortic stenosis *(AS, left)* and hypertrophic obstructive cardiomyopathy *(HOCM, right)*. Post-PVC in AS has a larger gradient, slow upstroke, larger pulse pressure, and preserved aortic (Ao) waveform. In contrast, post-PVC HOCM tracings show a larger gradient, smaller pulse pressure, vertical Ao pressure upstroke, and spike-and-dome pattern of Ao pressure. *LV,* Left ventricle.

4 — Invasive Hemodynamics 285

Table 4.4

Provocative Tests for Hypertrophic Cardiomyopathy.[a]	
Drug or Maneuver	**Mechanism Increasing Ao-LV Gradient**
Drugs	
Isoproterenol	Increased myocardial contractility, decreased blood pressure
Amyl nitrite	Decreased systemic arterial pressure (peripheral vasodilatation), reflex increasing sympathetic tone, decreased venous return, and increased myocardial contractility
Nitroglycerin	Decreased venous return, decreased CO, and increased narrowing of LVOT
Maneuvers	
Extrasystole (PVC)[a]	Postextrasystolic increase in myocardial contractility and decreased pulse pressure
Valsalva maneuver	Decreased venous return, decreased LV volume, and increased narrowing of outflow tract

Ao, Aortic; *CO,* cardiac output; *LV,* left ventricular; *LVOT,* left ventricular outflow tract; PVC, premature ventricular contraction.

[a]Stroke volume and systemic arterial pulse pressure decrease in the postextrasystolic beat (the Brockenbrough-Braunwald-Morrow effect).

Aortic Regurgitation

The characteristic hemodynamic feature of Ao regurgitation is wide pulse pressure, brisk Ao (femoral) pressure upstroke, and rapid filling of LV diastolic pressure. Often there is marked overshoot of the FA pressure. Figures 4.35, 4.36, and 4.37 illustrate simultaneous Ao and LV pressures in several patients with different degrees of Ao regurgitation. In Figure 4.36 the large and prominent a wave shows the effect of first-degree AV block (long P–R interval, *arrows*) on the LV pressure. Figure 4.37 illustrates the physiology of the Ao-LV gradient in diastole. No atrial contribution of LV pressure is present.

Hemodynamically severe Ao regurgitation is indicated by rapidly increasing LV diastolic pressure with near equilibration of Ao and LV pressure at end diastole (Figs. 4.36 and 4.37). Chronic Ao regurgitation leads to a wide pulse pressure, but this pressure may not be wide when the lesion is acute.

Mitral Regurgitation

In mitral regurgitation (Fig. 4.38), large v waves in the PCW tracing represent LV volume transmitted backward through an incompetent

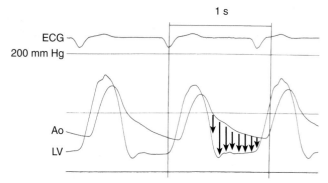

Fig. 4.35 Hemodynamic tracing in a patient with aortic *(Ao)* insufficiency (and minimal aortic stenosis [AS]), showing the Ao–left ventricular *(LV)* diastolic gradient *(arrows)* that are important for coronary perfusion. (Note the loss of the a wave because of paced rhythm.) *ECG,* Electrocardiogram.

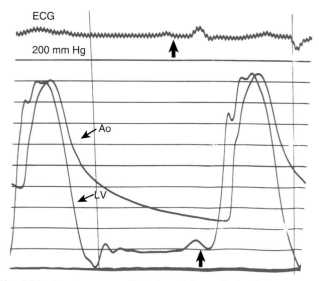

Fig. 4.36 Simultaneous aortic *(Ao)* and left ventricular *(LV)* pressures in a patient with Ao insufficiency. Note the absence of a systolic pressure gradient. The time delay in the Ao pressure upstroke indicates that femoral sheath pressure is used. The presence of a large and early a wave *(thick bottom arrow)* occurs with P–R interval prolongation *(top thick arrow).* ECG, Electrocardiogram.

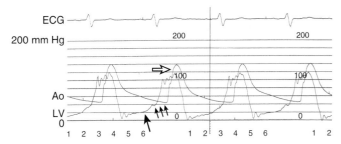

Fig. 4.37 Severe aortic *(Ao)* regurgitation shown by rapidly increasing left ventricular *(LV)* diastolic pressure *(lowest closed arrow)* and end-diastolic equilibration of Ao and LV pressure *(three small arrows)*. Peripheral arterial pressure overshoot or amplification is caused by forceful LV ejection and compliant arterial system. *(open arrow)* (In this case, Ao pressure was matched with femoral arterial [FA] sheath pressure.) *ECG,* Electrocardiogram. (From Kern MJ, Aguirre FV. Interpretation of cardiac pathophysiology from pressure waveform analysis: aortic regurgitation. *Cathet Cardiovasc Diagn.* 1992;26:232-240.)

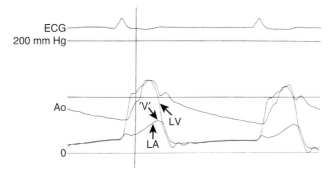

Fig. 4.38 Hemodynamic tracings in a patient with mitral regurgitation, characterized by a giant v wave *(downward arrow)* in left atrial *(LA)* *(arrow up)* pressure. This v wave corresponds to marked increase in flow and volume into the LA. *Ao,* Aortic pressure; *ECG,* electrocardiogram; *LV,* left ventricular pressure *(arrow pointing leftward)*.

mitral valve. The LA v wave occurs on the downstroke of LV pressure. V waves occur anytime there is a decrease in LA compliance, and thus are not specific for mitral regurgitation.

Figure 4.39 shows large v waves with a persistent LV-PCW gradient in patients with mixed mitral regurgitation and stenosis. Left ventriculography confirms significant mitral regurgitation. The slope of the v waves in mitral regurgitation and stenosis is flatter

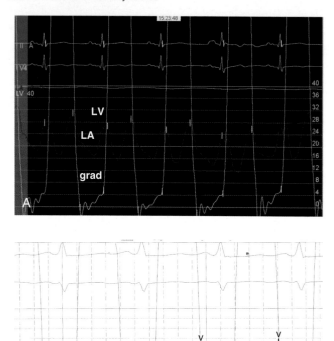

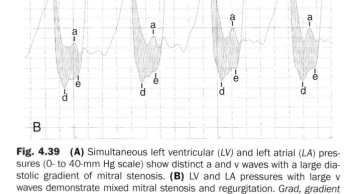

Fig. 4.39 **(A)** Simultaneous left ventricular (*LV*) and left atrial (*LA*) pressures (0- to 40-mm Hg scale) show distinct a and v waves with a large diastolic gradient of mitral stenosis. **(B)** LV and LA pressures with large v waves demonstrate mixed mitral stenosis and regurgitation. *Grad, gradient between LV and LA.*

than that in which large v waves are associated with isolated mitral regurgitant flow alone.

Mitral Stenosis

In mitral stenosis (see Fig. 4.39), LV and PCW pressures show the diastolic pressure gradient, indicating the severity of LA outflow obstruction. The a wave on beat 1 is associated with a normal v wave. On the following beat, atrial activity is delayed and follows the QRS, contributing to a giant v wave (36 mm Hg). The augmented filling increases the mitral valve gradient, which is influenced by HR. When the rhythm is irregular (as in AF), calculations of gradients should be made from the average of 10 beats. Figure 4.40 illustrates the effect of R–R cycle length on the mitral stenosis gradient. In some patients with mitral stenosis, balloon catheter valvuloplasty may be used to open a narrowed mitral orifice.

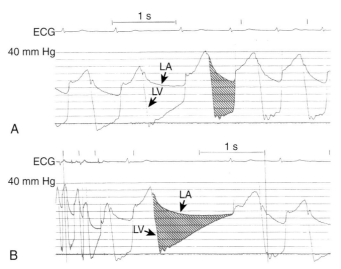

Fig. 4.40 Influence of heart rate (HR; diastolic period) on mitral valve gradient. The mitral stenosis gradient changes with HR (R–R interval). **(A)** A short R–R interval is associated with a gradient *(shaded area)* of 22 mm Hg. **(B)** A long R–R interval has a mean gradient of 29 mm Hg. When computing mean valve area in atrial fibrillation (AF), average is 10 beats. *ECG,* Electrocardiogram; *LA,* left atrial pressure; *LV,* left ventricular pressure. (From Kern MJ, Aguirre F. Interpretation of cardiac pathophysiology from pressure waveform analysis: mitral valve gradients: Part I. *Cathet Cardiovasc Diagn.* 1992;26: 308-315.)

Constrictive Pericarditis

Constrictive pericarditis limits filling of the heart by the confining pericardium. The RV fills at the expense of the LV, with the septum pushing into the LV during RV filling (e.g., inspiration). Typical hemodynamic findings include Kussmaul sign (an inspiratory increase in RA pressure), an elevated RA pressure with an M or W configuration, and a dip and plateau pattern of early rapid diastolic filling, with abrupt cessation of further caused by pericardial constraint (Fig. 4.41). Discordance of LV/RV systolic pressures during respiration is the most specific hemodynamic finding, establishing a diagnosis of constrictive pericarditis.

In Figure 4.42, matching elevated diastolic pressures with an early dip followed by a plateau during diastole (on the first beat) is the characteristic pattern. Often, the classic dip-and-plateau configuration appears only during slow HRs. Tachycardia and respiratory effort obscure the pattern, but matching RV and LV pressures during diastole is consistent. The most specific and sensitive sign that can differentiate constrictive from restrictive physiology is the

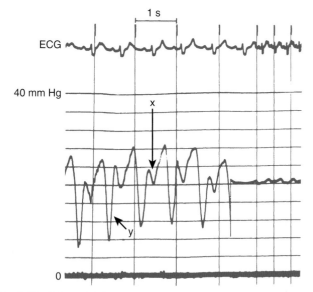

Fig. 4.41 Right atrial (RA) pressure showing pattern of constrictive physiology with large y descent and smaller x descent. Mean RA pressure is 20 mm Hg. *ECG*, Electrocardiogram.

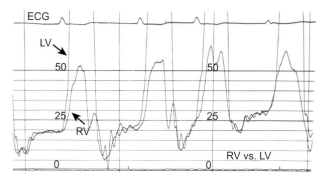

Fig. 4.42 Simultaneous left ventricular *(LV)* and right ventricular *(RV)* pressure tracing in a patient with constrictive pericarditis. Matching diastolic pressures is one of the hallmarks of this condition. However, dynamic respiratory variation of systolic pressures is diagnostic in differentiating constriction from restrictive cardiomyopathy. *ECG,* Electrocardiogram.

dynamic respiratory variations in RV and LV systolic pressures. RV/LV systolic pressures that increase and decrease in a concordant manner are findings of restrictive cardiomyopathy, whereas discordant responses during respiration of the RV/LV systolic pressures are the hallmark of constrictive physiology (Fig. 4.43). RA pressure shown in Figure 4.44 demonstrates the characteristic pattern of prominent y descent with a classic M or W configuration of constrictive physiology. These waveforms are the altered x and y troughs resulting from impaired ventricular filling. Myocardial restrictive heart disease or heart failure also shows this pattern occasionally.

Hemodynamics of Tamponade

In contrast to constrictive physiology waveforms, observe the RA pressure in a patient with cardiac tamponade (Fig. 4.45). High pericardial pressure blunts all diastolic filling waveforms. Tamponade physiology has an elevated RA pressure with blunted y descents, reflecting impairment in early diastolic filling and the life-threatening nature of this disorder. The arterial pressure shows pulsus paradoxus (an exaggerated [>20 mm Hg] inspiratory decrease in arterial pressure). In tamponade, two-dimensional (2D) echocardiography shows the pericardial fluid and diastolic RA and RV chambers collapse as a result of periodic high pericardial pressure acting on the RA/RV filling patterns (see Chapter 7).

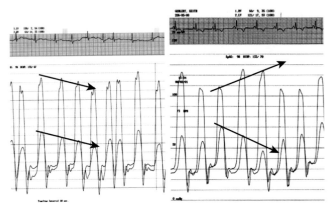

Fig. 4.43 Dynamic respiratory variation in constrictive and restrictive physiology. Normal respiratory activity results in a parallel decrease in right ventricular (RV)/left ventricular (LV) systolic pressures. *Left:* RV/LV systolic pressures move together with respiration in a concordant manner, a finding highly consistent with restrictive cardiomyopathy. (Left side, arrows depict parallel change in LV/RV systolic pressures.) *Right:* RV/LV systolic pressures move discordantly during respiration, a finding highly specific for constrictive physiology and constrictive pericardial disease. (Right side, arrows depict discordant change in LV/RV systolic pressures.)

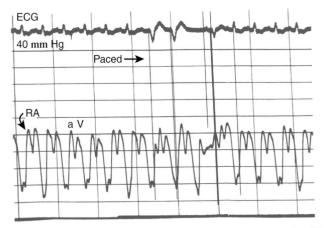

Fig. 4.44 Right atrial *(RA)* pressure in a patient with constrictive pericarditis showing abnormally elevated pressure with a classic M configuration. The elevated pressure with exaggerated y descent is also seen in cardiomyopathy. *ECG*, Electrocardiogram. *a*, a wave; v.

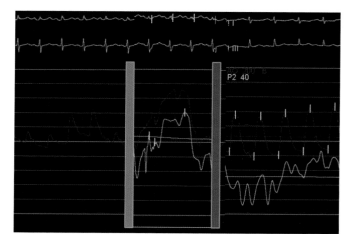

Fig. 4.45 *Left:* Arterial pressure shows pulsus paradoxus (inspiratory decrease >10 mm Hg of systolic pressure). *Center:* Atrial, pericardial, and aortic (Ao) pressures in a patient with pericardial tamponade. Before pericardiocentesis, right atrial (RA) pressure blunted x and y descents. *Right:* After pericardiocentesis, pulsus paradoxus is absent and RA waveform is lower and more phasic.

Hypertrophic Cardiomyopathy

HCM, an inherited autosomal dominant heart disease with a prevalence of 1 in 500 individuals, is characterized by myocardial hypertrophy and fibrosis in the absence of a secondary cause (i.e., hypertension or valvular heart disease). Symptoms are primarily caused by diastolic dysfunction and/or obstruction of flow across the left ventricular outflow tract (LVOT) from septal hypertrophy and systolic anterior motion of the mitral valve.

The degree of LVOT gradients in HCM depends both on loading conditions and LV contractile function. During each cardiac cycle, myocardial contraction promotes bulging of the interventricular septum, which narrows the LVOT and creates Venturi forces that drag the anterior leaflet of the mitral valve into the LVOT, thereby worsening the magnitude of LVOT obstruction. In addition, HCM patients often have a displaced anterior mitral valve leaflet that is further pulled into the LVOT during ventricular systole, leading to poor mitral leaflet coaptation and subsequent mitral regurgitation. Therefore, increased cardiac contractility (i.e., exercise, inotropes), reduced afterload (i.e., vasodilator therapy), or reduced preload (i.e., diuretics or dehydration) can all increase the LVOT gradient. An LVOT gradient >30 mm Hg is associated with symptom progression and identifies potential candidates for septal reduction therapy by surgical myectomy or alcohol septal ablation.

In most patients, resting LVOT obstruction can be identified by 2D echocardiography. For patients without LVOT obstruction at rest, exercise echocardiography is the preferred method for provoking LVOT gradients. Noninvasive methods to provoke LVOT gradients include exercise, Valsalva maneuver, or pharmacologic provocation with amyl nitrate or isoproterenol.

Invasive hemodynamic evaluation of HOCM is reserved for preoperative evaluation along with coronary angiography or in cases where a discrepancy between symptoms and noninvasive testing exits. First, RHC establishes CO, severity of pulmonary hypertension, and biventricular filling pressures. Next, resting intracavitary gradients are measured within the LV. Depending on the technique used, precise determination of the LVOT gradient can be challenging. End-hole catheters may become entrapped in the myocardium and catheters with side holes may produce erroneous pressure measurements. In most cases, retrograde LV catheterization using a pigtail catheter across the Ao valve is used with care to keep the side holes along the distal shaft under the obstructed region. Pigtail catheters can lead to underestimation of LVOT gradients.

Alternative catheters for intracavitary gradient measurements include a multipurpose catheter with side holes or the HALO catheter with multiple side holes around a perpendicular ring that prevents catheter entrapment. If a resting LVOT gradient >50 mm Hg is identified, further provocative testing is not required. If no resting LVOT gradient is established, a PVC is provoked by the intracavitary catheter. Postextrasystolic potentiation enhances contractility associated with the post-PVC beat, leading to four findings associated with obstructive HCM: (1) increased LVOT gradient, (2) rapid Ao upstroke, (3) narrowed Ao pulse pressure, and (4) spike-and-dome configuration to the Ao waveform (the Brockenbrough-Braunwald-Morrow effect). In contrast, post-PVC waveforms associated with AS (fixed LVOT) obstruction will exhibit only an increased LVOT gradient. If no LVOT gradient is observed after a PVC, perform Valsalva maneuver to reduce LV preload, thereby narrowing the LVOT and augmenting any LVOT gradient. If an LVOT remains undetected and suspicion for obstructive HCM is high, perform hemodynamics with exercise to increase contractility and reduce afterload or introduce pharmacologic challenge with isoproterenol (enhanced inotropy) or amyl nitrate (decreased afterload) (Figs. 4.46, 4.47, and 4.48).

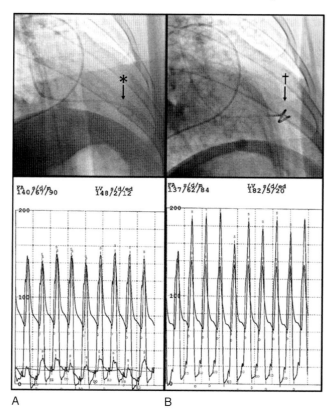

A   B

Fig. 4.46 Proper left ventricular *(LV)* catheter placement. **(A)** Pigtail catheter entrapment leads to an erroneous lack of an intracavitary gradient in a patient with known obstructive hypertrophic cardiomyopathy (HCM). **(B)** In the same patient with a HALO catheter at the LV apex, a 50-mm Hg, dynamic intracavitary gradient is revealed. ∗ indicates a pigtail catheter with potential for entrapment and erroneous pressure measurement. + indicates use of Halo catheter which cannot be entrapped and has accurate pressure signal.

Invasive Measures of Ventricular Performance: Pressure and Volume Recordings

In 1914, Ernest Starling extended findings from Otto Frank and defined the Frank-Starling mechanism, which describes the ability of the heart to increase SV in response to increases in LV

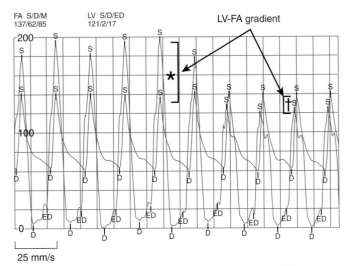

FA S/D/M
137/62/85

LV S/D/ED
121/2/17

LV-FA gradient

25 mm/s

Fig. 4.47 Intracavitary pull-back gradient. Retraction of a HALO catheter reveals an intracavitary gradient from the left ventricular *(LV)* apex *(*)* to just below the aortic (Ao) valve (†; subvalvular) consistent with hypertrophic obstructive cardiomyopathy (HOCM). *FA,* Femoral artery.

pressure or volume. Numerous observations have shown that during acute or chronic heart failure, small changes in LV pressure or volume can lead to hypotension or pulmonary congestion (Fig. 4.49). At each stage of heart failure (i.e., acute heart failure, stable chronic heart failure, and decompensated heart failure/ cardiogenic shock), therapy is directed at improving SV and reducing intracardiac volume and pressure overload, while maintaining an adequate mean arterial pressure to support end-organ tissue perfusion.

During the past four decades, specialized pigtail catheters, known as *conductance catheters*, that simultaneously measure ventricular pressure and volume have been developed to quantify ventricular function and the effect of therapeutic interventions. At present, these catheters are primarily reserved for research purposes but are used more frequently to provide clinically relevant hemodynamic data. By applying a constant electric current across multiple electrodes, the catheter converts the electrical conductance of blood within the LV into volume measurements. A solid-state transducer simultaneously measures LV pressure, and a real-time measurement of pressure-volume relationships across the cardiac cycle can be obtained (Fig. 4.50).

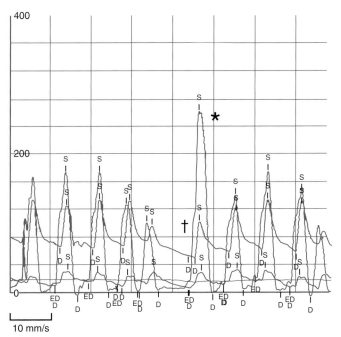

Fig. 4.48 Postextrasystolic potentiation (the Brockenbrough effect). The beat following a premature ventricular contraction (PVC) shows a significant increase in the left ventricular outflow tract (LVOT) gradient *(*)* and a narrowing of the pulse pressure on the aortic (Ao) tracing *(†)*.

These data points provide an advanced measure of hemodynamic conditions associated with acute and chronic cardiac injury (Fig. 4.51) and are now more commonly applied as a method to understand the impact of drug and device therapy on changes in cardiac structure and function.

Invasive Hemodynamics with Exercise and Pharmacologic Challenges

Symptoms associated with cardiovascular disease are often absent at rest and provoked by exertion. For this reason, exercise

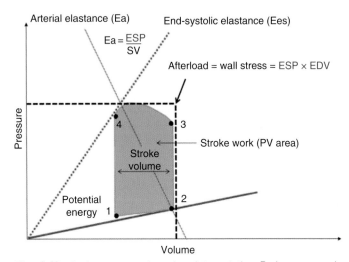

Fig. 4.49 Basic pressure-volume loop interpretation. Each pressure-volume *(PV)* loop represents one cardiac cycle. Beginning at the end of isovolumic relaxation *(1)*, left ventricular (LV) volume increases during diastole *(1 to 2)*. At end diastole *(2)*, LV volume is maximal and isovolumic contraction begins *(2 to 3)*. At the peak of isovolumic contraction, LV pressure exceeds aortic (Ao) pressure and blood begins to eject from the LV into the aorta *(3)*. During this systolic ejection phase, LV volume decreases until Ao pressure exceeds LV pressure and the Ao valve closes, which is known as the end-systolic pressure-volume (ESPV) point *(4)*. Stroke volume *(SV)* is represented by the width of the PV loop as the difference between end-systolic and end-diastolic volumes *(1 to 2)*. Load-independent contractility, also known as *end-systolic elastance (Ees)*, is defined as the maximal slope of the ESPV point under various loading conditions, known as the ESPV relationship (ESPVR). Effective *arterial elastance (Ea)* is defined as the ratio of end-systolic pressure and SV. Under steady-state conditions, optimal LV pump efficiency occurs when Ea:Emax approaches 1. Ea is a component of afterload, which is defined as the resistance to LV ejection throughout systole and can be represented as the product of *end-systolic pressure (ESP)* and *end-diastolic volume (EDV)*. (Courtesy Navin Kapur, MD.)

testing in the cardiac catheterization laboratory can unmask hemodynamic abnormalities that explain exertional symptoms resulting from coronary insufficiency, systolic heart failure, impaired diastolic function, valvular heart disease, and pericardial disease. During exercise, a normal physiologic response includes an increase in oxygen consumption by skeletal muscle and increased oxygen extraction from arterial blood. To match this rising oxygen demand, HR and contractile function increase

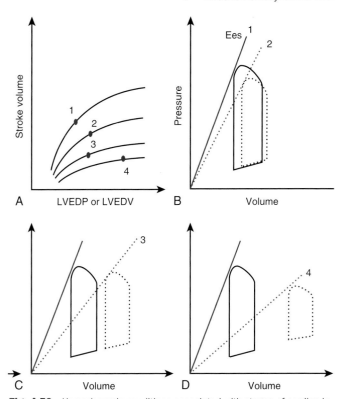

Fig. 4.50 Hemodynamic conditions associated with stages of cardiac injury and treatment profiles. **(A)** Frank-Starling curves represent the relationship (slope) between stroke volume (SV) (or cardiac output [CO]) and left ventricular end-diastolic pressure *(LVEDP)* or left ventricular end-diastolic volume *(LVEDV)*. **(B)** to **(D)** Pressure volume (PV) loops represent the relationship between left ventricular (LV) pressure and LV volume. **(A)** to **(D)** Resting conditions are represented by slope *1* and solid-lined PV loops. Increased LVEDP or LVEDV is associated with increased SV. **(B)** Acute cardiac injury reduces the Frank-Starling curve (slope *2*) and end-systolic elastance *(Ees; dashed line)* and increases end-diastolic volume and pressure. **(C)** Chronic systolic heart failure is associated with a reduced Frank-Starling curve (slope *3*) and Ees. Patients with compensated systolic heart failure may demonstrate preserved SV (width of the PV loop), increased LVEDV, and normal or mildly increased LVEDP. Increased LVEDP or LVEDV are associated with small increases in SV. **(D)** Decompensated systolic heart failure or cardiogenic shock is associated with reduced Ees and a flat Frank-Starling curve (slope *4*). In this condition, increased LVEDP or LVEDV are not associated with increased SV. (Courtesy Navin Kapur, MD.)

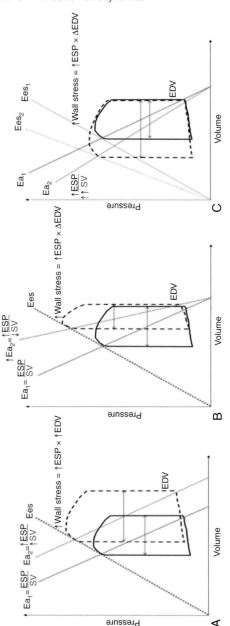

Fig. 4.51 Impact of altered loading conditions on ventricular pressure and volume. **(A)** Increasing preload augments left ventricular (*LV*) stroke volume (*SV*) (*horizontal arrows*) and increases both end-systolic pressure (*ESP*) and end-diastolic volume (*EDV*) without changing elastance at end-systolic elastance (*Ees*) or arterial elastance (*Ea*). The net effect is increased LV wall stress (i.e., afterload) as a result of increased ESP and EDV. **(B)** Vasopressors increase ESP and reduce SV without affecting EDV or Ees. Both Ea and LV wall stress are increased because of elevated ESP. **(C)** Inotropes increase myocardial contractility (Ees), ESP, and SV without affecting EDV. Ea is decreased as a result of increased SV, but LV wall stress is increased because of increased ESP. Inotropes also increase heart rate (HR) and promote myocardial oxygen demand. *Solid lines,* Baseline conditions (*1*); *dashed lines,* modulated conditions (*2*). (Courtesy Navin Kapur, MD.)

resulting in an augmented delivery of oxygen through increased cardiac CO. Assuming that lung function is normal, arterial oxygen saturation remains normal, whereas venous oxygen saturation decreases (because of increased consumption by skeletal muscle). This net increase in the AVO_2 difference correlates with an increase in CO.

Exercise may be categorized as dynamic (bicycle ergometry; repeated arm or leg lifts) or static (isometric hand grip). Both dynamic and static exercise increases HR, CO, and systemic arterial pressure, with either reduced or preserved peripheral vascular resistance. Hemodynamic measurements using either type of exercise should be first made under resting conditions, then during peak exercise. An adequate response to exercise includes:

1. Normal ventilatory responses (i.e., arterial oxygen extraction)
2. Normal HR increases in response to an increase in CO
3. Normal ventricular volume responses (i.e., decrease in cardiac filling pressures because of higher CO and increase in diastolic relaxation)
4. Adequate metabolic substrate use (i.e., appropriate use of glucose as an energy source without generating lactic acid)

Dynamic Exercise

Dynamic exercise measures the ability of the cardiovascular system to supply oxygen in keeping with the demands of the heart. Oxygen consumption and workload increases should be parallel until the maximum oxygen consumption for the patient's size is reached. Dynamic exercise in the catheterization laboratory requires simultaneous right- and left-heart pressure measurements at rest and during exercise. Most commonly, a supine bicycle that allows for quantification of exercise in watts is attached to the catheterization table. The patient's oxygen consumption is also measured and compared with hemodynamic responses. Supine exercise differs from normal upright exercise in several ways: (1) Ventricular volumes are larger when the patient is supine rather than upright; (2) HR and diastolic arterial pressure are higher the patient is upright rather than supine; (3) pulmonary and intracardiac filling pressures are lower when the patient is upright; (4) SV increases by 100% with maximal exercise when the patient is upright and only 20% to 50% when the patient is supine; and (5) both upright and supine exercise is normally associated with increases in left ventricular end-diastolic volume (LVEDV) and decreases in end-systolic volume (ESV), with a concomitant increase in LV ejection fraction. In patients with coronary artery disease (CAD), these findings may not occur.

Methodology for the performance of a dynamic exercise test in the catheterization laboratory can be:

1. With the patient in a supine position, obtain resting hemodynamic data. For supine cycle ergometry, record resting hemodynamics with passive leg elevation before initiation of exercise.

2. Start exercise using either supine cycle ergometry or outstretched arm adduction weight (4 to 5 lb) lifting. Patients performing leg exercise can cycle at 60 rpm, starting at a 20-watt workload and increasing by 10-watt increments in 3-minute stages to maximum tolerated levels.

3. For patients performing arm exercise, increase repetition frequency gradually to subjective fatigue. HR and hemodynamic changes including CO can be recorded after 2 minutes of low-level exercise (20 watts), after 4 minutes, and at peak exercise, and during 1 and 5 minutes of recovery with legs still elevated if using supine cycle ergometry (Borlaug et al. 2010).

Analyze data with respect to change in hemodynamics (i.e., valve gradients), CO, and oxygen consumption. Patients may be unable to exercise because of leg weakness, depressed cardiac function, peripheral vascular disease, or severe deconditioning. These factors may preclude determination of accurate exercise results in the catheterization laboratory and should be considered before undertaking the study.

Measurements of Response to Exercise

1. CO, a useful measurement for studying practically all types of heart disease, predicts a normal response and allows categorization of a given patient's response.

   a. Dexter index: The predicted cardiac index (CI) with exercise is equal to $2.99 \times 0.0059 \times$ measured O_2 consumption index with exercise. The measured CI is the CO divided by body surface area (BSA). The normal Dexter index equals the measured CI with exercise, divided by the predicted CI. The result should be >1.

   b. Normal exercise factor: For every 100-mL/min increase in O_2 consumption with exercise, the CO should increase by at least 600 mL/min. Thus, normal exercise factor = mL/min CO divided by mL/min O_2 consumption ≥ 6.

   Note: Exercise factor is calculated directly from observed changes in CO and O_2 consumption; it is not indexed to BSA.

2. Note appropriate increases in arterial blood pressure and HR.

3. Compute LV volumes (useful in myopathy, coronary, and valvular heart disease). With exercise, changes in LVEDV and LVEDP

(more commonly used) may be plotted against observed changes in some parameter of LV systolic function (SV or SW) to define a modified LV function curve.

4. Recording changes in filling pressures or valvular gradients are useful in myopathy, coronary, and valvular heart disease. In particular, patients with symptoms of heart failure and preserved systolic function demonstrate significant perturbation of diastolic filling pressures and CO with provocative exercise testing.

Isometric Exercise

Isometric exercise consists of skeletal muscle contraction without shortening. In the cardiac catheterization laboratory, isometric exercise is commonly performed using a handgrip with a graded hand dynamometer. Measurements of hemodynamics and ventricular function are obtained during sustained handgrip at a predetermined range (15% to 50% of the maximal handgrip contraction) for a period of 3 to 4 minutes. The size of the involved muscle group is unimportant, provided that maximal voluntary contraction is maintained to increase oxygen demand during the isometric exercise period. Isometric exercise is easy to perform and to repeat and requires inexpensive equipment. It does not involve body motion that may interfere with hemodynamic measurements. An involuntary Valsalva maneuver may occur during unsupervised isometric exercise. Careful monitoring, patient cooperation, and practice in the use of the handgrip dynamometer will minimize false hemodynamic information. In patients with CAD, isometric exercise rarely precipitates ischemia but may induce new LV wall motion abnormalities, a decrease in LV ejection fraction, and an increase in ESV with no change in diastolic volume. SV and CO may decline during isometric exercise. In patients with CHF, HR and systemic pressure may rise appropriately with a fall in SV and CO, resulting in an increase in LVEDV and PA pressure.

Pharmacologic Testing

Treatment with vasoactive drugs is another approach to study cardiovascular function using invasive hemodynamics in the catheterization laboratory. Changes in preload, afterload, and contractility have a profound impact on ventricular function (see Fig. 4.51). Altering loading conditions can be helpful when evaluating patients with valvular heart disease. For example, in patients with stage D2 low-output/low-gradient AS, low-dose dobutamine stress testing with echocardiography or invasive hemodynamic measurements is recommended to help distinguish patients with moderate or severe AS in the setting of primary myocardial dysfunction.

Vasodilator testing with invasive hemodynamics is an important part of the evaluation for patients with primary or secondary pulmonary hypertension. In primary pulmonary hypertension (PPH), vasodilator testing is used to identify potential responders to therapy with calcium channel blockers and to establish prognosis. In these cases, RHC is required for the diagnosis of PPH, which is defined by a mean pulmonary artery pressure (mPAP) >25 mm Hg, a PCWP or LVEDP <15, and a pressure-volume relationship (PVR) >3 Wood units. Vasodilator testing is performed with increasing exposure to vasodilators, such as epoprostenol, adenosine, or inhaled nitric oxide. An acute response to vasodilator testing is defined as a decrease in mPAP by at least 10 mm Hg to an absolute level less than 40 mm Hg without a decrease in CO.

Provocative testing is also an important part of the evaluation for patients with advanced systolic heart failure who are being considered for orthotopic heart transplant. Relative contraindications to OHTx include a PVR ≥5, a pulmonary vascular resistance index (PVRI) ≥6, and a transpulmonary gradient (TPG) ≥16. A PA systolic pressure ≥60 mm Hg and any of the aforementioned elevations in pulmonary pressures are associated with increased mortality after OHTx. For these reasons, RHC is required in all OHTx candidates and should be repeated annually until transplantation or every 3 to 6 months if the patient has documented pulmonary hypertension. Vasodilator testing is performed to evaluate for potentially reversible secondary pulmonary hypertension resulting from pulmonary venous congestion and left-sided heart failure. Vasodilator testing is recommended in potential OHTx candidates with a pulmonary artery systolic pressure (PASP) ≥50, TPG ≥15, or PVR ≥3. Ideally, patients should have a PCWP <25 before testing to limit contribution from ongoing pulmonary venous congestion. Agents (such as nitroglycerine, nipride, inhaled nitric oxide, epoprostenol, or milrinone) are often used to assess pulmonary pressures in patients with advanced heart failure. If acute vasodilator testing fails, patients are often admitted for 48 to 72 hours of continuous infusion therapy with milrinone and diuretics to optimize pulmonary pressures. In select cases, acute mechanical support can be used to reduce left-heart filling pressures and to evaluate reversibility of secondary pulmonary hypertension.

Basic Electrocardiography in the Cardiac Catheterization Laboratory

Basic electrocardiography may be unfamiliar to the new catheterization laboratory technician or nurse. This section reviews the fundamentals of electrocardiography as used in the cardiac catheterization laboratory for monitoring patients.

Cardiac Electrical System

Myocardial contraction is triggered by electrical activity. For every beat on the ECG, a corresponding pressure pulse usually occurs from myocardial contraction. The heart's electrical system has specialized tissue for the origination and transmission of electrical impulses. The normal sequence of electrical activation is shown in Figure 4.52 and consists of: sinoatrial node, atrial tissue, AV node, bundle of His, bundle branches, Purkinje fibers, and ventricular myocardium.

Electrocardiogram

The ECG is a graphic recording of electrical impulses that are generated by depolarization (contraction) and repolarization (relaxation) of the myocardium. The standard ECG includes six limb leads and six chest leads. The proper placement of electrodes for recording the 12-lead ECG is shown in Figures 4.53 and 4.54.

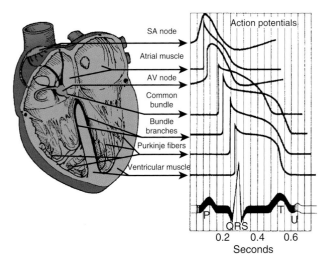

Fig. 4.52 Genesis of electrocardiogram (ECG) and pathways through the heart. *AV,* Atrioventricular; *SA,* sinoatrial. (Modified from the CIBA Collection of Medical Illustrations, Vol. 5.)

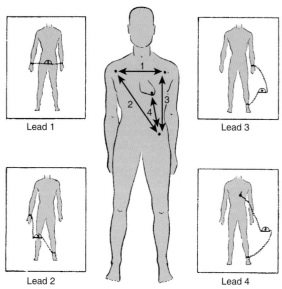

Fig. 4.53 Standard limb leads and one precordial lead. (From Marriott HLJ. *Practical Electrocardiography.* 7th ed. Baltimore: Williams and Wilkins; 1983.)

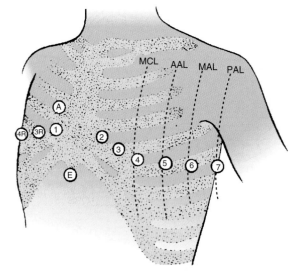

Fig. 4.54 Precordial points for chest leads. (From Marriott HLJ. *Practical Electrocardiography.* 7th ed. Baltimore: Williams and Wilkins; 1983.)

The ECG 12 leads reflect different electrical views of the heart depolarization and repolarization. Typically, certain leads are associated with electrical activity from specific parts of the myocardium. Leads II, III, and aV_F reflect electrical activity in the inferior wall of the heart; leads I and aV_L and chest leads V_5 and V_6, reflect electrical activity in the lateral wall of the heart; chest leads V_1 and V_2, reflect electrical activity in the septal region of the heart; and V_3 and V_4, reflect electrical activity in the anterior wall of the heart. Electrical activity from the posterior wall of the heart is not directly recorded, and ischemia, injury, and necrosis are reflected by depolarization and repolarization abnormalities on the anterior surface of the heart (leads V_1 to V_3). In inferior-posterior myocardial infarction, ST segment, T-wave changes, and Q waves are opposite in direction from an anterior myocardial infarction. During ischemia, instead of ST depression, ST elevation occurs in leads V_1 to V_3. During acute injury, ST depression occurs. During infarction, a pathologic R wave rather than a Q wave occurs in these leads.

Components of the Electrocardiogram

Figures 4.55 and 4.56 show the components of the electrocardiogram.

P Wave

The sinus node is normally the pacemaker of the heart because the cells of the sinus node possess the greatest spontaneous automaticity (ability to initiate an impulse). As the electrical waves travel through the atrium, a P wave is produced on the surface ECG, which represents an electrical contraction (depolarization) of the atria. Mechanical contraction of the atria follows, which contributes to ventricular filling. From the atria, the impulse travels through the AV node and the His-Purkinje system and results in electrical activation of the ventricle. The P–R interval is the interval from the beginning of the P wave to the onset of the QRS and reflects conduction time from the sinoatrial node through the atria, AV node, and His-Purkinje system.

QRS Complex

After the P wave, the next tracing on the ECG usually is the QRS complex, which represents ventricular depolarization. The electrical activation of the ventricle results in myocardial contraction (systole).

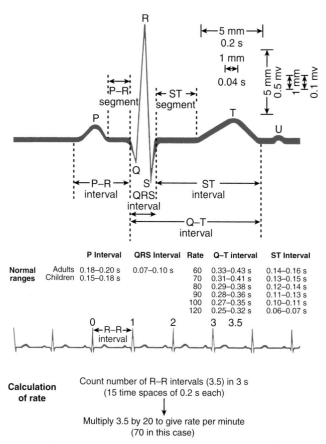

		P Interval	QRS Interval	Rate	Q–T interval	ST Interval
Normal ranges	Adults	0.18–0.20 s	0.07–0.10 s	60	0.33–0.43 s	0.14–0.16 s
	Children	0.15–0.18 s		70	0.31–0.41 s	0.13–0.15 s
				80	0.29–0.38 s	0.12–0.14 s
				90	0.28–0.36 s	0.11–0.13 s
				100	0.27–0.35 s	0.10–0.11 s
				120	0.25–0.32 s	0.06–0.07 s

Calculation of rate

Count number of R–R intervals (3.5) in 3 s
(15 time spaces of 0.2 s each)

↓

Multiply 3.5 by 20 to give rate per minute
(70 in this case)

Fig. 4.55 Components of the electrocardiogram (ECG) demonstrating normal intervals. (Modified from the CIBA Collection of Medical Illustrations, Vol. 5.)

ST Segment and T Wave

The QRS is followed by the ST segment and T wave, which represent repolarization of the ventricles and correspond to myocardial relaxation (diastole). The period from the end of the QRS complex to the beginning of the T wave is called the *ST segment*. Depression or elevation of this segment from baseline may be produced by ischemia (depression) or acute injury (elevation).

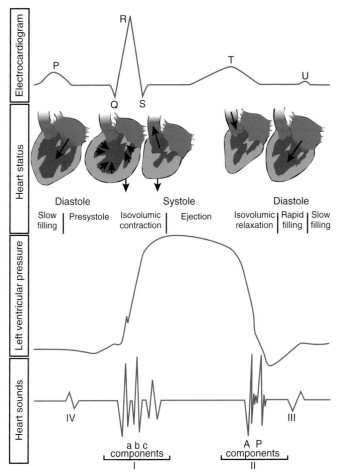

Fig. 4.56 Electrical and mechanical activity sequence of the heart. (Modified from the CIBA Collection of Medical Illustrations, Vol. 5.)

Abnormal Rhythms

During sinus rhythm, there is usually a regular rhythm with a normal sequence of activation. Premature beats are those that occur before the next expected beat. PVCs arise from abnormal electrical activity in the ventricles, and the configuration of a

PVC is usually a wide, bizarre QRS complex (Fig. 4.57A). PVCs that occur from a single focus are referred to as *unifocal PVCs*. PVCs that arise from different areas of the ventricles have different morphologies and are referred to as *multifocal PVCs*. VT is defined as the occurrence of three or more PVCs in a row (see Fig. 4.57B). A PVC may result in a reduced pressure pulse because of the abnormal activation sequence of the ventricle and a lack of coordination between atrial and ventricular contraction. During sustained VT, blood pressure may drop dramatically. Ventricular fibrillation is the most disorganized and hemodynamically compromising arrhythmia that can occur (see Fig. 4.57C). During ventricular fibrillation, electrical activities are chaotic and uncoordinated so that no effective ventricular contraction takes place. As a result, no pulse or CO occurs and clinical death results.

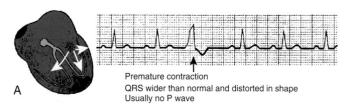

Premature contraction
QRS wider than normal and distorted in shape
Usually no P wave
A

Rate >120: Ventricular tachycardia

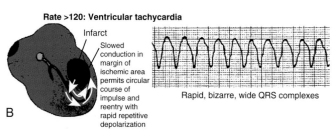

Infarct
Slowed conduction in margin of ischemic area permits circular course of impulse and reentry with rapid repetitive depolarization

Rapid, bizarre, wide QRS complexes
B

Ventricular fibrillation

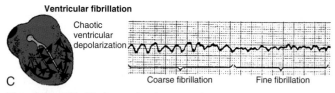

Chaotic ventricular depolarization

Coarse fibrillation   Fine fibrillation
C

Fig. 4.57 **(A)** Rhythm strip demonstrating a premature ventricular contraction (PVC). **(B)** Rhythm strip demonstrating a run of monomorphic ventricular tachycardia. **(C)** Rhythm strip demonstrating ventricular fibrillation. (Modified from Scheidt S. Basic electrocardiography: abnormalities of electrocardiographic patterns. *Clin Symp.* 1984;36:2-32.)

Typical Electrocardiographic Changes Seen in the Cardiac Catheterization Laboratory

Changes in the ST segment and T wave of the ECG may indicate a lack of blood flow to the myocardium through the coronary arteries. This lack of blood flow, referred to as *ischemia,* results in oxygen deprivation to the myocardium. If ischemia persists, tissue damage or death (necrosis) may occur. Dead tissue is referred to as *infarcted tissue.* ECG changes of ischemia and infarction are illustrated in Figures 4.58 and 4.59.

Ischemia can result in many different ECG changes. Ischemia affecting the entire depth of the myocardium (transmural) is detected as deep symmetric T-wave inversion. T-wave inversion can be seen in many conditions unrelated to ischemia (intracranial trauma, pulmonary embolism, and myocardial contusion). Acute T-wave changes occurring during anginal symptoms are specific for ischemia. Horizontal ST depression or downsloping ST segments are the hallmarks of subendocardial ischemia or, in many cases, infarction. Reversible depression favors ischemia, however. Nonspecific ST and T-wave changes and normalization of T-wave abnormalities over findings on a baseline ECG of a pain-free patient are also ECG findings consistent with ischemia.

ECG findings of acute infarction occur in a stepwise temporal fashion. The earliest phase of infarction is associated with tall upright T waves that are referred to as *hyperacute T waves.* These T-wave changes are usually followed shortly by the development of ST-segment elevation in the region where myocardial damage is occurring. Conversely, reciprocal ST-segment depression can be noted in the ECG leads recording from the opposing surface of the heart. In an acute inferior myocardial infarction, ST-segment elevation is present in inferior leads (II, III, and aV_F), whereas ST-segment depression is recorded simultaneously in anterior leads (I, aV_L, V, and V_2). Within hours of the onset of myocardial infarction, Q waves appear as a result of damage that occurs throughout all layers of the myocardium, resulting in a transmural or Q-wave myocardial infarction. Myocardial necrosis results in an electrically silent segment that fails to contribute to the normal electrical forces of the heart during cardiac depolarization. An ECG lead recording over a segment of infarcted myocardium detects electrical forces moving away from the dead region, resulting in a negative Q wave. Infarctions that are confined to the subendocardial region do not result in Q-wave formation and are termed *non–Q-wave* or *non–ST elevation myocardial infarctions.*

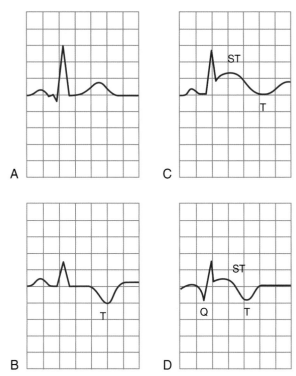

Fig. 4.58 Electrocardiogram (ECG) changes indicative of ischemia, injury, and infarction (necrosis) of the myocardium. **(A)** Normal ECG. **(B)** Ischemia indicated by inversion of the T wave. **(C)** Ischemia and current of injury indicated by T-wave inversion and ST-segment elevation. The ST segment may be elevated above or depressed below the baseline, depending on whether the tracing is from a lead facing toward or away from the infarcted area and depending on whether epicardial or endocardial injury occurs. Epicardial injury causes ST elevation in leads facing the epicardium. **(D)** Ischemia, injury, and myocardial necrosis. The Q wave indicates necrosis of the myocardium. (Reproduced with permission from Urden L, Stacy K, Lough M. Cardiovascular disorders. In: *Priorities in Critical Care Nursing.* St. Louis: Elsevier; 2008.)

Before a cardiac catheterization is performed, obtain a baseline 12-lead ECG; the ECG can be used for comparison if symptoms develop during the procedure. During the catheterization, monitor one to three ECG leads continuously to evaluate for rhythm disturbances or ST-segment and T-wave changes that may indicate alterations in myocardial blood supply. During coronary

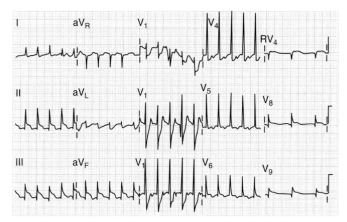

Fig. 4.59 Fifteen-lead electrocardiogram (ECG) with inferior, lateral, posterior, and right ventricular acute myocardial infarction (AMI). The standard 12-lead ECG reveals the typical ST segment elevation (STE) in the inferior and lateral leads as well as ST segment depression (STD) with prominent R wave in the right precordial leads. Posterior AMI is indicated by both the right precordial STD with prominent R wave and the STE in posterior leads V8 and V9. Note that the degree of STE is less pronounced than that seen in the inferior leads because of a relatively longer distance from the posterior epicardium to surface leads. The right ventricular infarction is noted in this case using the simplified approach with only RV4, which demonstrates STE of relatively small magnitude. (Reproduced with permission from Marx et al. Acute coronary syndrome. In: J Marx, R Walls, R Hockberger. *Rosen's Emergency Medicine: Concepts and Clinical Practice.* 8 ed. Philadelphia: Elsevier; 2014.)

angioplasty, balloon inflation temporarily interrupts blood supply to the downstream myocardium. This interruption may result in reversible ischemia and transient ST-segment and T-wave changes. Persistent ST-segment elevation or depression may indicate ongoing ischemia or acute myocardial injury. Other situations encountered in the cardiac catheterization laboratory that may result in ST-segment or T-wave changes include injection of contrast media into a coronary artery, occlusion of an artery with a diagnostic catheter (engaging the ostium of the left main [LM] artery or RCA), improper or incomplete deflation of an angioplasty balloon catheter, dissection of a coronary artery, coronary artery spasm, and blockage of a side branch by the balloon catheter or thrombus.

Rhythm disturbances are encountered commonly during cardiac catheterization. During right-sided heart catheterization, atrial arrhythmias and PVCs can result from catheter irritation. Catheter trauma to the right bundle branch can occur while attempting to float a catheter into the RVOT. Although this situation often results in transient right bundle-branch block, complete heart block can be induced if preexisting left bundle-branch block is present. In this situation, the operator must be prepared to pace the RV until the right bundle recovers its function. PVCs and VT can be induced by LV irritation from the ventriculography catheter or during contrast media injection. Bradycardia, sinus arrest, VT, and ventricular fibrillation can result from contrast media injection of the coronary arteries (especially the RCA). Catheter-induced coronary spasm can result in ventricular fibrillation caused by impaired coronary blood flow. The treatment of catheter-induced arrhythmias is straightforward; removing the catheter from the LV cavity or the coronary artery ostium is often enough to terminate the arrhythmia. VT or fibrillation that persists requires immediate resuscitation. If arrhythmias persist, investigate other underlying causes, including ischemia or electrolyte abnormalities. Prophylactic use of antiarrhythmic drugs to suppress arrhythmias during cardiac catheterization is not recommended. Coronary spasm during cardiac catheterization may be reversed by intra-coronary infusion of nitroglycerin. Bradycardia and sinus node dysfunction can typically be reversed with vigorous coughing or the administration of atropine (see Chapter 3). Knowledge of and experience with the defibrillator in the cardiac catheterization laboratory are crucial (see Chapter 8).

Suggested Readings

Baim DS. *Grossman's Cardiac Catheterization, Angiography, and Intervention.* 7th ed. Philadelphia, PA: Lippincott Williams & Wilkins; 2006.

Brown LK, Kahl FR, Link KM, et al. Anatomic landmarks for use when measuring intra-cardiac pressure with fluid-filled catheters. *Am J Cardiol.* 2000;86:121-124.

Chatterjee K. The Swan-Ganz catheters: past, present, and future: a viewpoint. *Circulation.* 2009;119:147-152.

Cui W, Dai R, Zhang G. A new simplified method for calculating mean mitral pressure gradient. *Catheter Cardiovasc Interv.* 2007;70:754-757.

Doorey AJ, Gakhal M, Pasquale MJ. Utilization of a pressure sensor guide wire to measure bileaflet mechanical valve gradients: hemodynamic and echocardiographic sequelae. *Cath Cardiovasc Interv.* 2006;67:535-540.

Folland ED, Parisi AF, Carbone C. Is peripheral arterial pressure a satisfactory substitute for ascending aortic pressure when measuring aortic valve gradients? *J Am Coll Cardiol.* 1984;4:1207-1212.

Ford LE, Feldman T, Chiu YC, Carroll JD. Hemodynamic resistance as a measure of functional impairment in aortic valvular stenosis. *Circ Res.* 1990;66:1-7.

Goldstein JA, Harada A, Yagi Y, Barzilai B, Cox JL. Hemodynamic importance of systolic ventricular interaction, augmented right atrial contractility and atrioventricular synchrony in acute right ventricular dysfunction. *J Am Coll Cardiol.* 1990;16:181-189.

Gorlin R, Gorlin SG. Hydraulic formula for calculation of stenotic mitral valve, other cardiac valves, and central circulatory shunts. *Am Heart J.* 1951;41:1-29.

Grayburn PA. Assessment of low-gradient aortic stenosis with dobutamine. *Circulation.* 2006;113:604-606.

Hakki AH, Iskandrian AS, Bemis CE, et al. A simplified valve formula for the calculation of stenotic cardiac valve areas. *Circulation.* 1981;63:1050-1055.

Hurrell DG, Nishimura RA, Higano ST, et al. Value of dynamic respiratory changes in left and right ventricular pressures for the diagnosis of constrictive pericarditis. *Circulation.* 1996;93:2007-2013.

Kern MJ, ed. *Hemodynamic Rounds: Interpretation of Cardiac Pathophysiology from Pressure Waveform Analysis.* 3rd ed. New York, NY: Wiley-Liss; 2009.

Kern MJ, Aguirre FV. Interpretation of cardiac pathophysiology from pressure waveform analysis: pericardial compressive hemodynamics, Part I. *Cathet Cardiovasc Diagn.* 1992;25:336-342.

Kern MJ, Aguirre FV. Interpretation of cardiac pathophysiology from pressure waveform analysis: pericardial compressive hemodynamics, Part II. *Cathet Cardiovasc Diagn.* 1992;26:34-40.

Kern MJ, Aguirre FV. Interpretation of cardiac pathophysiology from pressure waveform analysis: pericardial compressive hemodynamics, Part III. *Cathet Cardiovasc Diagn.* 1992;26:152-158.

Nichols WW, O'Rourke MF, eds. Measuring principles of arterial waves. *In McDonald's blood flow in arteries: theoretical, experimental and clinical practices.* 3rd ed. Philadelphia, PA: Lea & Febiger; 1990:143-161.

Nishimura RA, Otto CM, Bonow RO, et al. 2014 AHA/ACC guideline for the management of patients with valvular heart disease: a report of the American College of Cardiology/American Heart Association Task Force on practice guidelines. *J Am Coll Cardiol.* 2014;63(22):e57-e185.

Omran H, Schmidt H, Hackenbroch M, et al. Silent and apparent cerebral embolism after retrograde catheterisation of the aortic valve in valvular stenosis: a prospective, randomised study. *Lancet.* 2003;361:1241-1246.

Parham W, Shafei AE, Rajjoub H, et al. Retrograde left ventricular hemodynamic assessment across bileaflet prosthetic aortic valves: the use of a high-fidelity pressure sensor angioplasty guidewire. *Cath Cardiovasc Interv.* 2003;59:509-513.

Reddy PS, Curtiss EI, Uretsky BF. Spectrum of hemodynamic changes in cardiac tamponade. *Am J Cardiol.* 1990;66:1487-1491.

Sagristà-Sauleda J, Angel J, Sambola A, Alguersuari J, Permanyer-Miralda G, Soler-Soler J. Low-pressure cardiac tamponade: clinical and hemodynamic profile. *Circulation.* 2006;114:945-952.

Peripheral Arterial Disease and Angiography

ANDREW JOHN KLEIN • SUBHASH BANERJEE •
DOUGLAS EMMET DRACHMAN

Peripheral arterial disease (PAD) encompasses a wide spectrum of systemic diseases including atherosclerosis, aneurysms, and vasculitis. The term *peripheral arterial disease* is most often used to describe the result of atherosclerosis in the arteries of the lower extremity, upper extremity, renal, mesenteric, and carotid arterial beds. Patients with PAD are at significant risk of cardiovascular morbidity and mortality, primarily as a result of stroke (from cerebrovascular atherosclerosis) and myocardial infarction (from coronary atherosclerosis). Therefore, the cornerstone of PAD management is the focus on system atherosclerotic risk reduction, including smoking cessation, and control of hypertension (HTN), dyslipidemia, and diabetes. The prevalence of PAD increases with age. Of US individuals aged 40 to 59 years, 3% will develop PAD; in those aged 60 to 69 years, 8% will be affected; and in those above the age of 70 years, 19% will develop PAD.

Similar to angina in the coronary vessel, claudication—the symptom associated with PAD in the lower extremities—is related to the mismatch of blood supply relative to demand because of arterial stenosis or occlusion (Table 5.1). Present in 10% to 30% of patients with PAD, classic intermittent claudication is described as exertion-induced calf, thigh, or leg pain that abates with rest. Some patients (10%–30%) with PAD have atypical symptoms of claudication, perhaps due to altered sensation or neuropathy from diabetes, including leg weakness, a sense that the legs may give out, fatigue, numbness, or paresthesia. Patients with PAD may have significant impairment in quality of life, and functional decline has been shown to occur even in the absence of classic claudication symptoms.

Of note, only 1% to 4% of patients with PAD progress to the point of critical impairment of perfusion of the lower extremity resulting in rest pain, ulceration, or tissue loss. This condition of profound

Table 5.1

Clinical Presentation of Patients with Peripheral Arterial Disease.	
Clinical Presentation of Peripheral Artery Disease	
Asymptomatic	No obvious symptomatic complaint (but usually presents with a functional impairment)
Classic claudication	Lower-extremity symptoms are confined to the muscles with a consistent (reproducible) onset with exercise and relief with rest
Atypical leg pain	Lower-extremity discomfort that is exertional but does not consistently resolve with rest, consistently limited exercise at a reproducible distance, nor meets all Rose questionnaire criteria
Critical limb ischemia	Ischemic rest pain, nonhealing wound, or gangrene
Acute limb ischemia	The "six Ps," defined by the clinical symptoms and signs that suggest potential limb jeopardy: pain, pulselessness, pallor, paresthesias, paralysis, and poikilothermia

hypoperfusion of the lower extremity is termed *critical limb ischemia* (CLI). Individuals who manifest signs of CLI are at significant risk of the need of amputation unless revascularization is performed and pulsatile blood flow is restored to the foot. Patients with CLI may describe a pain, ache, or numbness in the leg at rest, worsened with elevation of the leg, and relieved with dependent positioning, such as dangling the leg off the edge of the bed. CLI patients have poor outcomes, with an estimated 25% risk of one-year mortality, predominantly because of major adverse cardiovascular and cerebrovascular events. The three risk factors that most dramatically increase the risk of CLI are tobacco use, diabetes, and advancing age.

Patients undergoing evaluation for known or suspected cardiovascular disease should also undergo a complete review of systems to assess for all forms of PAD including the following:

· Impaired ambulation as a result of cramping, fatigue, aching, numbness, or pain; it is helpful to note the patient's primary site(s) of discomfort, typically in the buttock, thigh, calf, or foot, along with the relationship of such discomfort to rest or exertion.

· Poorly healing or nonhealing wounds of the legs or feet

· Pain at rest, localized to the lower leg or foot, associated with upright or recumbent positions

Box 5.1 Physical Examination Findings of Peripheral Artery Disease.

Limb examination includes the following:

- Absent or diminished femoral or pedal pulses (especially after exercising the limb)
- Arterial bruits
- Hair loss
- Poor nail growth (brittle nails)
- Dry, scaly, atrophic skin
- Dependent rubor
- Pallor with leg elevation after 1 minute at 60 degrees (normal color should return in 10 to 15 seconds; longer than 40 seconds indicates severe ischemia)
- Ischemic tissue ulceration (punched-out, painful, with little bleeding), gangrene

- Abdominal pain provoked by eating and associated with weight loss
- Family history of a first-degree relative with an abdominal aortic aneurysm (AAA)

Physical examination for PAD may disclose the following (see Box 5.1):

- Diminished or absent pulses (all should be assessed with Doppler if needed)
- Bruits (carotid, supraclavicular, abdominal, and femoral)
- Muscle atrophy
- Dependent rubor and elevation pallor of the feet
- Signs of CLI: hair loss, smooth/shiny skin, dystrophic nails, coolness, pallor, or cyanosis of the foot
- Pulsatile abdominal and/or popliteal masses (aneurysms)

It is important to differentiate between other processes with similar symptoms, such as degenerative disc disease or spinal stenosis (pseudoclaudication). In some instances, patients may describe pain that persists while standing still or that is relieved while continuing to walk or leaning forward. These symptoms are less characteristic of PAD and indicative of pseudoclaudication. Diabetic neuropathy, deconditioning, and muscular strain may be difficult to distinguish from PAD. The two most common classification schemes for PAD are Rutherford and Fontaine classifications (Tables 5.2 and 5.3).

Table 5.2

Rutherford Classification Scheme of Peripheral Arterial Disease.		
Grade	Category	Clinical Symptoms
0	0	Asymptomatic
I	1	Mild claudication
	2	Moderate claudication
	3	Severe claudication
II	4	Ischemic rest pain
	5	Minor tissue loss
III	6	Major tissue loss

Table 5.3

Fontaine Classification Scheme of Peripheral Arterial Disease.	
Stage	Clinical Symptoms
I	Asymptomatic
IIa	Mild claudication
IIb	Moderate to severe claudication
III	Rest pain
IV	Ulcer or gangrene

Noninvasive Diagnostic Testing

With a class I indication in the Peripheral Artery Disease guidelines, the most useful and cost-effective test to diagnose PAD is the ankle-brachial index (ABI). The study is performed by applying a blood pressure (BP) cuff to the calf, then measuring BP at the ankle using a continuous-wave Doppler probe. Ankle pressures at the dorsalis pedis and posterior tibial artery (PTA) pressures are recorded. The process is then repeated with the cuff on the biceps and the Doppler on the brachial artery, quantifying the brachial pressure. The ABI is then calculated by dividing the higher ankle pressure by the higher of the two brachial pressures. A normal ABI is between 0.9 and 1.4. An ABI after exercise is very useful for those patients who have classic symptoms of claudication and/or decreased common femoral pulses and a normal ABI at rest. Resting ABI may be insensitive for detecting mild aortoiliac disease and is not designed to define the degree of functional limitation. In some patients (e.g., those with end-stage renal disease [ESRD] or diabetes mellitus [DM]) with secondary medial calcification, infrapopliteal vessels may become noncompressible. The noncompressible nature may limit the accuracy of the ABI and may lead to the elevated ankle pressure and corresponds to an ABI >1.4. In these cases, a toe-brachial index (TBI) may be considered. The magnitude of ABI reduction has been linked to overall mortality in a U-shaped distribution, with increasing mortality associated with ABIs <1.0 and >1.4. An abnormal ABI in patients with established coronary artery disease (CAD) and DM is associated with an incremental risk of adverse cardiovascular outcomes.

Another useful noninvasive vascular assessment is the segmental limb pressure (SLP) evaluation, measuring blood pressure at the thigh, calf, ankle, transmetatarsal, and digits. Identifying the location in the leg where BP abruptly diminishes relative to the brachial pressure determines the corresponding level of arterial obstruction. Additionally, an arterial pressure gradient of >20 mm Hg implies significant obstructive disease. Analogous and often obtained simultaneously, pulse volume recordings (PVRs) may also aid in the determination of arterial stenosis severity and location. SLPs record a pressure and PVRs record a noninvasive arterial waveform at the same anatomic levels. Analyzing the amplitude and morphology of the arterial waveform provides insight into the presence and severity of obstruction.

Limb Morbidity and Patient Mortality

The natural history of PAD with respect to limb morbidity and patient morbidity/mortality varies among patients with and without claudication. Most patients with claudication (~70%) will have constant stable symptoms for the next 5 years; approximately 10% to 30% will report progressive worsening of symptoms; and few (2% to 4%) will progress to CLI. In contrast, morbidity/mortality is much greater. In individuals with PAD who develops claudication after the age of 55 years, there is a 5-year mortality of 25% to 30%, with the majority (75%) of these deaths attributed to cardiovascular causes. Another 20% of these patients will suffer a nonfatal cardiovascular event. In contrast, in CLI patients there is a primary amputation rate of between 10% to 40%, mortality of 20% at 1 year, 40% to 70% at 5 years, and 80% to 95% at 10 years, mainly from cardiovascular causes.

Noninvasive Imaging for Anatomic Assessment

There are four methods that are commonly used to delineate arterial anatomy, each of which has advantages and disadvantages.

These include (1) duplex ultrasound, (2) computed tomography angiography (CTA), (3) magnetic resonance angiography (MRA), and (4) invasive angiography and digital subtraction angiography (DSA).

Duplex ultrasound is useful to diagnose the anatomic location and degree of stenosis. Duplex is frequently used to evaluate infrainguinal vessels and can provide a detailed image of stenosis including the anatomic location within the leg. Renal, iliac, and infrapopliteal vessels can also be imaged using duplex ultrasound, but this is often time-consuming, technique-dependent, and may not be feasible in some patients because of obese habitus or bowel gas obscuring vascular structures in the abdomen and pelvis. Duplex ultrasound is recommended for routine surveillance after femoral-popliteal or femoral-tibial/pedal bypass.

CTA of the extremities may be used to diagnose anatomic location and presence of significant stenosis in patients with lower-extremity, renal, upper-extremity, and carotid stenosis. CTA may be considered as a substitute for MRA for those patients with contraindications to MRA (claustrophobia or presence of pacemaker/implantable cardioverter defibrillator). CTA is noninvasive but confers some risk of contrast-induced nephropathy and poses a small risk of radiation exposure to the patient. CTA imaging of the infrapopliteal vasculature may have limited resolution, and heavy calcification of the vessels may obscure luminal stenosis, making accurate interpretation challenging.

MRA may provide detailed anatomic location and degree of arterial stenosis without the use of radiation or iodinated contrast. MRA most commonly requires the intravenous administration of gadolinium as a contrast agent, which is contraindicated in patients with an estimated glomerular filtration rate (eGFR) <60 ml/min, because of the associate risk of nephrogenic systemic fibrosis (NSF) and nephrogenic fibrosing dermopathy. Alternative, newer imaging agents, including ferumoxytol (Feraheme), may be considered in patients with chronic kidney disease (CKD). MRA may sometimes overestimate the severity of arterial stenosis.

Invasive vascular angiography has long been considered the gold standard for anatomic imaging. Angiography inherently provides a two-dimensional (2D) image of a three-dimensional (3D) structure. In some instances, eccentric lesions may require multiple angiographic views to determine stenosis severity. Like CTA, invasive angiography requires the use of iodinated contrast, and therefore confers a risk of contrast-induced nephropathy (CIN), particularly in individuals with CKD. To reduce the contrast load and risk of CIN, a 50/50 mixture of contrast and saline may be used for most peripheral angiography. If the use of iodinated contrast is not clinically feasible, gadolinium or CO_2 angiography may also be considered. When angiography identifies an arterial stenosis of indeterminate severity, assessing a pressure gradient has been considered as a potential surrogate for the physiologic significance of a lesion. Some operators may use a narrow caliber (i.e., 4 F) end-hole catheter to measure a translesional pressure gradient; others may prefer the use of a 0.014-inch pressure wire. Assessment of the translesional pressure gradient at rest or following the induction of hyperemia with the administration of peripheral vasodilating medications may also elucidate the hemodynamic impact—and potentially the clinical relevance—of an arterial stenosis. Intravascular ultrasound (IVUS) or optical coherence tomographic imaging may provide additional, detailed anatomic data that may help define the extent and severity of arterial disease and morphologic characteristics such as the presence of thrombus or calcium.

DSA may provide better resolution of vascular structures than conventional angiography by eliminating adjacent nonvascular elements from the image acquired. Since the peripheral arteries are relatively static structures, DSA is technically feasible in this distribution, although the patient may need to stop breathing during image acquisition of vascular structures in the thorax and in the abdomen/pelvis to reduce the impact of motion artifact.

Endovascular Revascularization

Overview

Arterial revascularization, whether performed with surgical or endovascular techniques, is reserved for patients who experience lifestyle-limiting symptoms of claudication, rest pain, or tissue loss. Individuals who present with claudication should embark on a supervised exercise program and should receive guideline-directed medical therapy, with consideration of pharmacotherapy for claudication (cilostazol) before being considered for arterial revascularization. In individuals who present with symptoms caused by aortoiliac disease, endovascular revascularization may be considered a first-line therapeutic option. Current guidelines recommend endovascular procedures for individuals with a vocational or lifestyle-limiting disability as a result of intermittent claudication, when clinical features suggest a reasonable likelihood of symptomatic improvement with endovascular intervention and (1) there has been an inadequate response to exercise or pharmacological therapy and/or (2) there is a very favorable risk-benefit ratio (e.g., focal aortoiliac occlusive disease). Revascularization, however, is not a substitute for guideline-directed medical therapy, which reduces cardiovascular morbidity and mortality. Moreover, outcomes from two recent randomized clinical trials indicate that the combination of endovascular therapy (EVT) plus supervised exercise therapy (SET) may provide the best functional outcomes for individuals with lifestyle-limiting claudication.

In individuals who present with CLI, the potential benefit for revascularization is most pronounced. In patients with ankle pressures <40 mm Hg and toe pressures <30 mm Hg, ulcerations will not heal without revascularization: the metabolic requirements for wound healing and for the prevention of infection are much higher than the basal state required to maintain intact skin integrity without ulceration. Without revascularization, loss of skin integrity increases risk of infection, gangrene, and tissue loss.

There is a prevailing practice that emphasizes restoration of blood flow to the angiosome (the infrapopliteal vessel that directly perfuses the affected region of the foot) as a more effective strategy than restoring blood flow indirectly through a different vessel. In some instances, it is not possible to provide direct in-line flow; supplying collateral flow from the peroneal artery or via the metatarsal arch may still be effective, but meticulous observation is critical for wound-healing success.

For patients with CLI, revascularization is an essential element for limb salvage. The choice of whether to pursue an endovascular or surgical approach depends on patient- and institution-specific features. In addition, the revascularization approach may depend on the technique that will provide the most robust straight-line flow, incurring the lowest risk for the patient. Patient comorbidities, anatomic features, presence of surgical targets and venous conduit, physician preference, and overall candidacy for safe performance and recovery from surgery must all be considered in this decision. Endovascular options are minimally invasive and, when compared with surgery, confer a lower risk of perioperative stress and adverse cardiovascular events. Endovascular therapy has historically been plagued by high restenosis rates. Restenosis may have limited clinical impact, however, if the vessel stays open long enough to promote wound healing. In the Bypass versus Angioplasty in Severe Ischemia of the Leg (BASIL) trial, there was no difference in amputation-free survival for up to 3 years among patients treated with an endovascular-first (as compared with a surgical-first) strategy at 3 years. Although surgical bypass has been long held as the gold standard treatment for patients with CLI, endovascular approaches may emerge dominant in the coming decade. Currently, the choice of revascularization approach remains patient and institution specific.

Endovascular therapy offers several distinct advantages over surgical revascularization, including (1) reduced morbidity and mortality (same-day or short-stay procedure), (2) ease of repeat procedure if needed, (3) future surgery not precluded in optimal outcomes, (4) general anesthesia unnecessary, and (5) decreased infection rates. A small arteriotomy, compared with the large wound from an open surgical approach, confers a lower risk of infection and typically permits return to normal activity within 24 to 48 hours after an uncomplicated procedure. This has led to widespread adoption of an endovascular-first approach, depending on the anatomical substrate and patient.

Endovascular therapy, however, is associated with risk for vascular injury (vascular dissection, perforation, abrupt closure, or thrombosis), bleeding (access, retroperitoneal, and potentially gastrointestinal from dual antiplatelet therapy), and exposure to radiation and nephrotoxic contrast. In addition, depending on the vascular bed, endovascular therapy has a high rate of restenosis and need for repeat revascularization. The Trans-Atlantic Inter-Society Consensus (TASC II) document provides anatomic and lesion guidance on which revascularization strategy may be most efficacious for a particular lesion. In general, TASC A and B lesions are felt to be amenable to endovascular therapy, whereas more complex lesions such as long occlusions (TASC C and D) might be better served with surgical revascularization. This document, however, was generated before the advent of technologies that, in experienced hands, permit successful crossing and treatment of even the most complex lesions using advanced endovascular techniques and is generally considered outdated. Each vascular bed (Fig. 5.1) and the corresponding angiographic techniques and data for revascularization, are reviewed in detail in the following sections.

Appropriate Use Criteria (AUC)

In 2014, The Society for Cardiovascular Angiography and Interventions (SCAI) developed the first expert consensus document establishing appropriate use of peripheral vascular intervention for the renal, iliac, femoropopliteal, and infrapopliteal arterial beds. This document was updated in 2017 and provides operators guidance for when and how to revascularize lesions in these territories. As has become customary when considering coronary intervention in the era of AUC documents, operators considering peripheral intervention should be familiar with the appropriate indications for revascularization and should document the rationale for considering intervention in detail.

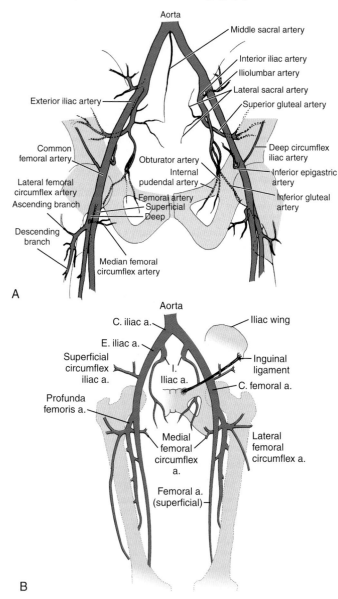

Fig. 5.1 Schematic diagram of the iliac **(A)** and femoral **(B)** arterial systems. a., Artery; *C.*, common; *E.*, exterior.

Iliac Interventions

As noted, the TASC classification was generated for aortoiliac lesions (Fig. 5.2), with general recommendations for an endovascular approach for TASC A and B lesions and a surgical approach for the more complex TASC C and D lesions. This classification system provides a simple schema to categorize lesion complexity. The evolution of endovascular technology and outcome data, however, has rendered the guidelines less relevant to contemporary clinical practice. In fact, recent expert consensus documents from the SCAI advocates for an endovascular-first approach to most aortoiliac lesions, with surgery recommended for endovascular failures. Current American College of Cardiology/American Heart Association (ACC/AHA) guidelines recommend endovascular revascularization of aortoiliac disease when a favorable risk-benefit ratio is present, depending on patient- and lesion-specific determinants.

In contemporary practice, most iliac occlusions and complex lesions can be treated with endovascular technique with high procedural success rates and excellent long-term patency. Two recent meta-analyses confirmed that technical success rates for aortoiliac intervention exceed 90%, and confer 4- to 5-year primary patency rates of 60% to 86%, secondary patency rates of 80% to 98%, and limb salvage rates of 98%.

Aortoiliac lesions are generally treated with stent insertion, since stenting may minimize vessel recoil and prevent abrupt occlusion. However, a provisional stenting strategy may also be used in simple lesions. This approach has been shown to be safe and cost-effective over a 5-year period. The current ACC/AHA guideline supports primary stenting over provisional stenting of the common and external iliac arteries with a class-I recommendation (level of evidence B) and should likely be considered at the preferred approach in complex iliac lesions.

Technical Details

When considering revascularization for lower extremity PAD, using preprocedural noninvasive imaging may aid planning a favorable access and treatment strategy for these lesions. The preferred site for arterial access depends on several factors, including (1) location of the target lesion(s), (2) presence/absence of any lesions in the contralateral iliac artery, (3) need to treat infrainguinal vessels, (4) presence of common femoral artery (CFA) disease, (5) angulation of the aortoiliac bifurcation, (6) severity of target lesion (occluded or not), and (7) availability of radial or brachial artery access. When treating unilateral disease within the proximal iliac system (e.g., the common iliac artery), ipsilateral

Type-A lesions

- Unilateral or bilateral stenosis of CIA
- Unilateral or bilateral single short (≤3 cm) stenosis of EIA

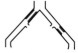

Type-B lesions

- Short (≤3 cm) stenosis of infrarenal aorta
- Unilateral CIA occlusion
- Single or multiple stenosis totaling 3 to 10 cm involving the EIA, not extending into the CFA
- Unilateral EIA occlusion not involving the origins of internal iliac or CFA

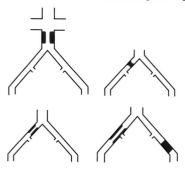

Type-C lesions

- Bilateral CIA occlusions
- Bilateral EIA stenosis 3 to 10 cm long, not extending into the CFA
- Unilateral EIA stenosis extending into the CFA
- Unilateral EIA occlusion that involves the origins of internal iliac and/or CFA
- Heavily calcified unilateral EIA occlusion with or without involvement of origins of internal iliac and/or CFA

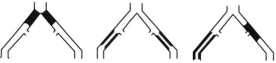

Fig. 5.2 Trans-Atlantic Inter-Society Consensus (TASC) classification of aortoiliac lesions. *AAA,* Abdominal aortic aneurysm; *CFA,* common femoral artery; *CIA,* common iliac artery; *EIA,* external iliac artery. (Reproduced with permission from Norgren L, Hiatt WR, Dormandy JA, et al. Inter-society consensus for the management of PAD [TASC II]. *J Vasc Surg.* 2007;45[suppl S]:S5-S67.)

Type-D lesions

- Infrarenal aortoiliac occlusion
- Diffuse disease involving the aorta and both iliac arteries requiring treatment
- Diffuse multiple stenosis involving the unilateral CIA, EIA, and CFA
- Unilateral occlusions of both CIA and EIA
- Bilateral occlusions of EIA
- Iliac stenosis in patients with AAA requiring treatment and not amenable to endograft placement or other lesions requiring open aortic or iliac surgery

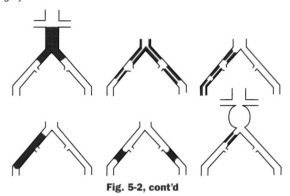

Fig. 5-2, cont'd

access is preferable to permit direct delivery of equipment. A contralateral approach is possible but will often be met with challenges of establishing adequate coaxial support to deliver a balloon/stent to a lesion that is proximal in the common iliac artery.

In contrast, if the target lesion is in the distal common or external iliac artery, contralateral access may be preferred, particularly in situations where external iliac disease extends distally to the common femoral region, compromising ipsilateral sheath placement. If entire reconstruction of the aortoiliac bifurcation is required, bilateral femoral access permits simultaneous bilateral iliac stent placement and kissing balloon postdilatation. More than one access site (a second site could be femoral or brachial/ radial) may be required to approach chronic total occlusions (CTOs) (Fig. 5.3) in order to facilitate both antegrade and retrograde crossing and for better visualization of the extent of occlusion. Initial arterial access via the radial or brachial artery is also an attractive option, but lesion location and equipment length should be taken into account during treatment planning.

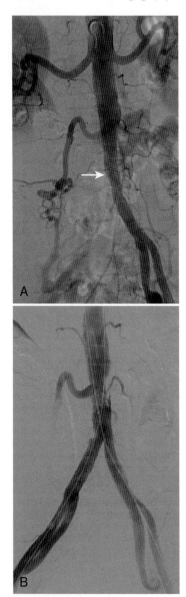

Fig. 5.3 **(A)** Totally occluded right common iliac artery (origin indicated by *white arrow*). **(B)** Right iliac artery after successful angioplasty and stenting.

Table 5.4

Most Useful Angiographic Views for Different Vascular Territories.	
Artery or Vascular Territory	**Angiographic View (Degrees)**
Aortic arch	30 to 60 LAO (with slight cranial angulation)
Brachiocephalic vessels (origin)	30 to 60 LAO
Subclavian	AP, ipsilateral oblique with caudal angulation
Vertebral origin	AP, ipsilateral oblique with cranial angulation
Carotid extracranial	Lateral, AP, ipsilateral, 45 oblique
Renal arteries (origin)	AP, 5 to 25 LAO
Mesenteric arteries (origin)	Lateral or steep RAO
Iliac artery	Contralateral, 20 to 45 oblique
CFA, SFA, and PFA arteries	Ipsilateral, 30 to 60 oblique
Femoropopliteal	AP, ipsilateral, 20 to 30 oblique
Infrapopliteal trifurcation and runoff	AP

AP, Anteroposterior; *CFA,* common femoral artery; *LAO,* left anterior oblique; *PFA,* profunda femoral artery; *RAO,* right anterior oblique; *SFA,* superficial femoral artery.

Angiographic Technique

Initial DSA angiography (with a breath hold) of the iliac arteries should be performed in the contralateral oblique, using either a pigtail or omniflush catheter with or without power injection (Table 5.4). Contralateral oblique imaging opens up the common iliac and bifurcation into the external and internal iliac arteries. In the setting of iliac occlusions, the pigtail should be proximal enough in the aorta (i.e., near the level of L4 to L5) to opacify all of the lumbar vessels that typically provide collaterals through various branches. The imaging should be engaged long enough to permit the outflow from collateral vessel and determine whether the occlusion involves the CFA and/or lateral circumflex iliac vessel. If the CFA is not involved and the lateral circumflex iliac or another side branch is patent, ipsilateral access can often be obtained under roadmap function with use of these side branches for wiring to provide enough support to place a sheath. This then permits a retrograde approach that affords greater support for advancement of interventional equipment.

Stent Types

Two types of stents are available for endovascular interventions. Balloon-expandable (BE) stents offer greater precision of placement and superior radial strength; they are therefore better suited for calcified vessels but may be less desirable in segments that involve excessive tortuosity. They are often used to treat common iliac lesions and with aortoiliac kissing stents. Self-expanding (SE) stents, characterized by their flexibility and ability to conform to varying vessel diameters, are the optimal choice for vessel size mismatch across the lesion. These stents have less radial strength compared with BE stents, but in vascular segments inherently prone to flexion or extrinsic compression or in tortuous vessels, the superior flexibility of SE stents may outweigh the compromise in terms of radial strength. Recent data comparing these two stent types in the aortoiliac arterial bed suggest that SE stents may have an enhanced patency rate over BE. There has been debate on whether stent architecture or composition (i.e., nitinol vs. stainless steel) has any effect on restenosis rates. However, the CT Perfusion to Predict Reponse to Recanalization in Ischemic Stroke Project (CRISP) trial failed to show any differences in clinical outcomes 1 year between nitinol (S.M.A.R.T. Nitinol Stent System; Cordis Corporation, Miami Lakes, FL) and stainless steel (Wallstent, Boston Scientific Corp., Watertown, MA) iliac artery SE stents.

Polytetrafluoroethylene (PTFE)-covered stents are also available in BE and SE formats. Whereas covered stents were previously reserved for the treatment of iliac aneurysms, arteriovenous (AV) fistulae, and iatrogenic perforations, recent studies suggest that covered stents may be used for primary treatment of stenotic lesions as well. The comparison of covered versus bare expandable stents (Covered versus Balloon Expandable Stent Trial [COBEST]) for the treatment of aortoiliac occlusive disease trial demonstrated a significantly lower restenosis rate with the use of the covered stent when compared with bare-metal stents. In a subgroup analysis of these data, the outcomes from treatment of TASC C and D lesions with covered stents were superior to those treated with bare-metal stents, although in part this finding might be attributed to operator confidence in providing higher-pressure balloon postdilatation following covered-stent placement, resulting in greater luminal gain. One disadvantage of expanded PTFE (ePTFE)-covered stents, however, is the slightly reduced deliverability because of the scaffold stiffness and the need for larger sheaths, although this has recently changed with 6-F compatible covered stents. PTFE-covered stents may also occlude any spanned side braches, including major vessels, such as the internal iliac artery and/or major collaterals, potentially obliterating collateral flow in the event of stent occlusion.

Anticoagulation

Unfractionated heparin (UFH) is most commonly used for intraprocedural anticoagulation during aortoiliac intervention and offers the benefit of acute reversibility (using protamine sulfate) in the event of serious adverse bleeding events, such as iliac perforation. Direct thrombin inhibitors, such as bivalirudin, have been used for peripheral intervention but are more costly, are irreversible, and have not achieved widespread adoption.

Procedural Techniques

After selection of the vascular access site and placement of a sheath (4 to 8 F or larger), wiring techniques are similar to other interventional procedures. It is imperative that operators be familiar with equipment compatibility among stents, balloons, crossing catheters, and covered stents, because they may use 0.035-, 0.018-, and 0.014-inch systems. For the greatest degree of support and trackability, especially if vessel tortuosity or calcification is encountered, 0.035-inch wires may provide the best option. Small profile systems, compatible with 4-F to 6-F sheaths, are available for balloon and stent treatment of most aortoiliac lesions, if desired. In clinical situations where the potential for vessel perforation is a concern, it may be advisable to use a 7-F to 8-F sheath system, to permit the delivery of PTFE-covered stents. Larger caliber sheaths are often required for the delivery of specialized crossing and reentry catheters, which may be necessary to complete complex interventions in totally occluded vessels, and may improve procedural success rates to more than 90%.

Complications of Iliac Endovascular Intervention

Although major complications during iliac interventional procedures are rare, the interventional team must always be vigilant for evidence of contrast reaction, arterial perforation, dissection, embolization, and access site complications. The two most dangerous complications are distal embolization (DE) and iliac perforation. DE has been reported to occur between 0.4% and 9% and may be treated with mechanical or rheolytic thrombectomy, balloon inflation, stent placement, and, occasionally, surgical embolectomy.

One of the most acutely potentially catastrophic complications is iliac artery perforation or rupture, the incidence of which ranges from 0.5% to 3%. As proceduralists continue to address increasingly complex lesions, the risk of major complications such as iliac perforation and rupture correspondingly increases. During balloon inflations, patients should be monitored for the report of pain, especially during postdilatation of stents, since pain may indicate stretching of the adventitia, which confers the potential risk of vessel rupture. Given the fact that the retroperitoneal space may rapidly expand with blood if the iliac artery is ruptured, which can lead to exsanguination and potentially fatal consequences, the operator must keep at the ready a full complement of covered stents and aortic occlusion balloons during any iliac intervention. Special attention should also be paid to sheath and guidewire compatibility of occlusion balloons and covered stents. All iCAST covered stents are 7-F sheath compatible. Viabahn covered stents: 7 to 8 mm: require 8-F sheath; 9 mm: 9 F; 10 to 11 mm: 11F; and 13 mm: 12 F compatible. Coda balloon need a14-F sheath and Tyshak balloons 18 to 25 mm, a minimum 9-F sheath.

Perforation may result from manipulation of guidewires, reentry devices, crossing catheters, or during balloon/stent deployment. The report of acute low back or abdominal pain, especially during balloon inflation, should indicate to the operator the potential for impending vessel rupture. If there is a concern for rupture, careful attention should be paid to the arterial pressure waveform. If a precipitous drop in pressure occurs, an angioplasty balloon should be inflated proximal to the possible site of rupture to tamponade the bleeding. Once tamponade is attained, an appropriately sized covered stent should be considered. There is rarely time to proceed with open surgical repair in these patients, but if the patient is stable, this may be also considered if technically necessary.

Femoropopliteal Interventions

Compared with intervention in the aortoiliac distribution, the outcomes following endovascular treatment of the femoropopliteal segment have considerably higher rates of restenosis. There are several pathophysiologic differences that explain this discrepancy in outcomes: (1) Femoropopliteal atherosclerosis is often more diffuse, heavily calcified, or totally occluded than are lesions in the iliac segments; (2) the femoropopliteal segment is uniquely exposed to major extrinsic forces, including repetitive flexion, torsion, and compression along its length; and (3) the engineering challenge is great for creating a scaffold or platform that can withstand the biologic nature and physical forces unique to the femoropopliteal segment.

In the TASC II document (Box 5.2), the complexity of femoropopliteal disease is categorized as A, B, C, or D, reflecting severity on the basis of lesion length, presence of total occlusion, and territory involved. Although more severe TASC C and D lesions have historically been considered best amenable to surgical revascularization, recent advances in endovascular technique

Box 5.2 Trans-Atlantic Inter-Society Consensus Classification of Femoropopliteal Lesions.

Type-A Femoropopliteal Lesions

- Single stenosis <10 cm in length
- Single occlusion <5 cm in length

Type-B Femoropopliteal Lesions

- Multiple lesions (stenosis or occlusions), each <5 cm
- Single stenosis or occlusion, <15 cm, not involving the infrageniculate popliteal artery
- Single or multiple lesions in the absence of continuous tibial vessels to improve inflow for a distal bypass
- Heavily calcified occlusion <5 cm in length
- Single popliteal stenosis

Type-C Femoropopliteal Lesions

- Multiple stenosis or occlusions totaling >15 cm with or without heavy calcification
- Recurrent stenosis or occlusions that need treatment after two endovascular interventions

Type-D Femoropopliteal Lesions

- Chronic total occlusions of CFA or SFA (>20 cm, involving the popliteal artery)
- Chronic total occlusion of popliteal artery and proximal trifurcation vessels

Norgren L, Hiatt WR, Dormandy JA, et al: Inter-society consensus for the management of peripheral arterial disease (TASC II). *J Vasc Surg.* 2007;45[suppl S]:S5-S67.

CFA, Common femoral artery; *SFA,* superficial femoral artery.

and device technology have dramatically improved acute procedural success rates with endovascular treatment. Despite these advances, however, the long-term patency following endovascular therapy remains suboptimal. Appropriate treatment decisions for disease in the femoropopliteal territory require careful consideration of patient, lesion, and operator-specific factors. Patient factors include age, systemic comorbidity, availability of endogenous conduit, and whether disease is associated with CLI versus claudication. Important anatomic features include extent of disease, involvement of points of flexion less amenable to stent treatment and historically preserved for bypass anastomosis (common femoral and popliteal arteries), and presence of calcification. Operator experience with advanced techniques may also play an important role in procedural outcomes and durability.

Endovascular therapy of the femoropopliteal segment has historically been hampered by high rates of restenosis. Balloon angioplasty has been associated with a 63% rate of restenosis after 1 year. BE stents, subject to extrinsic compression and chronic deformation, are not mechanically suitable for use in the femoropopliteal segment and should be reserved for rare occasions where other modalities have failed. Nitinol SE stents, with shape memory and flexibility, have enjoyed greater success in the femoropopliteal segment.

As demonstrated in the coronary arteries, locally delivered antirestenotic therapy also reduces restenosis following treatment of the femoropopliteal segment. In the Zilver PTX trial, 2-year primary patency was 83.4% following paclitaxel-eluting stent deployment compared with 64.1% following bare-metal stent use. The polymer coated SE paclitaxel-eluting stent has recently been shown to be noninferior for the primary endpoint of 1-year primary patency to the Zilver PTX, that is polymer free. Drug-coated balloons have revolutionized femoropopliteal revascularization with the ability to deliver antirestenotic therapy without the need to implant a permanent metal scaffold. The patency rates of DCBs versus PTA alone mark an exceptional improvement in durability, with a recently published 65% patency following DCB at 36 months versus <40% using conventional PTA.

Stent-graft systems (ePTFE covered SE stents) may be useful in the treatment of stenosis, iatrogenic perforation, and aneurysmal disease in the femoropopliteal segment. Edge restenosis within the graft may portend future graft thrombosis. Although the Viabahn stent graft is US Food and Drug Administration (FDA) approved for the treatment of superficial femoral artery (SFA) lesions, comparative studies with bare-metal stents in complex TASC C and D have not shown an advantage to Viabahn use over nitinol stents at 3 years.

Technologies, such as atherectomy, cryoplasty, cutting balloon, and laser atherectomy, may offer niche-specific advantages to managing particular femoropopliteal lesions, but no randomized comparative data exist that demonstrate improved outcomes compared with conventional balloon angioplasty and stenting. The one setting where laser atherectomy has been shown to be effective and is FDA approved is in the arena of femoropopliteal in-stent restenosis.

Atherectomy removes obstructive plaque and can be used in conjunction with angioplasty and stenting or as a stand-alone technique (Figs. 5.4, 5.5, and 5.6). Atherectomy devices can be divided into either excisional (removal of plaque) or ablative (disintegration or fragmentation of plaque). These devices provide the opportunity to reduce plaque volume, which may provide advantages in traditional no-stent zones (common femoral and popliteal

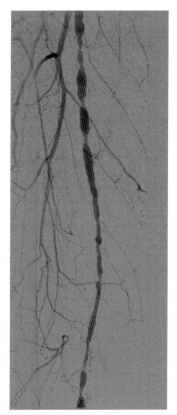

Fig. 5.4 Right superficial femoral artery (SFA) with significant serial stenosis.

artery) (Figs. 5.7 and 5.8), in lesions with bulky plaque (optimization of stent and/or balloon expansion), and in complex lesions involving the bifurcation of vessels where plaque prolapse may compromise flow to an adjacent segment.

In the femoropopliteal segment, there are a number of potential devices that can be used to revascularize the vessel and vary from balloon angioplasty to drug-coated stents. The myriad of devices is often overwhelming while comparative-effectiveness data are generally lacking. Operators should be aware of the risks and benefits of each device available and refer to recently published consensus data to facilitate selecting the appropriate device and approach.

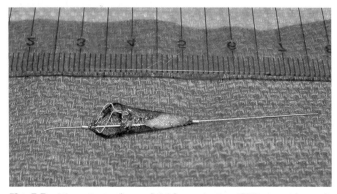

Fig. 5.5 Atherectomy of superficial femoral artery (SFA) plaque (some is caught in the distal protection device/basket).

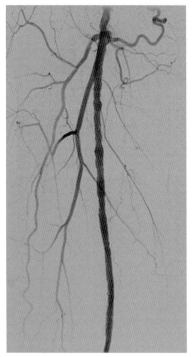

Fig. 5.6 Postatherectomy angiogram of right superficial femoral artery (SFA).

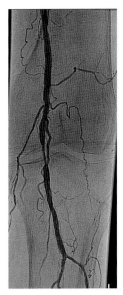

Fig. 5.7 Popliteal artery stenosis.

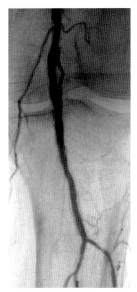

Fig. 5.8 Postangioplasty angiogram of popliteal artery.

Table 5.5

Arterial Access for Different Vascular Territories.	
Vascular Access	**Target Vessel(s) to Revascularize**
Retrograde CFA	Aortic arch vessels, renal, and mesenteric arteries
Contralateral CFA	Contralateral iliacs, CFA, PFA, SFA, and popliteal arteries
Antegrade CFA	Mid to distal femoral, popliteal, and infrapopliteal
Brachial/radial artery	Renal (caudal takeoff), mesenteric, and iliac arteries
Retrograde popliteal artery	SFA and iliac artery
Retrograde pedal	Infrapopliteal, popliteal, SFA

CFA, Common femoral artery; *PFA,* profunda femoral artery; *SFA,* superficial femoral artery.

Technical Considerations

Selection of arterial access site (Table 5.5) for endovascular treatment of the femoropopliteal segment depends on lesion location, presence of concomitant iliac or infrapopliteal disease, patient-specific variables, and operator proficiency. Most often, the preferred approach is retrograde access from the contralateral CFA, with advancement of a sheath over the iliac bifurcation. This strategy permits treatment of iliac artery disease and allows familiar access techniques to be used. The crossover approach may be hampered by inadequate length of interventional equipment if treatment of the infrapopliteal distribution is required, and attenuation of one-to-one torque in cases with acute angulation of the iliac bifurcation. In the absence of iliac and CFA disease, for patients in whom infrapopliteal or distal femoropopliteal disease is the target, an antegrade common femoral approach may be beneficial. Straight-line access and proximity of the access platform to lesion substrate improves wire torque and catheter manipulation. The benefits of antegrade access are attenuated by a higher risk of bleeding and the relatively greater degree of difficulty compared with retrograde femoral access. In cases of complex occlusion with bridging collaterals or in lesions recalcitrant to antegrade recanalization, retrograde access via the popliteal or pedal arteries may be considered. Transradial access is gaining popularity for iliac interventions; however, in most patients, catheter lengths of 135 or 150 cm do not have adequate reach to treat diseased segments beyond the proximal or mid-superficial femoral artery.

Angiographic Technique

As in other vascular distributions, the use of DSA, a large flat-panel detector plate, and appropriate collimation optimizes image quality and reduces radiation exposure. The bifurcation of superficial and profunda femoris arteries is best visualized in 45-degree ipsilateral oblique angulation. Sometimes contralateral oblique imaging is helpful when imaging a suspected ostial SFA occlusion. The main course of the femoropopliteal artery is best imaged in a straight anteroposterior (AP) projection, or perhaps 15 to 30 degrees of ipsilateral oblique, in order to display the infrapopliteal trifurcation. Imaging eccentric lesions may require tailored angulations. Baseline and postintervention runoff angiography is recommended in order to exclude iatrogenic DE.

Anticoagulation

Femoropopliteal interventions are most often performed with UFH because it may be rapidly reversed if necessary. The optimal target activated clotting time (ACT) is between 250 and 300 seconds. Bivalirudin has been used with increasing frequency in endovascular interventions, but it is more expensive and not immediately reversible.

Procedural Technique

The particular technique used to cross a femoropopliteal stenosis depends on lesion, patient, and operator-specific parameters. Support catheters are commonly used in conjunction with 0.035-, 0.018-, or 0.014-inch guidewires. CTOs pose a unique challenge and may be addressed with a variety of techniques. In some lesions, it may be possible to pass a wire in an antegrade fashion through the occlusion from true lumen to true lumen; in other cases, a subintimal approach may be required, advancing a prolapsed or knuckled wire in the subintimal plane parallel to the reconstituted lumen and then reentering the true lumen using an angled wire or a dedicated CTO reentry device. The overall success rate of crossing even complex lesions (TASC C and D) is approximately 85% to 95% among experienced operators.

Complications of Femoropopliteal Endovascular Interventions

Because DE may occur during interventional procedures, many advocate the use of distal embolic protection strategies in cases with only one-vessel infrapopliteal runoff, particularly in the context of CLI. If DE is observed, treatment options may include mechanical or rheolytic thrombectomy, balloon inflation, stent placement, and occasionally surgical embolectomy. Evaluate the possibility of DE before and after every femoropopliteal intervention with comprehensive runoff angiography.

During balloon inflations, stent placement, or atherectomy, the creation of AV fistulae is not uncommon. Large AV fistulae can be treated with nitinol SE stents that direct blood flow straight to the foot, permitting most of these fistulae to heal on their own. They can also be treated with placement of a PTFE stent graft (Viabahn stent).

Vessel perforation or rupture is a feared complication and can lead to compartment syndrome if not treated quickly. Most wire perforations can be managed conservatively, whereas larger perforations must be immediately treated with balloon tamponade. Prolonged balloon inflations (5 to 10 minutes) with or without reversal of heparin can seal most perforations. If this fails, consider placement of a PTFE stent graft (Viabahn stent) with possible surgical referral. Overall, most such complications can be treated percutaneously.

Stent and vessel thrombosis after femoropopliteal endovascular revascularization has been reported in randomized trials and multicenter registries and ranges between 3% and 4% at 1 year. This probably highlights a complex interplay of vascular anatomy, endovascular devices, and adjunctive antithrombotic and antiplatelet medications that remains to be elucidated.

Infrapopliteal Interventions

Disease involving the infrapopliteal vessels may be highly variable in its anatomic features, response to conventional endovascular techniques, and clinical importance to the patient. Significant controversy remains regarding the optimal management of patients with infrapopliteal disease. The term *infrapopliteal* refers to vessels that include the anterior tibial (AT); tibioperoneal trunk; PTA; peroneal, medial, and lateral plantars; and metatarsal arch arteries. These vessels are relatively small in caliber and are often diffusely diseased or occluded. These anatomic features render them recalcitrant to endovascular techniques, but technology breakthroughs have improved outcomes. Such breakthroughs include the development of improved guidewire technology that permits crossing of long CTOs; long, low-profile angioplasty balloons that minimize the development of luminal disruption or dissection even when treating very long CTOs; increased operator familiarity and dexterity with transpedal access and retrograde wire techniques to cross CTO segments where antegrade crossing was unsuccessful; and the future promise of drug-eluting therapies to reduce restenosis following successful endovascular treatment.

In contrast to patients with iliac and femoropopliteal disease, for whom the majority of endovascular treatments are performed to relieve claudication, those with infrapopliteal disease typically undergo revascularization only for advanced clinical stages of disease, such as CLI. Such patients often present with rest pain and/or tissue breakdown and ulceration (Rutherford IV to VI) because of arterial insufficiency. The technical and therapeutic goal in patients with CLI caused by infrapopliteal disease is to reestablish straight-line pulsatile

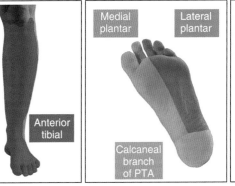

Fig. 5.9 Angiosome concept. Three main arteries supply six angiosomes of the foot and ankle. *Left*: The anterior tibial artery (*ATA*) becomes the dorsalis pedis artery that supplies the dorsum of the foot and dorsum side of the toes. *Middle*: Three main branches of the posterior tibial artery (*PTA*) supply distinct portions of the sole: the calcaneal branch to the heel, the medial plantar artery to the medial, and the lateral plantar artery to the lateral mid foot and the forefoot. The PTA supplies the plantar side of the toes, the web spaces between the toes, the sole of the foot, and the inside of the heel. *Right*: The peroneal artery (*PA*) supplies the lateral border of the ankle and the outside of the heel. (From Iida O, Soga Y, Hirano K, et al. Long-term results of direct and indirect endovascular revascularization based on the angiosome concept in patients with critical limb ischemia presenting with isolated below-the-knee lesions. *J Vasc Surg.* 2012;55:363-370.)

blood flow to the foot (see Fig. 5.3), specifically the region of the foot supplied by one particular infrapopliteal vessel. It has been demonstrated that restoring perfusion to the affected angiosome (Fig. 5.9) is more effective than restoring indirect flow through a different infrapopliteal vessel that does not directly perfuse the ulcerated territory.

Although endovascular treatment of infrapopliteal disease has high rates of restenosis, the temporary reestablishment of pulsatile flow to the foot is often sufficient to promote wound healing. Even if restenosis of the treated segments occurs, the impact of wound healing and limb salvage may remain durable. As a result, this treatment paradigm for CLI has evolved: Reestablish straight-line flow to the foot (even if long-term patency is limited), because this may have profound impact on wound healing and limb salvage.

Technical Considerations

In many ways, the technical approach to infrapopliteal disease mirrors strategies perfected in the coronary distribution with arteries of similar caliber. The majority of interventions is performed using 0.014-inch wires, low-profile angioplasty balloons, occasional use of atherectomy techniques, and—in rare cases of highly recalcitrant stenosis or flow-limiting dissection—coronary stent systems, including drug-eluting stents.

In cases of pure infrapopliteal disease, antegrade arterial access from the ipsilateral CFA may provide the most effective platform for intervention. Delivery of a long sheath to the distal popliteal artery may limit contrast use and permits excellent wire torque and catheter handling through these complex segments. Ipsilateral retrograde, or transpedal, access is gaining popularity, because it provides opportunity to address lesions where the proximal cap of a CTO may not readily be traversed in an antegrade fashion. Care should be taken when accessing the dorsalis pedis or PTAs, however, because disruption of these vessels may compromise the only remaining outflow to the foot. Although beyond the scope of this chapter, pedal access is often obtained using smaller needle/wire systems (e.g., micropuncture) and mimics radial access. When used in conjunction with an antegrade femoral sheath, a small caliber wire is advanced (often through a microcatheter system) from the transpedal access site and is then snared and externalized from the femoral access point, permitting the rest of the intervention to be performed in antegrade fashion. At the conclusion of the procedure, the microcatheter is removed from the transpedal access site with manual compression, taking care to monitor pedal vessel patency.

Debulking strategies (such as atherectomy, rotational atherectomy, orbital atherectomy, laser atherectomy, and cutting balloon atherectomy) may have niche-specific application for infrapopliteal disease. Indications may include removal of plaque from a complex bifurcating segment to prevent tissue prolapse or compromise of an adjacent vessel; desire to reduce likelihood of dissection in a no-stent zone; and reduction of the burden of calcified plaque that may be recalcitrant to conventional PTAs. Outcomes of debulking strategies have not been compared with PTAs in rigorous randomized-controlled fashion. Take care to protect against DE with any intervention, especially debulking strategies that have a higher incidence of DE.

Acute Limb Ischemia

Rarely, patients with PAD may present with acute limb ischemia (ALI). The "six Ps" characterizes cardinal manifestations of ALI: pain, pallor, pulselessness, paresthesia, paralysis, and poikilothermia (coolness). ALI should be addressed with urgency, such as with that of acute myocardial infraction, and it has been classified by presenting symptoms (Table 5.6). ALI is the "heart attack equivalent in

Table 5.6

Rutherford Classification Scheme for Acute Limb Ischemia.						
Class	Category	Prognosis	Sensory Loss	Muscle Weakness	Arterial Doppler	Venous Doppler
I	Viable	No immediate limb threat	None	None	Audible	Audible
IIA	Threatened: Marginal	Salvageable if treated promptly	Minimal to none	None	+/− audible	Audible
IIB	Threatened: Immediate	Salvageable if treated immediately	More than just toes	Mild to moderate	Rare audible	Audible
III	Irreversible	Limb loss or permanent damage	Profound	Profound	None	None

Modified from Rutherford RB, Baker JD, Ernst C, et al. Recommended standards for reports dealing with lower extremity ischemia: revised version. *J Vasc Surg.* 1997;26:517–538.

the leg." In the absence of reperfusion, permanent impairment of neurologic and motor function may occur within 6 hours. Physical examination and detection of arterial and venous Doppler signals can be extremely helpful in rapidly establishing the diagnosis of a viable, marginally or immediately threatened, and a non-viable lower extremity in ALI. Minimal sensory loss with no muscular weakness is the hallmark of a marginally threatened limb, and the presence of muscle weakness identifies an immediately threatened limb. An anesthetic limb with profound muscle weakness and no audible venous Doppler signals suggests a non-viable extremity in ALI. Upon identification of ALI, initiate heparin infusion immediately and implement plans for urgent revascularization. ALI often results from acute arterial embolization and is often caused by a cardioembolic event in the context of atrial fibrillation, from a hypercoagulable state, or artery-to-artery embolus from a more proximal aneurysm. Acute stent or graft thrombosis may also lead to ALI.

Immediately consider surgical or catheter-based therapy. Invasive angiography followed by either catheter-directed thrombolysis with tissue-plasminogen activator or mechanical/rheolytic thrombectomy is often performed. Technological advances now permit pulse spray thrombolysis, where the clot is sprayed with a thrombolytic agent that is permitted to dwell for 20 to 60 minutes, and rheolytic thrombectomy is then performed. There is also the option to use ultrasound-assisted thrombolysis using specialized infusion catheters. In some centers, surgical thrombectomy is performed as initial therapy, and if this fails, surgical bypass occurs. Regardless of revascularization approach, all patients must be monitored post revascularization for the development of compartment syndrome, which can result from hyperemic tissue swelling. In severe cases, swelling—constrained within the fascial compartments of the leg— may lead to permanent nerve injury with sensory and motor loss if surgical fasciotomy is not performed. This underscores the need for collaboration between specialists with endovascular skills and those with open surgical skills for the treatment of patients with ALI.

Renal Artery Disease

Renal artery stenosis (RAS) is widely prevalent and confers a risk for adverse events both in terms of organ-specific as well systemic vascular outcomes. The presence of RAS is commonly identified at the time of coronary angiography. In five studies involving 2178 patients undergoing coronary angiography, concomitant renal angiography identified more than 50% RAS in 19% of the patients, 17.4% of which were bilateral; more than 75% stenosis was identified in 4.8% of these patients, 0.8% of which were bilateral.

> ## Box 5.3 Clinical Clues to the Diagnosis of Renal Artery Stenosis.
>
> Accelerated, resistant, or malignant HTN
> Early-onset (<30 years) HTN or severe late-onset (>55 years) HTN
> Development of new azotemia or worsening renal function after administration of ACE inhibitor or ARB
> Sudden unexplained pulmonary edema
> Unexplained renal dysfunction
> Multivessel CAD
> Refractory angina
> Unexplained CHF

ACE, Angiotensin-converting enzyme; *ARB,* angiotensin receptor blocker; *CAD,* coronary artery disease; *CHF,* congestive heart failure; *HTN,* hypertension.

Atherosclerosis represents the most common etiologic factor in RAS. For patients identified as having severe RAS, nearly 15% will progress to total occlusion; if the RAS is bilateral, this may lead to dialysis-dependent ESRD. The presence and severity of atherosclerotic disease in the renal arteries may serve as an indicator of the severity of systemic atherosclerosis and, therefore, the overall risk of adverse cardiovascular events. A linear relationship has been identified between the severity of RAS and mortality.

Three key categories of clinical findings may indicate the presence of RAS (Box 5.3): (1) presence of drug-resistant HTN (requiring the administration of four antihypertensive medications including a diuretic) or the abrupt onset, marked acceleration, or presence of malignant HTN; (2) organ-specific manifestations including the presence of an atrophic kidney (<7 to 8 cm), discrepancy in renal sizes (>1.5 cm), or unexplained renal failure following administration of angiotensin-converting enzyme (ACE) inhibitor or angiotensin receptor blocker (ARB) therapy; and (3) cardiovascular manifestations, including unexplained pulmonary edema or congestive heart failure (CHF) and refractory angina.

Although atherosclerosis comprises nearly 90% of all cases of RAS, vasculitis and fibromuscular dysplasia (FMD) may also involve the renal artery and may produce a stenosis. Atherosclerotic stenosis lesions typically involve the aorta surrounding the renal artery ostium, the ostium itself, and the proximal third of the main renal artery. FMD usually involves the distal two-thirds of the main renal artery or its branches. Vasculitides (involving medium sized vessels, such as polyarteritis nodosa) impact the entire vessel. FMD should be suspected in individuals with early-onset HTN below 30 years of age, particularly in females.

Table 5.7

Screening Tests for Renal Artery Stenosis.		
Test	**Advantage(s)**	**Disadvantage(s)**
Duplex ultrasound	High sensitivity Operator/experience dependent	Difficult specificity in obese patients
MRA	Good sensitivity and specificity Operator/experience dependent	Increased false positives Not useful if stents are present Potential for NSF
CTA	Good sensitivity and specificity Useful to visualize stents	Ionizing radiation Iodinated contrast
Captopril renal artery scintigraphy	Good specificity	Poor sensitivity (~10% to 25% false negative)
Renal vein renin	Lateralizing renin predicts treatment response	Poor sensitivity/ specificity Invasive
Renal catheter-based angiography	High sensitivity and specificity	Invasive

CTA, Computed tomography angiography; *NSF*, nephrogenic systemic fibrosis (also called nephrogenic fibrosing dermopathy); *MRA*, magnetic resonance angiography.

Noninvasive Testing

Patients clinically suspected to have RAS should be referred for noninvasive assessment. Currently, the most effective modalities to screen for RAS include renal duplex ultrasound (RADUS), MRA, and CTA (Table 5.7). The sensitivity and specificity of RADUS are both technician and reader dependent; but, when effectively performed, the studies provide anatomic and functional data including renal size, echogenicity of the renal cortex, and insight into the microvascular disease state including the renal resistive index (RI). The renal RI, calculated by the formula RI = peak systolic velocity (PSV) − end-diastolic velocity (EDV)/PSV or 1 − (EDV/maximal systolic velocity) × 100, indicates the severity of microvascular renal resistance and has been used to predict whether revascularization of the main renal artery will confer benefit. The appropriate cutoff value and the utility of using the RI calculation remain controversial. RADUS may offer valuable anatomic and physiologic information following renal artery stenting and is the preferred methodology for poststent surveillance.

CTA and MRA may also be highly effective strategies to image the renal arteries, but they carry significant limitations. CTA requires the administration of potentially nephrotoxic iodinated contrast, exposes patients to radiation, and may not effectively discriminate extravascular calcium from intraluminal stenosis. MRA frequently overestimates the degree of RAS and, when performed using gadolinium, may confer a risk of nephrogenic systemic sclerosis in patients with advanced renal disease. Recent developments in MRA technique provide the opportunity for imaging vascular territories without the use of gadolinium but are not yet widely available. Captopril renal artery scintigraphy may have specific utility in identifying patients with unilateral RAS but is not effective in patients with abnormal GFR, and it is therefore not recommended. Measurement of plasma renin levels is not typically pursued, because elevated levels are neither a specific nor sensitive indicator of renovascular HTN.

Catheter-Based Angiography

Catheter-based renal angiography remains the gold standard for imaging renal arteries and may be required to establish the diagnosis of RAS when noninvasive findings are ambiguous. Catheter-based angiography has a low rate of complications, but careful technique must be used to reduce the risks of atheroembolization, contrast-induced nephropathy, and vascular complications. Although retrograde femoral access is most commonly used, a brachial or radial approach may be easier in circumstances where the renal artery origin is angulated downward, as may commonly be the case. Acute angulation of the renal artery origin may require specialized catheters for effective engagement. Nonselective angiography of the renal arteries is often performed by placing a pigtail, omniflush, tennis racket, or universal catheter in the abdominal aorta at the level of T12/L1, using a power injection of dilute iodinated contrast and DSA. Nonselective imaging identifies the location and number of renal arteries and may provide critical insight into the disease status of the aorta, particularly if complex protruding atherosclerotic lesions are imperative to avoid during catheter manipulation. A slight left anterior oblique (LAO) projection (10 to 20 degrees) may provide the best orthogonal image of the renal artery ostia, limiting overlap with the aorta. Alternative angiographic techniques include the use of carbon dioxide or gadolinium as the contrast agent.

Selective renal arterial cannulation and angiographic imaging provide the greatest amount of detail. Using an LAO 10- to 20-degree projection may enable cannulation and optimal imaging of both renal artery ostia in 75% of cases. The most appropriate catheter for selective renal artery angiography depends on anatomic features in the vessel. Soft-tipped atraumatic catheters and guidewires may reduce the risk of vascular complications. Commonly used catheters include the internal mammary (IMA), JR4, cobra, renal double curve, hockey stick, multipurpose, or SOS Omni. When brachial access is used for a downward angulated renal artery, advance a 6-F to 7-F, 90-cm long vascular sheath (Shuttle, Raabe, Balkan, or Ansel; Cook Medical, Bloomington, IN) over the guidewire and position in the suprarenal abdominal aorta. Advance a 5-F to 6-F IMA catheter, multipurpose, or JR4 through the long sheath and engage the renal artery (Figs. 5.10, 5.11 and 5.12).

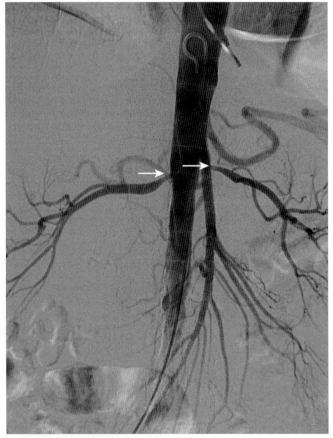

Fig. 5.10 Aortogram showing bilateral renal artery stenosis (RAS) (*arrows*).

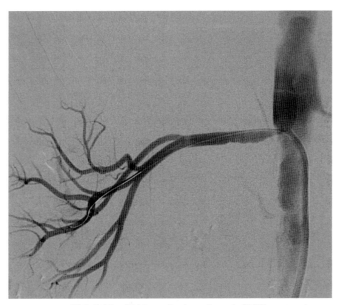

Fig. 5.11 Right renal artery stenosis (RAS).

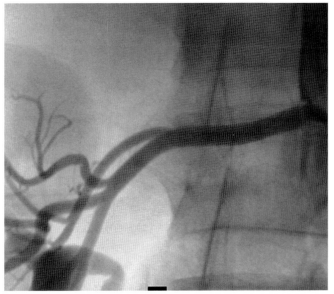

Fig. 5.12 Angiogram of right renal artery after stenting.

Assessment of Renal Artery Stenosis Significance

Standard selective angiography provides a limited 2D view of the renal artery. Because many clinical trials, predicated on the identification of RAS using angiographic measurement, have yielded discordant data on the clinical benefit of renal artery revascularization, there has been great interest in developing reliable strategies to predict those patients who will most likely benefit from renal artery revascularization. In patients with RAS resulting from FMD, it has been well validated that PTA alone is sufficient to disrupt the webs of tissue responsible for causing the stenosis and is often highly effective to reduce associated HTN (Fig. 5.13). However, in patients with atherosclerotic disease, debate persists regarding who will most benefit from revascularization. Similar to the practice in CAD, there has been a recent movement to define significant RAS, not by

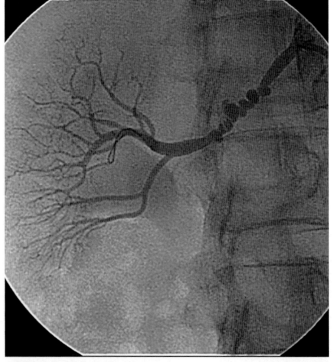

Fig. 5.13 Angiogram demonstrating fibromuscular dysplasia (FMD) of the renal artery. (Courtesy Dr. Michael Jaff.)

anatomic severity, but rather by physiologic impact using pressure wire evaluation with induction of hyperemia. Of note, adenosine should not be used in the renal vasculature for the induction of vasodilation because it can paradoxically provoke renal artery vasoconstriction. The optimal vasodilator for the renal vasculature is papaverine, which must be used with heparin-free saline, because the combination of these two drugs leads to formation of a precipitate that may provoke microvascular injury. Some studies have evaluated the use of other vasodilators, including dopamine. A hemodynamically significant RAS is characterized by *one* of the following conditions: (1) resting pressure distal to stenosis/pressure in the aorta (Pd/Pa) <0.90, (2) hyperemic Pd/Pa called *fractional flow reserve* (FFR) for the coronary circulation <0.80, (3) hyperemic mean gradient >20 mm Hg, (4) hyperemic systolic gradient >20 mm Hg, and (5) minimal luminal area (MLA) by IVUS imaging of 8.6 mm^2 or less. Given the limitations of angiography, any intermediate stenosis should be assessed using one of these techniques.

Renal Artery Revascularization

Indications for renal artery revascularization include facilitation of BP control in patients with resistant HTN, preservation of renal function, or reversal of end-stage renal failure or prevention of a decline in renal function in selected patients. Renal artery stenting has also been shown to improve functional class in patients with unstable angina and CHF.

Large-scale randomized clinical trials (including DRASTIC, ASTRAL, and STAR), testing the efficacy of renal artery revascularization versus medical management, have concluded that renal artery stenting does not confer significant benefit compared with medical therapy. Significant methodologic flaws have limited translation of these results to general clinical practice. The most recent CORAL trial enrolled patients with relatively mild clinical indications (patients took two antihypertensive medications), and physiologic assessment of lesion severity was not required. Considering these limitations, renal artery revascularization produced modest improvement in BP control during these clinical trials. Further prospective randomized studies with physiologic determination of stenosis severity may provide greater insight in determining those patients who may benefit from renal artery revascularization.

Subclavian and Brachiocephalic Intervention

Upper-extremity arterial insufficiency resulting from obstructive disease of the major aortic arch vessels affects up to 7% of individuals in select populations. Atherosclerotic disease most commonly involves the ostium or proximal segments of the subclavian and brachiocephalic arteries; in other conditions, such as FMD, large vessel vasculitides (e.g., Takayasu arteritis, giant cell arteritis), thoracic outlet syndrome, or radiation-induced disease may cause lesions in more distal locations.

Symptoms of subclavian obstruction include arm claudication with fatigue, paresthesia, or pain during exertion. The presence of stenosis may first be identified by discrepant BP readings between arms, with a lower BP recorded on the affected side. Proximal left subclavian stenosis may also impede antegrade flow through the left vertebral artery, resulting in symptoms of vertebro-basilar insufficiency that may manifest as diplopia or vertigo with left arm exertion, known as *subclavian steal*. In patients with left or right internal mammary (LIMA or RIMA) bypass grafting for coronary artery bypass graft (CABG) surgery, the presence of proximal subclavian stenosis may result in angina during arm exercise or periods of physiologic subclavian steal.

Noninvasive Testing

In patients with suspected obstructive disease of the upper extremities, CTA or MRA may be helpful to confirm the diagnosis and provide anatomic insight. Imaging studies permit assessment of arch anatomy and degree of atherosclerotic burden and may be helpful for procedural planning if revascularization is considered. Duplex ultrasound may be used to evaluate vertebral artery flow on the affected side. Reversal of vertebral flow found on Duplex characterizes subclavian steal physiology. Presence of the steal phenomenon alone does not warrant revascularization unless the disease involves the left subclavian artery and the LIMA is intended for use in CABG surgery. To confirm the diagnosis of subclavian steal syndrome (vs. phenomenon alone), patients must have symptoms of vertebral-basilar insufficiency (VBI), angina, or arm claudication.

Invasive DSA may provide enhanced anatomic detail. Arch aortography using a pigtail catheter placed into the ascending aorta at 40 degrees LAO defines the origins of the great vessels and permit selective angiography if needed. The determination of translesional pressure gradients to determine the significance of intermediate lesions involving the arch vessels may be diagnostic of important stenosis. Selective canalization of the vessels may be performed using a variety of specialized catheters; in cases where prolonged catheter manipulation is required, anticoagulation is recommended.

Revascularization

Revascularization of the brachiocephalic and subclavian arteries is indicated for the presence of significant symptoms or empirically if a LIMA is required as a conduit for CABG surgery. Endovascular treatment of the subclavian and brachiocephalic arteries is successful in more than 95% of cases. Surgical bypass is possible but has a comparatively high rate of complications, including cranial nerve palsy, lymphocele, and morbidity related to the need to enter the chest cavity. To date, there have been no trials comparing outcomes with open surgical revascularization and endovascular therapy in subclavian and innominate artery distribution.

The optimal approach to upper-extremity revascularization depends on lesion location and arch anatomy. The femoral approach is most often used, although brachial or radial access may facilitate treatment of CTOs, where it may be difficult to localize the vessel's origin from the aortic arch or maintain adequate catheter support to cross the occlusion. Radial access is gaining popularity and most BE stent platforms up to 8 mm may be delivered through 6-F sheath systems and postdilated up to 10 mm with 6-F compatible balloons. Simultaneous femoral and arm access may permit embolic protection of the vertebral artery or carotid in the case of innominate intervention or in cases where complex proximal plaque is felt to pose a particularly high risk of DE.

Aorto-ostial and proximal lesions are generally treated with BE stents, because radial force is desirable, precision of deployment is imperative, and this territory is not exposed to extrinsic compression. For lesions located in the more distal portions of these vessels, SE stents may be preferred to accommodate extremity movement and the propensity for flexion, extrinsic compression, and other forces that could result in stent deformation.

Atheroembolization, although uncommon, is a devastating complication that occurs from using the direct route to cerebral circulation through the vertebral artery. Some operators advocate for the use of cerebral embolic protection at the time of treatment for bulky subclavian or brachiocephalic lesions. No large study has evaluated the safety or efficacy of this approach, but given the unknown timing of vertebral flow reversal, some operators recommend embolic protection. In the rare event of acute thrombotic occlusions of the arch vessels, embolic protection to vertebral and axillary arteries seems prudent, because more DE may occur at the time of instrumentation.

Carotid Disease

In the United States, cerebrovascular disease remains the third leading cause of death and represents a significant cause of morbidity and health care expenditure. Approximately 800,000 individuals develop a new or recurrent stroke each year, of whom two-thirds are first-time events and one-third are recurrent. Although 80% of strokes are ischemic in origin and result from long-standing HTN, 20% to 25% are the result of atherosclerotic disease of the carotid artery. The risk of stroke from carotid artery plaque itself depends on both the severity of narrowing and characteristics of the plaque biology (i.e., whether a prior stroke or transient ischemic attack [TIA] has occurred from an unstable lesion).

The highest risk of recurrent stroke occurs in the context of symptomatic severe carotid lesions of 70% to 99% as established by angiography. These data, described in the North American Symptomatic Carotid Endarterectomy Trial (NASCET), firmly established that the risk of recurrent ipsilateral stroke at a 2-year follow-up was 26%. In less severe but symptomatic stenosis (50% to 69%), the 5-year risk of any ipsilateral stroke was 22.2%. The highest risk of stroke occurred early after the index event, highlighting the importance of early revascularization. Although medical therapy at the time of NASCET was limited, the benefit of early revascularization of symptomatic patients with carotid disease is now well established.

Asymptomatic patients enrolled in the Asymptomatic Carotid Surgery Trial (ACST) with a carotid stenosis more than 60% (determined by ultrasound) were found to have a stroke risk of 11% at 5-year follow-up. In contrast to symptomatic patients, who have a high risk of recurrent stroke early after an index event, the risk of stroke in asymptomatic patients was constant during the 5-year period, implying that revascularization in these patients may be considered on a more elective basis.

Diagnostic Testing

Duplex ultrasonography is the standard test used to assess coronary artery stenosis (CAS). Numerous criteria have been established to assist in the diagnosis of severe carotid stenosis. In most cases, greater than 80% stenosis correlates with PSV of 300 to 400 cm/s, an EDV greater than 100 cm/s, and a ratio of internal carotid artery/common carotid artery (ICA/CCA) systolic velocity of more than 4:1. Other features, such as the presence of contralateral occlusion, diminished cardiac output from severe left ventricular (LV) dysfunction, valvular pathology such as aortic stenosis, and concomitant CCA stenosis, may render these measurements less reliable. MRA and CTA may also facilitate the identification of CAS. Still, catheter-based angiography remains the gold standard for evaluating carotid stenosis. Angiography provides information on vessel anatomy, plaque morphology, flow characteristics, and presence of collateral circulation. These parameters are particularly useful in predicting the safety of carotid endarterectomy (CEA) or carotid artery stenting. However, angiography also carries risks of vascular complications including cerebrovascular accident (CVA), which should be carefully considered.

Carotid and Cerebral Angiography

Carotid and cerebral angiography is most commonly performed from the femoral artery approach. However, in some cases, right radial or brachial arterial access may be preferred. Regardless of approach, meticulous procedural technique must be used during carotid and cerebral angiography. It is recommended that anticoagulation with heparin be achieved to prevent catheter- and/or wire-related thrombosis and embolism. Careful flushing and back bleeding of every catheter must be performed to prevent air or thromboembolism. In most cases, selective angiography of the great vessels should not be completed without first performing a nonselective angiogram of the aortic arch.

Standard baseline arch aortography may be performed using a pigtail catheter with power injection (typical volume of 40 cc) in a LAO 30- to 40-degree orientation. There should be limited foreshortening of the catheter. This position permits visualization of the origins and proximal segments of the great vessels and enables determination of arch type, which may indicate any potential technical challenges related to performing selective carotid angiography.

The aortic arch typically gives rise to the brachiocephalic trunk, the left CCA, and the left subclavian artery. The brachiocephalic trunk usually bifurcates into the right subclavian artery and right CCA. In 20% to 30% of the population, the brachiocephalic trunk and left CCA share a common origin. The aortic arch can be classified into three types, defined by Myla and described by Uflacker et al., on the basis of the distance of the origin of the great vessels from the top of the arch (Fig. 5.14). The widest diameter of the left common carotid is used as a reference vessel. In a type-I arch, all great vessels originate within one diameter length (diameter length of the widest portion of the left common

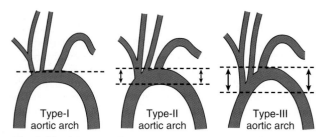

Fig. 5.14 Schematic diagram showing classification of aortic arch.

carotid) from the top of the arch; in a type-II arch, all great vessels originate within two diameter lengths from the top of the arch; and in a type-III arch, the great vessels originate within more than two diameter lengths from the top of the arch (see Fig. 5.9). In addition, a small segment of the population has the left carotid artery originating from the innominate artery. This is known as a bovine arch (Fig. 5.15). Given the potential variability in arch configuration and the marked impact that anomalous configurations have on procedural technique, arch aortography is a critical first step.

Various-shaped catheters are available for selective carotid and vertebral artery angiography. The catheters can be divided into three groups: passive, intermediate, and active shape designs. Use of a particular category of catheter will depend on the type of aortic arch and the geometry of the origins of the great vessels. Passive catheters, such as headhunter, multipurpose, vertebral, and Bernstein, are used to access the great vessels in patients with a type-I aortic arch. Intermediate catheters, including the Vitek (Cook, Inc., Medical, Bloomington, IN) and JB 1–3; (Cordis Corp., Hialeah, FL), require more manipulation than passive catheters and are ideal for type-II aortic arches. Active catheters including the Simmons Sidewinder and Newton catheter are useful for type-II or -III arches but must be shaped in the ascending aorta and therefore may introduce the opportunity for release of atheroemboli. A practical way to shape these catheters requires advancing them into the aortic arch over a wire (an angled Glidewire is recommended). With removal of the wire, the catheter may then be retracted and the tip positioned in the left subclavian artery. Further rotation will allow the catheter to prolapse into the ascending aorta. The catheter can then be manipulated into each specific great vessel.

Following the review of arch aortography, selection of an appropriate catheter, and assurance that systemic anticoagulation

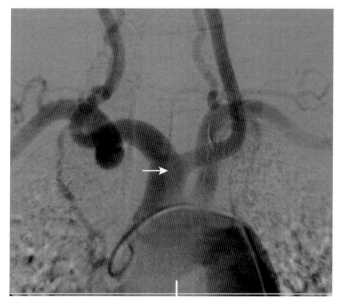

Fig. 5.15 Bovine arch angiogram demonstrating the left common carotid arising from the innominate artery (*arrow*).

has been achieved, the great vessels may then be engaged. The right anterior oblique (RAO) view allows visualization of the origins of the right common carotid, right subclavian, and right and left vertebral arteries (Figs. 5.16 and 5.17). The LAO view allows visualization of the left common carotid and left subclavian and innominate arteries. Following selective engagement of the common carotid from the arch (or innominate), wiring of the common carotid is often required to allow the catheter to be advanced and appear in the field of view for quantitative angiography of carotid bifurcation. Take care with any wire or catheter advancement to prevent the catheter from jumping forward into the lesion. Angiography performed from the proximal or middle portion of the common carotid (if not diseased) is usually sufficient. Once the diagnostic catheter is in place, angiography of the carotid bifurcation in the AP, lateral, and ipsilateral oblique (45 degrees) is obtained. The carotid artery is classically divided into four segments: cervical, petrous (often washed out in appearance as the artery courses through the petrous bone), cavernous, and supraclinoid.

With the catheter selectively in each carotid artery, obtain intracranial imaging in both the AP cranial and lateral projections.

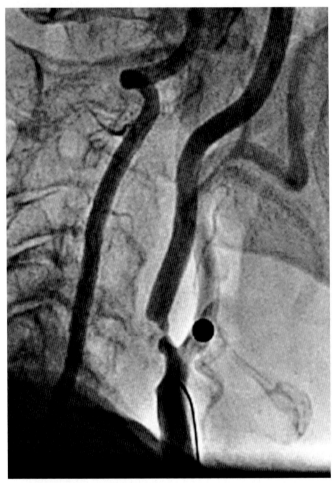

Fig. 5.16 Ulcerated plaque in internal carotid artery (ICA).

Although additional discussion is beyond the scope of this chapter, any operator performing selective carotid and intracranial angiography should be familiar with the anatomy of the major cerebral vessels and branches and should recognize congenital variations as well as the presence or absence of collateral vessels when intracranial disease is present.

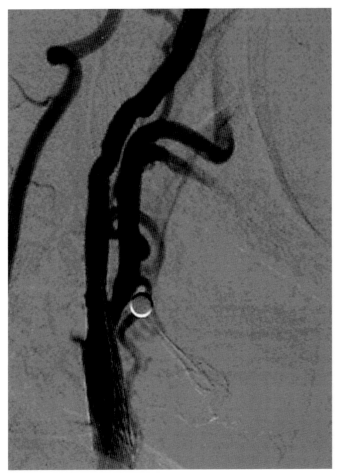

Fig. 5.17 Poststent angiogram of internal carotid artery (ICA).

Vertebral Artery Disease

In contrast to carotid disease, the optimal management of vertebral artery stenosis is less well known, in large part because the manifestations of vertebral disease may be ambiguous and underappreciated. Vertebral arteries provide the blood supply to the posterior aspect of the brain, including the cerebellum. Ischemic insults to this area may manifest with dizziness, ataxia, diplopia, hemiparesis, and bilateral lower-extremity weakness and numbness. The vertebral arteries merge together to form the basilar artery; occlusion of the basilar artery presents as locked-in syndrome, in which the patient may only control lateral movement of the eyes.

The primary cause of posterior circulation strokes is embolization from the heart, aorta, or proximal aspect of the vertebral arteries themselves. Transient ischemia of the posterior circulation may also occur in the context of inflow vessel (subclavian or innominate artery) stenosis or occlusion, where flow is further compromised by transient reduction in BP, or during episodes where steal physiology reduces antegrade flow, classically with strenuous use of the ipsilateral arm.

Atherosclerosis represents the most common cause of vertebral artery stenosis, primarily concentrated at the vessel origin. Other, less common causes of vertebral artery stenosis include arterial dissection (usually traumatic), FMD, migraine, and vasculitides, such as Takayasu and giant cell arteritis. The diagnosis of VBI is often quite challenging because of vague and indistinct symptoms. The location of the arteries and their intercervical course make duplex ultrasonography challenging. The best tests for assessing vertebral arteries include CTA, MRA, and invasive angiography.

Vertebral arteries most commonly arise from the proximal portion of the subclavian artery, although in 5% of patents, the left vertebral may arise directly from the arch. Classically, the vertebral artery is divided into four segments, designated V1 to V4. The V1 section is the one most affected by atherosclerosis and extends from the origin to the point at which the vessel enters the transverse foramina of the vertebra (C5 to C6) where it then becomes the V2 section. From the intervertebral foramina, the vertebral courses behind C2 extracranially (the V3 section) and then enters the skull through the foremen magnum, where it is then called the *V4 segment*. This final portion enters the brain and merges with the contralateral vertebral artery to form the basilar artery. It is common to find a size discrepancy between the two vertebral arteries, with the left often the larger of the two. The larger vertebral is often referred to as the dominant vessel.

Traditionally, treatment of symptomatic vertebral artery disease has been surgical using one of the following approaches: (a) transection of the vertebral artery above the stenosis with reimplantation into the ipsilateral subclavian or carotid artery, (b) vertebral artery endarterectomy, and (c) vein patch angioplasty. These surgeries are associated with high morbidity and mortality (10%–20%). Currently, endovascular neurointerventional approaches are being increasingly pursued at specialized centers. Data to support this revascularization strategy are currently limited.

Conclusion

Peripheral arterial disease is prevalent and encompasses a wide spectrum of disorders. Clinicians must be vigilant for vascular disease, since the diagnosis confers high risk of adverse cardiovascular events. Once diagnosed, the mainstay of treatment for PAD is medical therapy, focused on the modification of cardiovascular risk factors. Exercise therapy may substantially improve symptoms of claudication, but for the select patients who fail conservative therapy, there are a growing number of endovascular and surgical therapeutic options. Through keen understanding of clinical and anatomic features and appreciation of the range of therapeutic strategies, we may tailor our approach to optimize outcomes for our patients.

Suggested Readings

Adam DJ, Beard JD, Cleveland T, et al. Bypass versus angioplasty in severe ischaemia of the leg (BASIL): multicenter, randomised controlled trial. *Lancet*. 2005;366:1925-1934.

Banerjee S, Sarode K, Mohammad A et al. Femoropopliteal artery stent thrombosis: report from the Excellence in Peripheral Artery Disease Registry. *Circ Cardiovasc Interv*. 2016;9:e002730.

Barnett HJ, Taylor DW, Eliasziw M, et al. Benefit of carotid endarterectomy in patients with symptomatic moderate or severe stenosis. North American symptomatic carotid endarterectomy trial collaborators. *N Engl J Med*. 1998;339:1415-1425.

Bates ER, Babb JD, Casey DE, Jr, et al. ACCF/SCAI/SVMB/SIR/ASITN 2007 clinical expert consensus document on carotid stenting: a report of the American College of Cardiology Foundation Task Force on Clinical Expert Consensus Documents (ACCF/SCAI/SVMB/SIR/ASITN Clinical Expert Consensus Document Committee on Carotid Stenting). *J Am Coll Cardiol*. 2007;49:126-170.

Bonaca MP, Scirica BM, Creager MA, et al. Vorapaxar in patients with peripheral artery disease: results from TRA2° P-TIMI 50. *Circulation*. 2013;127:1522-1529, 1529e1-e6.

Brott TG, Halperin JL, Abbara S, et al. 2011 ASA/ACCF/AHA/AANN/AANS/ACR/ASNR/CNS/SAIP/SCAI/SIR/SNIS/SVM/SVS guideline on the management of patients with extracranial carotid and vertebral artery disease: executive summary: a report of the American College of Cardiology Foundation/American Heart Association Task Force on Practice Guidelines, and the American Stroke Association, American Association of Neuroscience Nurses, American Association of Neurological Surgeons, American College of Radiology, American Society of Neuroradiology, Congress of Neurological Surgeons, Society of Atherosclerosis Imaging and Prevention, Society for Cardiovascular Angiography and Interventions, Society of Interventional Radiology, Society of Neuro Interventional Surgery, Society for Vascular Medicine, and Society for Vascular Surgery. Developed in collaboration with the American Academy of Neurology and Society of Cardiovascular Computed Tomography. *J Am Coll Cardiol*. 2011;57:1002-1044.

Brott TG, Hobson RW II, Howard G, et al. Stenting versus endarterectomy for treatment of carotid artery stenosis. *N Engl J Med*. 2010;363:11-23.

Cooper CJ, Murphy TP, Cutlip DE, et al. Stenting and medical therapy for atherosclerotic renal-artery stenosis. *N Engl J Med*. 2014;370:13-22.

Criqui MH, Langer RD, Fronek A, et al. Mortality over a period of 10 years in patients with peripheral arterial disease. *N Engl J Med*. 1992;326:381-386.

Dake MD, Ansel GM, Jaff MR, et al. Sustained safety and effectiveness of paclitaxel-eluting stents for femoropopliteal lesions: two-year follow-up from the Zilver PTX randomized and single-arm clinical studies. *J Am Coll Cardiol*. 2013;61:2417-2427.

Dawson DL, Cutler BS, Meissner MH, Strandness Jr DE. Cilostazol has beneficial effects in treatment of intermittent claudication: results from a multicenter, randomized, prospective, double blind trial. *Circulation*. 1998;98:678-686.

Diener HC, Bogousslavsky J, Brass LM, et al. Aspirin and clopidogrel compared with clopidogrel alone after recent ischaemic stroke or transient ischaemic attack in high-risk patients (MATCH): randomised, doubleblind, placebo-controlled trial. *Lancet*. 2004;364:331-337.

Endarterectomy for asymptomatic carotid artery stenosis. Executive Committee for the asymptomatic carotid Atherosclerosis Study. *JAMA*. 1995;273:1421-1428.

Gerhard-Herman MD, Gornik HL, Barrett C, et al. 2016 AHA/ACC Guideline on the management of patients with lower extremity peripheral artery disease: executive summary: a report of the American College of Cardiology/American Heart Association Task Force on Clinical Practice Guidelines. *J Am Coll Cardiol*. 2017;69: 1465-1508.

Geraghty PJ, Mewissen MW, Jaff MR, Ansel GM. Three-year results of the VIBRANT trial of VIABAHN endoprosthesis versus bare nitinol stent implantation for complex superficial femoral artery occlusive disease. *J Vasc Surg*. 2013;58:386-395.

Hirsch AT, Haskal ZJ, Hertzer NR, et al. ACC/AHA 2005 Practice Guidelines for the management of patients with peripheral arterial disease (lower extremity, renal, mesenteric, and abdominal aortic): a collaborative report from the American Association for Vascular Surgery/Society for Vascular Surgery, Society for Cardiovascular Angiography and Interventions, Society for Vascular Medicine and Biology, Society of Interventional Radiology, and the ACC/AHA Task Force on Practice Guidelines (Writing Committee to Develop Guidelines for the Management of Patients with Peripheral Arterial Disease): endorsed by the American Association of Cardiovascular and Pulmonary Rehabilitation; National Heart, Lung, and Blood Institute; Society for Vascular Nursing; TransAtlantic Inter-Society Consensus; and Vascular Disease Foundation. *Circulation*. 2006;113:e463-e654.

Jenkins JS, Patel SN, White CJ, et al. Endovascular stenting for vertebral artery stenosis. *J Am Coll Cardiol*. 2010;55:538-542.

Jongkind V, Akkersdijk GJ, Yeung KK, Wisselink W. A systematic review of endovascular treatment of extensive aortoiliac occlusive disease. *J Vasc Surg*. 2010;52:1376-1383.

Klein AJ, Feldman DN, Aronow HD, et al. SCAI expert consensus statement for aortoiliac arterial intervention appropriate use. *Catheter Cardiovasc Interv*. 2014;84: 520-528.

Klein AJ, Pinto DS, Gray BH, et al. SCAI expert consensus statement for femoral-popliteal arterial intervention appropriate use. *Catheter Cardiovasc Interv*. 2014;84: 529-538.

Laird JR, Katzen BT, Scheinert D, et al. RESILIENT Investigators. Nitinol stent implantation versus balloon angioplasty for lesions in the superficial femoral artery and proximal popliteal artery: twelve-month results from the RESILIENT randomized trial. *Circ Cardiovasc Interv*. 2010;3:267-276.

Leesar MA, Varma J, Shapira A, et al. Prediction of hypertension improvement after stenting of renal artery stenosis: comparative accuracy of translesional pressure gradients, intravascular ultrasound, and angiography. *J Am Coll Cardiol*. 2009;53: 2363-2371.

Morrow DA, Braunwald E, Bonaca MP, et al. Vorapaxar in the secondary prevention of atherothrombotic events. *N Engl J Med*. 2012;366:1404-1413.

Murphy TP, Cutlip DE, Regensteiner JG, et al. Supervised exercise versus primary stenting for claudication resulting from aortoiliac peripheral artery disease: six-month outcomes from the claudication: exercise versus endoluminal revascularization (CLEVER) study. *Circulation*. 2012;125:130-139.

Norgren L, Hiatt WR, Dormandy JA, et al. Inter-Society Consensus for the Management of Peripheral Arterial Disease (TASC II). *J Vasc Surg*. 2007;45(suppl S):S5-S67.

North American Symptomatic Carotid Endarterectomy Trial collaborators, Barnett HJM, Taylor DW, et al. Beneficial effect of carotid endarterectomy in symptomatic patients with high-grade carotid stenosis. *N Engl J Med*. 1991;325:445-453.

Patel SN, White CJ, Collins TJ, et al. Catheter-based treatment of the subclavian and innominate arteries. *Catheter Cardiovasc Interv*. 2008;71:963-968.

Rooke TW, Hirsch AT, Misra S, et al. 2011 ACCF/AHA focused update of the guideline for the management of patients with peripheral artery disease (updating the 2005 guideline): a report of the American College of Cardiology Foundation/American Heart Association Task Force on Practice Guidelines: developed in collaboration with the Society for Cardiovascular Angiography and Interventions, Society of Interventional Radiology, Society for Vascular Medicine, and Society for Vascular Surgery. *Catheter Cardiovasc Interv*. 2011;79:501-531.

Sacco RL, Adams R, Albers G, et al. Guidelines for prevention of stroke in patients with ischemic stroke or transient ischemic attack: a statement for healthcare professionals from the American Heart Association/American Stroke Association Council on Stroke: co-sponsored by the Council on Cardiovascular Radiology and Intervention: the American Academy of Neurology affirms the value of this guideline. *Stroke*. 2006;37:577-617.

Scheinert D, Katsanos K, Zeller T, et al. A prospective randomized multicenter comparison of balloon angioplasty and infrapopliteal stenting with the sirolimus eluting stent in patients with ischemic peripheral arterial disease. *J Am Coll Cardiol*. 2012;60:2290-2295.

Scheinert D, Scheinert S, Sax J, et al. Prevalence and clinical impact of stent fractures after femoropopliteal stenting. *J Am Coll Cardiol*. 2005;45:312-315.

Schillinger M, Sabeti S, Loewe C, et al. Balloon angioplasty versus implantation of nitinol stents in the superficial femoral artery. *N Engl J Med*. 2006;354:1879-1888.

Selvin E, Erlinger TP. Prevalence of and risk factors for peripheral arterial disease in the United States: results from the National Health and Nutrition Examination Survey, 1999-2000. *Circulation*. 2004;110:738-743.

Stewart KJ, Hiatt WR, Regensteiner JG, Hirsch AT. Exercise training for claudication. *N Engl J Med*. 2002;347:1941-1951.

Tepe G, Zeller T, Albrecht T, et al. Local delivery of paclitaxel to inhibit restenosis during angioplasty of the leg. *N Engl J Med*. 2008;358:689-699.

Tetteroo E, van der Graaf Y, Bosch JL, et al. Randomised comparison of primary stent placement versus primary angioplasty followed by selective stent placement in patients with iliac-artery occlusive disease. Dutch Iliac Stent Trial Study Group. *Lancet*. 1998;351:1153-1159.

Warfarin Antiplatelet Vascular Evaluation Trial Investigators, Anand S, Yusuf S, et al. Oral anticoagulant and antiplatelet therapy and peripheral arterial disease. *N Engl J Med*. 2007;357:217-227.

Willigendael EM, Teijink JA, Bartelink ML, Peters RJ, Büller HR, Prins MH. Smoking and the patency of lower extremity bypass grafts: a meta-analysis. *J Vasc Surg*. 2005;42:67-74.

Yadav JS, Wholey MH, Kuntz RE, et al. Protected carotid-artery stenting versus endarterectomy in high-risk patients. *N Engl J Med*. 2004;351:1493-1501.

Ye W, Liu CW, Ricco JB, Mani K, Zeng R, Jiang J. Early and late outcomes of percutaneous treatment of TransAtlantic Inter-Society Consensus class C and D aorto-iliac lesions. *J Vasc Surg*. 2011;53:1728-1737.

Interventional Cardiology Procedures

SANTIAGO GARCIA • MORTON J. KERN • MICHAEL LEE
• PAUL SORAJJA

Percutaneous coronary and structural heart disease interventional techniques are commonly performed after diagnostic angiography for patients with ischemic and structural (e.g., valvular or atrial septal defects [ASDs]) heart disease. The *Interventional Cardiac Catheterization Handbook,* a companion book to this volume, expands on the concepts presented in this chapter and provides a more detailed foundation for indications, contraindications, and complications of interventional cardiology techniques. Tables 6.1 and 6.2 list diagnostic and therapeutic interventional procedures performed in the catheterization laboratory.

Percutaneous Coronary Interventions

Coronary balloon angioplasty was first performed in 1977. Up to that time, coronary artery bypass graft (CABG) surgery was the only alternative to medical treatment of coronary artery disease. During CABG, a segment of leg vein, arm artery, and/or chest wall artery is attached to the heart to detour blood around the narrowed portion (i.e., stenosis) of a coronary artery. Percutaneous transluminal coronary angioplasty (PTCA) (with the introduction of stents, PTCA is now called *percutaneous coronary intervention* [PCI]) provided an alternative to CABG. Without surgery, PCI selectively enlarges the narrowed portion of the artery by the insertion of a long thin balloon to open the blocked artery. Rarely used by themselves today, coronary balloons are now used to predilate the lesion and facilitate the delivery of coronary stents (metal mesh-like stainless steel or metal alloy implants) and with other devices (such as, cutters, grinders, lasers, and aspiration catheters) to treat a wide variety of artery problems.

Table 6.1

Diagnostic and Therapeutic Procedures in the Cardiac Catheterization Laboratory.	
Diagnostic Procedures	**Therapeutic Procedures**
Coronary angiography	PCIs (balloon, stents, rotablator, cutting balloon, and so on)
Ventriculography	Valvuloplasty, TAVR, mitral clip
Hemodynamics	ASD, PFO, PDA, VSD shunt closure
Shunt detection	Thrombolysis, thromboaspiration
Aortic and peripheral angiography	Coil embolization
Pulmonary angiography	Pericardiocentesis, window
Coronary hemodynamics	
Endomyocardial biopsy	

ASD, Atrial septal defect; *PCI,* percutaneous coronary intervention; *PDA,* patent ductus arteriosus; *PFO,* patent foramen ovale; *TAVR,* transcatheter aortic valve replacement; *VSD,* ventricular septal defect.

Table 6.2

Applications of Percutaneous Coronary Intervention Devices.				
Special Lesion Type	**Stent**	**Cutting Balloon**	**Rotablator**	**Thrombus Aspiration**
Type A	+++	+	±	−
Complex	++	++	+	−
Ostial	++	++	+	−
Diffuse	+	+	++	−
Total occlusion	++	+	−	−
Calcified bifurcation	±	++	+++	−
SVG focal	+++	±	±	−
SVG diffuse	+	±	−	−
SVG thrombotic	±	−	−	++
Complication	+++	−	±	±
Acute occlusion	++	−	−	±
Thrombosis	+	−	−	+++
Perforation	@	−	−	−

+++, Highly applicable; ++, somewhat helpful; +, applicable; ±, marginally applicable depending on status; −, not applicable; @, covered stent; *SVG,* saphenous vein graft.

These methods are collectively referred to as PCI. The nomenclature is informative:

· *Percutaneous* refers to the nonsurgical insertion of a catheter into the body through a small puncture site in the skin, usually into an artery.

- *Coronary* identifies the specific artery to be dilated.
- *Intervention* denotes the technique for remodeling a blood vessel through the introduction of an expandable stent, balloon catheter, or other specialized tools for treating a diseased artery.

Figure 6.1 shows the process of performing PCI. A guiding catheter is seated in the coronary ostium. A thin, steerable guidewire is introduced into the coronary artery to traverse the stenosis into the distal aspect of the artery. A balloon angioplasty catheter, which is considerably smaller than the guiding catheter, is inserted through the guiding catheter and positioned (in the artery) across the stenotic area by tracking it over the guidewire. The balloon or stent is on the PCI catheter. After correct positioning within the area to be treated, the balloon on the PCI catheter is inflated at 10 to 16 atmospheres (atm) for periods ranging from 10 to 30 seconds. The inflation and deflation of the balloon stent in the blocked artery

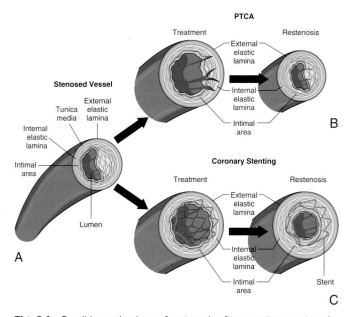

Fig. 6.1 Possible mechanisms of restenosis after percutaneous transluminal coronary angioplasty *(PTCA)* and coronary stenting. **(A)** Atherosclerosis. **(B)** PTCA to left and restenosis following PTCA on right. **(C)** Coronary stenting to left and restenosis of stent to right. (Reproduced with permission from Monahan FD, et al. Coronary artery disease and dysrhythmias. In: Monahan, F. D., & Phipps, W. J. *Phipps' Medical-Surgical Nursing: Health and Illness Perspective.* 8th ed. St. Louis: Mosby; 2007.)

restores blood flow to an area of the heart previously deprived by the stenosed artery. After successful stent implantation, patients usually stay overnight in the hospital and are discharged the following morning. Same-day discharge has emerged as an alternative option for low-risk patients. This strategy was associated with lower costs and was preferred by patients. Patients can usually resume their normal routine within several days.

How Do Balloon Angioplasty and Stents Work?

Several theories regarding the mechanisms of angioplasty have been proposed.

Disruption of Plaque and Arterial Wall

The major effective mechanism of balloon angioplasty involves a balloon that inflates and exerts pressure against the plaque and arterial wall, fracturing and splitting the plaque. The concentric lesion fractures and splits at its thinnest and weakest point, whereas an eccentric lesion splits at the junction of the plaque and the arterial wall. Dissection, or separation of the plaque from the medial wall, releases the splinting effect that is caused by the lesion and results in a larger lumen. This is the major effective mechanism of balloon angioplasty.

Loss of Elastic Recoil

Balloon dilation thins and stretches the medial wall, causing the medial wall to lose its elastic properties. The degree of elastic recoil loss is affected by the balloon-to-artery size ratio. Over time (1 to 6 weeks), the artery may re-narrow as a result of elastic recoil, which is prevented by placement of a stent in the artery.

Redistribution and Compression of Plaque Components

Shear pressures cause denudation or stripping of endothelial cells and the extrusion or pushing out of plaque components. Molding of the softer lipid material may occur, but this effect accounts for a small part of the overall effect of angioplasty.

Mechanism of Stents

Stents scaffold the lumen and plaque open, holding back dissection flaps, stopping vessel recoil, and re-narrowing the lumen.

Restenosis is the re-narrowing of the vessel after treatment by balloon and stent, leading to recurrence of myocardial ischemia and potentially a return of anginal symptoms. Significant restenosis is not considered a true complication, but it is an event that may require retreatment with PCI or CABG surgery. Restenosis is caused mostly by intimal hyperplasia and rarely by vessel recoil after stenting. Typically, restenosis occurs during the initial 6 months after PCI. The in-stent restenosis rate is <10% with drug-eluting stents.

Stent thrombosis is the abrupt formation of a blood clot inside the stent, which is potentially catastrophic and can lead to myocardial infarction (MI) or death. The incidence of stent thrombosis is 1% to 2%. It is more likely to occur if dual antiplatelet therapy (i.e., aspirin and clopidogrel or other $P2Y_{12}$ platelet inhibitors) is prematurely discontinued or the stent is suboptimally expanded.

The indications, contraindications, and complications of PCI are listed in Box 6.1.

Equipment

PCI equipment consists of three basic elements: guiding catheter, balloon-stent catheter, and coronary guidewire (Fig. 6.2).

Box 6.1 Indications, Contraindications, and Complications of Percutaneous Coronary Intervention.

Indications for Percutaneous Coronary Intervention

Angina pectoris causing sufficient symptoms despite optimal medical therapy
Mild angina pectoris with objective evidence of ischemia (by abnormal stress testing or physiology) and high-grade lesion (>70% diameter narrowing) of a vessel supplying a large area of myocardium
Unstable angina or NSTEMI
STEMI as primary therapy or in patients who have persistent or recurrent ischemia after failed thrombolytic therapy
Angina pectoris after CABG
Restenosis after successful PCI
LV dysfunction with objective evidence of viability of a vessel supplying the myocardium
Arrhythmia secondary to ischemia

Contraindications for Percutaneous Coronary Intervention[a]

Unsuitable coronary anatomy
Extremely high-risk coronary anatomy in which closure of vessel would result in patient death
Bleeding diathesis
Patient noncompliance with dual antiplatelet therapy and unwillingness to follow post-PCI instructions
Multiple in-stent restenosis
Patients who cannot give informed consent

Continued on following page

> **Box 6.1   Indications, Contraindications, and Complications of Percutaneous Coronary Intervention.** (Continued)
>
> **Complications Associated with Percutaneous Coronary Intervention**
>
> Death (<1%)
> MI (<3% to 5%)
> Stent thrombosis (~1%)
> Emergency CABG (<1%)
> Abrupt vessel closure (0.8%)
> Coronary artery perforation (<1%)
> All complications that can occur during cardiac catheterization, including access site bleeding, pseudoaneurysm, AV fistula, ischemic vascular complications, stroke, allergic reaction to contrast media, and renal failure.

AV, Atrioventricular; *CABG,* coronary artery bypass graft; *LV,* left ventricular; *MI,* myocardial infarction; *NSTEMI,* non-ST segment elevation myocardial infarction; *PCI,* percutaneous coronary intervention; *STEMI,* ST-segment elevation myocardial infarction.
[a]If PCI is the only life saving procedure, risk versus benefit is weighed and the contra-indication become

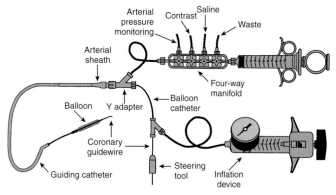

Fig. 6.2 Components of percutaneous coronary intervention (PCI) equipment. (From Freed M, Grines C, Safian RD. *The New Manual of Interventional Cardiology.* Birmingham, MI: Physicians' Press; 1996.)

Guiding Catheter

A special large-lumen catheter is used to guide the coronary balloon catheter to the vessel that has the lesion to be dilated (Fig. 6.3). Compared with a diagnostic catheter, a guiding catheter has a thinner wall and larger lumen, which allows contrast injections and accommodates interventional equipment. A guiding catheter is stiffer than a diagnostic catheter to provide support for

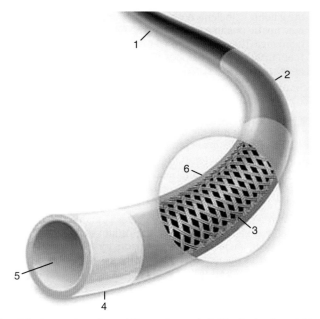

Fig. 6.3 Illustration of a guiding catheter. *1,* Stiffer body; *2,* variable softer primary curve; *3,* wire braiding; *4,* atraumatic tip; *5,* large lumen (optional radiopaque marker); *6,* lubricous coating. (Courtesy Boston Scientific Corporation, Boston, MA.)

advancing the balloon-stent catheters into the coronary artery. It responds differently to manipulation than a diagnostic catheter. The guiding catheter tip is not tapered, occasionally blocking the ostium and causing pressure dampening while engaging the coronary ostium. A 6-F guiding catheter is generally used. Some catheters have relatively shorter and more flexible tips than others, theoretically to decrease catheter-induced trauma. Others may have side holes to help maintain blood flow during PCI. Larger guiding catheters (7 F or 8 F) may be necessary for kissing balloons/stents, rotablator burrs >2 mm, and some cutting balloons. The guiding catheter comes in many different shapes for femoral and radial approaches. Guide catheters are shaped for specific anatomic variations.

Functions of the Guiding Catheter

The three major functions of a guiding catheter during PCI include:

1. Balloon-stent catheter delivery: The guiding catheter is the delivery device of the balloon catheter to the coronary artery. If

the guiding catheter is not seated properly in a coaxial manner, it may not be possible to advance the balloon stent across the stenotic area. The guiding catheter is seated in the coronary artery (cannulation) and provides the necessary backup support or platform to push the balloon/stent catheter across the stenosis.

Several terms that are commonly used when referring to guiding catheters are important:

- *Backing out:* The guiding catheter is ejected from the coronary ostium into the aortic root when pressure is applied to the balloon in an attempt to cross the lesion. This is caused by an insufficient support position or a tight stenosis.
- *Strong backup:* A stable support position of the guiding catheter at the orifice of the coronary ostium provides the necessary platform to advance the balloon across the lesion.
- *Deep seating:* The guiding catheter is manipulated over the balloon catheter shaft past the ostium and further into the vessel to increase backup support for crossing difficult lesions. This maneuver is typically used as a last resort because of the increased risk of guiding catheter–induced dissection of the proximal vessel.

2. Contrast injection: The guiding catheter permits visualization of the target by contrast administration with or without the balloon catheter in place. Some large PCI devices may block adequate contrast injection, which makes the procedure more difficult.

3. Pressure monitoring: The guiding catheter lumen measures aortic pressure for determination of the transstenotic pressure gradient for physiologic lesion assessment, ostial lesions (pressure wave damping), and hypotension during prolonged ischemia.

Balloon Angioplasty and Stent Delivery Catheters

Technologic refinements of balloon catheters have dramatically improved the success rate of PCI. There are two principal types of balloon-stent catheters: (1) over the wire (OTW) angioplasty PCI systems and (2) rapid-exchange (RX; monorail) PCI catheters.

Over the Wire Angioplasty Percutaneous Coronary Intervention Systems

An OTW angioplasty PCI catheter (Fig. 6.4) has a central lumen throughout the length of the catheter for the guidewire and a separate lumen for balloon inflation. This catheter is approximately 145 to

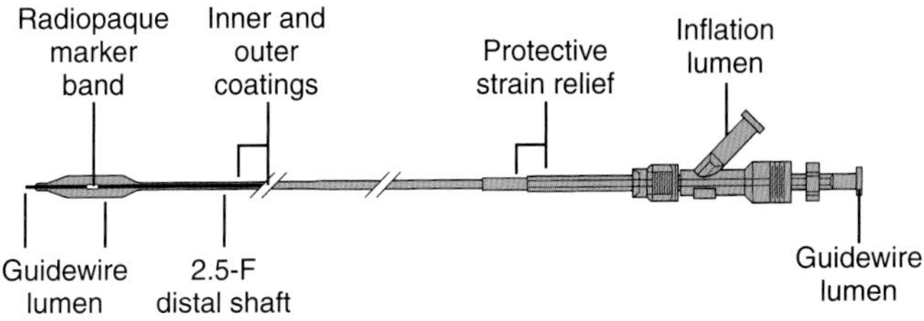

Fig. 6.4 Schematic design of a typical over the wire (OTW) angioplasty balloon catheter. The guidewire extends the entire length of the catheter.

155 cm long and can be used with a long or short guidewire, usually 0.014 inch.

This catheter can accept multiple guidewires, which allows for exchanging of additional devices that may require stronger, stiffer guidewires. Maintenance of distal wire position beyond the target stenosis is paramount in coronary angioplasty. For an OTW balloon catheter, the guidewire can be extended to help maintain distal position while the balloon catheter is withdrawn completely over the guidewire to permit another balloon catheter to be exchanged and introduced over the same guidewire for additional dilations. A 300-cm exchange wire is commonly used.

One disadvantage of an OTW angioplasty balloon catheter is that a primary operator and an experienced assistant are required to perform catheter exchanges. A technique to make balloon catheter exchanges easier involves a balloon inside the guide catheter inflated to fix a 155-cm guidewire in place, which permits OTW catheters to be exchanged without using a 300-cm guidewire. Dedicated trapping balloons have been introduced to facilitate balloon catheter exchanges.

Rapid-Exchange (Monorail) Percutaneous Coronary Intervention Catheter

An RX balloon catheter is the most popular catheter used today and allows a single operator to exchange PCI catheters unassisted. It differs from OTW PCI catheters in that only a variable length of the shaft has two lumens (Fig. 6.5). One lumen is for balloon inflation and the other, which extends through only a portion of the catheter shaft, houses the guidewire. Because only a limited portion of the balloon requires dual lumens, the catheter shafts can be made smaller than OTW systems.

An RX balloon catheter eliminates the need for a long exchange guidewire and permits an operator to maintain distal guidewire position without the aid of an assistant.

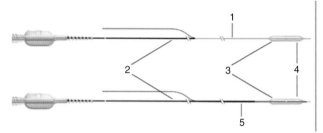

Fig. 6.5 Schematic design of a typical rapid-exchange (RX) angioplasty balloon catheter. The guidewire extends through the distal part of the catheter, allowing for single-operator use. 1- Shaft, 2- Inflation lumen, 3- Proximal shoulder of the balloon catheter, 4- Distal shoulder of the balloon catheter, 5- Inflation lumen with guidewire in place. (Courtesy Boston Scientific Corporation, Boston, MA.)

Limitations of a monorail catheter include the need for excellent guiding catheter support and more operator skill for the complexity in manipulating the guidewire, balloon catheter, and guiding catheter. Blood loss during removal of the monorail balloon catheter at the rotating hemostatic valve can be a problem but can be reduced with better technique and attention to the Y connectors.

The advantages and limitations of OTW and RX balloon catheters are listed in Table 6.3.

Procedural Details for Percutaneous Coronary Intervention

After crossing the lesion with the balloon catheter, the balloon is inflated and deflated using a hand-held syringe device with a

Table 6.3

Advantages and Limitations of Angioplasty Balloon Catheter Types.		
Type	**Advantages**	**Limitations**
Over the wire (OTW)	• Distal wire position • Accepts multiple wires; distal port for pressure, contrast injection	• Needs two people for exchanging balloon catheter/stent
Rapid exchange (RX; monorail)	• Ease of use; single-operator system • Enhanced visualization	• Needs good guide support • Blood loss at Y valve during exchanges; inability to change wire

pressure gauge. Balloon catheter sizes range from 1.5 to 5 mm in diameter (size of the inflated balloon) for coronary arteries and are larger for peripheral arteries. Balloon diameter is selected according to the angiographic size of the vessel to be dilated. The plastic materials of balloon catheter construction determine the flexibility of the catheter shaft and balloon characteristics (e.g., burst pressure and actual diameter under different pressure levels). Special-purpose coronary balloon catheters are available for specific types of lesions. A noncompliant high-pressure balloon is commonly used to optimize stent implantation results to achieve full stent expansion and strut apposition. Balloon lengths vary from 10 to 38 mm in length. A cutting balloon is a special balloon catheter with three to four atherotomes (or blades) that run longitudinally on the balloon to score the lesion in a more controlled fashion.

Angioplasty Guidewires

Coronary angioplasty guidewires are small-caliber (0.010-inch to 0.014-inch diameters) steerable wires that are typically 170 to 190 cm long. They are advanced into the coronary artery or branches beyond the lesion to be dilated. The flexible tip may be shaped by the operator to negotiate side branches and tortuous artery curves. The balloon-stent catheter is advanced over the wire and, after artery dilation, removed from the artery with the wire remaining in place beyond the dilated lesion. Extra-long guidewires (300 cm) are used to exchange OTW balloon catheters. Tip flexibility and torque control characteristics of these coronary guidewires vary. Generally, the softer wires are safer and easier to advance into tortuous branches, whereas the stiffer wires give better torque control and may be useful for crossing difficult or total occlusions. Hydrophilic wires, which have special coatings to cross subtotally or totally occluded stenoses better, generally carry a higher risk of perforation if the tip position is not kept in the major vessel lumen and dissection if the guidewire is advanced under an intimal flap.

Exchange and Extension Guidewires

An exchange guidewire is similar to the standard 180 cm guidewire mentioned previously except that its length is 280 to 300 cm. This long wire replaces the initial wire when the exchange of an OTW balloon catheter is necessary. Alternatively a 120- to 145-cm extension wire can be connected to the end of the initial guidewire to allow balloon catheter exchanges.

Other Equipment

Y Connector (Adjustable Hemostasis Device)

The Y connector, which comes with a rotating or spring-controlled valve, is an accessory device that minimizes back-bleeding while the balloon/stent catheter is inserted into and removed from the guiding catheter. This device allows the injection of contrast media and pressure monitoring through the guiding catheter, regardless of balloon catheter position.

Inflation Device

A disposable syringe device is used to inflate the balloon on the balloon catheter with precise measurement of the inflation pressure in atmospheres, generally ranging from 4 to 20 atm. Although stents may be inflated at 10 to 18 atm, the balloon is typically inflated with sufficient pressure to compress the plaque caused by stenosis and fully expand the dumbbell, or indentation, at the waist of the partially inflated balloon. Occasionally, hard, resistant stenoses (calcium or fibrosis) may require high pressures (>14 atm) to expand the dumbbell indentation. Needless balloon overinflation increases the risk of coronary dissection and perforation.

Torque (Tool) Device

A small cylindrical pin vise clamp slides over the proximal end of the angioplasty guidewire, permitting the operator to perform fine manipulations of the guidewire by turning the torque tool in a clockwise or counterclockwise direction. Figure 6.6 shows examples of the inflation device, Y connectors, guidewire introducers, and torque tool.

Clinical Procedure

The clinical procedure for PCI is:

I. Clinical and angiographic indications for proceeding with PCI should be confirmed. Noninvasive testing for ischemia is recommended in patients with atypical anginal symptoms or chest pain syndrome without evidence of clinical ischemia. Before PCI, the following procedures can be performed to obtain objective evidence of ischemia: electrocardiogram (ECG) (for evidence of resting ischemia or recent infarction); stress perfusion imaging or stress echocardiography (either exercise or pharmacologic); or for lesions of uncertain significance, in-laboratory translesional physiology assessment

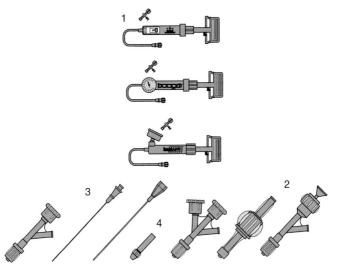

Fig. 6.6 Examples of balloon inflation device and Y connectors, wire introducer needles, and torque tool. 1- Inflation device; 2- Y-adapter with hemostatic valve (Tuohy); 3- Wire introducer; 4- Torquer device. (Reprinted with permission from Meritt Medical Systems, Inc. All rights reserved.)

(with the use of fractional flow reserve [FFR] or instantaneous wave-free ratio [iFR]).

II. Pre-PCI preparation

1. Patient preparation should include placement of ECG electrodes, pacer/defibrillator pads, and intravenous (IV) line. Make sure you have a list of the patient's current medications and a signed informed consent form.

2. Perform patient and family teaching, including explaining the procedure, anticipated results, and potential for complications.

3. Give cardiothoracic surgery consultation for high-risk patients and those with multivessel disease (especially patients with diabetes), left main disease, or left ventricular (LV) dysfunction.

4. Do a laboratory blood work check, including complete blood cell and platelet counts and measurements of international normalized ratio (INR), partial thromboplastin time (PTT), electrolytes, blood urea nitrogen, and creatinine.

III. Patient preparation in catheterization suite

1. ECG (inferior and anterior wall leads): Use ECG with 12 leads (radiolucent).

2. Skin preparation: Prepare inguinal area for femoral artery or wrist for radial artery.

3. Consider femoral venous access for high-risk patients or those with acute MI, rotablator, or thrombus aspiration device. Most PCI procedures can also be performed from the radial approach, with lower bleeding risk obviating the need for a vascular closure device (VCD). Venous access for temporary pacing is no longer routine.

4. Antiplatelet therapy: Aspirin (325 mg orally). Failure to administer aspirin before PCI is associated with a two to three times higher acute complication rate, including acute MI and stent thrombosis. Clopidogrel (600 mg orally) or other $P2Y_{12}$ platelet inhibitors, such as prasugrel or ticagrelor, if patient presents with acute coronary syndrome (ACS), should be routinely given before or immediately after PCI.

5. Anticoagulation: Heparin (70- to 100-mcg/kg bolus or lower if glycoprotein [GP] IIb/IIIa blocker is used) with a target activated clotting time (ACT) >250 seconds. Bivalirudin is an alternative to heparin, with reports of lower bleeding risk in some patients.

6. Consider GP IIb/IIIa blockers in patients with complicated procedures associated with thrombus or MI with large thrombotic burden.

7. Give Versed (1 mg IV) and Fentanyl (25 to 100 mcg IV) for sedation.

8. For patients allergic to contrast media, give prednisone (60 mg, 13 hours, 7 hours, and 1 hour before cardiac catheterization). Diphenhydramine (25 to 50 mg IV or orally) and H_2 blockers are used in some centers.

IV. Guiding coronary angiograms (after 100 to 200 mcg of nitroglycerin IC)

1. Define coronary anatomy and collateral supply (if any).

2. Store guiding shots to use as reference roadmap for balloon-stent positioning.

3. Select device size as judged from known guide catheter diameter to select the balloon-stent diameter.

   Note: 8 F = 2.87 mm, 6 F = 2 mm (size of PCI device based on distal artery normal reference segment; balloon/artery ratio <1:1.2)

V. PCI procedure

1. Select guiding catheter for angle of vessel takeoff and optimal backup support.

2. Ensure the guiding catheter is seated; coaxial alignment is best.

3. Advance guidewire beyond target stenosis to distal position in the vessel.

4. Insert balloon catheter through hemostasis Y valve on guiding catheter and advance into the stenosis, centering the balloon using radiopaque markers on balloon catheter.

5. Inflate balloon to expand fully and remove dumbbell indentation of lesion on underinflated balloon. Balloons and stents may be inflated for 10 to 30 seconds or longer, as tolerated. Then, deflate the balloon.

6. Exchange the balloon catheter for the stent catheter and repeat the process. Using a balloon first opens the vessel, providing pressure and flow to the distal vessel segment. This often enlarges the size of the vessel, possibly changing initial thinking regarding the best stent size.

7. Determine final result after intravascular ultrasound (IVUS) and optical coherence tomography (OCT) with or without high-pressure noncompliant balloon for optimal stent implantation.

VI. Assessment of PCI result

1. Check for enlarged artery lumen ($<10\%$ residual lesion) and good angiographic flow (thrombolysis in MI [TIMI] grade 3).

2. Full stent apposition is based on angiogram and/or IVUS.

3. Check for absence of adverse angiographic complications (e.g., thrombus, dissection, or perforation).

4. Make sure there is no residual ischemia (ECG changes with or without chest pain).

VII. Considerations for additional stenting

1. New lesion proximal or distal to stent (i.e., edge dissection) may require additional stenting.

2. Large dissection extending in either direction may require additional stenting.

3. Slow flow may require FFR or IVUS to establish cause (i.e., occult dissection).

VIII. Postprocedure angiograms and access site hemostasis

1. Remove guidewire for final images after administering additional intracoronary (IC) nitroglycerin. Leaving the guidewire in during final angiography may hold a dissection flap in place, which would be missed if the guidewire had not been removed.

2. For the femoral approach, perform femoral angiography before VCD selection (>30 degrees right anterior oblique [RAO] for right femoral artery or left anterior oblique [LAO] for left femoral artery). Avoid VCD in patients with scarring from previous procedures.

3. Alternatively, if no closure device is used, secure sheaths in place for later removal (2 hours) or when ACT is <160 seconds for manual hemostasis for arterial sheaths. Do not use prolonged (>6 hours) heparin infusions unless thrombus or other complications are present. Increased bleeding risk is associated with postprocedure heparin infusions.

4. For radial procedures, apply radial artery compression band with enough pressure to achieve patent hemostasis, maintaining good flow to hand. Remove band in 2 hours. Reapply if hemostasis is not achieved.

IX. Postprocedure outside laboratory

1. Teach about hospital course and bleeding problems, late complications, and restenosis.

2. Notify referring physician and care team in recovery area or critical care unit (CCU).

3. Use ECG and laboratory and telemetry monitoring of vital signs.

X. Post-PCI medications

1. The patient should take aspirin (325 mg orally daily for 1 month, then 81 mg/day indefinitely).

2. Prescribe clopidogrel (600-mg loading dose and 75 mg/day orally) for at least 4 weeks after stenting with a bare metal stent and 12 months with a drug-eluting stent. For patients with ACS, prescribe prasugrel (60-mg loading dose and 10 mg/day orally) or ticagrelor (180-mg loading dose and 90 mg/twice daily orally). Second-generation $P2Y_{12}$ receptor antiplatelet agents, such as ticagrelor or prasugrel, are commonly used as alternatives to clopidogrel.

3. Initiate statin drugs if not already prescribed.

4. Restart antihypertensive or antianginal medications depending on patient's clinical needs.

XI. Follow-up schedule
   1. Check access site on first office visit.
   2. Do *not* perform stress testing early after PCI or annually unless symptoms or other clinical indications appear.
   3. Repeat coronary angiography if symptoms or signs of ischemia are present early after PCI.
   4. Instruct patient to return gradually to activities of daily living.

Percutaneous Coronary Intervention Pharmacology

See Chapter 1 for more information about commonly used drugs in the catheterization laboratory.

Oral Antiplatelet Agents

All patients who undergo PCI receive aspirin (81mg to 325 mg/day), which should be administered >2 hours prior to the procedure with a loading dose of 162 or 325 mg. Current PCI guidelines recommend a loading dose of $P2Y_{12}$ inhibitor at the time of PCI. Options include clopidogrel 600 mg, prasugrel 60 mg, or ticagrelor 180 mg. The duration of dual antiplatelet therapy (DAPT) after stent implantation is usually 12 months. Shorter and longer DAPT durations have been proposed for patients with increased bleeding or thrombotic risks, respectively.

Some patients do not respond to clopidogrel because of a genetic predisposition. Clopidogrel is a prodrug and needs to be catalyzed to its active metabolite by the cytochrome P450 2C19 (CYP2C19) enzyme. Some patients are CYP2C19-poor metabolizers, leading to lower levels of the active metabolite of clopidogrel, less platelet inhibition, and increased risk of adverse cardiovascular events, including stent thrombosis, MI, and death.

As an alternate for patients with ACS, prasugrel (60-mg loading dose with 10 mg/day maintenance), a $P2Y_{12}$ receptor inhibitor, reduced the combined rate of death from cardiovascular causes, nonfatal MI, or nonfatal stroke but was associated with increased risk of bleeding complications. Contraindications include a history of stroke or transient ischemic attack, age $\geq$75 years, and weight <60 kg because of an increased risk of bleeding.

ACS patients after PCI who were treated with another antiplatelet agent, ticagrelor, showed improved clinical outcomes compared with clopidogrel. In addition to reduction in the combined endpoints of death from vascular causes, MI, or stroke, ticagrelor was associated with a reduction in mortality compared with clopidogrel. Rates of fatal or life-threatening bleeding were similar with clopidogrel. The loading dose is 180 mg (two 90-mg tablets) and 60 mg and then 90 mg every 12 hours.

Antithrombotic Agents

Heparin is a commonly used antithrombotic agent for PCI but is associated with a variety of limitations including variable anticoagulation responses, heparin resistance, need to monitor degree of anticoagulation, risk of heparin-induced thrombocytopenia, and activation of platelets.

Bivalirudin is a direct thrombin inhibitor and, when compared with heparin plus GP IIb/IIIa inhibitor, is associated with fewer bleeding complications across the full spectrum of patients with coronary artery disease who undergo PCI. The HORIZONS-AMI trial reported a reduction in 30-day mortality in ST-segment elevation myocardial infarction (STEMI) patients who underwent primary PCI with bivalirudin compared with heparin plus GP IIb/IIIa inhibitors. However, planned GP IIb/IIIa inhibition is not routinely used in elective PCI, and the use of this agent might explain the increased bleeding found in the heparin groups studied. The MATRIX study compared bivalirudin with heparin, without routine GP IIb/IIIa inhibitors, and found similar rates of ischemic and bleeding events.

Stenosis Assessment in the Catheterization Laboratory by Pressure Sensor Guidewire: Fractional Flow Reserve and Instantaneous Wave-Free Ratio

The ischemic potential of a questionable or intermediate (40% to 70%) lesion can be determined by FFR, which is the ratio of aortic pressure (from the guide catheter) to poststenotic pressure measured from the pressure guidewire beyond the stenosis during hyperemia (adenosine IV infusion or IC bolus).

There are five steps to measure FFR:

1. Set guide catheter pressure and guidewire pressure to atmosphere on the table (zero).
2. Advance the pressure guidewire to the central aortic position either at the tip of the guide just inside the coronary artery or in the aorta.

3. Match the pressures of the guidewire and guide catheter before the stenosis is crossed. This step is called *pressure normalization* or *equalization* and eliminates any small differences in pressures between the two systems.

4. Cross the lesions with the pressure wire 1 to 3 cm distally. Begin recording pressures.

5. Induce hyperemia, most often with IV adenosine. Measure both aortic and distal coronary pressures during adenosine-induced hyperemia (preferred: 140 mcg/kg/min $\times$ 3 to 4 minutes or, alternatively, IC 30 to 50 mcg for right coronary artery [RCA] and 50 to 100 mcg for left coronary artery [LCA]).

6. Compute FFR, the distal coronary pressure (Pd)/proximal aortic pressure (Pa) ratio at maximal hyperemia.

FFR reflects the percentage of normal blood flow through the stenosis. A normal value is 100% or 1.0. The FFR is an accurate reflection of the ischemic potential of a stenosis. Before PCI in the patient example in Figure 6.7B, the Pa of 145/68 mm Hg is obtained through the guiding catheter. The Pd, measured from the sensor angioplasty guidewire, is 110/50 mm Hg. During IC administration of adenosine, the hyperemic mean pressures (74 mm Hg/102 mm Hg) are used, yielding an FFR of 0.72 (FFR <0.75 is associated with inducible ischemia). The resting gradient (Pd/Pa) was insignificant and did not correlate with inducible ischemia.

After PCI, the gradient between proximal and distal artery pressures is decreased or abolished. An FFR of >0.90 is considered a very successful result. Normal arteries have FFR >0.94. In this patient after PCI, the FFR is 0.98 (see Fig. 6.7C).

A low FFR (<0.80), especially if the angiographic result is suboptimal, is an indication for further treatment, often with stenting. FFR is critically important when the operator is in doubt about the clinical significance of any lesion. The use of adjunctive imaging and diagnostic techniques during PCI is presented in Box 6.2. Remember that IVUS or optical coherence tomographic imaging measures anatomy, not flow, and can be used to assess the anatomic (but not physiologic) severity of the stenosis and confirms optimal stent implantation.

The iFR has recently emerged as an alternative to FFR. The iFR is a pressure-only measurement that takes an alternative approach to assessing stenosis severity. iFR focuses on the period in diastole when coronary resistance is minimal and constant (wave-free period). Under such conditions, pressure and flow are directly proportional, which allows for measurements of pressure gradients without the need for pharmacological vasodilation (Fig. 6.8). Coronary revascularization guided by iFR (cutoff 0.89) is comparable to coronary revascularization guided by FFR (cutoff 0.80) with regard to important clinical outcomes (death, non-fatal MI, and unplanned revascularization). It is possible to measure both iFR and FFR using the same specialty wire.

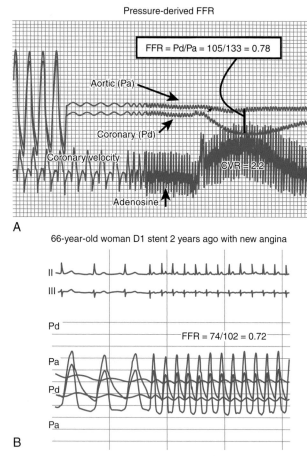

Pressure-derived FFR

FFR = Pd/Pa = 105/133 = 0.78

Aortic (Pa)

Coronary (Pd)

Coronary velocity

CVR = 2.2

Adenosine ↑

A

66-year-old woman D1 stent 2 years ago with new angina

II

III

Pd

FFR = 74/102 = 0.72

Pa

Pd

Pa

B

Fig. 6.7 Use of fractional flow reserve *(FFR)*. **(A)** Proximal guide catheter pressure *(Pa)* and distal coronary pressure *(Pd)* and coronary flow velocity at rest and after intracoronary (IC) adenosine *(bottom arrow)*. Hyperemia widens gradient and decreases Pd when velocity is maximal (coronary vasodilatory reserve *[CVR]* = 2.2), FFR = Pd/Pa = 105/133 = 0.78, above the ischemic threshold value (0.80). **(B)** Patient example: Before percutaneous coronary intervention (PCI), FFR = 0.72.

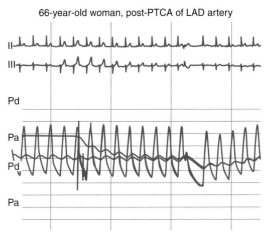

66-year-old woman, post-PTCA of LAD artery

C

Fig. 6.7, cont'd (C) After PCI, FFR = 0.98. *LAD,* Left anterior descending; *PTCA,* percutaneous transluminal coronary angioplasty.

Box 6.2 Diagnostic and Imaging Adjuncts to Percutaneous Coronary Intervention.

Fractional Flow Reserve

Indication: Coronary lesion assessment (any location) when hemodynamic significance is unknown or in doubt. Angiographic lesions, especially eccentric or of intermediate severity (40% to 70% diameter narrowed) are the most commonly assessed.

Derivation: FFR, Q_{sten}/Q_{normal} at maximal hyperemia; normal, theoretically same artery without stenosis. *Q,* Flow; *sten,* stenotic artery.

$$Q_{sten} = P_{sten}/resistance_{sten},$$

$$Q_{normal} = P_{aorta}/resistance_{sten}, \text{ then}$$

$$Q_{sten}/Q_{normal} = P_{sten}/P_{aorta}$$

Hence,

$$FFR = P_{distal\ to\ stenosis}/P_{aorta}$$

Complete derivation includes venous pressure (Pv) because:[a]

$$FFR = P_{distal\ to\ stenosis} - Pv/P_{aorta} - Pv$$

Features: Nonischemic threshold range >0.75 to 0.80, normal value of 1.0 for every artery and every patient, epicardial lesion specific, linear relation with relative maximum blood flow, independent of hemodynamic alterations, value that accounts for total myocardial blood flow, including collaterals, highly reproducible, high spatial resolution (pressure pull back recording).

Continued on following page

| **Box 6.2** | **Diagnostic and Imaging Adjuncts to Percutaneous Coronary Intervention.** (Continued) |

Coronary Flow Velocity Reserve

Indication: Used to assess microcirculation when insignificant epicardial lesions do not explain chest pain syndromes.

Derivation: CFVR, $Q_{hyperemia}/Q_{base}$. Q, Velocity if cross-sectional area unchanged during hyperemia.

Features: Nonischemic threshold range of CFR >2.0; coronary flow reserve in unobstructed vessels assesses microvascular integrity, useful for studies of coronary endothelial function, accurate estimation of volumetric flow when vessel cross-sectional area is available.

Intravascular Ultrasound Imaging and Optical Coherence Tomography

Indications:

- Evaluation of lesion severity at a location difficult to image by angiography, in a patient with a positive functional study and a suspected flow-limiting stenosis.
- Assessment of a suboptimal angiographic result after PCI
- Diagnostic and management of coronary disease after cardiac transplantation
- Assessment of the adequacy of deployment of coronary stent, including the extent of stent apposition and determination of the minimal luminal diameter within the stent
- Determination of plaque location and circumferential distribution
- Determination of the mechanism of stent restenosis or thrombosis (inadequate expansion vs. neointimal proliferation) and to enable selection of appropriate therapy (plaque ablation vs. repeat balloon expansion)
- Preinterventional assessment of lesion characteristics of hazy lesions (e.g., calcification) as a means of selecting an optimal revascularization device

CFR, Coronary vasodilatory reserve; *CFVR,* coronary flow velocity reserve; *FFR,* fractional flow reserve; *PCI,* percutaneous coronary intervention.
[a]See Pijls et al.

Stent Implantation

Stents are used in nearly all PCIs. Decisions regarding drug-coated, bare metal, or bioabsorbable stents are individually tailored. There are several different designs for stents (Fig. 6.9).

Compared with balloon angioplasty, stenting produces a larger minimal luminal diameter, maintains arterial patency, and reduces restenosis with excellent long-term results. Stents improve long-term results compared with balloon angioplasty in nearly every angiographic subset examined. Stenting reduces the incidence of acute recoil, abrupt vessel closure, and the need for

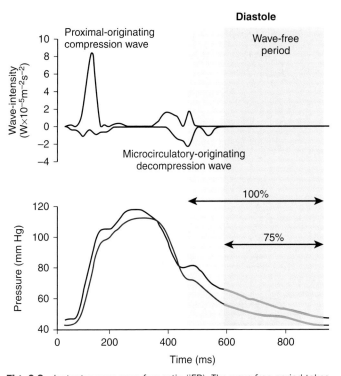

Fig. 6.8 Instantaneous wave-free ratio (iFR). The wave-free period takes 75% of diastole and is characterized by minimal and constant coronary resistance allowing for adenosine-free assessment of translesional gradients. (From Sen Sayan, Asrress KN, Nijjer S, Petraco R, et al. Diagnostic classification of the instantaneous wave-free ratio is equivalent to fractional flow reserve and is not improved with adenosine administration. *J Am Coll Cardiol.* 2013;61;1409-1420.)

emergency CABG previously associated with plain old balloon angioplasty. Drug-eluting stents reduce the rates of restenosis compared with bare metal stents and are generally used if there are no contraindications for prolonged dual antiplatelet therapy.

Although bioabsorbable vascular scaffolds (BVS) have promising characteristics, early clinical application has demonstrated a higher risk of stent thrombosis prompting the manufacturer to withdraw the product from the US market shortly after receiving US Food and Drug Administration (FDA) approval.

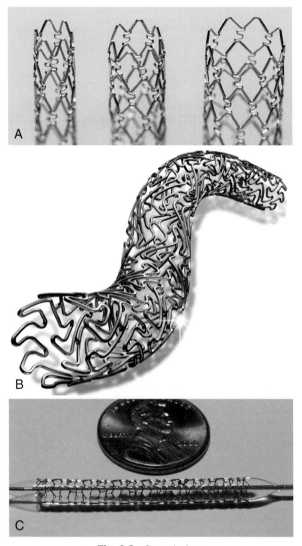

Fig. 6.9 Stent designs.

Contraindications to Stenting

Contraindications are divided into two types: clinical and anatomic factors. Relative contraindications based on patient factors include:

1. Inability to take dual antiplatelet therapy.
2. Inability to dilate the lesion fully.
3. Hypersensitivity to stent material.
4. History of bleeding or other conditions that preclude anticoagulation during PCI.
5. Noncardiac surgery required within 2 weeks.

Figures 6.10 and 6.11 are case examples of PCI.

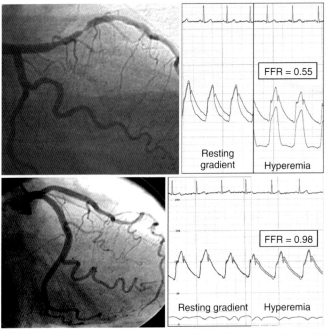

Fig. 6.10 Single-vessel stenting. *Top:* Left anterior descending (LAD) artery with a 90% narrowing, significant hemodynamic gradient, and low fractional flow reserve *(FFR)* before percutaneous coronary intervention (PCI). *Bottom:* Post-PCI result with 0% angiographic residual and normalization of translesional pressure. (Courtesy Drs. Bernard De Bruyne and Nico Pijls.)

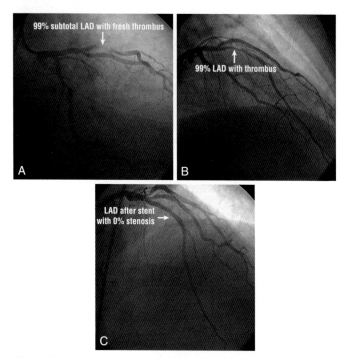

Fig. 6.11 Percutaneous coronary intervention (PCI) for acute ST-segment elevation myocardial infarction (STEMI) of left anterior descending *(LAD)* artery. **(A)** LAD in right anterior oblique (RAO) cranial projection showing thrombotic narrowing. **(B)** LAD in anteroposterior (AP) cranial projection. **(C)** Post-PCI of LAD after stenting for STEMI.

Coronary Atherectomy

Because atherosclerotic plaque remains in the artery after balloon dilation, physical removal of the plaque from inside the coronary artery was thought to improve procedural and clinical results. Atherectomy devices are still in use for this purpose: the high-speed rotablator for coronary calcified plaque (Fig. 6.12), the directional atherectomy catheter (DCA) for peripheral vascular disease, and the Diamond 360 orbital atherectomy system for coronary and peripheral applications.

Rotational Atherectomy (Rotablator)

The rotablator is made of an olive-shaped steel burr (1.25 to 2.5 mm in diameter; Fig.6.13A) that is embedded with microscopic

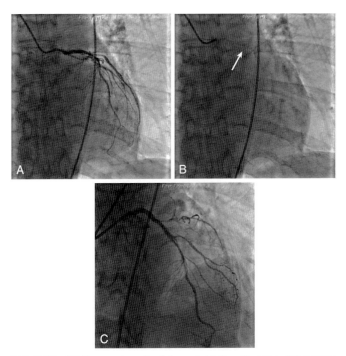

Fig. 6.12 **(A)** Severe stenosis of the ostial left main artery. **(B)** Heavily calcified left main artery. **(C)** After rotational atherectomy, final angiographic results after percutaneous coronary intervention (PCI) with drug-eluting stent.

diamond particles in the front half and rotated on a torque wire at up to 200,000 rpm by an external air turbine. The device is inserted through 6-F to 9-F guiding catheters over a special 0.009-inch stainless-steel guidewire. Continuous pressurized heparinized saline (with or without emulsifiers) is infused through the device to aid lubrication and heat dissipation. After the burr is placed just proximal to the lesion, the system is activated, and the burr is advanced through the lesion in a slow, steady pecking manner. The abrasive surface of the burr selectively ablates (pulverizes) hard calcified plaque while sparing the softer normal wall (differential cutting). Several burr passes are performed up to 30 seconds per run before removal of the burr and a decision for a larger burr or balloon inflation is made. Definitive therapy with stenting is almost always performed. The maximum burr diameter should be no larger than 70% of the normal arterial luminal diameter.

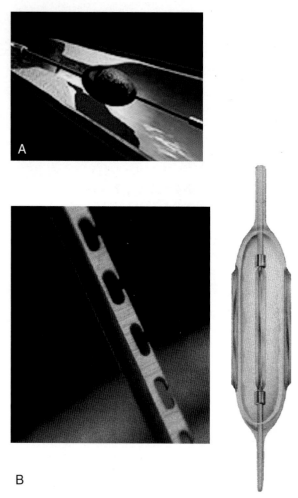

Fig. 6.13 **(A)** Rotablator burr. **(B)** Cutting balloon with microatheratome blades.

The rotablator is most suitable for rigid calcified and long lesions in which stent delivery success is likely to be low. The goal of rotational atherectomy is plaque modification of resistant lesions. Randomized comparisons for use of rotablator indicate no restenosis advantage but better procedure success in the calcified small vessel or long lesion subset.

A specific complication of the rotablator is a temporary no-reflow phenomenon, with creatinine kinase enzyme or troponin increase in some patients. This problem may necessitate insertion of a prophylactic pacemaker wire, especially for dominant right coronary lesions. Other potential complications are coronary artery dissection and perforation.

Orbital Atherectomy (Diamondback 360-Degree Orbital Atherectomy System)

An eccentric diamond-coated crown on the end of a drive-shaft is advanced over a 0.014-inch proprietary guidewire (ViperWire). During atherectomy runs, the crown moves centrifugally to modify calcified coronary plaques, as the crown orbits, the debulking area increases, and with increments in speed, the area increases further. The device is powered by a pneumatic drive console. On average, the minimal lumen diameter increases by 2 mm after atherectomy, which facilitates stent delivery in 98% of cases.

Cutting Balloon

The cutting balloon is equipped with microatherotomes to incise the plaque at three or four points along its circumference (see Fig. 6.13B). This scoring or cutting of the plaque is purported to produce more controlled and better dilation. The cutting balloon is commonly used for ostial lesions or in-stent restenotic lesions.

Thrombus Aspiration Systems

IC thrombus can be aspirated manually with several available manual aspiration catheters (Fig. 6.14) or a high-pressure mechanical rheolytic thrombectomy system (AngioJet, Boston Scientific, Maple Grove, MN). The AngioJet catheter uses high-pressure water jets directed backward into the catheter to create a strong suction at the space near the tip, which effectively evacuates and macerates thrombus (Fig. 6.15).

The clinical efficacy of manual aspiration thrombectomy catheters is mixed, with one trial (TAPAS) showing reduced mortality in patients with MI who undergo primary PCI. Another trial showed no benefit (INFUSE AMI). A full discussion of these devices can be found elsewhere (see Suggested Readings at the end of this chapter).

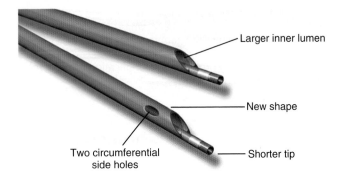

Fig. 6.14 Manual thrombus aspiration catheters.

Peripheral Arterial Balloon Angioplasty

Peripheral arterial disease is a common manifestation of atherosclerosis and often present in patients who undergo cardiac catheterization for coronary artery disease. Generally, peripheral arterial disease can be managed conservatively, although some patients require revascularization therapy (either via surgery or peripheral intervention). Certain anatomic considerations often make a patient a better candidate for one procedure as opposed to the other. In peripheral arterial disease, discrete localized lesions are usually treated best by balloon angioplasty (see Chapter 5), whereas diffuse disease and long total occlusions are often treated better with bypass surgery. A team approach involving input from the vascular interventionalist and vascular surgeon results in optimal treatment for the patient. Nomenclature for the peripheral vessels below the diaphragm is shown in Figure 6.16.

Indications

Indications for peripheral arterial revascularization include (1) intermittent (lifestyle-limiting) claudication for more than 6 months and (2) critical limb ischemia (pain at rest, nonhealing ulcer, and tissue loss). Revascularization is elective in nondiabetic patients and those who smoke with intermittent claudication, because (1) it does not affect long-term survival and (2) the incidence of severe limb-threatening ischemia is low because of distal vessel patency.

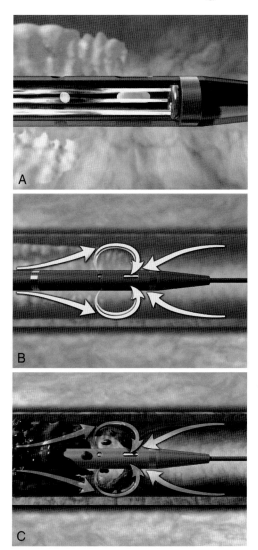

Fig. 6.15 Rheolytic thrombus aspiration catheter (AngioJet, Boston Scientific, Maple Grove, MN). **(A)** High-pressure water jet is directed from the tip back into the catheter lumen. **(B)** Jet creates Venturi suction at the top and **(C)** can aspirate material.

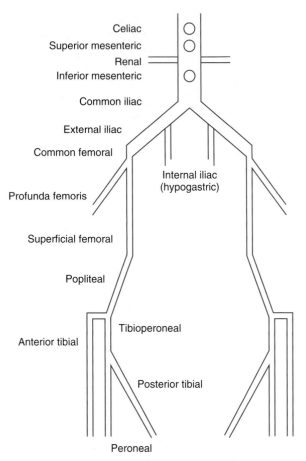

Celiac
Superior mesenteric
Renal
Inferior mesenteric
Common iliac
External iliac
Common femoral
Internal iliac (hypogastric)
Profunda femoris
Superficial femoral
Popliteal
Tibioperoneal
Anterior tibial
Posterior tibial
Peroneal

Fig. 6.16 Peripheral vascular interventional sites of the lower extremities. (Courtesy CJ White, SR Ramee, and TJ Collins, Ochsner Health System, New Orleans, LA.)

Vascular Access Technique for Lower Extremity Angioplasty

1. Antegrade, common femoral: The common femoral artery is entered above the midpoint of the femoral head. Most superficial femoral artery (SFA)–profunda bifurcations are below this

point and permit access to ipsilateral SFA, profunda, popliteal, and below-the-knee vessels.

2. Retrograde, common femoral: Access of the ipsilateral iliac artery permits a contralateral approach to iliac SFA and below-the-knee lesions.

3. Brachial-axillary (radial with extra long catheters) access requires extra-long catheters and balloons (120 to 145 cm). Access is used when bilateral iliofemoral vessels are occluded.

4. Popliteal: Retrograde access for SFA occlusions avoids the proximal cap and minimizes the likelihood of entering side branches in total occlusions. There is risk of joint space (knee) injury.

5. Tibial: Retrograde access for tibial occlusions avoids the proximal cap.

Angiography

1. Cardiac catheterization laboratory equipment (Digital subtraction angiography should be considered for noncoronary imaging.)
   - Image intensifier, 9-inch mode
   - Digital imaging subtraction to reduce radiation exposure
   - Cineframe rates show flow dynamics (helpful in assessing collaterals)
   - Speed of 15 frames/s is adequate

2. Abdominal aortogram
   - Catheter positioned above or at the level of renal arteries (L1 or L2 disk space)
   - Contrast medium injection, 15 mL/s × 3 s or 20 mL/s × 2 s
   - Pan to iliofemoral vessels
   - Lateral plane for celiac, superior mesenteric, or inferior mesenteric artery origins
   - LAO 20 degrees for renal artery origins

3. Selective iliofemoral angiography with runoff to feet
   - Catheter positioned in proximal common iliac artery
   - Simmons, SOS Omni Selective Catheter (AngioDynamics, Latham, NY), VCF, Cobra (Terumo Medical, Somerset, NJ), internal mammary, or pigtail catheters used
   - Contrast medium injection, 6 to 8 mL/s × 4 to 6 s

- Lateral angulation of image intensifier at 30 degrees (SFA-profunda bifurcation)
- Pan from common iliac artery to foot vessels
- Chapter 5 provides illustrations of common peripheral vascular interventions and complications

Figure 6.17 shows an example of renal artery stenting.

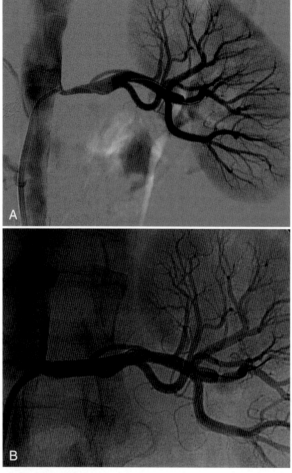

Fig. 6.17 Cineframe of left renal artery before **(A)** and after **(B)** renal artery stenting.

Structural Heart Disease: Valvuloplasty and Percutaneous Valve Replacement

Percutaneous techniques as alternatives to surgery for the treatment of valvular and congenital heart disease were introduced in the early 1980s and have undergone dramatic advances. Today, we have a large spectrum of therapeutic interventions to address problems once confined to the cardiothoracic surgeon (Fig. 6.18).

This section addresses balloon valvuloplasty for aortic and mitral valves in adults, transcatheter aortic valve replacement (TAVR) for adult aortic stenosis, MitraClip (Abbott Vascular, Redwood City, CA) for mitral regurgitation (MR), patent foramen

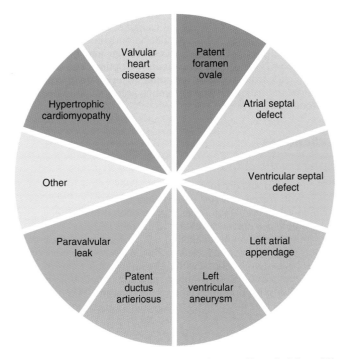

Fig. 6.18 Spectrum of structural heart disease. (From Steinberg DH, Staubach S, Franke J, et al. Defining structural heart disease in the adult patient: current scope, inherent challenges and future directions. *Eur Heart J Suppl.* 2010;12(Suppl E), E2-E9.)

ovale (PFO)/ASD closure devices, left atrial appendage (LAA) closure devices, and alcohol septal ablation for hypertrophic obstructive cardiomyopathy (HOCM). This review is not intended to be comprehensive but merely a source of introductory information regarding some of the available devices and techniques that may be encountered in catheterization laboratories across the country.

Percutaneous Balloon Mitral Valvuloplasty

For mitral stenosis, balloon mitral valvuloplasty is an excellent alternative to surgical commissurotomy or valve replacement and, in selected patients, considered to be the initial mechanical treatment of choice. Percutaneous balloon mitral valvuloplasty (PBMV) for the treatment of mitral stenosis has been studied extensively and, when successful, yields marked immediate hemodynamic improvement and sustained clinical benefit. Prospective comparisons of PBMV with surgical commissurotomy in selected patients have shown similar hemodynamic and clinical results in follow-up. Clinical success is high and complication rates are low. However, not all patients are optimal candidates for PBMV. Echocardiography is essential to evaluate mitral valve structure and to exclude LA thrombus before making decisions to proceed with PMBV.

Indications

Symptomatic Mitral Stenosis

Patients with isolated symptomatic mitral stenosis or stenosis combined with mixed valvular disease, less than moderate MR, and suitable valvular characteristics can be offered PBMV because of comparable risk and relative ease of the procedure.

Immobile, severely thickened, and fused or calcified valve leaflets may not respond well to PBMV. However, patients with symptoms of mitral stenosis with these unfavorable characteristics who are not candidates for surgery may still benefit from the procedure. PBMV is contraindicated in the presence of atrial thrombus, which is best detected by transesophageal echocardiography (TEE).

Procedure

Antegrade transseptal access to the mitral valve with use of a single, specially designed balloon catheter (Inoue balloon) (Fig. 6.19) is the easiest and most reliable method for LA access. Because of

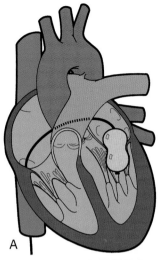

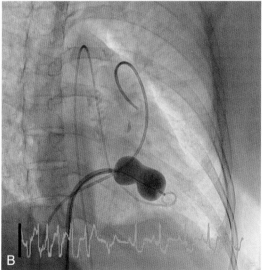

Fig. 6.19 **(A)** Diagram of Inoue balloon catheter in position across the mitral valve during mitral valvuloplasty. **(B)** Cineangiogram frame of Inoue balloon catheter in position across the mitral valve during mitral valvuloplasty. Front and back portions of balloon are inflated, creating a dog-bone shape that self-positions the balloon in the mitral orifice. The balloon continues to be inflated until the waist is eliminated. Transmitral pressure gradient must be checked before increasing inflation volume on the next balloon expansion.

its single-balloon design and relative ease in crossing the mitral valve, use of the Inoue balloon generally requires less fluoroscopic and procedural time than previously used double-balloon techniques.

After baseline hemodynamic measurements are obtained, transseptal catheterization is performed (see Chapter 7). Experienced operators perform the puncture mid to low on the septal wall to avoid a high puncture, because this location presents great difficulty in crossing the mitral valve and positioning the balloon catheter.

Dilating the Interatrial Septum. After crossing the atrial septum with the catheter and placement of the exchange guidewire, a 6-mm to 8-mm balloon is used to dilate the septum allowing easy passage of the larger dilation catheters. The residual small ASD is not generally clinically important.

Inoue Balloon Technique. The Inoue balloon catheter has a unique design that allows inflation of the distal part of the balloon to facilitate crossing the mitral valve. Once across the mitral valve, a step-wise incremental valve dilation can be performed using a calibrated inflation syringe. Selection of balloon size is based on patient height. After LA access is obtained, the interatrial septum is dilated, and the Inoue balloon is tracked over the special guidewire into the left atrium. The distal balloon tip is floated across the mitral valve, steered with a stylet. The partially inflated balloon is withdrawn to engage the mitral valve leaflets and then fully inflated to achieve commissural splitting. The transmitral pressure gradient and an echocardiographic assessment of commissural splitting and any regurgitation have been recommended after each dilating step to assess the need for continued larger balloon dilations to safely obtain the maximum mitral orifice possible without producing MR.

After the last inflation, LA-LV pressure and right-sided oxygen saturation (to detect left-to-right shunting at the atrial septal level) are measured. The average decrease in mitral valve gradient is approximately 50% to 75% of the baseline gradient, and the increase in valve area is usually around 100% (average 2 cm^2), leading to a doubling of the cardiac output. Figure 6.20 shows a hemodynamic case example of PBMV.

Complications

Procedural and hospital mortality are rare (0% to 2%) and usually the result of ventricular perforation. Complications of transseptal puncture, such as hemopericardium or tamponade, are also rare

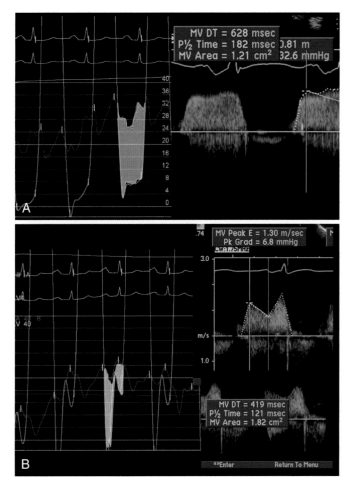

Fig. 6.20 **(A)** Directly measured left atrial (LA)-left ventricular (LV) gradient and transmitral Doppler flow velocity before a percutaneous balloon mitral valvuloplasty (PBMV) shows a gradient of 32 mm Hg. **(B)** After PBMV, the LA-LV gradient is 8, with corresponding reduction in Doppler flow velocity and no mitral regurgitation (MR).

(<2%). Systemic emboli may occur in 1% to 2% of patients. MR increases in 20% to 50% of patients but significantly (by more than one angiographic grade) in only 8% to 10% of patients. Significant MR may appear late after PBMV. MR severe enough to require valve replacement occurs in 0.9% to 3% of patients after PBMV and is usually the result of noncommissural tearing of the mitral leaflets or chordal rupture. An ASD with left-to-right shunting is detectable in 8% to 87% of patients (depending on the sensitivity of the method used for detection); most of these defects have shunt fractions of <1.4 to 1, are clinically unimportant, and decrease or disappear during follow-up.

Follow-Up

The symptomatic status of the patient generally improves immediately and during follow-up. Short-term symptomatic improvement is present in most patients. Long-term results (≥5 years) remain positive in well-selected patients. In such patients, event-free 5-year survival is >80%. Patients with more deformed valves and higher echocardiographic scores have a higher rate of restenosis. The incidence of restenosis and long-term outcome after PBMV is comparable to closed mitral commissurotomy in selected patients.

MitraClip for Mitral Regurgitation

The standard of care for treatment of severe degenerative MR is surgical mitral valve repair or replacement. The MitraClip (Fig. 6.21) is the most widely used percutaneous repair system, duplicating a stitched edge-to-edge technique to create a smaller double-orifice valve. The MitraClip system has been evaluated in EVEREST I and II studies and the COAPT trial.

Indications

Presently, the MitraClip Delivery System is indicated for the percutaneous reduction of significant symptomatic mitral regurgitation (MR ≥3) because of primary abnormality of the mitral apparatus (degenerative MR) in patients who have been determined to be at prohibitive risk of mitral valve surgery by a heart team (Class IIb). The use of MitraClip for the treatment of functional mitral regurgitation was found to be life-saving and reduced heart failure hospitalization in the COAPT trial, and is likely to be approved for this use in the United States.

MitraClip Procedure

The MitraClip procedure is performed with the patient under general anesthesia and with the use of fluoroscopy and TEE for device guidance. The right femoral vein is accessed and an 8-F sheath is commonly inserted. Right-heart catheterization is optional.

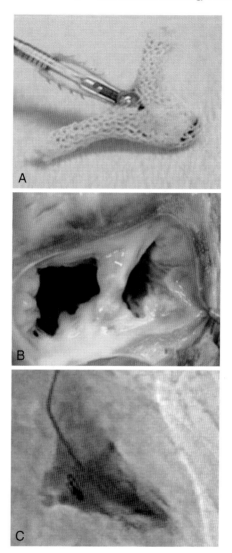

Fig. 6.21 **(A)** MitraClip (Abbott Laboratories, Abbott Park, IL, Abbott Vascular). **(B)** Approximation of anterior and posterior mitral valve leaflets as effected by the MitraClip. **(C)** Ventriculogram in systole with MitraClip in place, showing minimal mitral regurgitation (MR). (From Steinberg DH, Staubach S, Franke J, et al. *Eur Heart J Suppl.* 2010;12:E2-E9.)

Transseptal puncture follows using standard technique via the right femoral vein at a height of 4.0 cm to 4.5 cm above the mitral valve in a posterior superior orientation. Heparin is then given with a goal ACT of >300 seconds. The steerable guide catheter is 24 F proximally and 22 F at the atrial septum. The transseptal sheath is exchanged for the guide catheter and tapered dilator. The clip delivery system is advanced through the guide catheter and into the left atrium. Controls on the guiding catheter allow deflection of the distal tip. The clip delivery system has two dials that permit medial-lateral and anteroposterior steering. Using fluoroscopic and echocardiographic guidance, the MitraClip is steered until axially aligned and centered over the origin of the regurgitant jet. The clip is opened to extend the two arms and then advanced into the LV below the mitral leaflets. The clip is retracted so that each leaflet is grasped by an extended arm and then closed to coapt the mitral leaflets. The inner portion of the clip has two grippers adjacent to each arm to secure the leaflets as the clip is closed. Leaflet insertion into the clip and MR reduction are assessed by two-dimensional and Doppler echocardiography. If reduction in MR is not adequate, the clip can be reopened to release the leaflets and the clip repositioned. After adequate reduction of MR has been achieved, the clip is deployed and the delivery system and guide catheter are removed.

In patients who are at high risk from surgery, the MitraClip percutaneous mitral valve repair system is a safe and effective treatment option that reduces MR, has a favorable impact on LV remodeling, improves symptoms, and reduces hospitalizations for heart failure.

A full discussion of the indications, contraindications, complications, and outcomes is provided in the *Interventional Cardiac Catheterization Handbook*.

Transcatheter Aortic Valve Replacement

The advent of TAVR provided an option for those previously unable to undergo surgical AVR. Indications for TAVR have expanded to intermediate- and high-risk patients, and trials targeting low-risk patients have recently been completed.

Evaluation for TAVR is very detailed and includes determination of any coronary artery disease, LV dysfunction, presence of concomitant medical comorbidities (chronic obstructive pulmonary disease [COPD], renal insufficiency, carotid disease), assessment of the patient's frailty, and determination of the degree of peripheral vascular disease. The workup requires transthoracic echocardiography (TTE) and/or, cardiac catheterization with coronary angiography and pulmonary function testing, carotid duplex imaging, and body computed tomography (CT) angiography. CT is the imaging modality of choice for the preprocedural workup of the TAVR patient and assists in device size selection and route of placement. Preprocedural evaluation of vascular access with CT angiography is an important step to determine suitability for a transfemoral (TF) or alternative access (subclavian, aortic, transapical carotid or caval) for TAVR.

Standard for TAVR is a hybrid operating room/catheterization laboratory for simultaneous fluoroscopy guided catheter manipulation and conversion to open surgery, if needed. The room should be large enough to accommodate a team consisting of cardiac anesthesiologists, echocardiographers, cardiac surgeons, and interventional cardiologists.

Two valves for TAVR are currently available in the United States: the balloon-expandable Edwards SAPIEN XT and 3 systems and the self-expanding Medtronic Evolut R and PRO (Fig. 6.22). These third-generation valves (SAPIEN 3 and Evolut PRO) have device enhancements that mitigate paravalvular regurgitation. In addition, the Commander delivery system has a dual articulating piece that enables coaxiality and facilitates valve delivery in tortuous anatomy.

Procedural Details

Large-bore vascular access is obtained followed by guidewire crossing of the aortic valve most commonly without balloon valvuloplasty (Fig. 6.23). Delivery of the valve catheter is performed under fluoroscopic guidance and positioned across the aortic valve. An aortogram identifies calcific aortic and valvular landmarks and overall valve position before deployment (Fig. 6.24). Once position is confirmed, usually using fluoroscopy, rapid pacing is initiated to halt ventricular ejection. Once achieved, the valve can be deployed using fluoroscopic and echocardiographic guidance. Post deployment, echocardiography is necessary to assess accurately for either valvular or paravalvular (PVL) aortic regurgitation, ventricular function, mitral valve function, and complications, such as annular rupture, pericardial effusion, or tamponade. An immediate assessment can be helpful in identifying a potential complication of the valve deployment (Fig. 6.25). Procedural risks of TAVR are summarized in Box 6.3. TAVR under monitored anesthesia care (minimalistic approach) is associated with similar safety and superior outcomes in properly selected patients and is gaining traction in the interventional community.

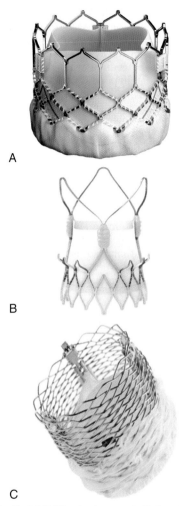

A

B

C

Fig. 6.22 The Evolut R **(A)** valve has a polyethylene terephthalate fabric skirt sewn to the bottom portion of the interior and exterior of the frame (sealing skirt). The ACURATE neo valve is a self-expanding supra-annular valve **(B)** and LOTUS Edge valve system **(C)** is mechanically expanded, fully retrievable valve. (Courtesy Edwards Lifesciences LLC, Irvine, CA. Edwards, Edwards Lifesciences, Edwards SAPIEN, SAPIEN, SAPIEN XT and SAPIEN 3 are trademarks of Edwards Lifesciences Corporation.)

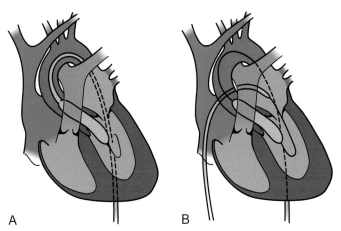

Fig. 6.23 Diagram of two techniques of aortic balloon valvuloplasty. **(A)** Retrograde approach; **(B)** antegrade, transseptal approach.

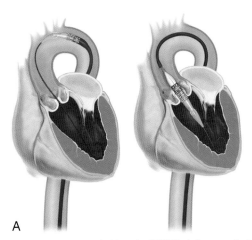

A

Fig. 6.24 **(A)** Positioning of Edwards SAPIEN delivery catheter in the ascending aortic before crossing the aortic valve. Note the delivery catheter with the enclosed valve position in the aortic root across the previously dilated aortic valve. *Continued*

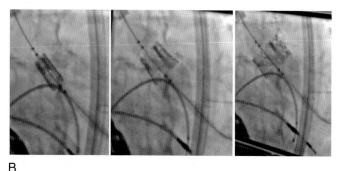

B

Fig. 6.24, cont'd (B) Frames from cineangiogram of Edwards SAPIEN valve being deployed. Note expansion of the stent valve to its full diameter in bottom frame (26 mm). (Fig. 6.24A from Webb JG, Altwegg L, Masson JB, et al. A new transcatheter aortic valve and percutaneous valve delivery system. *J Am Coll Cardiol.* 2009;53(20):1855-1858; with permission from Edwards Lifesciences Corporation. All rights reserved. Fig. 6.24B reprinted with permission from the *Cath Lab Digest*. Copyright HMP Communications.)

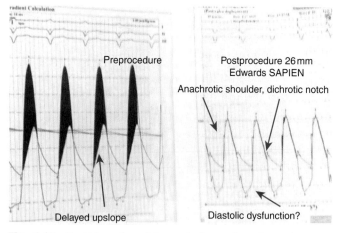

Fig. 6.25 Hemodynamics of transcatheter aortic valve replacement (TAVR). *Left:* Preprocedure with 80 mm Hg *(black areas),* slow upstroke, and moderated left ventricular end-diastolic volume (LVEDP). *Right:* Post-TAVR shows elimination of left ventricular (LV)-aortic (Ao) gradient and restoration of anachrotic shoulder and dichrotic notch. There is some increase in LVEDP. (Reprinted with permission from *Cath Lab Digest*. Copyright, HMP Communications.)

Box 6.3 **Transcatheter Aortic Valve Replacement**
Procedural Risks.

- Stroke
- Vascular complications
- Conduction system abnormalities
- Valvular insufficiency
- Coronary ostial compromise

Structural Heart Disease: Atrial Septal Defects and Patent Foramen Ovale Closure

Most full service catheterization laboratories treat ASDs and PFO with specific closure devices used by experienced operators. In brief, the technique involves placing an 8-F or 9-F sheath across the defect (Fig. 6.26). An appropriately sized closure device (Fig. 6.27) is delivered to the left atrium. The device is partially deployed, pulled back into the septal defect, and the right-sided disk is deployed, capturing the atrial septum. The procedure is monitored continuously by either TEE or intracardiac echocardiography. Postprocedure care involves removal of the large

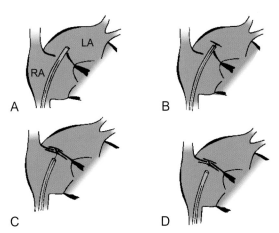

Fig. 6.26 Method of atrial septal defect (ASD)/patent foramen ovale (PFO) closure. **(A)** Delivery catheter is placed across PFO. **(B)** The left atrial (*LA*) disk is deployed. **(C)** The PFO device is pulled back into the defect, and the right atrial (*RA*) disk is deployed. **(D)** After confirmation of atrial defect tissue capture, the device is released.

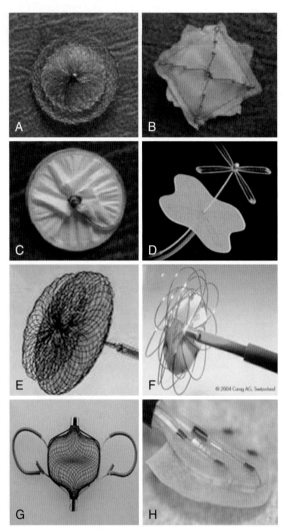

Fig. 6.27 Various patent foramen ovale (PFO) closure devices. **(A)** AMPLATZER PFO Occluder (St. Jude Medical, St. Paul, MN). **(B)** NMT Septal Occluder (NMT Medical, Inc., Boston, MA). **(C)** GORE HELEX Septal Occluder (W.L. Gore & Associates, Inc., Flagstaff, AZ). **(D)** Premere (St. Jude Medical, St. Paul, MN). **(E)** Occlutech PFO Occluder (Occlutech, Jena, Thuringia, Germany). **(F)** Soly-safe (Swissimplant AG, Solothurn, Switzerland). **(G)** SeptRx (Secant Medical, Perkasie, PA). **(H)** PFx (Cierra, Redwood City, CA). (From Steinberg DH, et al. *Eur Heart J Suppl.* 2010;12:E2-E9.)

ASD OCCLUDER   PFO OCCLUDER

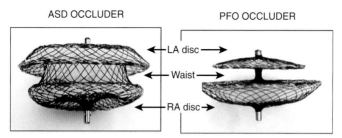

Fig. 6.28 *Left:* AMPLATZER atrial septal defect *(ASD)*. *Right:* Patent foramen ovale *(PFO)* occluders. Note the difference in left atrium *(LA)* disk size and diameter of the connecting waist. *RA,* Right atrium.

venous sheath and treatment with aspirin and clopidogrel for 6 to 12 months.

The long-term results of RESPECT, CLOSE, and REDUCE trials confirmed lower stroke rates with PFO closure compared with medical therapy in appropriately selected patients. (Fig. 6.28).

Left Atrial Appendage Closure

Patients with atrial fibrillation are at risk of stroke, presumably because of thrombus formation in the LAA. Patients are commonly treated with chronic oral anticoagulants but are at risk of life-threatening bleeding complications, including intracranial hemorrhage. An alternative to chronic oral anticoagulation is occlusion of the LAA to prevent thrombus formation.

The LAA closure device placement procedure may be done under local or, most commonly, general anesthesia using a standard transseptal catheterization technique. The procedure usually lasts approximately 1 hour, and the patient is typically discharged the day after the procedure.

Before placement, a transesophageal echocardiogram is used to measure the LAA to determine the device size suitable for implantation. After the interatrial septum is crossed using a standard transseptal access system, the LAA access sheath system is advanced over a guidewire into the left atrium. The access sheath is then advanced into the distal portion of the LAA over a pigtail catheter. The LAA device delivery system is prepped, inserted into the access sheath, and slowly advanced under fluoroscopic guidance followed by deployment into the LAA. Device release criteria are confirmed via fluoroscopy and before releasing the device. After release, the catheters are removed, and venous access hemostasis is obtained.

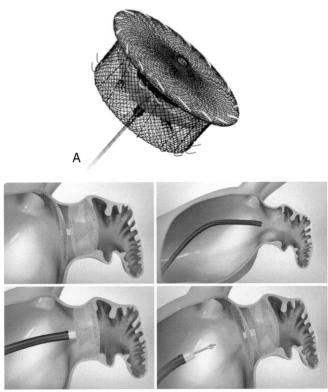

Fig. 6.29   Left atrial appendage (LAA) occluders. **(A)** WATCHMAN (Boston Scientific, Marlborough, MA). **(B)** AMPLATZER Amulet device (St. Jude Medical, St. Paul, MN). Amplatzer and Amulet are trademarks of Abbott or its related companies. Reproduced with permission of Abbott © 2019. All rights reserved.

The WATCHMAN device (Fig. 6.29; Boston Scientific, Marlborough, MA) was not inferior to warfarin for reducing the risk of the composite endpoint of cardiovascular mortality, all stroke and systemic embolization, and all causes of mortality and cardiovascular mortality. Currently the device is indicated for thromboembolic prevention in patients with nonvalvular atrial fibrillation who are poor candidates for long-term anticoagulation. Other devices such as AMPLATZE Amule (St. Jude Medical/

Abbott, St. Paul, MN) are currently being compared with WATCH-MAN (Fig. 6.29B).

Alcohol Septal Ablation for Hypertrophic Obstructive Cardiomyopathy

In some patients, symptoms of dyspnea, presyncope, chest pain, or syncope are caused by HOCM. In this entity, there is obstruction of flow across the left ventricular outflow tract (LVOT) by septal hypertrophy and systolic anterior motion of the mitral valve. For patients with symptoms refractory to medical therapy or who are either high risk or not candidates for surgical myectomy, a controlled septal MI can be produced by injecting alcohol into the septal artery with angioplasty techniques. This nonsurgical septal mass reduction method is called *alcohol septal ablation* for HOCM.

In brief, a small balloon catheter is inserted into the septal artery with standard angioplasty techniques and alcohol is instilled. This causes the septal muscle to infarct, become noncontractile, and scar, which eliminates the LVOT gradient.

Criteria for alcohol septal ablation for HOCM include (1) refractory symptoms on maximal medical therapy, (2) septal thickness of ≥1.8, (3) outflow tract gradient >30 mm Hg at rest or >50 mm Hg with provocation (e.g., premature ventricular contraction [PVC] or Valsalva maneuver, amyl nitrate challenge), and (4) LVOT gradient localized to the proximal region of the ventricular septum with obstruction demonstrated by echocardiogram. Other considerations should be the absence of moderate MR with no organic abnormalities of the mitral valve and no indication for cardiac surgery that is either in need of treatment or might explain the symptoms.

Technique of Alcohol Septal Ablation

Complete hemodynamic and angiographic study should precede alcohol-induced septal ablation. The right and left femoral arteries and veins are cannulated. A 5-F pigtail (carefully positioned for accurate hemodynamic data) or Halo ventriculography catheter is positioned in the LV. A 6-F Judkins left 4-cm guide catheter is inserted into the left coronary ostium from the contralateral artery. A 5-F balloon-tip pacemaker is positioned in the right ventricle for pacing if complete heart block is induced. In some patients, an internal jugular vein is selected for pacer insertion if more than 48 hours of temporary pacing is necessary. A pulmonary artery catheter may provide more hemodynamic data and cardiac output. After the catheters are positioned, coronary arteriography identifies the large septal artery originating in the proximal left anterior descending (LAD) artery. The echocardiography technician performs imaging of the LV septum and LVOT gradient. Heparin, 40 U/kg as a bolus, is administered because manipulations of angioplasty guidewires and catheters may induce thrombus. Heparin is discontinued after the procedure. Analgesia with fentanyl or a similar agent is given intravenously before septal cannulation and occlusion.

A 0.014-inch angioplasty guidewire is used to enter the largest, most proximal septal artery. A large double 45-degree bend on the angioplasty guidewire facilitates entry into the 90-degree origin of the septal branch. A 2-mm × 10-mm OTW balloon catheter is advanced into the septal artery and inflated. Angiography is performed to show that the balloon is located properly within the septum and it occludes antegrade septal flow. The guidewire is removed with the balloon, occluding the septal artery. A small amount of contrast material is injected into the septal balloon (1) to ensure no reflux of contrast material or, later, alcohol and (2) to opacify the septal artery and subbranch distribution. Subselective septal artery branch ablation may render hemodynamic results equivalent to those with complete septal artery ablation with a lower rate of heart block. After x-ray contrast imaging of the septum, echocardiographic microbubble contrast material is diluted, and 0.5 to 1 mL is injected into the septal artery. Echo contrast imaging allows visualization of the distribution of blood to the septum, hopefully corresponding to the site of LVOT obstruction. This is best seen on four-chamber, long-axis, and two-chamber echocardiographic views. In addition, this technique identifies those patients in whom the septal artery empties into the RV or perfuses the inferior wall and apex, which might be infarcted by alcohol runoff.

After echocardiographic confirmation of correct septal branch occlusion, 1 to 2 mL of 98% denatured alcohol is delivered slowly for 3 minutes into the septal artery, followed by a 5-minute observation period. Complete heart block may occur, with the need for temporary pacing. Chest pain with alcohol instillation is a common occurrence. LVOT pressures are obtained continuously before, during, and after alcohol septal ablation. The LVOT gradient is often abolished immediately with the septal infarction. After a

5-minute observation period, the balloon catheter is aspirated and then the balloon deflated. Suction is kept on the catheter lumen as the catheter is withdrawn from the LAD. Coronary angiography is repeated. Final hemodynamics are again measured. In most cases, the LV outflow gradient is abolished; 10% to 20% of patients may need permanent ventricular pacing. A modest MI occurs with creatinine phosphokinase elevation of 500 to 2000 units. Patients are monitored in the hospital for 4 to 5 days after the procedure to ensure absence of late heart block. Examples are shown in Figures 6.30 through 6.32.

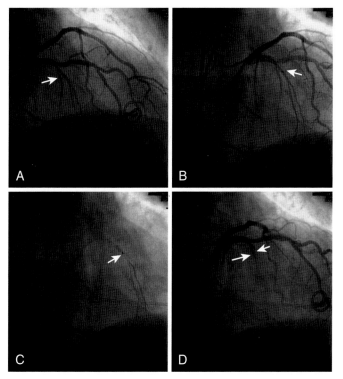

Fig. 6.30 **(A)** Coronary angiogram of left anterior descending (LAD) and first and second septal arteries *(arrow)*. **(B)** A small angioplasty balloon is placed *(arrow)* and its position verified by echocardiographic and radiographic contrast imaging. **(C)** Selective x-ray contrast injection into septal artery through occlusion balloon *(arrow)*. **(D)** After alcohol (1 to 2 mL) is instilled, the balloon is deflated and removed. The angiogram shows cutoff of a thrombosed first septal artery *(arrows)*.

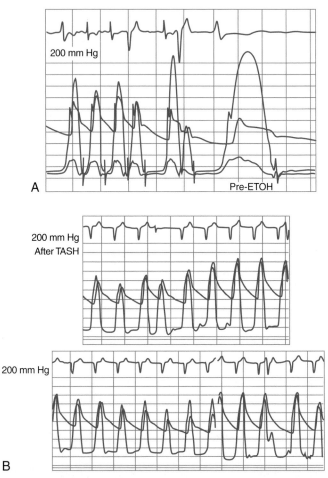

Fig. 6.31 Hemodynamics of left ventricular (LV) and aortic pressures. **(A)** Before transcoronary ablation of septal hypertrophy *(TASH) (pre-ETOH)* for hypertrophic cardiomyopathy. **(B)** After TASH during Valsalva maneuver. *ETOH,* Ethyl alcohol.

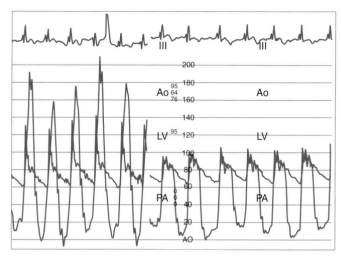

Fig. 6.32 Hemodynamics of hypertrophic cardiomyopathy before *(left)* and after *(right)* transcoronary ablation of septal hypertrophy (TASH). *Ao,* Aortic; *LV,* left ventricle; *PA,* pulmonary artery.

Suggested Readings

Boden WE. Optimal medical therapy with or without PCI for stable coronary artery disease. *N Engl J Med.* 2007;356:1503-1516.

Carroll JD, Saver JL, Thaler DE. Closure of patent foramen ovale versus medical therapy after cryptogenic stroke. *N Engl J Med.* 2013;368:1092-1100.

Chiam PT, Ruiz CE. Percutaneous transcatheter aortic valve implantation: assessing results, judging outcomes, and planning trials: the interventionalist perspective. *JACC Cardiovasc Interv.* 2008;1:341-350.

Davies JE, Sen S, Escaned J. Instantaneous Wave-free ratio versus fractional flow reserve. *N Engl J Med.* 2017;377:1597-1598.

de Bruyne B, Bartunek J, Sys SU, et al. Simultaneous coronary pressure and flow velocity measurements in humans: feasibility, reproducibility and hemodynamic dependence of coronary flow velocity reserve, hyperemic flow versus pressure slope index and fractional flow reserve. *Circulation.* 1996;94:1842-1849.

Dehmer GJ, Blankenship JC, Cilingiroglu M, et al. SCAI/ACC/AHA expert consensus document: 2014 update on percutaneous coronary intervention without on-site surgical backup. *J Am Coll Cardiol.* 2014;63:2624-2641.

Feldman T, Foster E, Qureshi M, et al. *The EVEREST II Randomized Controlled Trial: three year outcomes.* Miami, FL: Transcatheter Cardiovascular Therapeutics; October 22-26, 2012.

Holmes DR, Jr, Mack MJ, Writing Committee. Transcatheter valve therapy: a professional society overview from the American College of Cardiology Foundation and the Society of Thoracic Surgeons. *J Am Coll Cardiol.* 2011;58(4):445-455.

Inglessis I, Landzberg MJ. Interventional catheterization in adult congenital heart disease. *Circ.* 2007;115:1622-1633.

Kern MJ, Lerman A, Bech JW, et al. Physiological assessment of coronary artery disease in the cardiac catheterization laboratory: a scientific statement from the American Heart Association Committee on Diagnostic and Interventional Cardiac Catheterization, Council on Clinical Cardiology. *Circulation.* 2006;114:1321-1341.

Leon MB, Smith CR, Mack M, et al. Transcatheter aortic-valve implantation for aortic stenosis in patients who cannot undergo surgery. *N Engl J Med.* 2010;363(17):1597-1607.

Leon MB, Smith CR, Mack MJ, et al. Transcatheter or surgical aortic-valve replacement in intermediate-risk patients. *N Engl J Med.* 2016;374:1609-1620.

Lincoff AM, Bittl JA, Harrington RA, et al. Bivalirudin and provisional glycoprotein IIb/IIIa blockade compared with heparin and planned glycoprotein IIb/IIIa blockade during percutaneous coronary intervention: REPLACE-2 randomized trial. *JAMA.* 2003;289:853-863.

Mas JL, Derumeaux G, Guillon B, et al. Patent foramen ovale closure or anticoagulation vs. antiplatelets after stroke. *N Engl J Med.* 2017;377:1011-1021.

Meier B, Kalesan B, Mattle HP, et al. Percutaneous closure of patent foramen ovale in cryptogenic embolism. *N Engl J Med.* 2013;368:1083-1091.

Oyama J, Lee MS. Unprotected left main PCI: status report 2013. *J Invasive Cardiol.* 2013;25:478-482.

Pijls NH, De Bruyne B, Peels K, et al. Measurement of fractional flow reserve to assess the functional severity of coronary-artery stenoses. *N Engl J Med.* 1996;334:1703-1708.

Reardon MJ, Van Mieghem NM, Popma JJ, et al. Surgical or transcatheter aortic-valve replacement in intermediate-risk patients. *N Engl J Med.* 2017;376:1321-1331.

Saver JL, Carroll JD, Thaler DE, et al. Long-term outcomes of patent foramen ovale closure or medical therapy after stroke. *N Engl J Med.* 2017;377:1022-1032.

Smith CR, Leon MB, Mack MJ, et al. Transcatheter versus surgical aortic-valve replacement in high-risk patients. *N Engl J Med.* 2011;364(23):2187-2198.

Sorajja P, Vemulapalli S, Feldman T, et al. Outcomes with transcatheter mitral valve repair in the United States: an STS/ACC TVT Registry report. *J Am Coll Cardiol.* 2017;70:2315-2327.

Steinhubl SR, Berger PB, Mann JT 3rd, et al. Early and sustained dual oral antiplatelet therapy following percutaneous coronary intervention: a randomized controlled trial. *JAMA.* 2002;288(19):2411-2420.

Stone GW, McLaurin BT, Cox DA, et a.: Bivalirudin for patients with acute coronary syndromes. *N Engl J Med.* 2006;355:2203-2216.

Stone GW, Witzenbichler B, Guagliumi G, et al. Bivalirudin during primary PCI in acute myocardial infarction. *N Engl J Med.* 2008;358:2218-2230.

Thourani VH, Kodali S, Makkar RR, et al. Transcatheter aortic valve replacement versus surgical valve replacement in intermediate-risk patients: a propensity score analysis. *Lancet.* 2016; 387:2218-25.

Tonino Pim AL, De Bruyne B, Pijls NHJ, et al. Fractional flow reserve versus angiography for guiding percutaneous coronary intervention. *N Engl J Med.* 2009;360:213-224.

Wallentin L, Becker RC, Budaj A, et al. Ticagrelor versus clopidogrel in patients with acute coronary syndromes. *N Engl J Med.* 2009;361(11):1045-1057.

Webb JG, Wood DA. Current status of transcatheter aortic valve replacement. *J Am Coll Cardiol.* 2012;60(6):483-492.

Wiviott SD, Braunwald E, McCabe CH, et al. Prasugrel versus clopidogrel in patients with acute coronary syndromes. *N Engl J Med.* 2007;357:2001-2015.

Yusuf S, Zhao F, Mehta SR, et al. Effects of clopidogrel in addition to aspirin in patients with acute coronary syndromes without ST-segment elevation. *N Engl J Med.* 2001;345(7):494-502.

The Electrophysiology Laboratory and Electrophysiologic Procedures

SCOTT W. FERREIRA • ALI A. MEHDIRAD

During the past two decades, the dedicated electrophysiology laboratory has evolved into a highly specialized procedure room where a variety of procedures are offered, ranging from diagnostic electrophysiologic (EP) studies, curative catheter ablation procedures, implantation of loop recorders, and pacemakers, defibrillators, and resynchronization therapy devices to extraction of chronic in-dwelling leads.

The electrophysiologic study (EPS) is an invasive procedure that involves the placement of multipolar catheter electrodes at various intracardiac sites. Electrode catheters are routinely placed in the right atrium (RA), across the tricuspid valve annulus in the area of the atrioventricular (AV) node and His bundle (a special part of the conduction system), in the right ventricle (RV), in the coronary sinus, and sometimes in the left ventricle (LV; Fig. 7.1). The general purposes of EPS are to characterize the EP properties of the conduction system, to induce and to analyze the mechanism of arrhythmias, and to evaluate the effects of therapeutic interventions. Invasive EP techniques and procedures are routinely used in the clinical management of patients who have supraventricular and ventricular arrhythmias (Box 7.1). In today's laboratory, computer-generated electroanatomical maps are very much a part of the jargon, and even a novice must be able to recognize the color-coded activation patterns of common arrhythmias shown later in this chapter. Individuals seeking a more in-depth discussion of the procedures and concepts described should refer to the Suggested Readings section later in this chapter.

Equipment

An EP laboratory is equipped with radiographic imaging systems, a recording and monitoring system, a stimulator, and all drugs and equipment required for advanced cardiovascular life support (ACLS)

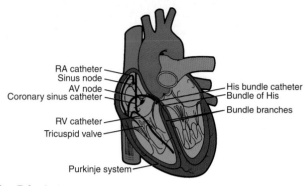

Fig. 7.1 Catheter positions for routine electrophysiologic study (EPS). Multipolar catheters are positioned in the high right atrium *(RA)* near the sinus node, area of the atrioventricular *(AV)* node and His bundle, right ventricular *(RV)* apex, and coronary sinus.

Box 7.1 Clinical Applications of Electrophysiologic Studies.

Diagnostic

- Diagnose SND
- Determine site of AV nodal block
- Define cause of syncope of unclear origin
- Differentiate VT from SVT in cases of wide-complex tachycardia
- Define mechanism of SVT or VT and map site of origin of tachycardia

Therapeutic

- Guide drug therapy for sustained VT, aborted sudden death, or SVT
- Select appropriate candidates for cardioverter-defibrillator and antitachycardia pacing therapy
- Test efficacy of device therapy for ventricular tachyarrhythmias
- Select appropriate candidates for catheter ablative and surgical therapy
- Test efficacy of ablative and surgical therapies

Interventional

- AV nodal ablation or modification for AF
- Ablation for atrial tachycardia and atrial flutter
- AV nodal modification (slow-pathway or fast-pathway ablation)
- Accessory pathway ablation in WPW syndrome
- Ablation of VT

Prognostic

- Risk stratification in asymptomatic WPW syndrome
- Risk stratification in patients after myocardial infarction
- Risk stratification in patients with nonsustained VT

AF, Atrial fibrillation; *AV,* atrioventricular; *SVT,* supraventricular tachycardia; *SND,* sinus node dysfunction; *VT,* ventricular tachycardia; *WPW,* Wolff-Parkinson-White.

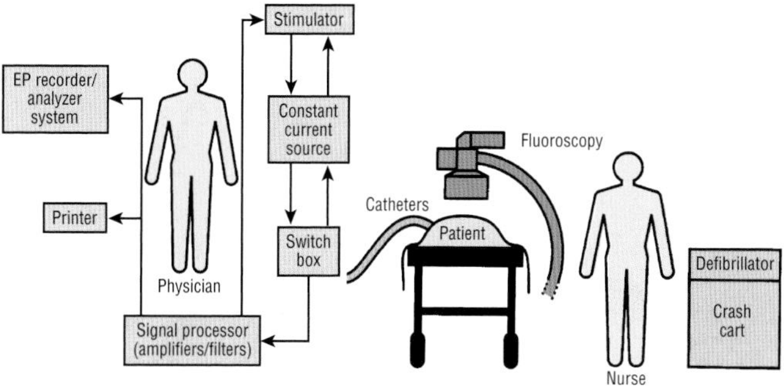

Fig. 7.2 General setup of the equipment used for electrophysiologic studies (EPSs). *EP*, Electrophysiologic.

(Fig. 7.2). Although a dedicated laboratory would be preferable, in many institutions, these procedures are performed in the cardiac hemodynamic-angiographic catheterization laboratory. If used for pacemaker and defibrillator implantation procedures, the room should have air filtering equivalent to that in a surgical operating room.

Although expensive and elaborate equipment cannot substitute an experienced and careful operator, the use of inadequate equipment may prevent adequate amounts of data from being collected and can make all the difference between success and failure. The arrhythmia targeted determines which equipment is required. A complete evaluation of most arrhythmias that may require activation mapping necessarily involves the use of multiple catheters, several recording channels, a programmable stimulator, and sophisticated and computerized three-dimensional (3D) mapping systems. Thus, an appropriately equipped laboratory should provide all of the equipment necessary for the most detailed study.

Electrode Catheters

Diagnostic Catheters

The hallmark feature of an EP catheter is the presence of at least two ring electrodes that can be used for bipolar and unipolar pacing and recording of local myocardial electrical activity. The material used to construct these catheters may be of the woven Dacron variety or synthetic materials, such as plastic or polyurethane. The number of electrodes in these catheters can vary between 2 and 20, interelectrode spacing between 2 and 20 mm, and thickness between 4 F and 7 F. The shape of these catheters can vary on the basis of the structures that they are designed to map: the crista terminalis, His bundle, coronary sinus, or pulmonary vein ostium. Typical EP catheters are shown in Figure 7.3.

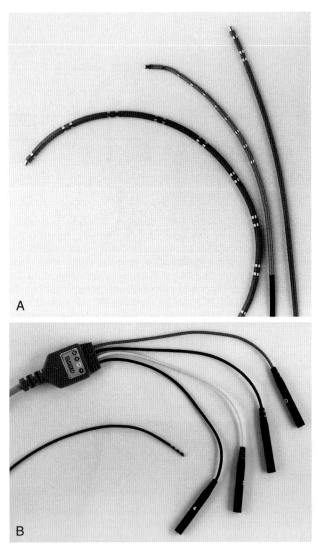

Fig. 7.3 **(A)** Several types of multipolar catheters used in routine electrophysiologic studies (EPSs). Note the difference in the number of electrodes and in spacing between the electrodes among the various catheters. **(B)** Proximal end of a quadripolar electrode catheter. The number on each pin corresponds to the electrode position at the tip of the catheter, with *D* representing the most distal electrode.

Ablation Catheters

Ablation catheters of various designs allow the operator to map and to deliver energy in a very precise manner. These catheters vary with respect to the length of the ablation/tip electrode, which can range from 3.5 to 10 mm in length. Figure 7.4 shows commonly used ablation catheters. Notice that the tip of the catheter can be deflected to allow the arrhythmogenic myocardium to be reached. Conventionally, the tip of the ablation catheter is longer than the electrode of a diagnostic catheter to prevent overheating of the ablation electrode with consequent coagulum formation. Prevention of overheating of the ablation electrode can also be achieved by actively cooling with saline irrigation.

Electroanatomical Mapping Catheters

In the mid 1990s, a novel technology termed *nonfluoroscopic electroanatomical mapping* revolutionized the practice of interventional EP. Electroanatomical mapping systems integrate three functionalities: (1) nonfluoroscopic catheter localization in 3D space, (2) 3D display of activation sequences and electrogram voltage, and (3) integration of this electroanatomical information with noninvasive images of the heart (i.e., computed tomography, magnetic resonance images, or ultrasound images [image fusion]). Two leading mapping systems are available and most laboratories

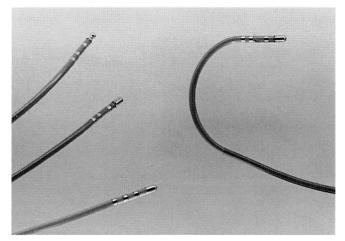

Fig. 7.4 Specialized large-tip catheter electrodes designed for ablative procedures.

use one or both. They are (1) the CARTO 3 system, manufactured by Biosense Webster, Inc., and (2) the NavX system, manufactured by St. Jude Medical.

CARTO 3. In the mid 1990s, Biosense Webster, Inc. created a catheter that has the appearance of a standard ablation catheter with a magnetic sensor within the shaft near the tip. Together with a reference sensor, it can be used to map precisely the 3D spatial location of the catheter (Fig. 7.5). The electroanatomical mapping system is called the *CARTO 3 system* and consists of the reference and catheter sensor, an external ultra-low magnetic emitter (Figs. 7.6 and 7.7), and a processing unit. The amplitude, frequency, and phase of the sensed magnetic fields contain information to solve the algebraic equations, yielding the precise locations (see Fig. 7.6) in three dimensions (x, y, and z axes) and orientation of the catheter tip sensor (roll, pitch, and yaw). An electrogram can also be recorded simultaneously in space, and an electroanatomical map can be generated. The catheter can also be moved without fluoroscopy, thus decreasing radiation exposure. An example of atrial tachycardia arising from a focal point that was mapped and ablated successfully with the use of the CARTO 3 system is shown in Fig. 7.7 for focal tachycardia. A left anterior oblique (LAO) view of an electroanatomical map of the right and left atria

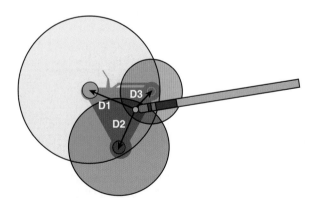

Fig. 7.5 Illustration of the principles of operation of the CARTO 3 system; specifically, how catheter location is determined. The location pad, fixed beneath the patient table, is constructed of three coils that generate ultra-low magnetic fields (1, 2, and 3 kHz). The emitted fields possess well-known temporal and spatial distinguishing characteristics that code the mapping space around the patient's chest. Sensing of the magnetic field by the location sensor (passive) enables determination of the location and orientation of the catheter in 6 degrees of freedom.

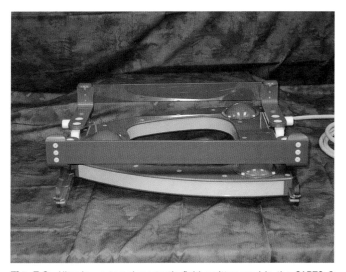

Fig. 7.6 Ultra-low external magnetic field emitter used in the CARTO 3 system. This device is placed below the patient. The system comprises a miniature passive magnetic field sensor located at the tip of the catheter, external ultra-low magnetic field emitter, and processing unit. The system uses the magnetic technology to determine accurately location and orientation of the catheter in 6 degrees of freedom (x, y, z, roll, pitch, and yaw) and simultaneously records the intracardiac local electrogram from its tip. The three-dimensional (3D) geometry of the chamber is reconstructed in real time with the electrophysiologic (EP) information, which is color-coded and superimposed on the electroanatomical map.

is shown as well as the coronary sinus. The activation data seen with the color scale show the arrhythmia to arise from the ostium of the coronary sinus.

NavX. The NavX system uses three low-amplitude high-frequency current fields that are generated in three axes over the patient's thorax to compute the position of an electrode in the thorax relative to a reference electrode that can be placed in the heart or on the patient's thorax. On the basis of these measurements, the system then displays the position of any EP catheter. The advantage of this system is that multiple catheters can be displayed, and unlike the CARTO 3 system, they are not limited to the products of a single manufacturer. Figure 7.8 shows an example of an LAO cranial view of an electroanatomical map of the left atrium *(LA, purple*

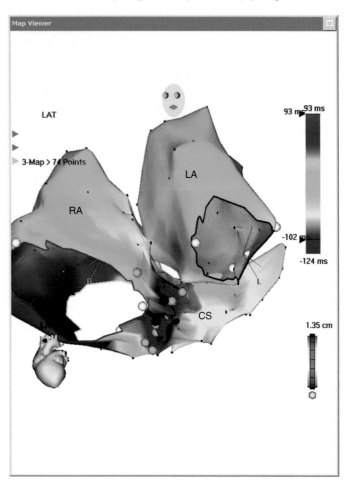

Fig. 7.7 Focal tachycardia image showing an electroanatomical map of right and left atria *(RA; LA)* along with the coronary sinus *(CS)*. The activation sequence pattern of an atrial tachycardia is shown. *Red:* sites of early activation. *Blue* and *purple:* late sites. The activation pattern shows a focal arrhythmia arising from the anterior lip of the coronary sinus ostium. *Maroon dots:* sites where catheter ablation was performed. *LAT,* Lateral.

shell) along with the four pulmonary veins and the left atrial appendage *(LAA, green)* constructed with NavX. Also seen are the coronary sinus catheter, tip of the ablation catheter, and a circular mapping catheter. This map was performed in a patient undergoing catheter ablation of atrial fibrillation (AF).

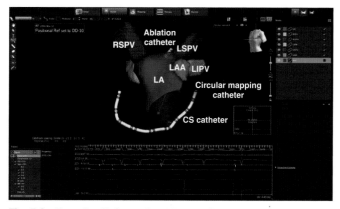

Fig. 7.8 Example of left anterior oblique (LAO) cranial view of an electro-anatomical map of the left atrium *(LA, purple shell)* along with the four pulmonary veins and left atrial appendage *(LAA, green)* constructed with NavX. Also seen are the coronary sinus catheter, the tip of the ablation catheter, and a circular mapping catheter. This map was performed in a patient undergoing catheter ablation of atrial fibrillation (AF). *CS,* Coronary sinus; *LIPV,* left interior pulmonary vein; *LSPV,* left superior pulmonary vein; *RSPV,* right superior pulmonary vein. (EnSite, Velocity, Quartet, SJM Confirm, and St. Jude Medical are trademarks of St. Jude Medical, Inc. or its related companies. Reproduced with permission from St. Jude Medical, © 2015. All rights reserved.)

Junction Box and Recording Apparatus

The junction box and recording apparatus consists of pairs of numbered multiple pole switches matched to each recording and stimulation channel and permits the ready selection of any pair of electrodes for stimulation or recording. Current computer junction boxes come in banks of 8 or 16. Nowadays, the signal processor (filters and amplifier), visualization screen, and recording apparatus are incorporated as a single unit in the form of a computerized system. GE Healthcare, EP Med Systems (St. Jude Medical), and Bard Electrophysiology manufacture popular systems. Eight to 14 amplifiers should be available to process surface electrocardiogram (ECG) leads simultaneously with multiple intracardiac electrograms. The number of amplifiers can be as many as 128 in some systems. Intracardiac recordings must be displayed simultaneously, with at least three surface ECG leads. Most computers allow several pages to be stored, with one page displaying a 12-lead ECG. Thus, an operator can always have a 12-lead ECG recorded simultaneously while observing intracardiac electrogram data. The amplifiers used for recording intracardiac electrograms must have the ability to have gain modification and to alter both high and low band pass filters to permit appropriate attenuation of the incoming signals. For example, the His bundle electrogram is most clearly visualized when the signal is filtered between 30 and 40 Hz (high pass) and 400 and 500 Hz (low pass; Fig. 7.9). In addition, assessing unipolar electrograms also requires acquiring open filters (0.05 to 500 Hz).

Stimulation Apparatus

Most EPSs require a complex programmable stimulator that has (1) a constant current source, (2) minimal current leakage, (3) the ability to pace at a wide range of cycle lengths (100 to 2000 ms) from at least two simultaneous sites, (4) the ability to introduce multiple extrastimuli, and (5) the ability to synchronize the stimulator to appropriate electrograms during spontaneous and paced rhythms. The stimulator is equipped with dials or switches by

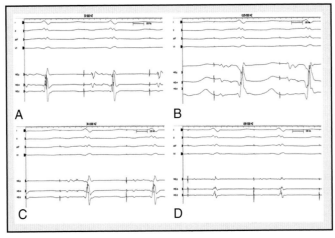

Fig. 7.9 Effect of filtering frequency on the His bundle electrogram. Pacing from the proximal coronary sinus is performed at a basic cycle length of 60 ms. In each of the four panels, surface leads I, II, aV$_F$, and V$_1$ are shown. A recording catheter is placed in the standard position to record the His bundle electrogram; and recordings from the proximal, mid, and distal electrode pairs are displayed. **(A)** His bundle electrograms, where the signal is filtered between 30 Hz (high pass) and 500 Hz (low pass); **(B)** recording made between filter settings of 0.05 and 500 Hz; **(C)** recording made between 30 and 1000 Hz; **(D)** recording made between 100 and 500 Hz. The clearest recording of the His bundle electrogram occurs with a filtering of the signals below 30 Hz and above 500 Hz **(A)**.

which the pacing intervals and coupling intervals of the extra-stimuli may be adjusted (Fig. 7.10). A junction box that interfaces with the recording system and stimulator facilitates changes in the pacing site without the need to disconnect catheters. The stimulator should be able to deliver variable currents that can be accurately controlled, with a range from 0.1 to 10 mA. The ability to change pulse widths is also useful. The results of programmed stimulation can be influenced by the delivered current, and for consistency and safety, stimulation is generally performed at two and a half times diastolic threshold.

It is preferable that the stimulator, computerized data recorder, and other devices used in EP are permanently installed. Most laboratories use a stimulator and computer system that modifies all input signals and stores them in an optical disc. All equipment must be grounded, and other aspects of electrical safety must be ensured because even small amounts of leakage current can pass to the patient and potentially induce arrhythmias. A technical engineer must check the equipment so that leakage current remains <10 mA. Figure 7.2 shows an illustration of the organization of the relevant equipment required during an EPS.

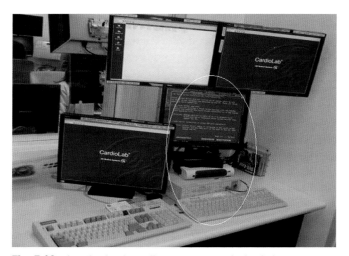

Fig. 7.10 Junction box/recording apparatus and stimulation apparatus. Image shows the Prucka CardioLab EP system. Also seen within the white oval is a computerized stimulator manufactured by Micropace. The junction box interfaces with the recording system and stimulator, thus allowing us to change the pacing site without the need to disconnect catheters.

Defibrillator

A functioning defibrillator should be available at the patient's side throughout all EPSs. A backup defibrillator is optimal in case of a rare but potentially disastrous failure of one defibrillator. Defibrillators should be tested before each study and equipped with an emergency power source. Many laboratories use commercially available R2 pads, which are placed on the patient before the EPS procedure begins. One pad is placed under the right scapula and the other on the anterior chest over the LV apex and connected to the defibrillator with an adapter. In rare instances in which transthoracic defibrillation fails to convert induced ventricular fibrillation (VF), emergency defibrillation through an intracardiac electrode catheter may be effective in terminating the arrhythmia (Fig. 7.11). It is our practice to have biphasic defibrillators in our laboratories.

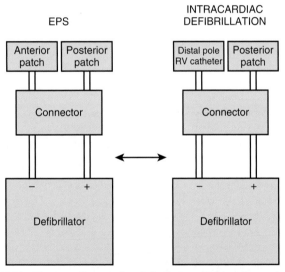

Fig. 7.11 Diagram of intracardiac defibrillation, which may be used when ventricular fibrillation (VF) is refractory to multiple transthoracic defibrillations. During the routine electrophysiologic study *(EPS)*, anterior and posterior skin patches are attached by a connector to a standard defibrillator. When multiple transthoracic high-energy shocks fail to terminate VF, the anterior patch may be disconnected and the distal pole of the right ventricular *(RV)* catheter attached to the defibrillator. High-energy shocks are delivered from the RV catheter to the posterior patch. (From Cohen TJ, Scheinman MM, Pullen BT, et al. Emergency intracardiac defibrillation for refractory ventricular fibrillation during routine electrophysiologic study. *J Am Coll Cardiol.* 1991;18:1280-1284.)

Because the physician's attention is often focused on the stimulator and electrograms, he or she relies heavily on the nurse to monitor the patient's condition and to communicate significant changes. The nurse usually sits between the patient and the cardioverter-defibrillator and crash cart. The nurse monitors the patient's blood pressure, heart rate (HR), rhythm, and oxygen saturation via a pulse oximeter; administers drugs for diagnostic and therapeutic interventions during EPS; and performs cardioversion or defibrillation when an induced hemodynamically unstable arrhythmia appears. Optimally, a second nurse is available during procedures to administer medications or assist in technical aspects of the procedure.

Implantation of Pacemakers, Defibrillators, and Resynchronization Therapy Devices

Pacemakers

Pacemakers, the original devices implanted for cardiac rhythm management, have the ability to provide electrical stimulation (pace) to the heart. They are indicated in patients who no longer have the intrinsic ability to provide adequate electrical stimulation to maintain a functional HR or complete conduction from the atria to the ventricles. They can be either single or dual chamber devices with a lead in the atrium, ventricle, or both, depending on the patient, pathology, and clinical scenario. Recently, a leadless pacemaker has been approved. This device is different from standard pacemakers in that the entire device is contained within the heart, which eliminates the need for a generator and a pocket, therefore reducing the risk of infection. These devices are single-chamber ventricular pacemakers implanted via the femoral vein and are an alternative for transvenous pacemakers for patients who only require ventricular pacing. (Fig 7.12)

A technique that has been showing benefit in recent research is that of His bundle pacing.

RV apical pacing causes interventricular dysynchrony, which can lead to adverse hemodynamics and progression to pacing induced cardiomyopathy (PCIM) in some patients. While biventricular pacing may be an option, it introduces a nonphysiologic ventricular activation sequence. Permanent His bundle pacing is an alternative option as it directly engages the His-Purkinje system, utilizing normal physiology to maintain synchronized ventricular activation.

Implantable Cardiac Defibrillators

Where pacemakers are used for bradycardic indications, defibrillators are designed to treat tachyarrhythmias, specifically ventricular

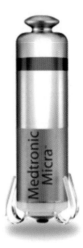

Fig. 7.12 Figure from Medtronic for Micra. (©2019 Medtronic. All rights reserved. Used with the permission of Medtronic.)

tachycardia (VT) and VF. These devices have all of the functions of a pacemaker, but in addition, they have the ability to defibrillate (shock) the heart. The primary difference in these devices in comparison with a pacemaker is the use of a high-voltage lead in the RV with an active "can" (pulse generator [PG]) to complete the defibrillation circuit. The lead has at least one shock coil and acts with the PG to provide a defibrillation wave front across the heart if the need arises. In addition, all current defibrillators have the ability to pace the ventricle rapidly (anti-tachycardia pacing [ATP]) to attempt to terminate ventricular tachyarrhythmias and to prevent the need for a shock.

In addition to transvenous defibrillators, there are also subcutaneous defibrillators (SICD) that have become available in recent years. With transvenous ICDs, insertion of electrodes into the central venous circulation and inside cardiac chambers can cause vascular obstruction, thrombosis, infection, and cardiac perforation. In addition, lead failure has been estimated to be up 20% in 10 years. The SICD consists of a 3-mm tripolar parasternal lead (12 F, 45 cm) connected to an electrically active pulse generator. The lead is vertically positioned in the subcutaneous tissue of the chest, parallel and 1 to 2 cm to the left sternal mid line. The pulse generator is positioned in the subcutaneous tissue of the left lateral chest. (Fig. 7.13). These devices are currently only capable of defibrillation and only have postshock (subcutaneous) pacing. They are not capable of performing any other pacing function,

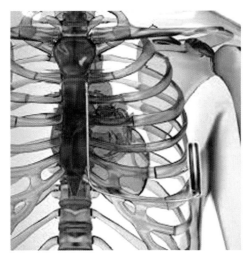

Fig. 7.13 Diagram of external subcutaneous pacing array system.

including ATP pacing to terminate arrhythmias or bradycardia pacing.

When a patient with an implantable cardiac defibrillator (ICD) undergoes a change in his or her antiarrhythmic drug regimen, the device may need to be tested, because changes in rate of tachycardia may necessitate reprogramming the device's rate detection criteria, and changes in the defibrillation threshold may be caused by certain medications.

Primary Prevention of Sudden Death

The survival rate after out-of-hospital cardiac arrest is extremely low, and attention has been directed at identifying high-risk patients who may benefit from prophylactic treatment as a means of primary prevention of sudden cardiac death. Two primary prevention trials indicated that patients with coronary disease, significant LV dysfunction (left ventricular ejection fraction [LVEF] 35% to 40%), spontaneous nonsustained VT, and inducible sustained ventricular arrhythmia by EPS experienced a survival benefit from prophylactic ICD implantation. There is no evidence that EPS-guided antiarrhythmic drug therapy is effective as preventive therapy for sudden cardiac death in high-risk individuals. A primary prevention trial, which did not require spontaneous or induced ventricular arrhythmias as entry criteria, concluded that prophylactic ICD implantation benefited patients with coronary artery disease and found an LVEF of less than 30%. This study suggests that poor LV function alone is a strong predictor of subsequent sudden cardiac death. Indications for implantation of pacemakers and ICDs are listed in Table 7.1.

Table 7.1

Indications for Pacemaker and Implantable Cardiac Defibrillator Implantation.	
Pacemaker	
SND	• SND with documented symptomatic bradycardia, including frequent sinus pauses that produce symptoms (class I, LE C)
	• Symptomatic chronotropic incompetence (class I, LE C)
	• Symptomatic sinus bradycardia that results from required drug therapy for medical conditions (class I, LE C)
	• Minimally symptomatic patients with chronic HR <40 bpm while awake (class IIb, LE C)
	• Not indicated for SND in asymptomatic patients (class III, LE C)
	• Not indicated for SND in patients for whom symptoms suggestive of bradycardia have been clearly documented to occur in the absence of bradycardia (class III, LE C)
	• Not indicated for SND with symptomatic bradycardia resulting from nonessential drug therapy (class III, LE C)
Acquired AV block in adults	• Third-degree and advanced second-degree AV block at any anatomic level associated with bradycardia with symptoms (including HF) or ventricular arrhythmias presumed to be due to AV block (class I, LE C)
	• Third- and advanced second-degree AV block at any anatomic level associated with arrhythmias and other medical conditions requiring drug therapy that results in symptomatic bradycardia (class I, LE C)
	• Third- and advanced second-degree AV block at any anatomic level in awake, symptom-free patients in sinus rhythm, with documented periods of asystole ≥3.0 s, any escape rate <40 bpm, or an escape rhythm that is below the AV node (class I, LE C)
	• Third- and advanced second-degree AV block at any anatomic level after catheter ablation of the AV junction (class I, LE C)
	• Third- and advanced second-degree AV block at any anatomic level associated with postoperative AV block that is not expected to resolve after cardiac surgery (class I, LE C)

Table 7.1

Indications for Pacemaker and Implantable Cardiac Defibrillator Implantation (Continued)

- Third- and advanced second-degree AV block at any anatomic level associated with neuromuscular diseases with AV block, such as myotonic muscular dystrophy, Kearns-Sayre syndrome, Erb dystrophy (limb-girdle muscular dystrophy), and peroneal muscular atrophy, with or without symptoms (class I, LV B)
- Second-degree AV block with associated symptomatic bradycardia regardless of the type or site of block (class I, LE B)
- Asymptomatic persistent third-degree AV block at any anatomic site with average awake ventricular rates of 40 bpm or faster if cardiomegaly or LV dysfunction is present or the site of block is below the AV node (class I, LE B)
- Second- or third-degree AV block during exercise in the absence of myocardial ischemia (class I, LE C)
- Persistent third-degree AV block with an escape rate >40 bpm in asymptomatic adult patients without cardiomegaly (class IIa, LE C)
- Asymptomatic second-degree AV block at intra- or infra-His levels found at EPS (class IIa, LE B)
- First- or second-degree AV block with symptoms similar to those of pacemaker syndrome or hemodynamic compromise (class IIa, LE B)
- Asymptomatic type-II second-degree AV block with a narrow QRS (class IIa, LE B)
- Neuromuscular diseases, such as myotonic muscular dystrophy, Erb dystrophy, and peroneal muscular atrophy with any degree of AV block (including first-degree AV block), with or without symptoms, because there may be unpredictable progression of AV conduction disease (class IIb, LE B)
- AV block in the setting of drug use and/or drug toxicity when the block is expected to recur even after the drug is withdrawn (class IIB, LE B)
- Not indicated for asymptomatic first-degree AV block (class III, LE B)
- Not indicated for asymptomatic type I second-degree AV block at the supra-His (AV node) level or that which is not known to be intra- or infra-Hisian (class III, LE C)
- Not indicated for AV block that is expected to resolve and is unlikely to recur (e.g., drug toxicity, Lyme disease, or transient increases in vagal tone or during hypoxia in sleep apnea syndrome in the absence of symptoms) (class III, LE B)

Continued on following page

Table 7.1

Indications for Pacemaker and Implantable Cardiac Defibrillator Implantation (Continued)

Chronic bifascicular block	• Advanced second-degree AV block or intermittent third-degree AV block (class I, LE B)
	• Type II second-degree AV block (class I, LE B)
	• Alternating bundle-branch block (class I, LE C)
	• Syncope not demonstrated to be caused by AV block when other likely causes have been excluded, specifically VT (class IIa, LE B)
	• Incidental finding at EPS of a markedly prolonged H–V interval (≥100 ms) in asymptomatic patients (class IIa, LE B)
	• Incidental finding at EPS of pacing-induced infra-His block that is not physiologic (class IIa, LE B)
	• In the setting of neuromuscular diseases, such as myotonic muscular dystrophy, Erb dystrophy, and peroneal muscular atrophy with bifascicular block or any fascicular block, with or without symptoms (class IIb, LE C)
	• Not indicated for fascicular block without AV block or symptoms (class III, LE B)
	• Not indicated for fascicular block with first-degree AV block without symptoms (class III, LE B)
After acute phase of MI	• Persistent second-degree AV block in the His-Purkinje system with alternating bundle-branch block or third-degree AV block within or below the His-Purkinje system after STEMI (class I, LE B)
	• Transient advanced second- or third-degree infranodal AV block and associated bundle-branch block. If block site is uncertain, an EPS may be necessary (class I, LE B)
	• Persistent and symptomatic second- or third-degree AV block (class I, LE C)
	• Persistent second- or third-degree AV block at the AV node level, even in the absence of symptoms (class IIb, LE B)
	• Not indicated for transient AV block in the absence of intraventricular conduction defects (class III, LE B)
	• Not indicated for transient AV block in the presence of isolated left anterior fascicular block (class III, LE B)
	• Not indicated in new bundle-branch block or fascicular block in the absence of AV block (class III, LE B)
	• Not indicated for persistent asymptomatic first-degree AV block in the presence of bundle-branch or fascicular block (class III, LE B)

Table 7.1

Indications for Pacemaker and Implantable Cardiac Defibrillator Implantation (Continued)

Hypersensitive carotid sinus syndrome and neuro-cardiogenic syncope	• Recurrent syncope caused by spontaneously occurring carotid sinus stimulation and carotid sinus pressure that induces ventricular asystole of >3 s (class I, LE C) • Syncope without clear, provocative events and with a hypersensitive cardioinhibitor response of ≥3 s (class IIa, LE C) • Significantly symptomatic neurocardiogenic syncope associated with bradycardia documented spontaneously or at the time of tilt-table testing (class IIb, LE B) • Not indicated for a hypersensitive cardioinhibitory response to carotid sinus stimulation without symptoms or with vague symptoms (class III, LE C) • Not indicated for situational vasovagal syncope in which avoidance behavior is effective and preferred (class III, LE C)
After cardiac transplantation	• Persistent inappropriate or symptomatic bradycardia not expected to resolve and for other class I indications for permanent pacing (class I, LE C) • When relative bradycardia is prolonged or recurrent, which limits rehabilitation or discharge after postoperative recovery from cardiac transplantation (class IIb, LE C) • Syncope after cardiac transplantation even when brady-arrhythmia has not been documented (class IIb, LE C)
Recommendations for permanent pacemakers that automatically detect and pace to terminate tachycardias	• Symptomatic recurrent SVT that is reproducibly terminated by pacing when catheter ablation and/or drugs fail to control the arrhythmia or produce intolerable side effects (class IIa, LE C) • Not indicated in the presence of an accessory pathway that has the capacity for rapid anterograde conduction (class III, LE C)
Pacing to prevent tachycardia	• Sustained pause-dependent VT with or without Q–T prolongation (class I, LE C) • High-risk patients with congenital LQTS (class IIa, LE C) • For prevention of symptomatic, drug-refractory, recurrent AF in patients with coexisting SND (class IIb, LE B) • Not indicated for frequent or complex ventricular ectopic activity without sustained VT in the absence of LQTS (class III, LE C) • Not indicated for torsades de pointes VT resulting from reversible causes (class III, LE A)
Pacing to prevent AF	• Not indicated for the prevention of AF in patients without any other indication for pacemaker implantation (class III, LE B)

Continued on following page

Table 7.1

Indications for Pacemaker and Implantable Cardiac Defibrillator Implantation (Continued)

Recommendations for pacing in patients with HCM	• SND or AV block in patients with HCM as described previously in guidelines (class I, LE C) • Medically refractory symptomatic patients with HCM and significant resting or provoked LV outflow tract obstruction (class IIa, LE A) • Not indicated for patients who are asymptomatic or whose symptoms are medically controlled (class III, LE C) • Not indicated for symptomatic patients without evidence of LV outflow tract obstruction (class III, LE C)
Recommendations for permanent pacing in children, adolescents, and patients with congenital heart disease	• Advanced second- or third-degree AV block associated with symptomatic bradycardia, ventricular dysfunction, or low cardiac output (class I, LE C) • SND with correlation of symptoms during age-inappropriate bradycardia; the definition of bradycardia varies with patient age and expected HR (class I, LE B) • Postoperative advanced second- or third-degree AV block that is not expected to resolve or that persists for at least 7 days after cardiac surgery (class I, LE B) • Congenital third-degree AV block with a wide QRS escaped rhythm, complex ventricular ectopy, or ventricular dysfunction (class I, LE B) • Congenital third-degree AV block in an infant with a ventricular rate <55 bpm or with congenital heart disease and a ventricular rate <70 bpm (class I, LE C) • Congenital heart disease and sinus bradycardia for the prevention of recurrent episodes of intraatrial reentrant tachycardia; SND may be intrinsic or secondary to antiarrhythmic treatment (class IIa, LE C) • Congenital third-degree AV block beyond the first year of life with an average HR <50 bpm, abrupt pauses in ventricular rate that are two or three times the basic cycle length, or association with symptoms caused by chronotropic incompetence (class IIa, LE B) • Sinus bradycardia with complex congenital heart disease with a resting HR <40 bpm or pauses in ventricular rate >3 s (class IIa, LE B) • Congenital heart disease and impaired hemodynamics caused by sinus bradycardia or loss of AV synchrony (class IIa, LE C) • Unexplained syncope in the patient with prior congenital heart surgery complicated by transient CHB with residual fascicular block after a careful evaluation to exclude other causes of syncope (class IIa, LE B)

Table 7.1

Indications for Pacemaker and Implantable Cardiac Defibrillator Implantation (Continued)

- Transient postoperative third-degree AV block that reverts to sinus rhythm with residual bifascicular block (class IIb, LE C)
- Congenital third-degree AV block in asymptomatic children or adolescents with an acceptable rate, narrow QRS complex, and normal ventricular function (class IIb, LE B)
- Asymptomatic sinus bradycardia after biventricular repair of congenital heart disease with a resting HR <40 bpm or pauses in ventricular rate >3 s (class IIb, LE C)
- Not indicated for transient postoperative AV block with return of normal AV conduction in an otherwise asymptomatic patient (class III, LE B)
- Not indicated for asymptomatic bifascicular block with or without first-degree AV block after surgery for congenital heart disease in the absence of prior transient complete AV block (class III, LE C)
- Not indicated for asymptomatic type I second-degree AV block (class III, LE C)
- Not indicated for asymptomatic sinus bradycardia with the longest relative risk interval <3 s and a minimum HR >40 bpm (class III, LE C)

Implantable Cardiac Defibrillator

- Survivors of cardiac arrest caused by VF or hemodynamically unstable sustained VT after evaluation to define cause of event and exclude any completely reversible causes (class I, LE A)
- Structural heart disease and spontaneous sustained VT, whether hemodynamically stable or unstable (class I, LE B)
- Syncope of undetermined origin with clinically relevant, hemodynamically significant sustained VT or VF induced at EPS (class I, LE B)
- LVEF ≤35% caused by prior MI, at least 40 days after myocardial infarction, and NYHA functional class II or III (class I, LE A)
- Nonischemic dilated cardiomyopathy, LVEF ≤35%, and NYHA functional class II or III (class I, LE B)
- LV dysfunction caused by prior MI or at least 40 days after myocardial infarction, LVEF ≤30%, and NYHA functional class I (class I, LE A)
- Nonsustained VT caused by prior MI, LVEF ≤40%, and inducible VF or sustained VT at EPS (class I, LE B)
- Unexplained syncope, significant LV dysfunction, and nonischemic dilated cardiomyopathy (class IIA, LE C)
- Sustained VT and normal or near-normal ventricular function (class IIA, LE C)
- HCM with one or more major risk factors for sudden cardiac death (class IIA, LE C)

Continued on following page

Table 7.1

Indications for Pacemaker and Implantable Cardiac Defibrillator Implantation (Continued)

- Prevention of sudden cardiac death, with ARVC or ARVD and one or more risk factors for sudden cardiac death (class IIA, LE C)
- Reduction of sudden cardiac death, with LQTS, syncope, and/or VT while receiving β-blockers (class IIa, LE B)
- Nonhospitalized and awaiting transplantation (class IIA, LE C)
- Brugada syndrome and prior syncope (class IIA, LE C)
- Brugada syndrome and documented VT that has not resulted in cardiac arrest (class IIa, LE C)
- Catecholaminergic polymorphic VT, syncope, and/or documented sustained VT while receiving β-blockers (class IIa, LE C)
- Cardiac sarcoidosis, giant cell myocarditis, or Chagas disease (class IIa, LE C)
- Nonischemic heart disease, LVEF ≤35%, NYHA functional class I (class IIb, LE C)
- LQTS and risk factors for sudden cardiac death (class IIb, LE B)
- Syncope and advanced structural heart disease with thorough invasive and noninvasive investigation failing to define cause (class IIb, LE C)
- Familial cardiomyopathy associated with sudden death (class IIb, LE C)
- LV noncompaction (class IIb, LE C)
- Not indicated in those without reasonable expectation of survival, with acceptable functional status for at least 1 year even after meeting ICD implantation criteria specified in class I, IIa, and IIb recommendations above (class III, LE C)
- Symptomatic sustained VT in association with congenital heart disease, with prior hemodynamic and EP evaluation; catheter ablation or surgical repair may offer possible alternatives in carefully selected patients (class I, LE C)
- Congenital heart disease with recurrent syncope of undetermined origin in the presence of either ventricular dysfunction or inducible ventricular arrhythmias at EPS (class IIa, LE B).
- Recurrent syncope associated with complex congenital heart disease and advanced systemic ventricular dysfunction after thorough invasive and noninvasive investigations have failed to define a cause (class IIb, LE C)

AF, Atrial fibrillation; *AV,* atrioventricular; *AVRC,* arrhythmogenic right-ventricular cardiomyopathy; *AVRD,* arrhythmogenic right-ventricular dysplasia; *bpm,* beats per minute; *CHB,* complete heart block; *EP,* electrophysiologic; *EPS,* electrophysiologic study; *HCM,* hypertrophic cardiomyopathy; *HF,* heart failure; *HR,* heart rate; *ICD,* implantable cardiac defibrillator; *LE,* level of evidence; *LQTS,* long QT syndrome; *LV,* left ventricle; *LVEF,* left ventricular ejection fraction; *MI,* myocardial infarction; *NYHA,* New York Heart Association; *QRS,* Q, R, and S waves; *SND,* sinus node dysfunction; *STEMI,* ST-segment elevation myocardial infarction; *SVT,* supraventricular tachycardia; *VF,* ventricular fibrillation; *VT,* ventricular tachycardia.

Cardiac Resynchronization Therapy

In the mid 1990s, a new tool was developed to assist in the management of patients with systolic heart failure (HF): biventricular pacing to improve systolic function. Since that time, the use of cardiac resynchronization devices has become a mainstay of an EP practice. These devices have undergone numerous refinements with time, and as clinical trials have been published, the patient population that can benefit from such therapy has greatly expanded (Fig. 7.14). This section provides a broad overview of cardiac resynchronization therapy (CRT) as a common procedure performed in the EP laboratory.

Theory

HF remains an extensive and expensive problem in the United States, and the majority of HF patients have systolic dysfunction. As systolic dysfunction becomes progressively worse, both mechanical and electrical remodeling occurs. The electrical component manifests in the QRS duration. As QRS duration increases, morbidity and mortality levels from systolic dysfunction significantly increase. The electrical delay often leads to delayed activation of the LV. Because of this delay in activation, the septal wall is not held stable by simultaneous contraction of the LVs and RVs, leading to a less efficient contraction. This has led to the advent of cardiac resynchronization devices to allow for pacing of both chambers to resynchronize the contraction and stabilize the septum for a more effective LV contraction.

Clinical response to CRT is variable and 30% of patients are considered "nonresponders." One of the most important correctable causes for lack of response to CRT is suboptimal coronary sinus lead position. As a result, multisite pacing (MSP) has been developed, which may be one way to improve the number of nonresponders in an appropriately selected patient population.

Implantation Procedure

The primary difference in implanting a CRT device compared with standard pacemakers and defibrillators is in the placement of an LV lead in a branch of the coronary sinus. This adds an additional level of complexity to the standard implant procedure, and thus, knowledge of the coronary sinus anatomy is essential. Given that cardiac electrophysiologists routinely place catheters in the coronary sinus for EPSs, they are very experienced in the intricacies of working in this vessel and are natural implanters for these devices. The coronary sinus is often accessed via the axillary vein and a long sheath

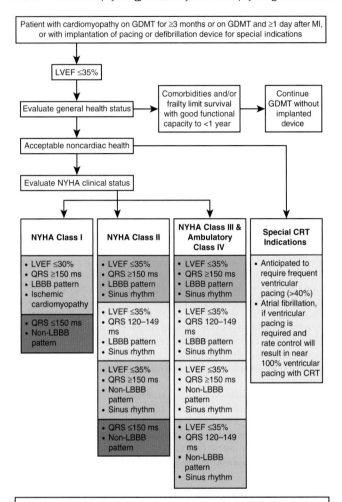

Patient with cardiomyopathy on GDMT for ≥3 months or on GDMT and ≥1 day after MI, or with implantation of pacing or defibrillation device for special indications

→ LVEF ≤35%

→ Evaluate general health status → Comorbidities and/or frailty limit survival with good functional capacity to <1 year → Continue GDMT without implanted device

→ Acceptable noncardiac health

→ Evaluate NYHA clinical status

NYHA Class I
- LVEF ≤30%
- QRS ≥150 ms
- LBBB pattern
- Ischemic cardiomyopathy

- QRS ≤150 ms
- Non-LBBB pattern

NYHA Class II
- LVEF ≤35%
- QRS ≥150 ms
- LBBB pattern
- Sinus rhythm

- LVEF ≤35%
- QRS 120–149 ms
- LBBB pattern
- Sinus rhythm

- LVEF ≤35%
- QRS ≥150 ms
- Non-LBBB pattern
- Sinus rhythm

- QRS ≤150 ms
- Non-LBBB pattern

NYHA Class III & Ambulatory Class IV
- LVEF ≤35%
- QRS ≥150 ms
- LBBB pattern
- Sinus rhythm

- LVEF ≤35%
- QRS 120–149 ms
- LBBB pattern
- Sinus rhythm

- LVEF ≤35%
- QRS ≥150 ms
- Non-LBBB pattern
- Sinus rhythm

- LVEF ≤35%
- QRS 120–149 ms
- Non-LBBB pattern
- Sinus rhythm

Special CRT Indications
- Anticipated to require frequent ventricular pacing (>40%)
- Atrial fibrillation, if ventricular pacing is required and rate control will result in near 100% ventricular pacing with CRT

Colors correspond to the class of recommendations in the ACCF/AHA Table 1.

Benefit for NYHA class I and II patients has only been shown in CRT-D trials, and although patients may not experience immediate symptomatic benefit, late remodeling may be avoided along with long-term HF consequences. There are no trials that support CRT pacing (without ICD) in NYHA class I and II patients. Thus, it is anticipated that these patients would receive CRT-D unless clinical reasons or personal wishes make CRT pacing more appropriate. In patients who are NYHA class III and ambulatory class IV, CRT-D may be chosen, but clinical reasons and personal wishes may make CRT pacing appropriate to improve symptoms and quality of life when an ICD is not expected to produce meaningful benefit in survival.

Fig. 7.14 Indications for biventricular pacing. *ACCF/AHA,* American College of Cardiology Foundation/American Heart Association; *CRT,* cardiac resynchronization therapy; *CRT-D,* cardiac resynchronization therapy defibrillator; *GDMT,* guideline-determined medical therapy; *HF,* heart failure; *ICD,* implantable cardiac defibrillator; *LBBB,* left bundle-branch block; *LVEF,* left ventricular ejection fraction; *MI,* myocardial infarction; *NYHA,* New York Heart Association. (From Tracy CM, Epstein AE, Darbar D, et al. ACCF/AHA/HRS focused update incorporated into the ACCF/AHA/HRS 2008 guidelines for device-based therapy of cardiac rhythm abnormalities: a report of the American College of Cardiology Foundation/American Heart Association Task Force on Practice Guidelines and the Heart Rhythm Society. *J Am Coll Cardiol.* 2013;61:e6-e75.)

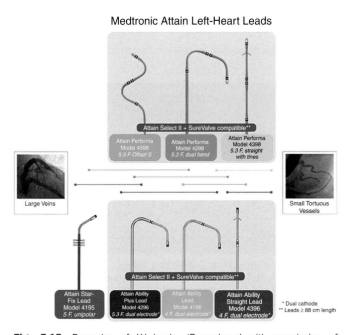

Fig. 7.15 Examples of LV leads. (Reproduced with permission of Medtronic, Inc.)

is passed into the coronary sinus to deliver the lead. LV leads are designed to be wedged into a branch vessel of the coronary sinus, and the lead tip usually has a cant or tab to help maintain the location of the lead (Figs. 7.15, 7.16, and 7.17). Once a lead is advanced and located in a branch of the coronary sinus, the sheath is split and

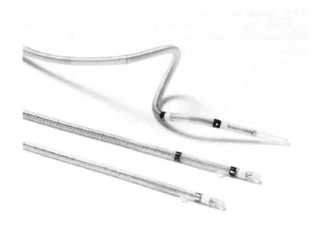

Fig. 7.16 Examples of LV leads. (From Boston Scientific Corporation.)

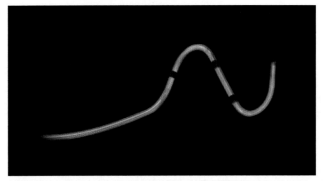

Fig. 7.17 Example of an LV lead. (EnSite, Velocity, Quartet, SJM Confirm, and St. Jude Medical are trademarks of St. Jude Medical, Inc. or its related companies. Reprinted with permission of St. Jude Medical, © 2015. All rights reserved.)

removed. The lead is sutured in place and can interface with a CRT defibrillator (CRT-D) or CRT pacemaker (CRT-P) PG.

Not only is it necessary to find a branch vein of the coronary sinus to accept the lead, location of the lead is also very important. Subgroup analyses of many major trials have investigated the importance of lead location and found that patients obtain the most benefit from a basilar location on the posterior or lateral LV.

Anterior placement of the lead has no benefit because of the lack of distance between LV and RV pacing (apical RV) locations, so true resynchronization does not occur. In addition, an apical placement of the lead has been shown to be harmful because patients tend to benefit less on subgroup analyses.

With the higher complexity of implanting a LV lead comes a higher level of complications from the procedure. Procedure times tend to be longer for CRT device implantation when compared with dual chamber devices. In addition, a third lead increases the risk of short-term and long-term mechanical problems. Lead dislodgement occurs at a higher rate because of the passive mechanisms used to retain the lead in place. Often, the number of possible branches available is limited in any given patient who can accept a lead, and pacing thresholds can frequently be elevated compared with acceptable thresholds for RA and RV leads. Diaphragmatic stimulation can also be a problem, because branches from the coronary sinus can traverse very near the phrenic nerve, which can allow stimulation from the LV lead. However, even with the higher level of complications, the benefit from such resynchronization therapy can be substantial and in most patients these additional risks are easily justified.

Implantable Cardiac Monitors

The use of implantable cardiac monitors has recently grown in popularity as the size of devices has been reduced and the implantation procedure simplified. Implantable cardiac monitors, also known as *loop recorders*, can record and store arrhythmias. They are implanted subcutaneously and generally have a battery life of approximately 3 years. Such devices can be useful for patients with rare symptoms, in whom traditional monitoring is unlikely to provide a diagnosis, or with patients unwilling or unable to wear traditional noninvasive monitors. A relatively new indication for these monitors has been in the area of cryptogenic stroke. A significant portion of cryptogenic strokes is caused by asymptomatic paroxysmal AF. The implantable cardiac monitor provides a method of monitoring these patients for AF. A diagnosis of this arrhythmia would change therapy for a stroke with the initiation of anticoagulation (Figs. 7.18 and 7.19).

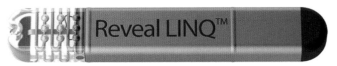

Fig. 7.18 Example of an implantable cardiac monitor. (Reproduced with permission of Medtronic, Inc.)

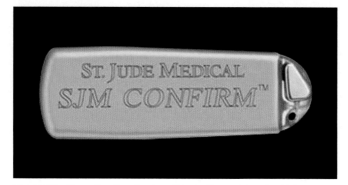

Fig. 7.19 Example of an implantable cardiac monitor. (EnSite, Velocity, Quartet, SJM Confirm and St. Jude Medical are trademarks of St. Jude Medical, Inc. or its related companies. Reprinted with permission of St. Jude Medical, © 2015. All rights reserved.)

Facilities, Personnel, and Equipment

In earlier days, surgeons in the operating room performed pacemaker implantation. As the device underwent progressive miniaturization, the procedure could be performed without a thoracotomy and moved to the catheterization laboratory. The skills required also evolved to include the ability to cannulate a central vein and place the lead against the appropriate myocardial location. With the advent of implantable defibrillators and resynchronization therapy devices, the operating physician needed to be adept at cannulating the coronary sinus and other coronary venous branches, manipulating over the wire leads, and comfortable inducing VF during a procedure. The need to perform high-quality coronary sinus venograms in multiple planes reinforced the shift from operating room to EP laboratory.

The support personnel required for an implant procedure are the same as for EPSs and ablations. They include a scrub nurse or technician familiar with the operating physician's preferences, a circulating nurse, and an individual responsible for electrical testing. It is useful to have a cardiovascular radiology technician. The presence of a nurse to administer conscious sedation depends on whether an anesthesiologist or nurse anesthetist is present during the procedure. In some institutions, deep sedation for testing defibrillation thresholds is administered by the electrophysiologist.

In the EP lab, a representative of the pacemaker or defibrillator manufacturer is often present for clinical support. A well-trained representative has experience and knowledge of the company's products, and their support is very helpful in achieving a good procedural outcome. However, responsibility for all aspects of the procedure remains with the operating physicians. Consideration of procedural liability dictates no hands-on involvement of nonhospital employees participating in more than a consultative role.

Pacemaker Systems Analyzer

For implantation of pacemakers and defibrillators, a pacemaker systems analyzer (PSA) is crucial. Because the circuitry replicates that of the PG, the PSA will accurately predict the performance of this generator. During our implants, we use the PSA provided by the manufacturer. The physician credentialing for pacemaker and defibrillator implantation procedures is controversial and in the recent past has also been contentious. Studies show that in patients undergoing defibrillator implantation, as a group, electrophysiologists are associated with fewer complications and better outcomes than cardiologists or thoracic surgeons.

Surgical Type of Sterile Environment

Early concerns about sterility are well founded. A defibrillator or pacemaker is a foreign body that will remain in place for several years, and hence, infection is a primary concern. Generally, the operating room is considered to be a highly sterile area and offers the best protection from infection. The catheterization laboratory is considered to be an intermediate sterile and high-traffic area but offers the advantage of high-quality radiography with high-resolution images, multiple projections, and image magnifications, along with the fact that these laboratories are fully equipped with all of the necessary catheters, sheaths, and wires that may be required. The right combination for device implantation is a dedicated EP laboratory, in which the ventilation system meets standards for operating rooms, and a rigid protocol for aseptic techniques.

The importance of adequate lighting for these procedures cannot be overemphasized. Many such procedures are performed on patients in whom antiplatelet and antithrombotic agents are not interrupted. To prevent pocket hematomas, it is important to be able to visualize the PG pocket. Although not always available in every laboratory, a high-intensity headlamp is particularly useful, especially when inspecting the pocket for bleeding vessels.

An electrocautery-surgery device involves the use of a pen that delivers alternating current in the radiofrequency range and creates resistive heating of tissues; it can be used for making incisions or achieving hemostasis.

Preprocedural Nursing Considerations

Patient Preparations

The evening before and morning of device implantation procedures, patients are instructed to scrub and wash their neck, shoulders, and chest with a chlorhexidine-containing soap. Preoperative skin cleansing with chlorhexidine-alcohol is superior to cleansing with povidone-iodine for prevention of surgical site infection, especially with *Staphylococcus aureus* after clean-contaminated surgery. Male patients have their chest hairs clipped before the procedure, and all patients should fast for at least 6 hours before. Although the administration of prophylactic antibiotics is controversial, we administer intravenous (IV) antibiotics immediately before the procedure. The IV line is started on the same side as the planned procedure to facilitate venography, if necessary.

Anticoagulation Issues

Device implantation in the anticoagulated patient has been controversial but is less so nowadays. Of late, several investigations have demonstrated the safety of performing implantation procedures without interrupting warfarin (Coumadin). In fact, it is safer to continue Coumadin than to bridge the patient with heparin before and after the procedure. We continue maintenance anticoagulation for implant procedures, especially if the patient has AF or prosthetic valves. The use of heparin postimplant is associated with increased bleeding.

   The use of novel oral anticoagulants is relatively new. However, there has been some recent data demonstrating that device implantation on uninterrupted anticoagulation with these medications is likely to be safe with minimal increase in bleeding complications. For patients undergoing implantation of a cardiac device, it is our practice to continue the use of these medications in the perioperative period.

Pacemaker Troubleshooting

1. Failure to deliver output
2. Failure to capture
3. Oversensing
4. Undersensing
5. Pacemaker-mediated tachycardia (PMT)

> ### Box 7.2 Gathering Information for Effective Pacemaker Troubleshooting.
>
> 1. Indication(s) for pacing
> 2. Implantation date of each component
> 3. Pacemaker/leads model
> 4. Current programmed parameters
> 5. Battery voltage/impedance
> 6. Lead impedance(s)
> 7. Measured parameters
> 8. Chest x-ray if necessary

6. Lead dislodgement

7. Pacemaker syndrome

8. Runaway pacemaker

Before attempting to troubleshoot a pacemaker malfunction, understanding its normal function is essential, as is obtaining basic information about the patient, implanted pacemaker leads, and programmed parameters (Box 7.2). Believe it or not, considering that so many special features are available in different pacemakers, it is very easy to misinterpret normal pacemaker functions. Obtaining a thorough history is crucial to determine the course of a problem.

The presence or absence of symptoms or hemodynamic compromise determines the urgency for repairing a problem. If the patient is severely bradycardiac and a pacemaker programmer is unavailable, transcutaneous or temporary pacing may be lifesaving. If a pacemaker malfunction occurs shortly after implantation, consider poor lead placement, lead dislodgement, loose set screws, and lead reversal, rather than lead conductor/insulation fracture and battery depletion.

In most cases of pacemaker-driven tachycardia, application of a magnet will terminate the tachycardia. In very rare cases of a runaway pacemaker (caused by a major pacing circuit component failure), urgent surgical PG removal is necessary.

The majority of *pacemaker-driven tachycardia* by DDD or VDD devices is tracking AF or flutter at an upper tracking rate. Magnet placement over the PG drops the pacing rate to a magnet rate for that specific device until programmed parameters are changed (i.e., activating a mode switch feature or using nontracking modes, such as [DDI] or [VVI]). Tachycardia in sensor-driven pacemakers may simply be remedied by turning the sensor off.

Electrocardiogram Assessment

It is critical to understand the basic timing of a dual chamber pacemaker (Fig. 7.20).

1. Look for pacing spikes.
2. If spikes are present, measure rate interval, presence of evoked response (complete paced beats), fusion beats, and pseudofusion beats.

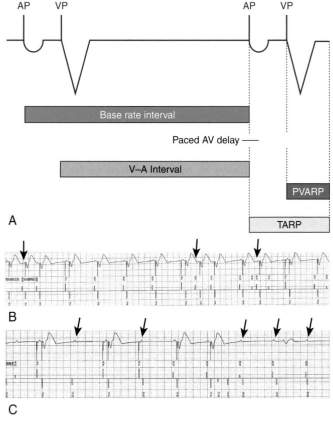

Fig. 7.20 **(A)** Basic timing in dual chamber pacemakers. **(B)** Atrial over-sensing, confirmed by marker channels showing atrial sensing (AS) markers without P waves. **(C)** Ventricular oversensing. (arrows in B, C, D and E point to p waves). Observe marker channel for ventricular sensing (VS) without a QRS.

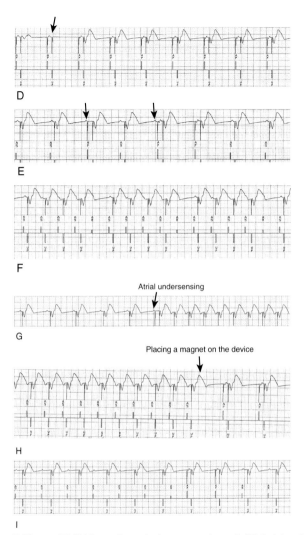

D

E

F

Atrial undersensing

G

Placing a magnet on the device

H

I

Fig. 7.20, cont'd (D) Loss of ventricular capture *(arrow).* **(E)** Atrial under-sensing; P waves without markers. **(F)** Pacemaker Wenckebach (WB). Occurs when the atrial rate increases but does not exceed the 2:1 block point. **(G)** Atrial undersensing. **(H)** Magnet makes the pacemaker pace in the atria and ventricle (DOO). *Arrow:* Placing of a magnet on the device. **(I)** Example of DDIR pacing mode: The response to sensing is to inhibit atrial output. No SAV is started, the ventricle is paced at the lower rate, and if after a V–A interval there is no AS, then AP/VP and PAV occur. DDIR is not appropriate for this patient due to a complete heart block (CHB). *AP, AS,* Atrial sensing; *AV,* atrioventricular; *PMT,* pacemaker-mediated tachycardia; *PVARP,* post-ventricular atrial refractory period; *SAV,* sensed atrioventricular; *TARP,* total atrial refractory period; *VP, V-A,* ventricular-atrial.

3. If absent, apply a magnet (mode will be switched to AAI/VOO or DOO) to see spikes.

Causes of Absent Pacing Output

1. PG output failure
2. Oversensing (can be diagnosed by applying a magnet)

   Placing a magnet on the PG is the next step. If spikes are seen, oversensing is the issue. If spikes are still absent, either the pacemaker is not putting out a pulse or the pulse does not reach the heart.

Pulse Generator Output Failure Causes

1. Battery depletion
2. Component failure
3. Electrocautery or defibrillator over or near the PG
4. Therapeutic radiation therapy over or near the PG

Noncapture Causes[a]

1. Low-output/high-capture threshold/exit block
2. Lead dislodgement
3. Lead conductor or insulation fracture
4. Loose set screws
5. Severe metabolic derangement or drugs

Undersensing Causes (Undersensing Causes Overpacing)

1. Poor lead positioning
2. Lead dislodgement

---

[a]Artificial noncapture: Pacing in the refractory period because of undersensing.

3. Lead conductor/insulation fracture
4. Infarction of tissue near lead tip
5. Safety pacing
6. DVI mode
7. Ectopies with short amplitude
8. Severe metabolic derangement
9. Defibrillation over or near pacemaker PG

Action needed: increase pacemaker sensitivity, change the sensing mode to unipolar mode, and, if necessary, repair or replace lead.

Oversensing Causes (Oversensing Causes Underpacing)

1. Myopotentials
2. Cross talk
3. Lead conductor/insulation fracture
4. Electromagnetic interference
5. T-wave oversensing and far-field sensing
6. Loose set screw

To repair, decrease the sensitivity. For T-wave oversensing and far-field sensing, we recommend prolonging the refractory period.

The sensing mode can be switched from the unipolar to bipolar setting. As is the case with unipolar sensing, the larger antenna is capable of causing oversensing. If leads are defective, lead repair or replacement is curative.

Pacemaker Syndrome

Pacemaker syndrome is seen in patients with normal sinus rhythm who have an inhibited VVI pacemaker or in those with dual chamber pacemakers if the atrial lead does not appropriately sense or capture the atrium.

Once atrial contribution/kick is lost, cardiac output diminishes and the patient may experience dyspnea, fatigue, palpitations, chest/neck/throat pulsations, and even syncope (as a result of atrial contraction against closed tricuspid and mitral valves [Cannon A waves]).

In patients with VVI pacemakers, we recommend allowing more time to be spent in intrinsic normal sinus rhythm by lowering the pacing rate. If this is not possible, upgrade to a dual chamber pacemaker. In patients with dual chamber pacemakers who have problems with atrial leads, reprogramming atrial lead parameters should resolve the issue; if not, atrial lead replacement is recommended.

Pacemaker-Mediated Tachycardia

Premature ventricular contraction (PVC), premature junctional contraction (PJC), or loss of atrial sensing or capture can cause PMT. With retrograde conduction of a ventricular ectopy to the atrium after completion of the postventricular atrial refractory period (PVARP), the retrograde "P" is sensed by the pacemaker, which in turn starts an AV delay after which a ventricular paced beat is forced. This beat can continue at the maximum rate of the upper tracking rate (PMT).

PMT can be terminated with the following actions:

1. Application of a magnet over the PG
2. Retrograde V–A conduction block
3. Programming a longer PVARP so that the retrograde P falls within the PVARP

Different manufacturers have different PMT remedies, such as PVARP extension for one beat after a PVC or DVI pacing for one beat after PVC.

Cross Talk

Cross talk occurs when the ventricular channel senses the atrial pacing spike and interprets it to be an intrinsic ventricular event, in which case ventricular output is inhibited. In patients who are pacemaker dependent and have no underlying escape mechanism, cross talk causes asystole, which may be fatal (on the ECG, an atrial spike can be seen followed by P waves without a ventricular output/pacing spike).

In some cases, simply programing the atrial impulse to lower amplitude or decreasing ventricular sensitivity can remedy the problem. At times, increasing the blanking period is necessary.

Safety pacing is another remedy for cross talk. Allow a brief period of ventricular sensing early after atrial pacing spike delivery (this interval follows the blanking interval). If an event is sensed during this interval, the pacemaker will force a ventricular paced beat with a short AV delay of 100 to 120 ms (Fig. 7.21).

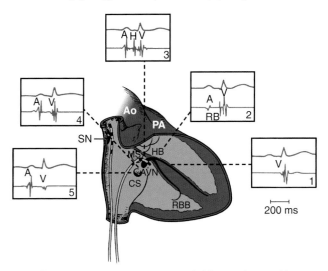

Fig. 7.21 Intracardiac electrograms recorded from various positions on a multipolar catheter positioned across the tricuspid valve. Numbers 1 to 5 refer to the intracardiac location of the catheters along with the corresponding electrograms; 1, most distal location recording a large ventricular electrogram and no atrial electrogram; 5, most proximal location displaying a large atrial electrogram with a small ventricular electrogram. The His potential is observed when the catheter is in the area of the tricuspid annulus and the atrial and ventricular electrograms recorded are approximately of equal size (position 3). A, Atrium; Ao, aorta; AVN, atrioventricular node; CS, coronary sinus; H, His; HB, His bundle; MS, membranous septum; PA, pulmonary artery; RB, right bundle; RBB, right bundle branch; SN, sinus node; V, ventricle. (From Grossman W. Cardiac catheterization and angiography. 2nd ed. Philadelphia: Lea & Febiger; 1974.)

Clinical Evaluations of the Patient Before Electrophysiology Procedures

The operating physician must comprehensively evaluate the patient before the study and plan the procedure on the basis of the specific needs of the individual patient. Whenever possible, review ECG documentation of the clinical event. Some or all of the procedures listed in Table 7.2 may be included in this evaluation.

Any potentially reversible arrhythmogenic factors, such as electrolyte abnormalities or decompensated congestive HF, should be corrected before the study is performed.

Table 7.2

Possible Components of Evaluation Before Electrophysiologic Testing.[a]	
Procedure	**Purpose**
History and physical examination	Identify signs and symptoms of cardiac or neurologic disease
	Identify factors known to exacerbate arrhythmias
	Determine details of syncopal events
Neurologic evaluation	Perform if history and physical examination suggest ruling out neurologic disease
Electroencephalogram	Rule out seizure disorder
Computed tomography/magnetic resonance imaging	Identify focal lesion
Carotid ultrasound	Identify significant cerebrovascular disease
12-lead ECG	Identify previous myocardial infarction
	Identify intraventricular conduction delays
	Identify prolonged Q–T interval
	Identify preexcitation syndromes
24- to 48-hour ambulatory ECG	Correlation of symptoms with ECG events
	Quantitation of ambient ectopy
	Identify diurnal variation in arrhythmia
Event recorder	Correlation of symptoms with ECG events
Head-up tilt-table testing	Diagnose vasovagal/vasodepressor syncope
Echocardiogram and radionucleotide ventriculography	Assessment of LV and RV size and function
	Detection of valvular pathology
Stress test (with or without perfusion scanning)	Detection of reversible ischemia
	Assessment of effects of catecholamines on arrhythmia induction
Cardiac catheterization	Definition of coronary anatomy

ECG, Electrocardiogram; *LV,* left ventricular; *Q–T,* interval from start of Q wave to end of T wave; *RV,* right ventricular.
[a]Selected procedures may vary depending on clinical presentation.

Discontinue all antiarrhythmic medications for at least five half-lives before the baseline study. For supraventricular tachycardia (SVT) studies, discontinue medications influencing AV nodal conduction (e.g., β-blockers, digoxin, and calcium channel blockers).

Premedication

The patient should have nothing by mouth after midnight except for essential cardiac medications, which may be taken with a small amount of water. The patient may be lightly sedated with IV diazepam or midazolam. In long diagnostic studies or in catheter ablation cases, more intensive levels of sedation are usually required. IV fentanyl and midazolam achieve somnolence in the patient during lengthy ablation procedures. However, excessive sedation may influence the ability to induce arrhythmias in some individuals.

Arterial and Venous Access

Routine diagnostic EPS involves stimulation and recording of electrical activity from the right side of the heart. Venous access may be obtained from the femoral, subclavian, internal jugular, or antecubital veins. A routine initial diagnostic EPS usually involves insertion of at least three catheters, most commonly via the femoral veins. These large veins easily permit the introduction of three 5-F to 8-F catheters per vein. The number of catheters required and venous access selected depend on the type of study being performed and the data being collected. Mapping of a left-sided bypass tract may necessitate catheterization of the left side of the heart for precise mapping.

For patients requiring beat-to-beat assessment of the hemodynamic effects of an induced arrhythmia, an arterial line may be placed. To evaluate completely a patient with Wolff-Parkinson-White (WPW) syndrome, the physician may have to access the LV for stimulation or recording of intracardiac electrical activity. If arterial catheterization is necessary, administration of IV heparin is mandatory. Patients undergoing prolonged studies involving venous access or those with a history of venous thromboembolism should also receive heparin.

Study Protocol

Although details of the protocol vary depending on the indication for the EPS and the information being obtained, most studies involve the recording and measurement of spontaneous intracardiac events and observation of the effects of programmed electrical stimulation. An initial study usually takes approximately 2 hours and depends on the complexity of the case. Possible components of the initial comprehensive EPS are listed in Box 7.3.

Box 7.3 Possible Components of Comprehensive Initial Electrophysiologic Study[a]

- Measurement of basic intervals
- Determination of sinus node function
- Determination of atrial, AV nodal, His-Purkinje, and ventricular conduction and refractoriness
- Identification of presence of dual AV nodal pathways
- Identification of presence, location, and electrical properties of accessory AV pathways
- Attempts to induce SVT
- Attempts to induce VT
- Determination of mechanism of induced arrhythmias
- Mapping of origin site(s) of induced arrhythmias
- Determination of effect of IV antiarrhythmic drugs on induced tachycardia
- Determination of efficacy of anti-tachycardia pacing for induced tachycardia

---

AV, Atrioventricular; *IV,* intravenous; *SVT,* supraventricular tachycardia; *VT,* ventricular tachycardia.
[a]The actual procedure varies depending on the individual case; not all parameters are assessed in all cases.

Positioning of Catheters

The RA is easily accessible by any venous access. The most common site for stimulation and recording is the high posterior lateral wall in the region of the sinus node. The potential is most easily found with a catheter introduced by the femoral approach and passed into the RA across the tricuspid valve and into the RV. The catheter is withdrawn across the tricuspid valve with the application of a slight degree of clockwise torque that tends to keep the catheter in contact with the septum (see Fig. 7.22). A hexapolar or octapolar catheter in the His position may be used so that electrical activity from multiple electrode pairs can be recorded, and the one showing the most stable and consistent His potential may be displayed. If multiple attempts to record a His potential with one catheter are unsuccessful, a differently shaped or steerable catheter with a deflectable tip may be used. In most patients, a His potential can be recorded successfully.

Usually, the LA is approached indirectly by recording in the coronary sinus. Cannulation of the coronary sinus os can be achieved from the femoral, left subclavian, or right or left internal jugular approaches. The appropriate position of the coronary sinus catheter is verified fluoroscopically in the LAO and right anterior oblique positions. The catheter curves upward toward the left shoulder in the LAO projection and is posteriorly oriented in the

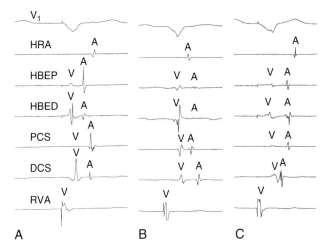

Fig. 7.22 Pattern of retrograde atrial activation. Electrograms from the high right atrium *(HRA)*, proximal His bundle *(HBEP)*, distal His bundle *(HBED)*, proximal coronary sinus *(PCS)*, distal coronary sinus *(DCS)*, and right ventricular apex *(RVA)* are shown. **(A)** Normal pattern of retrograde atrial activation through the atrioventricular (AV) node. **(B)** Sequence of retrograde atrial activation with a right-sided accessory pathway showing earliest activation in the HRA. **(C)** Sequence of retrograde atrial activation with a left-sided accessory pathway showing earliest activation in the DCS.

lateral projection. On the ECG, atrial and ventricular electrograms are recorded, with the timing of the LA electrograms appearing later than the high RA electrogram. Direct recording of electrical activity from the LA is possible in patients with a patent foramen ovale or atrial septal defect or by a transseptal approach.

In most baseline studies, a catheter is placed in the RV apex. For ventricular stimulation protocols, a second ventricular catheter is sometimes placed in the RV outflow tract, although most operators prefer to reposition the catheter from the apex to the outflow tract. The order in which the catheters are placed in the right side of the heart varies among operators, and no particular order is mandatory. In patients with a preexisting left bundle-branch block (LBBB), it is recommended that the RV apical catheter be positioned first to ensure adequate ventricular pacing in the event of catheter-induced trauma to the right bundle, which may result in complete heart block (CHB) while the His catheter is being positioned.

Catheterization of the LV may be necessary in patients with VT or preexcitation syndromes. The LV is most commonly accessed by the retrograde arterial approach for mapping procedures. Fluoroscopy that permits views in multiple planes is essential to ensure accurate positioning of the catheter. Stimulation may also be performed from the LV in cases in which patients with clinically documented sustained VT have arrhythmias that are noninducible with use of the standard protocol from the RV. To avoid inadvertent cannulation of the coronary arteries, the operator safely prolapses the catheter across the aortic valve. In patients with atrial septal defects, patent foramen ovale, or undergoing transseptal punctures, the LV may be approached through the LA and mitral valve.

Measurement of Conduction Intervals

After the catheters are positioned, basic conduction intervals are measured, including the basic sinus cycle length (A-to-A interval), P-wave duration, A–H interval, His spike duration, and H–V interval (Fig. 7.23). Measurements from the surface ECG, including the P–R, QRS, and Q–T intervals, are also recorded. Conduction interval measurements and refractory period measurements should be made at a paper speed of at least 100 mm/s in routine cases and at speeds of 100 to 200 mm/s in detailed mapping procedures. All

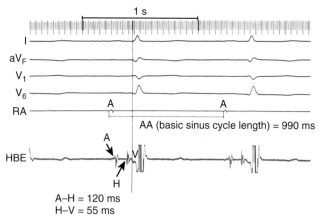

Fig. 7.23 Measurement of basic sinus cycle length and A–H and H–V intervals. *HBE,* His bundle electrogram; *RA,* right atrium.

Table 7.3

Pacing Interval Conversion Chart.[a]	
Pacing Interval (ms)	**Heart Rate (bpm)**
200	300
222	270
231	260
240	250
250	240
261	230
273	220
286	210
300	200
311	193
316	190
333	180
353	170
375	160
400	150
429	140
462	130
500	120
545	110
550	109
600	100
667	90
750	80
857	70
1000	60
1200	50
1500	40
2000	30

[a]Pulse-to-pulse interval (milliseconds) to beats per minute (bpm).

measurements of rate and conduction times are made in milliseconds. The pacing interval can be converted to HR by the following formula (Table 7.3): HR (beats per minute [bpm]) = 60,000/interval (ms).

The A–H interval represents conduction time from the low RA at the interatrial septum through the AV node to the His bundle and approximates AV nodal conduction time. The measurement is made from the earliest reproducible rapid deflection of the atrial electrogram on the His bundle recording to the onset of the His deflection on that electrogram (see Fig. 7.23). Normal values for adults are reported to range from 50 to 140 ms. The A–H interval is influenced strongly by the patient's autonomic tone and may vary by 50 ms during a study in a given patient. The A–H interval normally increases in response to increases in atrial pacing rates. It may also be altered by drugs that affect AV conduction, and the measurement may be influenced artificially by such factors as gain setting and position of the atrial catheter.

The H–V interval represents conduction time from the proximal His bundle to the ventricular myocardium. The measurement is made from the earliest deflection of the His spike on the His bundle recording to the earliest onset of ventricular activation, recorded from any intracardiac electrogram or surface ECG. Normal values range from 35 to 55 ms. In contrast to the A–H interval, the H–V interval normally remains relatively constant and is not significantly affected by variations in autonomic tone or atrial pacing rates.

Sequence of Activation

Determination of the sequence of antegrade and retrograde atrial activation during spontaneous rhythms, atrial pacing, ventricular pacing, and induced rhythms is essential in differentiating VT from SVT and in defining the reentrant circuit in SVT. The atrial activation normally begins in the high RA and spreads to the low RA and His bundle, with LA activation recorded from the coronary sinus catheter occurring significantly later. When ventriculoatrial conduction is present during ventricular pacing, the earliest retrograde atrial activity is recorded in the His bundle electrogram, followed by the RA and coronary sinus recordings. Abnormal or eccentric sequences of retrograde atrial activation occur in the presence of AV accessory pathways (Fig. 7.22). This is discussed in more detail in subsequent sections dealing with SVT and catheter ablation.

Programmed Electrical Stimulation

Programmed electrical stimulation involves observing the EP effects of incremental pacing and the introduction of programmed extrastimuli coupled to normal sinus rhythm or paced rhythms. The major purposes of programmed electrical stimulation are to characterize the EP properties of cardiac tissue and to induce and to analyze the mechanism of arrhythmias. The most commonly used types of pacing during the EPS are burst pacing, incremental pacing, and programmed stimulation. Fixed burst pacing involves the delivery of a series of impulses at a constant rate. A decremental burst consists of a series of impulses at progressively increasing rates. Programmed stimulation involves the coupling of premature extrastimuli to a short train (six to eight beats) of pacing or to sinus rhythm. The number of extrastimuli may vary from one to four. The pacing train is referred to as S_1, first extrastimulus as S_2, and second extrastimulus as S_3. Coupling intervals are decreased progressively and systematically by 10-ms decrements until an arrhythmia is induced or the first extrastimulus loses capture (the effective refractory period [ERP] of the tissue is reached).

Assessment of Sinus Node Function

Many studies begin with an evaluation of AV node function and assessment of atrial and AV nodal refractoriness. Assessment of sinus node function is no longer routinely performed because of the lack of sensitivity of the results. However, in studies performed to assess bradycardia or syncope, a sinus node recovery time measurement can be considered. Measurement of sinus node recovery time is performed by pacing the RA, most commonly near the region of the sinus node, at a slightly faster rate than the intrinsic sinus rate for approximately 30 seconds, then abruptly terminating pacing. Sinus node recovery time is the time from the last paced atrial complex on the RA recording to the return of the first sinus complex (Fig. 7.24). Generally, the slower the intrinsic sinus rate, the longer the sinus node recovery time. The absolute sinus node recovery time may be corrected for HR by subtracting the basic sinus cycle length (corrected sinus node recovery time). Normal values for absolute sinus node recovery time are up to 1.5 seconds and for corrected sinus node recovery time up to 550 ms. Secondary pauses are other indicators of sinus node dysfunction (SND).

Assessment of Atrioventricular Nodal and His-Purkinje System Function

AV nodal function is assessed by determining the point at which 1:1 AV conduction ceases and AV nodal Wenckebach (WB) begins. The normal response to incremental atrial pacing at progressively faster rates is to develop a longer AH interval and, ultimately, a block in the AV node (Fig. 7.25). Most normal individuals develop WB AV block at paced atrial cycle lengths of 500 to 350 ms (HRs of 120 to 170 bpm). AV nodal block does not usually occur during exercise when similar HRs are achieved, because catecholamines

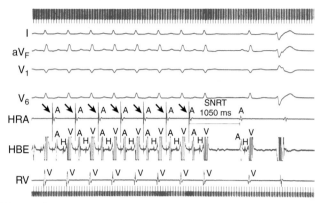

Fig. 7.24 Demonstration of a normal sinus node recovery time in a patient undergoing electrophysiologic study (EPS) for the evaluation of syncope of unknown cause. After a train of atrial pacing at a cycle length of 450 (approximately 133 bpm), 1050 ms elapsed before the return of sinus node activity. The absolute sinus node recovery time is 1050 ms. *HBE,* His bundle electrogram; *HRA,* high right atrium; *RV,* right ventricle; *SNRT,* sinus node recovery time.

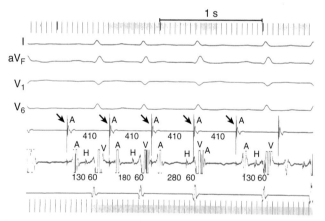

Fig. 7.25 Type-I second-degree atrioventricular (AV) block (Wenckebach [WB]) in the AV node induced by atrial pacing at a cycle length of 410 ms. Each paced atrial depolarization is followed by a progressively longer A–H interval until the fourth atrial depolarization is blocked in the AV node (no His depolarization is seen after the atrial electrogram). The A–H interval after the blocked atrial depolarization is shorter (130 ms) compared with the A–H interval preceding the block beat (280 ms). The H–V interval remains constant despite the progressive increase in A–H interval during the WB sequence.

enhance conduction through the AV node. The point at which WB AV block occurs in response to atrial pacing may be influenced by drugs that affect AV nodal conduction and by autonomic tone. WB AV block occurs at longer cycle lengths (slower pacing rates) in patients with enhanced vagal tone and at shorter cycle lengths (faster pacing rates) in patients with enhanced sympathetic tone. In contrast to the A–H interval, the H–V interval remains relatively constant during decremental atrial pacing, and block below His (intra-Hisian block) is considered pathologic at pacing cycle lengths >400 ms (rates <150 bpm).

Determination of Refractory Periods

The refractoriness of cardiac tissue is defined by the response of the tissue to the introduction of premature stimuli. For most routine EPSs, the ERP is defined as the longest coupling interval between the basic drive and the premature stimulus that fails to propagate through the tissue. Normal values for AV nodal, atrial, and ventricular refractory periods have been established (Table 7.4). The ERP of cardiac tissue may be affected by the current strength used, pacing rate, medications, and autonomic tone in the AV node.

Atrioventricular Nodal Function Curves

AV nodal function curves can be constructed by plotting the coupling interval of the premature stimulus (A_1A_2 interval) on the

Table 7.4

Normal Intervals and Refractory Periods.	
Parameter	**Normal Duration (ms)**
A–H	50–150
H–V	30–55
His	10–25
Atrial ERP	150–360
AV nodal ERP	230–430
HPS ERP	330–450
Ventricular ERP	170–290

AV, Atrioventricular; *ERP,* effective refractory period; *HPS,* His-Purkinje system.

horizontal axis versus the A–H interval (AV nodal conduction time) of the premature stimulus (A_2H_2 interval) on the vertical axis. In individuals without dual AV nodal pathways, a progressive and gradual increase occurs in the A–H interval before premature stimulus blocking in the AV node, and the function curve is continuous (Fig. 7.26). A sudden large increase (at least 50 ms) in the A–H interval (often referred to as a *jump*) in response to a small decrement (10 ms) in the coupling interval of the premature beat is evidence of functional dual AV nodal pathways (Fig. 7.27). This represents a shift from conduction over the fast AV nodal pathway to conduction over the slow AV nodal pathway (with a longer A–H interval), and the AV nodal function curve is discontinuous (see Fig. 7.26B). During programmed stimulation in patients with dual AV pathways, SVT is often initiated when the jump to the slow pathway occurs. Multiple extrastimuli may be used in patients with suspected or known SVT in an attempt to induce a clinically significant tachycardia. Drugs that modify refractoriness and conductive velocity in the AV node, such as isoproterenol or atropine, may be given in attempts to induce a clinically significant SVT.

Ventricular Stimulation

The safety and efficacy of programmed electrical stimulation in the diagnosis and treatment of patients with ventricular arrhythmias have been well established. The reported sensitivity and specificity of ventricular stimulation vary depending on the stimulation protocol used, presenting arrhythmia, and underlying cardiac disease. The sensitivity and specificity of programmed ventricular stimulation have been defined best in patients with coronary artery disease whose arrhythmia is spontaneous sustained monomorphic VT. In these individuals, the yield (and sensitivity) of the EPS increases with the addition of up to three extrastimuli; the addition of more extrastimuli provides little or no added benefit. In most patients, the clinical VT is initiated reproducibly by programmed electrical stimulation. The clinical significance of arrhythmias induced by programmed electrical stimulation must be interpreted with regard to the specific arrhythmia for which a patient is being evaluated. With more aggressive stimulation protocols, polymorphic VT or VF that may represent a nonclinical (or false-positive) response may be initiated. Even in normal individuals, at close coupling intervals of the extrastimuli (usually <180 ms), VF or polymorphic VT may be induced. In contrast, sustained monomorphic VT is considered a specific response to programmed electrical stimulation and generally occurs only in

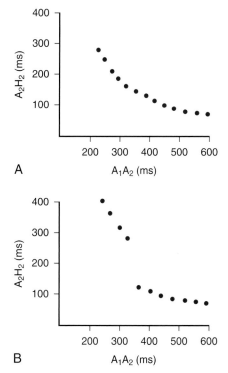

Fig. 7.26 **(A)** Normal atrioventricular (AV) nodal function curve in a patient without functional dual AV nodal pathways. In this graph, the conduction intervals (A_1A_2) are displayed on the x axis and the resulting A–H interval (A_2H_2) is displayed on the y axis. With progressively shorter coupling intervals, premature atrial beats are followed by progressively longer A–H intervals (A_2H_2), which represents progressive conduction delay in the AV node. The normal AV nodal conduction curve is smooth and continuous. **(B)** A typical AV nodal function curve in a patient with functional dual AV nodal pathways. Premature atrial impulses with longer coupling intervals conduct down the fast pathway and have short A–H intervals. With progressively earlier premature atrial impulses, the refractory period of the fast pathway is reached, and conduction shifts to the slow pathway. The jump from the fast pathway to the slow pathway is manifested by a sudden lengthening of the A_2H_2 interval and discontinuity in the AV nodal function curve. (A: from Forgoros RN. *Electrophysiologic Testing*. Cambridge, MA: Blackwell Scientific; 1991.)

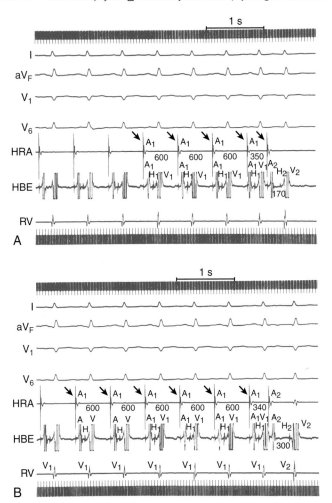

Fig. 7.27 A 130-ms jump in atrioventricular (AV) nodal conduction in a patient with functional dual AV nodal pathways. Premature atrial stimuli are coupled to a train of atrial pacing at a cycle length of 600 ms. **(A)** At a coupling interval of 350 ms, the premature atrial stimulus has an A–H interval of 170 ms. **(B)** At a coupling interval of 340 ms, the A–H interval of the premature impulse suddenly increases to 300 ms, representing a shift to the slow pathway. *HBE*, His bundle electrogram; *HRA*, high right atrium; *RV*, right ventricle.

Box 7.4   Ventricular Stimulation Protocol.

Standard Protocol

- Single extrastimulus coupled to ventricular pacing at cycle lengths of 600 and 400 ms from RV apex and RV outflow tract
- Double extrastimuli coupled to ventricular pacing at cycle lengths of 600 and 400 ms from RV apex and RV outflow tract
- Rapid ventricular pacing (400 ms to loss of 1:1 ventricular capture)
- Triple extrastimuli coupled to ventricular pacing at cycle lengths of 600 and 400 ms from RV apex and RV outflow tract

Additional Maneuvers That May Be Performed

- Extrastimuli may be coupled to sinus rhythm or other paced cycle lengths.
- A fourth extrastimulus may be coupled to ventricular pacing at cycle lengths of 600 and 400 ms from both RV sites.
- Stimulation may be performed at additional RV sites or from the LV.
- Isoproterenol may be infused and the stimulation protocol repeated.
- IV procainamide may be infused and the stimulation protocol repeated.

IV, Intravenous; *RV,* right ventricular.

---

patients with previous spontaneous VT or a pathologic substrate known to predispose to VT.

Although ventricular stimulation protocols vary slightly among different laboratories, the minimal complete protocol usually involves the introduction of three extrastimuli coupled to ventricular pacing at two cycle lengths from two RV sites, typically RV apex and RV outflow tract (Box 7.4). LV stimulation may be performed in some individuals who have documented sustained monomorphic VT but whose arrhythmia is noninducible from the RV. The yield is relatively low from LV stimulation, and LV stimulation may increase the morbidity of the procedure. In individuals with exercise-induced VT or catecholamine-dependent VT, isoproterenol may be infused and programmed stimulation repeated.

To perform the stimulation protocol, the operator systematically decreases the coupling interval between the last beat of the pacing train and the extrastimuli until the tissue reaches refractoriness (the first extrastimulus fails to capture) or an arrhythmia is induced (Fig. 7.28). If the patient is hemodynamically stable, a 12-lead ECG of the induced VT is recorded before attempts to terminate the tachycardia. The morphology of the VT is noted, and the cycle length is obtained. The most common method of terminating the VT is ventricular burst pacing at a cycle length less than that of the tachycardia. The cycle length of the burst pacing is decreased

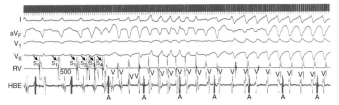

Fig. 7.28 Induction of sustained ventricular tachycardia (VT) with triple extrastimuli coupled to a train of ventricular pacing at 500 ms. During induced VT, atrial activity is dissociated from ventricular activity. This may be observed on the His channel *(HBE)* by the atrial electrogram *(A)* marching randomly through the tachycardia. *HBE,* His bundle electrogram; *RV,* right ventricle; *S1,* train; *S2,* first extrastimulus; *S3,* second extrastimulus; *S4,* third extrastimulus.

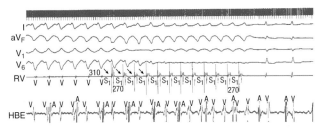

Fig. 7.29 Termination of monomorphic ventricular tachycardia (VT) with ventricular burst pacing at a rate faster than that of tachycardia. On the right ventricle *(RV)* channel, cycle length of monomorphic VT is measured at 310 ms. Ventricular burst pacing (indicated by *arrows* and S1) at a cycle length of 270 ms terminates the tachycardia. *HBE,* His bundle electrogram.

gradually until the tachycardia either terminates (Fig. 7.29) or accelerates and results in hemodynamic compromise, at which point cardioversion or defibrillation is performed on the patient. An initial 200-J biphasic shock is routinely used for sustained VT.

The most specific endpoint of the ventricular stimulation protocol is the induction of a sustained monomorphic VT that is identical to a patient's clinical VT. Sustained VT is commonly defined as VT lasting at least 30 seconds or requiring termination because of hemodynamic collapse before 30 seconds. Noninducibility by ventricular stimulation refers to the failure to induce sustained VT after the use of at least three extrastimuli at two pacing rates from two RV pacing sites. The arrhythmia may be noninducible on the initial EPS or may be rendered noninducible by antiarrhythmic drug therapy. Partial drug efficacy refers to significant lengthening (>100 ms) of the cycle length of the induced tachycardia or rendering a previously intolerable tachycardia hemodynamically stable.

Complications

Complications associated with diagnostic EPSs are low and mortality is extremely rare. Complications are usually associated with catheterization and catheter manipulation rather than stimulation and induction of arrhythmias. Reported complications include hemorrhage, venous thromboembolism (<1%), phlebitis (<1%), cardiac perforation and tamponade, and refractory VF. Hemothorax and pneumothorax, recognized complications, can occur when the subclavian or internal jugular venous approaches are used. Arterial catheterization increases associated morbidity, including vascular complications, stroke, systemic embolism, and protamine reactions. Most reported deaths have resulted from incessant VF and have occurred in patients with severe LV dysfunction, active myocardial ischemia, hypertrophic obstructive cardiomyopathy, or because of the proarrhythmic effect of drugs administered during the evaluation. Defibrillation through an intracardiac electrode is effective in situations in which transthoracic defibrillation fails and death might otherwise result. Pneumothorax, cardiac perforation/tamponade, and pocket and systemic infection are risks associated with implanting pacemakers and defibrillators.

Mortality is a real concern in patients undergoing extraction of chronic pacemaker and defibrillator leads. A special mention of the complications during and after catheter ablation of AF is necessary. In a worldwide survey of more than 8000 patients who underwent this procedure, Cappato et al. report an overall 4% incidence of major complications, such as pericardial effusion and tamponade, cerebrovascular events, pulmonary vein stenosis, and devastating consequences of a fistula developing between the LA and the esophagus. Pulmonary vein stenosis and atrioesophageal fistula can occur several weeks after the procedure.

Utility of Electrophysiologic Study for Specific Diagnosis

Sinus Node Dysfunction

The clinical applications of EPS in SND are limited. Although abnormal sinus node recovery times and sinoatrial conduction times have been reported to have a specificity of 90% to 100% in patients documented to have spontaneous SND, sensitivity is significantly less. In contrast to most induced tachyarrhythmias on EPS, it is difficult to correlate symptoms with an abnormal sinus node recovery time. In symptomatic patients with sinus bradycardia, an abnormal sinus node recovery time has been reported to predict which patients may benefit from cardiac pacing. The finding of an abnormal sinus node recovery time in an asymptomatic patient being studied for tachyarrhythmias may influence a decision to use certain medications.

Disorders of Atrioventricular Conduction

Abnormalities of AV conduction are classified as first-degree, second-degree, or third-degree AV blocks. Clues to the site of AV block can be derived by observing serial changes in the P–R interval in sequences of block that are <2:1 (i.e., 3:2 or 4:3), rate and duration of the QRS of the escape rhythm, and presence or absence of underlying intraventricular conduction delays on ECG. Compared with prolonged conduction in the AV node, conduction disease within or below the His bundle is associated with a high likelihood that complete AV block will develop. Complete AV block that occurs within or below the His bundle is associated with a slower and less stable escape rhythm than what occurs with complete AV block situated within the AV node. EPS can confirm the site of spontaneous AV block or conduction delay and assess the response of the conduction system to various pacing rates and the introduction of premature impulses. EPS may identify indications for permanent pacemaker implantation in individuals with syncope of unknown cause. Long H–V intervals (>80 to 100 ms) and block below the His bundle at atrial pacing rates of <150 bpm indicate disease in the His-Purkinje system and are associated with a relatively high incidence of subsequent CHB.

Sustained Ventricular Arrhythmias

For more than two decades, EPS was used to determine the efficacy of antiarrhythmic drug therapy in patients with sustained VT and survivors of cardiac arrest. This practice was based on the supposition that the (1) induced ventricular arrhythmia represents the patient's clinical arrhythmia and (2) inability to induce arrhythmia after drug treatment in a patient whose arrhythmia was previously inducible correlates with freedom from the clinical recurrence of the arrhythmia. The predictive accuracy of serial EPS is highest in patients with previous MI and spontaneous sustained monomorphic VT. There may be a significant number of false-negative results with EPS in patients with nonischemic cardiac disease or polymorphic VT or VF as a presenting clinical arrhythmia. Another important limitation of the technique is that even in patients whose arrhythmia is rendered noninducible by antiarrhythmic therapy, there is a significant clinical recurrence rate of sustained ventricular arrhythmia and cardiac arrest, reported to be as high as 50% for 4 years. Data indicate that survivors of cardiac arrest or sustained VT derive a significant survival benefit from an ICD compared with antiarrhythmic drug therapy. Most patients surviving a hemodynamically unstable ventricular arrhythmia receive an ICD without a preceding EPS. In rare cases, bundle-branch reentry tachycardia or AF with rapid ventricular response (in the setting of WPW syndrome) may precipitate a patient's cardiac arrest or unstable ventricular arrhythmia. If these circumstances are suspected, EPS may be useful because these arrhythmias are potentially curable by radiofrequency catheter ablation. In patients with hemodynamically stable monomorphic VT in whom ablative therapy is being considered, EPS is indicated.

Syncope of Unknown Cause

Syncope is a common clinical disorder, the workup of which can be expensive and nonproductive. The diagnostic use of EPS in patients with recurrent syncope has been reported to range from 12% to 79%. The reported abnormalities are listed in Box 7.5. The yield is highly dependent on the prevalence of structural heart disease

---

Box 7.5 Reported Abnormalities in Patients with Syncope on Electrophysiologic Study.

Sinus Node Dysfunction

Prolonged sinus node recovery time
Prolonged sinoatrial conduction time
Secondary pauses

Abnormalities of Atrioventricular Conduction

Prolonged AV nodal refractory period
Prolonged AV nodal WB cycle length
Prolonged H–V interval
Block induced within or below the His bundle

Induced Tachyarrhythmias

Rapid SVT
Sustained VT

AV, Atrioventricular; *SVT,* supraventricular tachycardia; *VT,* ventricular tachycardia; *WB,* Wenckebach.

in the population being studied. In patients with structurally normal hearts and no suggestion of ischemia, EPS has a low yield and an increased likelihood of false-positive results. In patients with a history of coronary artery disease and segmental wall motion abnormality or conduction disease on ECG, EPS has a relatively high yield and may rule out potentially life-threatening causes of syncope, such as sustained ventricular arrhythmia. In an unwitnessed syncope episode, the cause of the patient's syncope is never certain, and there is always the potential for inaccurately attributing the patient's syncope to an abnormality detected on EPS. It is desirable that a patient's symptoms be reproduced by induced arrhythmia.

Supraventricular Tachycardia

The treatment of SVT has undergone dramatic change because radiofrequency catheter ablation offers a high probability of cure with a low complication rate for many reentrant tachycardias. Although the relationship between the QRS complex and P waves on the 12-lead ECG may suggest the mechanism of SVT, performance of a detailed EPS is the only method of accurately characterizing the mechanism of tachycardia and defining the anatomic substrate.

The most often observed mechanism of narrow-complex SVT is atrioventricular nodal reentrant tachycardia (AVNRT), which usually involves slow- and fast-conducting pathways within or near the AV node. Although it was previously thought that AV nodal reentry occurred entirely within the compact AV node, experience from radiofrequency catheter ablation indicates that extranodal tissue may be involved in the reentrant circuit. Dual AV nodal pathways are characterized by discontinuous AV nodal conduction curves (see Fig. 7.26B). In typical AV nodal tachycardia, which constitutes more than 90% of AVNRT, antegrade conduction occurs over the slow pathway and retrograde conduction occurs up the fast pathway (slow-fast tachycardia) (Fig. 7.30). Retrograde ventriculoatrial conduction time is usually short, and atrial depolarization often occurs simultaneously with or immediately after ventricular depolarization. On surface ECG, the P waves are either not visible or occur in the ST segment with a short R–P interval.

Another common mechanism of SVT is AV reciprocating tachycardia, using an extranodal AV bypass tract (also referred to as an *accessory pathway*). The most common type of accessory pathway is the bundle of Kent, which occurs in WPW syndrome. The accessory pathway may be between the RA and ventricle or LA and ventricle. In an individual patient, an accessory pathway may be capable of antegrade conduction, retrograde conduction,

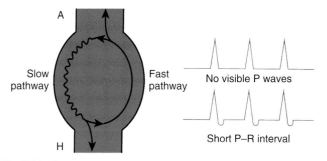

Common AVNRT
(antegrade slow–retrograde fast)

No visible P waves

Short P–R interval

Fig. 7.30 Schematic representation of the common form of atrioventricular nodal reentrant tachycardia *(AVNRT)*. In the typical form of AV nodal tachycardia, antegrade block occurs in the fast pathway, forcing antegrade conduction down the slow pathway. If antegrade conduction down the slow pathway is slow enough to allow retrograde conduction to occur up the previously refractory fast pathway, reentrant tachycardia ensues. Although previously it was thought that the limbs of the tachycardic circuit were contained within the compact AV node, more recent studies using radiofrequency ablation for AV nodal tachycardia suggest that perinodal tissue is contained in the reentrant circuit.

or both. Individuals with antegrade conduction over an accessory pathway exhibit a short P–R interval and a wide QRS complex because of ventricular preexcitation (this is also referred to as a *delta wave*). The axis of the delta wave and morphology of the QRS depend on the position of the accessory pathway and the amount of tissue depolarized through accessory pathway conduction compared with conduction over the normal AV node. During sinus rhythm, activation of the ventricle can occur over the accessory pathway and through the normal conduction pathway using the AV node. QRS morphology results from fusion of the two mechanisms of ventricular activation. Pathways capable of only retrograde conduction are referred to as *concealed pathways,* and no ventricular preexcitation (or delta wave) is present on the ECG.

WPW syndrome is characterized by the presence of ventricular preexcitation (short P–R interval and delta wave on ECG) and the clinical occurrence of arrhythmias. In patients with WPW syndrome, the most common type of SVT is orthodromic tachycardia, in which antegrade block occurs in the accessory pathway and a reentrant circuit is established with antegrade conduction occurring over the AV node and retrograde conduction up the accessory pathway (Fig. 7.31A, B). In orthodromic tachycardia, the QRS is narrow unless aberrancy occurs and there is a short R–P interval on the surface ECG. A less common type of tachycardia in patients with WPW syndrome is antidromic tachycardia, which is a reentrant tachycardia with antegrade conduction occurring over the accessory pathway and retrograde conduction through the AV node (Fig. 7.31C). Antidromic tachycardia is a regular wide-complex tachycardia that may resemble VT on surface ECG. Compared with the general population, patients with WPW syndrome have an increased incidence of AF, and conduction to the ventricle may occur over the accessory pathway and the AV node (Fig. 7.31D). The QRS morphology depends on the relative amount of conduction occurring through the accessory pathway compared with the normal conduction system. In patients with pathways capable of antegrade conduction and AF, rapid ventricular

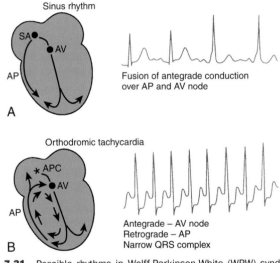

Fig. 7.31 Possible rhythms in Wolff-Parkinson-White (WPW) syndrome. Schematic representation of possible rhythms in a patient with an accessory atrioventricular (AV) bypass tract. **(A)** During sinus rhythm, the ventricle may be activated by conduction over the accessory pathway (AP) and through the normal AV conduction system. The QRS complex may be narrow if the ventricle is activated primarily by conduction through the AV node. The QRS complex is wide and preexcited if activation of the ventricle occurs primarily via the AP. **(B)** During orthodromic reentrant tachycardia, antegrade conduction occurs through the AV node and normal conduction system, whereas retrograde conduction occurs via the AP. The resulting tachycardia has a narrow QRS morphology.

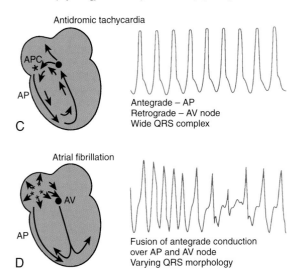

Fig. 7.31, cont'd (C) Antidromic tachycardia uses the AP as the antegrade limb of the reentrant circuit and the AV node and normal conduction system as the retrograde limb. The resulting tachycardia has a wide QRS complex. **(D)** When atrial fibrillation (AF) occurs in a patient with manifest accessory pathway, antegrade conduction to the ventricle may occur through the AV node or over the AP. Morphology of the QRS complex may be narrow and occurs primarily through the AV node, or wide and preexcited if conduction occurs over the accessory pathway. The morphology of the QRS complex may vary beat by beat during AF. *SA,* Sinoatrial.

responses may occur with a potential for degeneration to VF. During EPS in patients with WPW syndrome, it is important to induce AF and observe the shortest R–R interval that shows ventricular preexcitation to assess the antegrade ERP of the accessory pathway and the risk of sudden cardiac death. Patients who have WPW syndrome and are resuscitated from VF usually have inducible AF with a rapid ventricular response and shortest preexcited R–R interval of <250 ms. Programmed atrial stimulation with single premature extrastimuli defines the antegrade ERP of the accessory pathway. Programmed stimulation of the ventricle shows the retrograde conduction properties of the accessory pathway and defines retrograde ERP.

Catheter Ablation

Catheter ablation is an interventional discipline within EP whereby an arrhythmogenic focus or critical portion of an arrhythmia circuit is identified, localized, and subsequently destroyed by means of a percutaneous transcatheter technique. Arrhythmias that are currently amenable to ablative therapy include AF, atrial flutter, ectopic atrial tachycardias, SVTs caused by AV nodal reentry or accessory bypass tracts, and VT. Many modalities have been used for ablation. Historically, direct current energy was the initial energy source used for ablative procedures, dating back to the early 1980s.

More recently, radiofrequency energy has become the energy source most commonly used for ablative therapy. Radiofrequency energy uses a frequency range from 200 to 1200 kHz. Application of radiofrequency current causes tissue desiccation in a well-localized region at the point of catheter contact, resulting in a small discrete lesion approximately 0.5×0.5 cm^2. The localized nature of radiofrequency energy–induced lesions has made it the energy source of choice for most ablative procedures. Available technology allows regulation of temperature at the electrode-tissue interface, ensuring adequate contact and preventing sudden impedance rises. Other energy sources for ablation, such as microwave and ultrasound, are being investigated.

Indications for Ablation Therapy

Atrial Fibrillation

Catheter destruction of the AV junction has been used to treat patients with AF and rapid ventricular responses refractory to medical therapy. Patients who are intolerant of medical therapy and patients not desiring lifelong medical therapy are also candidates for this procedure, where CHB is created and a permanent ventricular pacemaker is required to normalize HR. Key points to remember when considering this procedure are:

1. Following the procedure, the patient is completely pacemaker dependent.

2. The procedure does not obviate the need for anticoagulation.

3. There is a risk of developing polymorphic ventricular arrhythmias soon after the procedure, and the ventricular pacing rate should be 90 bpm for the first 2 to 3 months after ablation.

Since 2005, ablation procedures have been developed in an attempt to eliminate AF. Initial attempts were to create linear lesions in the left and right atria, similar to the surgical (Maze) procedure. More recently, observations that pulmonary veins can be sites for electrical discharges that can initiate AF have created a revolution in interventional EP. In patients with paroxysmal AF, three important randomized clinical trials have shown that catheter ablation is superior to antiarrhythmic drug therapy (Pappone et al., Jais/Wilber et al., Wilber et al.). In these trials, freedom from AF was achieved in 63% to 93% of patients who underwent ablation, compared with 17% to 35% who were assigned to drug therapy. More than one ablation may be required to achieve success rates in the higher range. Predictors of success include absence of persistent AF, presence of smaller atria, age younger than 70 years, absence of significant atrial enlargement, and fibrosis. Ablation can be considered for patients with symptomatic AF despite antiarrhythmic drug therapy or intolerance to medications.

Atrial Flutter

In patients who present with atrial flutter, controlling the ventricular response and maintaining sinus rhythm with medications are more difficult than is the case in AF. Often, patients need polypharmacy, and many experience side effects of the medications. Generally, physicians are more likely to recommend ablation early on for patients who present with atrial flutter, especially if the reentrant circuit is felt to be in the RA.

Ectopic Atrial Tachycardias

Ectopic atrial tachycardia, also known as *automatic atrial tachycardia,* may be mapped and ablated. This procedure is now a front-line therapy for medically-resistant ectopic atrial tachycardias as a more economical and less invasive alternative to traditional surgical isolation procedures.

Atrioventricular Nodal Reentry Tachycardia and Wolff-Parkinson-White Syndrome

The usefulness of catheter ablation is described best in the category of reentrant tachycardias that includes the more common mechanisms of SVTs: AVNRT and tachycardias associated with accessory bypass tracts. The indication for catheter ablation in this group of arrhythmias includes recurrent symptomatic tachycardias. Ablation therapy has become a front-line therapeutic option for patients with paroxysmal SVT, obviating the need for therapy with antiarrhythmic agents. Another important indication for radiofrequency ablation is AF in the setting of an accessory pathway capable of conducting in an antegrade manner. These pathways have the potential for extremely rapid conduction, resulting in dangerously rapid ventricular responses with rates exceeding

250 bpm. In this clinical setting, degeneration to VF is possible. Patients with a history of syncope and an accessory pathway capable of antegrade conduction present another indication for curative ablation therapy.

Ventricular Tachycardia

VT presents a challenge in terms of applications of catheter ablation techniques. The extremely variable site of tachycardia origin and the diffuse nature of the arrhythmia circuit make localizing successful sites for energy application difficult. Initial ablation therapy in VT was undertaken in patients with recurrent VT and structurally normal hearts (idiopathic VT). Catheter mapping and ablation have abolished recurrent VT successfully with a remarkably low recurrence rate. However, only a small portion of patients have idiopathic VT with sustained recurrent VT. Other candidates for radiofrequency ablation are patients with nonischemic cardiomyopathy and bundle-branch reentry tachycardia. In these patients, ablation of the right bundle may eliminate VT.

Patients with severe cardiomyopathy represent most patients with recurrent VT. Patients with sustained hemodynamically stable VT and relatively well-maintained LV function seem to be the best candidates for mapping and ablation procedures.

Technical Aspects of Ablation Procedures

General Considerations

Before ablation procedures, the patient is prepared in a manner similar to that for a general EPS. All antiarrhythmic drugs are discontinued. Catheters are placed in the same manner as described earlier. When ablations that require retrograde approach via the aorta/LV are performed, activated coagulation times (ACTs) should be monitored regularly and full anticoagulation (ACTs >300 seconds) maintained throughout the procedure.

In addition to standard catheters, special steerable-tip catheters have been designed to facilitate mapping and ablation procedures (see Fig. 7.4). They are constructed with a large platinum tip (4 to 8 mm) that can produce adequate lesion size in the endocardial surface. An energy source is also necessary. In radiofrequency energy ablations, a generator capable of delivering a continuous unmodulated sine wave at approximately 500 kHz is standard. These generators also continuously monitor energy output and catheter impedance. The circuit is completed by a large indifferent skin electrode, usually positioned in the infrascapular region on the patient's back. A sophisticated electrogram monitoring and storage system is necessary for mapping and ablation procedures. Multiple computer-based multichannel recording systems are available that allow for real-time data analysis and facilitate the mapping-ablation procedure. Radiologic equipment capable of multiplane views is necessary for optimal catheter placement.

When the patient has been prepared properly and catheters have been placed, a baseline EPS is undertaken to document the properties and inducibility of the tachycardia. After characteristics of the tachycardia have been evaluated fully, the mapping and ablation procedures can begin. Techniques used in this part of the procedure are unique to the type of tachycardia to be studied. Specific mapping techniques are discussed here. When the optimal site for ablation has been localized, radiofrequency current is applied to the distal pole of the mapping catheter. Typically, current is applied during 30 to 60 seconds to achieve a target temperature of 60°C while rhythm and intracardiac electrograms are monitored closely (Fig. 7.32).

After ablation, there is typically a 20- to 30-minute waiting period during which repeat EPS is undertaken. This EPS is used to document successful ablation or signs of early recurrence. If no evidence of recurrent tachycardia is seen during approximately 20 minutes after ablation, the procedure can be terminated and

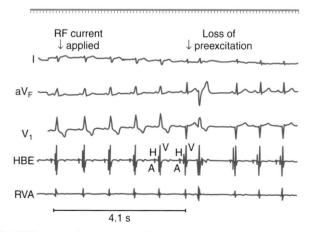

Fig. 7.32 Loss of preexcitation (delta wave) during application of radiofrequency current. Surface leads I, aV$_F$, and V$_1$ are displayed. Note the loss of the delta wave and lengthening of the P–R interval after 4.1 s of radiofrequency *(RF)* energy application, signifying successful ablation of the accessory pathway. *HBE,* His bundle electrogram; *RVA,* right ventricular apex electrogram.

the patient returned to their hospital room. For complex procedures, the patient should be hospitalized and observed with cardiac monitoring for approximately 24 hours after the procedure for early recurrence or new iatrogenic conduction abnormalities and procedure-related complications, such as pneumothorax, postprocedure fever, or vascular injury associated with the ablation procedure. Patients can typically be discharged the morning after the procedure with few physical limitations.

Atrioventricular Node Ablation

Our experience is to perform this procedure after a permanent pacemaker has been implanted. An 8-mm deflectable-tip electrode is placed across the tricuspid annulus and positioned where a prominent His potential is recorded. The catheter is slowly withdrawn into the atrium (Fig. 7.33). When the ablation catheter is positioned so that equal atrial and ventricular electrograms are recorded with a small His potential present, radiofrequency energy can be applied. Success is indicated by an accelerated junctional rhythm that is observed soon after the onset of radiofrequency energy delivery and is followed by high-degree AV block. Immediately after AV nodal ablation, the

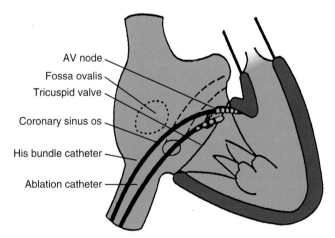

Fig. 7.33 Catheter position during atrioventricular (AV) junction ablation represented in the right anterior oblique view. The position of the His bundle recording catheter is used as a reference. The ablation catheter is positioned on the atrial side of the tricuspid valve just below the diagnostic catheter. (From Haines DE, Di Marco JP. *Curr Probl Cardiol.* 1992;27: 409-477.)

efficacy of radiofrequency-induced AV block is approximately 95%, with a 5% to 10% recurrence rate of AV conduction. Significant complications occur in 1% to 2% of patients. There also is a rare but recognized complication of sudden malignant ventricular arrhythmias occurring hours to days after AV node ablation. The mechanism is poorly understood but may be related to inhomogeneous dispersion of repolarization. This complication has largely been eliminated by programming the pacemaker rate to at least 90 bpm for the first several months.

Atrial Fibrillation

Initial ablation attempts consisted of focal ablation within the pulmonary veins, which had to be abandoned because of the development of pulmonic venous stenosis. Techniques then evolved into circumferential ablation around the ostium or antrum of the pulmonary veins, where electrical isolation of the veins is the key endpoint (Fig. 7.34). The procedure necessitates puncturing the interatrial septum with one or two sheaths; comfort with this technique of transseptal puncture is crucial. Catheters used include multipolar circular mapping catheters. Electroanatomical mapping (CARTO 3 and NavX) to recreate the anatomy of the atrium and pulmonary veins and guide ablation is extremely useful and considered the norm. Its use in the treatment of AF is mainly driven by safety considerations, such as shorter fluoroscopy and procedure times or visualization of structures that need to be protected during the procedure. The ablation process is illustrated in Figure 7.34. Figure 7.34A and B demonstrates the creation of electroanatomical maps of the LA and pulmonary veins using technology from the CARTO 3 or NavX systems. These images are used for ablation in a circumferential manner around the antral regions of the veins. The aim is to achieve electrical isolation of the veins as demonstrated in Figure 7.34C, where electrical silence is seen. Long-term success rates correlate with the ability to achieve electrical isolation of all four veins. Some of the technical challenges unique to this procedure include (1) the need to advance two sheaths into the LA, (2) anticoagulation with heparin to keep the ACT ≥350, and (3) the need to visualize the esophagus to limit the power of energy delivery adjacent to this structure. While performing ablation on the posterior LA wall, most operators monitor temperature in the esophagus with a temperature probe.

Atrial Flutter

Typical atrial flutter can be recognized by the ECG, which shows broad negative P waves with terminal positivity in leads II, III, and

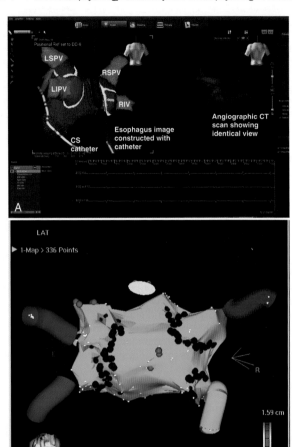

Fig. 7.34 **(A)** NavX map of the left atrium (LA; left posterior oblique view) along with the four pulmonary veins. A simultaneous volume-rendered reconstructed computed tomography *(CT)* scan of the same structure with an identical view as that of the NavX map is also depicted *(red)*. *Yellow dots and lines:* Locations at which radiofrequency energy applications were performed. *Maroon tube:* reconstructed esophagus to guide energy applications on the posterior LA wall. **(B)** Atrial fibrillation (AF) ablation CARTO 3. Cranial view of the LA *(teal)* and four pulmonary veins *(blue, purple, red, and green tubes)* created with the CARTO 3 system. The image was created to guide catheter ablation of AF. *Maroon dots:* Sites of radiofrequency energy application to achieve electrical isolation of pulmonary veins. In this map of the LA, no activation data are depicted.

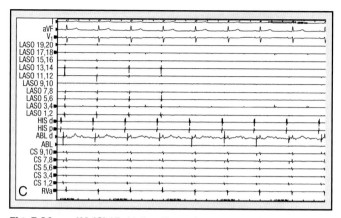

Fig. 7.34, cont'd (C) AF ablation. Figure demonstrates electrical isolation of the pulmonary vein achieved during catheter ablation of AF. A circumferential catheter is placed within the vein from which 10 electrograms are recorded (fourth through 13th tracings from the top). During circumferential ablation performed around the pulmonary vein ostium (similar to A and B), from the fifth beat onward, electrical silence is seen within the vein. *CS,* Coronary sinus; *LIPV,* left inferior pulmonary vein; *LSPV,* left superior pulmonary vein; *RIV,* right inferior vein; *RSPV,* right superior pulmonary vein. (A: EnSite, Velocity, Quartet, SJM Confirm and St. Jude Medical are trademarks of St. Jude Medical, Inc. or its related companies. Reprinted with permission of St. Jude Medical, © 2015. All rights reserved.)

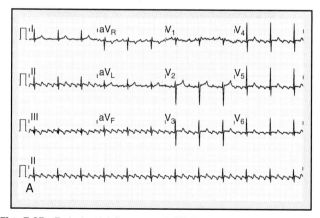

Fig. 7.35 Typical atrial flutter panel. **(A)** Typical 12-lead electrocardiogram (ECG). Broad negative P waves are seen with a terminal positivity in leads II, III, and aV_F. In addition, the P wave is negative in lead V_6 and is upright in lead V_1. *Continued*

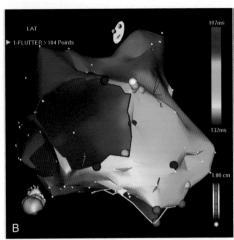

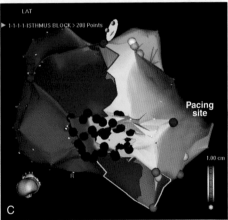

Fig. 7.35, cont'd (B) Typical atrial flutter is a reentrant arrhythmia around the tricuspid annulus. The electrical wave front traverses around the annulus in a counterclockwise manner, demonstrated by the color-coded activation sequences in the electroanatomical map using the CARTO 3 system. The map shows an left anterior oblique (LAO) caudal view of the right atrium (RA), tricuspid annulus, and "early meeting late," that is, red being adjacent to purple is very typical of a reentrant arrhythmia. **(C)** Electroanatomical map of the RA (LAO caudal view) and cavotricuspid isthmus, demonstrating a successful ablation for atrial flutter. After ablation, pacing is performed from the proximal coronary sinus *(red region)*. The CARTO 3 map demonstrates that the electrical impulse does not traverse the cavotricuspid isthmus. The achievement of conduction block across this structure correlates with long-term success. *Maroon dots:* Sites in the cavotricuspid isthmus at which catheter ablation was performed.

aV_F In addition, the P wave is negative in lead V_6 and is upright in lead V_1 (Fig. 7.35A). The presence of this ECG pattern almost always indicates a reentrant arrhythmia around the tricuspid annulus, with the direction of impulse propagation occurring in a counterclockwise fashion (see Fig. 7.35B). The narrowest part of the circuit with the slowest conduction properties tends to be the cavotricuspid isthmus, the site targeted during catheter ablation procedures. During the ablation procedure, the catheter is dragged from the tricuspid valve to the inferior vena cava and at each site where energy is delivered; the aim is to achieve transmural necrosis. At the end of ablation, the electrophysiologist will look to demonstrate the presence of bidirectional conduction block across this structure. In Figure 7.35C, conduction block is demonstrated as pacing medial to the RF line. Achievement of conduction block across this structure correlates with long-term success. Rarely, the ECG pattern may show P-wave polarity opposite to that seen in typical atrial flutter (Fig. 7.36A). In this situation, the reentrant circuit is the same as in typical counterclockwise flutter (i.e., around the tricuspid annulus) but the direction of impulse propagation is opposite. The LAO caudal view electroanatomical map of the RA (see Fig. 7.36B) shows that the impulse traverses around the cavotricuspid isthmus in a clockwise manner. The targeted site of ablation is still the cavotricuspid isthmus. In the era of AF ablation, atrial flutters are seen where the reentrant circuit is in the LA. A detailed discussion of LA flutters is beyond the scope of this chapter. At the end of the chapter, the reader is referred to additional reading on this topic.

Ectopic Atrial Tachycardia

Extensive mapping of the atria is crucial in ablation of ectopic atrial tachycardia. Initially, mapping used to take place with multipolar catheters, but in the current era, electroanatomical mapping is the norm (see Fig. 7.7). Activation mapping is performed to localize the region of earliest atrial activation. If during initial testing the tachycardia is localized to the LA, mapping is undertaken with a transseptal approach via a patent foramen ovale or transseptal puncture technique. For mapping the left side of the heart, meticulous anticoagulation must be maintained to reduce the risk of procedure-related embolic events.

Atrioventricular Nodal Reentrant Tachycardia

In AV nodal reentry, the circuit consists of slowly conducting and rapidly conducting pathways. Anatomically, these pathways are located in the perinodal interatrial septum and compact AV

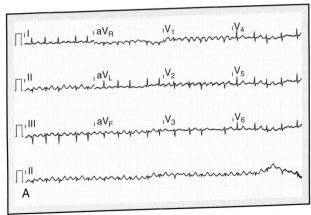

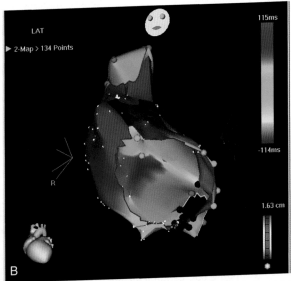

Fig. 7.36 (A) The 12-lead electrocardiogram (ECG) of clockwise atrial flutter. P waves are upright in leads II, III, aV$_F$, and V$_6$ and are negative in lead V$_1$ (the opposite of that seen in typical counterclockwise flutter). **(B)** Reentrant circuit is the same as that seen in typical counterclockwise flutter (i.e., around the tricuspid annulus, but the direction of impulse propagation is opposite). Left anterior oblique (LAO) caudal view electroanatomical map of the right atrium (RA) shows that the impulse traverses around the cavotricuspid isthmus in a clockwise manner. This is seen in only a minority of cases, and the targeted site of ablation is still the cavotricuspid isthmus.

node, respectively. The current approach to ablation for AV nodal reentry, termed *AV nodal modification*, is selective ablation of the slow pathway. In rare cases, a fast or intermediate pathway ablation must be performed for successful AV nodal modification.

Mapping of the slow pathway is performed around the inferior and posterior perinodal area in the posterior septal region of the RA, extending inferiorly to the os of the coronary sinus. Radiofrequency energy is delivered along the tricuspid annulus, where low-amplitude fragmented atrial electrograms are recorded (Fig. 7.37). Radiofrequency energy can be delivered during AVNRT or in sinus rhythm. Successful ablation is heralded by termination of the tachycardia when energy is delivered during SVT or by development of accelerated junctional rhythm when ablating in sinus rhythm.

Complete elimination of the slow pathway results in the inability to induce AVNRT or show conduction along the slow AV pathway. After ablation, routine programmed electrical stimulation is repeated to evaluate for the presence of slow-pathway conduction or inducible AV nodal reentry. If the slow pathway is not functional in the drug-free state, infuse isoproterenol to validate noninducibility. Success rates for AV nodal modification are ≥95%, and the risk of major complication is estimated to be 1% to 5%. Potential complications include iatrogenic high-degree AV block, pericarditis, cardiac

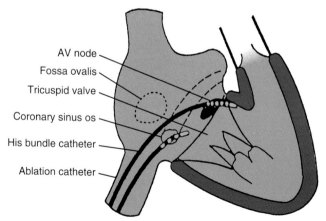

Fig. 7.37 Typical catheter position for ablation of the slow pathway for atrioventricular *(AV)* nodal reentry tachycardia. The ablation catheter is positioned on the atrial side of the tricuspid valve in the vicinity of the coronary sinus os. The ablation catheter is inferior and posterior to the His bundle catheter. (From Haines DE, Di Marco JP. *Curr Probl Cardiol.* 1992;27:409-477.)

perforation with tamponade, and vascular complications related to access. The estimated recurrence rate is 5%.

Accessory Pathways

The technique used for ablating accessory pathways is different depending on the location and the conduction properties of the accessory pathways. Before ablation, the patient undergoes a comprehensive EPS to determine the presence and electrical properties of accessory pathways. The pathways that conduct antegrade in sinus rhythm and exhibit a delta wave (manifest preexcitation) can be mapped during sinus rhythm. The general location of the accessory pathway can be identified by the axis of the delta wave on the 12-lead ECG. However, EPS and mapping are required to localize precisely the site of the accessory pathway. With a manifest accessory pathway, the mapping catheter is maneuvered slowly along the valve annulus to locate optimal electrode placement that will result in the earliest ventricular activation during sinus rhythm or atrial pacing (Fig. 7.38). Discrete electrical potentials from the accessory pathway have often been recorded at the successful ablation site and are referred to as *pathway potentials*. For pathways capable only of retrograde conduction, mapping is performed by determining the site of earliest retrograde atrial activity during ventricular pacing or induced orthodromic reciprocating tachycardia. Accessory pathways on the left side of the heart can be ablated by a transseptal approach using a patent foramen ovale, the Brockenbrough technique (Fig. 7.39), or the more conventional retrograde approach, in which the ablating catheter is prolapsed across the aortic valve (Fig. 7.40).

The overall success of radiofrequency ablation for accessory pathways depends on operator experience and location of the accessory pathway. Success rates of more than 95% are reported for left-sided pathways. Right-sided pathways are usually reported to be less successful, with efficacy rates of more than 90%. The complication rate for accessory pathway ablation is estimated to be 1% to 2%, and most complications result from catheter manipulation and not from delivery of radiofrequency energy. Complications include iatrogenic high-degree AV block (most commonly seen with anteroseptal accessory pathway ablations), pericarditis, cardiac perforation with tamponade, and vascular complications related to access associated with radiofrequency ablation of accessory pathways. Mortality is rare but has been reported to be approximately 0.3%. Complications, including procedure-related deaths, are higher in low-volume laboratories (<20 ablations/year) than in high-volume laboratories (>50 ablations/year). The estimated recurrence rate after ablation for an accessory pathway is 3% to 17%; the higher recurrence rates are seen with right-sided

PREABLATION   POSTABLATION

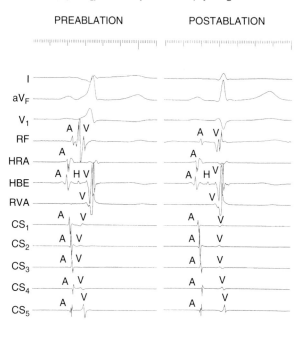

Fig. 7.38 Sequence of antegrade ventricular activation before and after radiofrequency ablation of a left-sided accessory pathway. Displayed are surface leads I, aV_F, and V_1. The earliest ventricular activation during sinus rhythm occurs in the midcoronary sinus (CS_2 to CS_3) region. Electrograms recorded from the ablating catheter at the successful ablation site radiofrequency (RF) show early ventricular activation and a short A-to-V interval. Shown at postablation is a normal sequence of antegrade activation. Note lengthening of the A-to-V interval in the coronary sinus electrograms and the electrogram recorded from the ablation catheter. CS1 to CS5, Recordings from the coronary sinus, with CS1 the most proximal coronary sinus recording and CS5 the most distal; HBE, His bundle electrogram; HRA, high right atrial electrogram; RVA, right ventricular apex electrogram.

accessory pathways. Patients who remain asymptomatic for 3 months after the procedure have an extremely low incidence of recurrence thereafter.

Ventricular Tachycardia

Several mapping techniques are used to target radiofrequency application during treatment for VT. These techniques are usually

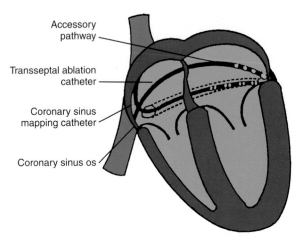

Fig. 7.39 Catheter position for ablation of a left free wall pathway using a trans-septal approach. The catheter is passed through a sheath that has been placed through the atrial septum and then positioned above the mitral valve annulus in close proximity to the accessory pathway located near the coronary sinus catheter. (From Haines DE, Di Marco JP. *Curr Probl Cardiol.* 1992;27:409-477.)

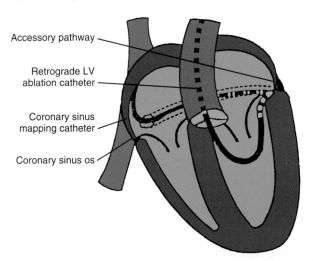

Fig. 7.40 Catheter position for ablation of left free wall accessory pathway via the retrograde approach. The ablation catheter is prolapsed across the aortic valve and positioned under the mitral valve leaflet, in close proximity to the accessory pathway located near the coronary sinus catheter. *LV,* Left ventricular. (From Haines DE, Di Marco JP. *Curr Probl Cardiol.* 1992; 27:409-477.)

used in combination to locate the optimal site of energy delivery. They can be used for idiopathic VTs (the most common being RV outflow tract tachycardia) or VTs associated with coronary artery disease. Initially, a gross estimation of tachycardia origin can be made from the 12-lead ECG of VT. This estimate helps to direct mapping efforts to the RV or LV and to specific regions within the appropriate ventricle.

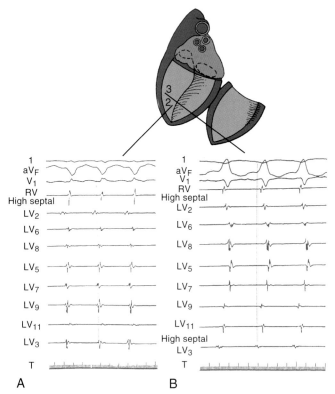

Fig. 7.41 Endocardial catheter mapping of two different ventricular tachycardia (VT) morphologies. **(A)** VT with a right bundle-branch morphology and right superior axis. A reference right ventricular *(RV)* catheter is shown along with multiple ventricular recordings. The earliest ventricular activation is recorded at LV₂, which corresponds with the RV apex. **(B)** VT with a left bundle-branch block (LBBB) pattern in right inferior axis. The earliest ventricular activation occurs near LV₃, which corresponds to the high-septal area. *T,* Time line. (From Josephson ME. Clinical cardiac electrophysiology: techniques and interpretations. Philadelphia: Lea & Febiger; 1993.)

During activation mapping, the mapping catheter is maneuvered to an endocardial location that shows the earliest activation time in tachycardia (Fig. 7.41). The presence of mid-diastolic potentials identifies optimal ablation sites. Pace mapping, in which pacing from the ablation catheter duplicates the QRS morphology of the clinical VT, is also used to identify the appropriate site for ablation energy application. After ablation, ventricular stimulation is undertaken again to ensure that the tachycardia is no longer inducible. Ablation of idiopathic VT seems to have a higher success rate (~85%) than ablation of VT associated with coronary artery disease (~60%). A survey by the North American Society of Pacing and Electrophysiology reported a low complication rate and mortality associated with radiofrequency catheter ablation, despite its use in a relatively high-risk patient population. VT associated with ischemic heart disease is an extremely variable entity and must be assessed on an individual basis.

Suggested Readings

Antiarrhythmics Versus Implantable Defibrillators (AVID) Investigators. A comparison of antiarrhythmic-drug therapy with implantable defibrillators in patients resuscitated from near-fatal ventricular arrhythmias. *N Engl J Med.* 1997;337:1576-1583.

Bristow MR, Saxon LA, Boehmer J, et al. Cardiac-resynchronization therapy with or without an implantable defibrillator in advanced chronic heart failure. *N Engl J Med.* 2004;350:2140-2150.

Calkins H, Yong P, Miller JM, et al. Catheter ablation of accessory pathways, atrioventricular nodal reentrant tachycardia, and the atrioventricular junction. *Circulation.* 1999;99:262-270.

Cappato R, Calkins H, Chen S, et al. Worldwide survey on the methods, efficacy, and safety of catheter ablation for human atrial fibrillation. *Circulation.* 2005;111: 1100-1105.

Cleland JG, Daubert JC, Erdmann E, et al. The effect of cardiac resynchronization on morbidity and mortality in heart failure. *N Engl J Med.* 2005;352:1539-1549.

Cohen TJ, Scheinman MM, Pullen BT, et al. Emergency intracardiac defibrillation for refractory ventricular fibrillation during routine electrophysiologic study. *J Am Coll Cardiol.* 1991;18:1280-1284.

Curtis JP, Luebbert JL, Wang Y, et al. Association of physician certification and outcomes among patients receiving an implantable cardioverter-defibrillator. *JAMA.* 2009;301: 1661-1670.

Da Costa A, Thevenin J, Roche F, et al. Results from the Loire-Ardéche-Drôme-Isère-Puy-de-Dôme (LADIP) trial on atrial flutter, a multicentric prospective randomized study comparing amiodarone and radiofrequency ablation after the first episode of symptomatic atrial flutter. *Circulation.* 2006;114:1676-1681.

Darouiche RO, Wall Jr, MJ, Itani KM, et al. Chlorhexidine-alcohol versus povidone-iodine for surgical-site antisepsis. *N Engl J Med.* 2010;362:18-26.

Feld GK, Fleck RP, Chen PS, et al. Radiofrequency catheter ablation for the treatment of human type 1 atrial flutter. Identification of a critical zone in the reentrant circuit by endocardial mapping techniques. *Circulation.* 1992;86:1233-1240.

Fogoros RN. *Electrophysiologic Testing.* Oxford, UK: Blackwell; 1991.

Forcinito M. Guidelines for clinical intracardiac electrophysiologic studies. A report of the American College of Cardiology/American Heart Association Task Force on Assessment of Diagnostic and Therapeutic Cardiovascular Procedures. (Subcommittee to Assess Clinical Intracardiac Electrophysiologic Studies). *J Am Coll Cardiol.* 1989;14:1827-1842.

Gepstein L, Hayam G, Ben-Haim SA. A novel method for nonfluoroscopic catheter-based electroanatomical mapping of the heart. In vitro and in vivo accuracy results. *Circulation.* 1997;95:1611-1622.

Haines DE, DiMarco JP. Current therapy for supraventricular tachycardia. *Curr Probl Cardiol.* 1992;27:409-477.

Haïssaguerre M, Jaïs P, Shah DC, et al. Spontaneous initiation of atrial fibrillation by ectopic beats originating in the pulmonary veins. *N Engl J Med.* 1998;339:659-666.

Horowitz LN, Kay HR, Kutalek SP, et al. Risks and complications of clinical cardiac electrophysiologic studies: a prospective analysis of 1,000 consecutive patients. *J Am Coll Cardiol.* 1987;9:1261-1268.

Jackman WM, Beckman KJ, McClelland JH, et al. Treatment of supraventricular tachycardia due to atrioventricular nodal reentry by radiofrequency catheter ablation of slow-pathway conduction. *N Engl J Med.* 1992;327:313-318.

Jackman WM, Wang X, Friday KJ, et al. Catheter ablation of accessory atrioventricular pathways (Wolff-Parkinson-White syndrome) by radiofrequency current. *N Engl J Med.* 1991;324:1605-1611.

Jaïs P, Cauchemez B, Macle L, et al. Catheter ablation versus antiarrhythmic drugs for atrial fibrillation: the A4 study. *Circulation.* 2008;118:2498-2505.

Josephson ME. *Clinical Cardiac Electrophysiology: Techniques and Interpretations.* Philadelphia, PA: Lea & Febiger; 1993.

Josephson ME, Maloney JD, Barold SS. Guidelines for training in adult cardiovascular medicine. Core cardiology training symposium (COCATS). Task Force 6: training in specialized electrophysiology, cardiac pacing and arrhythmia management. *J Am Coll Cardiol.* 1995;25:23-26.

Mason JW. A comparison of seven antiarrhythmic drugs in patients with ventricular tachyarrhythmias. Electrophysiologic Study versus Electrocardiographic Monitoring Investigators. *N Engl J Med.* 1993;329:452-458.

Moss AJ, Hall WJ, Cannom DS, et al. Improved survival with an implanted defibrillator in patients with coronary disease at high risk for ventricular arrhythmia. Multicenter Automatic Defibrillator Implantation Trial Investigators. *N Engl J Med.* 1996;335:1933-1940.

Moss AJ, Zareba W, Hall WJ, et al. Prophylactic implantation of a defibrillator in patients with myocardial infarction and reduced ejection fraction. *N Engl J Med.* 2002;346:877-883.

Pappone C, Augello G, Sala S, et al. A randomized trial of circumferential pulmonary vein ablation versus antiarrhythmic drug therapy in paroxysmal atrial fibrillation: The APAF study. *J Am Coll Cardiol.* 2006;48:2340-2347.

Pappone C, Rosanio S, Oreto G, et al. Circumferential radiofrequency ablation of pulmonary vein ostia: A new anatomic approach for curing atrial fibrillation. *Circulation.* 2000;102:2619-2628.

Scheidt S. *Basic Electrocardiography.* West Caldwell, NJ: Ciba-Geigy Pharmaceuticals; 1986.

Scheinman MM. Patterns of catheter ablation practice in the United States: results of the 1992 NASPE survey. North American Society of Pacing and Electrophysiology. *Pacing Clin Electrophysiol.* 1994;17:873-875.

Tracy CM, Akhtar M, DiMarco JP, et al. American College of Cardiology/American Heart Association clinical competence statement on invasive electrophysiology studies, catheter ablation, and cardioversion. *J Am Coll Cardiol.* 2000;36:1725-1736.

Waller TJ, Kay HR, Spielman SR, et al. Reduction in sudden death and total mortality by antiarrhythmic therapy evaluated by electrophysiologic drug testing: criteria of efficacy in patients with sustained ventricular tachyarrhythmia. *J Am Coll Cardiol.* 1987;10:83-89.

Wilber DJ, Pappone C, Neuzil P, et al. Comparison of antiarrhythmic drug therapy and radiofrequency catheter ablation in patients with paroxysmal atrial fibrillation: a randomized controlled trial. *JAMA.* 2010;303:333-340.

Wittkampf FH, Wever EF, Derksen R, et al. LocaLisa: new technique for real-time 3-dimensional localization of regular intracardiac electrodes. *Circulation.* 1999;99: 1312-1317.

Wittkampf FH, Wever EF, Vos K, et al. Reduction of radiation exposure in the cardiac electrophysiology laboratory. *Pacing Clin Electrophysiol.* 2000;23:1638-1644.

High-Risk Cardiac Catheterization

EMMANOUIL S. BRILAKIS • MICHAEL FORSBERG •
MICHAEL J. LIM

Diagnostic coronary angiography and percutaneous coronary intervention (PCI) may lead to complications, both acute (during the procedure or during the hospital stay) (Fig. 8.1) and long-term (such as restenosis or stent thrombosis). Acute complications include death, myocardial infarction, stroke or other thromboembolism, vascular complications, bleeding, need for emergency surgery, contrast reactions, radiation injury, and arrhythmias (Table 8.1).[1] An in-hospital complication is expected to occur in approximately 1 of 74 patients undergoing diagnostic catheterization, 1 of 22 patients without ST-segment elevation acute myocardial infarction (STEMI), and 1 of 8 patients undergoing PCI for STEMI (primary PCI).[1]

High-Risk Patient: Definition

Patients classified as high risk are more likely to die or have complications during cardiac catheterization than are other patients.[2] Numerous studies have summarized the clinical and anatomic characteristics of patients at high risk (Table 8.2).[3–7] Increased patient risk may be immediately obvious (for example in the acute myocardial infarction patient in cardiogenic shock) or less obvious (such as patients with high international normalized ratio [INR]).

High risk may be a function of the patient demographics (age, gender), cardiac and noncardial comorbidities, presentation, coronary anatomy, urgency of the procedure, and technique (Table 8.2). Several scores have been developed to predict the risk of acute and chronic complications during catheterization and PCI[3–7] and have been implemented in online calculators, such as the SCAI online calculator (http://www.scai.org/PCIRisk AssessmentTools/default.aspx).

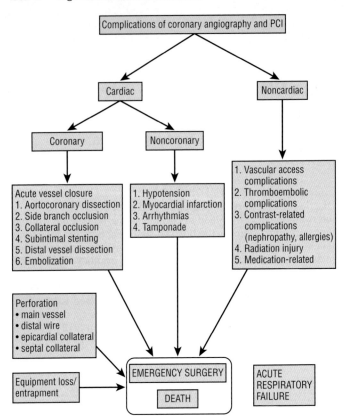

Fig. 8.1 Overview of acute complications of cardiac catheterization and percutaneous coronary intervention. (From Brilakis ES. *Manual of Coronary Chronic Total Occlusion Interventions. A Step-By-Step Approach.* 2nd ed. Elsevier; 2017.)

Prevention of Complications

Meticulous attention to the precatheterization patient assessment and recognition of potential risks decreases procedure-related complications.

The best complications are those that never occur.

Anonymous

Table 8.1

Procedure-Related Complications of Diagnostic Catheterization and Percutaneous Coronary Intervention from the NCDR.

	Diagnostic Catheterization Only Patients Without STEMI (n = 1,091,557)	PCI Patients Without STEMI (n = 787,980)	PCI Patients With STEMI (n = 153,268)
Complications (%)			
Any adverse event	1.35	4.53	12.4
Cardiogenic shock	0.24	0.47	3.87
Heart failure	0.38	0.59	3.46
Pericardial tamponade	0.03	0.07	0.15
CVA/stroke	0.17	0.17	0.56
% of total strokes that were hemorrhagic	9.16	15.6	19.7
New requirement for dialysis	0.14	0.19	0.63
In-hospital mortality			
Non–risk-adjusted	0.72	0.65	5.2
Non–risk-adjusted excluding CABG patients	0.60	0.62	
CABG performed during admission	7.47	0.81	
CABG Status			
Salvage/emergency	0.01/0.27	0.01/0.17	0.05/0.87
Urgent/elective	5.27/1.92	0.47/0.16	2.08/0.43
CABG Indication			
PCI failure without clinical deterioration		0.26	0.58
PCI complication		0.14	0.22
Bleeding Complications (%)			
Any bleeding event within 72 h of procedure	0.49	1.40	3.85
Any other vascular complication requiring treatment	0.15	0.44	0.62
RBC/whole-blood transfusion	N/R	2.07	5.61

From Dehmer GJ, Weaver D, Roe MT, et al. A contemporary view of diagnostic cardiac catheterization and percutaneous coronary intervention in the United States: a report from the CathPCI Registry of the National Cardiovascular Data Registry, 2010 through June 2011. *J Am Coll Cardiol.* 2012;60:2017-2031.

CABG, Coronary artery bypass grafting; *CVA,* Cerebrovascular accident; *NCDR,* National Cardiovascular Data Registry; *PCI,* percutaneous coronary intervention; *RBC,* red blood cell; *STEMI,* ST-segment elevation acute myocardial infarction.

Table 8.2

Variables Associated with Higher Risk During Cardiac Catheterization and Coronary Angiography.

Demographics

Age >60 years or <1 year
Female sex

Comorbidities: Non-cardiac

Poorly controlled hypertension
Diabetes mellitus
Renal insufficiency, including dialysis
Pulmonary disease (COPD, asthma, OSA)
Anemia ± bleeding diathesis, active bleeding, elevated INR,
    thrombocytopenia
Cerebrovascular disease
Severe peripheral vascular disease (vascular access difficulty is also included)
Very small or very large body habitus
High and low BMI
Frailty

Comorbidities: Cardiac

Severe left ventricular dysfunction (EF<30%)
Decompensated heart failure (especially NYHA class IV)
Pulmonary hypertension
Atrial/ventricular arrhythmias
Severe valvular disease
Prior PCI
Prior CABG

Medications

Erectile dysfunction drugs
Oral anticoagulants
Metformin
Insulin
Diuretics
IV contrast allergy

Presentation

Cardiac arrest
Cardiogenic shock
Acute myocardial infarction
Emergent procedure

Coronary Anatomy

Left main disease
Multivessel disease
Severe calcification
Tortuosity

Table 8.2

Variables Associated with Higher Risk During Cardiac Catheterization and Coronary Angiography. (Continued)

Saphenous vein graft lesion
Small vessel size
Chronic total occlusions
Bifurcations
Tortuosity
Spontaneous coronary dissection

Technique

Femoral access
Use of radiation

BMI, Body mass index; *CABG,* coronary artery bypass grafting; *COPD,* chronic obstructive pulmonary disease; *EF,* ejection fraction; *INR,* international normalized ratio; *IV,* intravenous; *NYHA,* New York Heart Association; *OSA,* obstructive sleep apnea.

Acute Vessel Closure

Several mechanisms can lead to acute vessel closure (Fig. 8.1), highlighting potential prevention strategies. Meticulous attention to pressure waveform (to avoid dampening) can minimize the risk for creating (and extending) an aortocoronary dissection. Protection of side branches (by inserting and jailing a guidewire) can reduce the risk of occlusion during bifurcation stenting.[8] Careful wire manipulation may decrease the risk of subintimal entry and dissection. Careful preparation of the manifold and back-bleeding of the catheter after wire removal, equipment exchanges, and use of the trapping technique may minimize the risk of air embolization.[9] A small air embolus usually resolves and does not often result in permanent damage. Significant air embolus to the coronary circulation can cause myocardial ischemia and circulatory collapse. Air aspiration should be promptly performed in such cases, together with administration of 100% oxygen (to help dissolve the air bubbles) and possibly use of intracoronary epinephrine and cardiopulmonary support.

Perforation

Coronary perforation can be classified according to location (large vessel, small vessel, septal and epicardial collateral perforation, Fig. 8.2) and according to severity (Ellis classification,[10] Box 8.1).[11] The risk of perforation may be minimized by avoiding use of oversized balloons and stents, careful use of atherectomy devices, and meticulous attention to distal guidewire position.

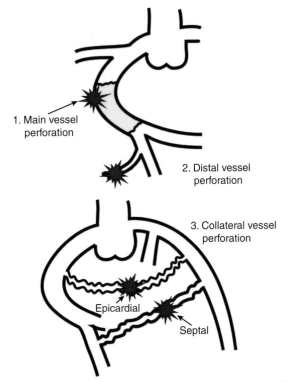

Fig. 8.2 Examples of the different types of coronary perforation. (From Brilakis ES. *Manual of Coronary Chronic Total Occlusion Interventions. A Step-By-Step Approach.* 2nd ed. Elsevier; 2017.)

Box 8.1   Ellis Classification of Coronary Perforations.

- Class 1: a crater extending outside the lumen only in the absence of linear staining angiographically suggestive of dissection.
- Class 2: Pericardial or myocardial blush without a ≥1 mm exit hole
- Class 3: Frank streaming of contrast through a ≥1 mm exit hole.
- Class 3-cavity spilling: Perforation into an anatomic cavity chamber, such as the coronary sinus, the right ventricle, etc.

From Ellis SG, Ajluni S, Arnold AZ, et al. Increased coronary perforation in the new device era. Incidence, classification, management, and outcome. *Circulation.* 1994;90:2725-2730.

The first step in the management of coronary perforation is to inflate a balloon rapidly to minimize blood extravasation into the pericardium (Fig. 8.3). In case of tamponade, emergency pericardiocentesis is performed. If pericardial bleeding continues after balloon inflation, use of a covered stent and fat or coil embolization are usually used to achieve hemostasis (Fig. 8.3). Anticoagulation should not be reversed until all equipment is removed from the coronary artery.[11]

Equipment Loss and Entrapment

Equipment loss or entrapment in the intravascular or intracoronary space may lead to emergency surgery for removal. Adequate lesion preparation is key for reducing the risk of stent loss or entrapment. In many cases, lost devices may not need to be retrieved: for example, lost stents can sometimes be deployed or crushed using another stent.[12]

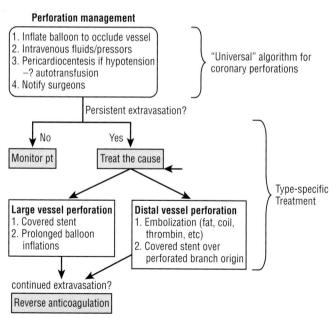

Fig. 8.3 Overview of the management of coronary perforations. (From Brilakis ES. *Manual of Coronary Chronic Total Occlusion Interventions. A Step-By-Step Approach.* 2nd ed. Elsevier; 2017.)

Hypotension

Hypotension may occur before, during, and after cardiac catheterization from a variety of conditions. Hypotension should be distinguished from pseudohypotension, for example when there is dampening of the pressure waveform because of deep catheter engagement or obstruction from thrombus/plaque. Correlation with noninvasive pressure can help make the diagnosis. If catheter obstruction is suspected, the catheter should be withdrawn without injection contrast or attempting to advance a guidewire through it (to minimize the risk for systemic thromboembolism).

Hypotension *during any stage of the procedure* may be caused by myocardial ischemia or cardiogenic shock that may require treatment with inotropic and vasopressor agents and with hemodynamic support devices.

Before cardiac catheterization, hypotension may be caused by hypovolemia induced by fasting before the procedure or diuretics.

During the procedure, hypotension may be caused by vasovagal reaction. Untreated vasovagal reactions with hypotension can lead to irreversible shock. Vasovagal reactions are often the result of pain at the vascular access site. In some elderly patients, a vagal reaction may occur without bradycardia and appear as unexplained hypotension. Hypotension that develops after coronary angiography or left ventriculography is generally transient, self-limited, and responds to IV fluids. Other considerations during the procedure include oversedation, IV contrast allergy, or vagal reaction from a full bladder. Nitroglycerin administration can also lead to hypotension.

During and after the procedure, hypotension may be caused by hypovolemia, myocardial ischemia, bleeding from the arterial access site, cardiac tamponade, or retroperitoneal hemorrhage. Any of these can present with bradycardia and hypotension and initially appear to be a vagal response.

Hypotension resulting from hypovolemia is treated with IV saline infusion. Patients often respond acutely to elevation (>30 degrees) of the legs (increased venous inflow, internal transfusion). Generally, several hundred milliliters of saline is required to restore adequate blood pressure in patients who have hypotension caused by hypovolemia. Preprocedure prevention of hypovolemia can be avoided by IV saline (>500 mL) for 4 to 6 hours before the start of the procedure.

For patients who have hypovolemia caused by hemorrhage, administration of blood products is necessary and hemostasis must be achieved as soon as possible. Care should be taken to prevent volume overload in patients with congestive heart failure. If a patient's volume status cannot be determined clinically, a pulmonary artery catheter and pulmonary capillary wedge pressure measurement may be necessary.

For patients with hypotension resulting from vasovagal or ischemia reaction, pharmacologic therapy may be necessary to restore adequate blood pressure. Atropine for vasovagal hypotension (0.5 mg IV every 3 minutes as needed) is used first. IV phenylephrine (0.1 to 0.3 mg) or an epinephrine bolus (1 mL of 1:10,000-U dilution) temporarily increases blood pressure to normal range while the staff member continues to assess the patient and prepare other vasopressors. For patients with prolonged hypotension or hypotension without hypovolemia, IV infusions of pressors may be initiated and can be titrated as needed. Dopamine starting at 5 mcg/kg/min or norepinephrine at 10 mcg/min can be titrated according to response.

Drug-induced hypotension should be addressed with agents that antagonize, ameliorate, or minimize the actions of the offending agent. Narcotic-induced hypotension can be treated with administration of naloxone (Narcan). The initial dose is 0.4 mg (1-mL ampule), which may be repeated every 2 to 3 minutes as needed. Hypotension (or hypoventilation) resulting from benzodiazepine administration can be treated with flumazenil (Romazicon). The initial dose is 0.2 mg (2 mL) administered over 30 seconds; additional doses of 0.2 mg (up to 1 mg) can be administered every 1 minute. Because of the sedatives' longer half-life than that of reversal agents, resedation can occur, and repeat doses can be given every 20 minutes, with a maximum dose of 3 mg/h.

Hypotension can result from negative inotropic, negative chronotropic, and vasodilator actions of calcium channel blockers. Vasodilator actions can be at least partially reversed by administration of calcium chloride (1 ampule, 13.6 mEq). Administration of glucagon (1 mg) may partially ameliorate the effects of β-blockers. If nitroglycerin-induced hypotension develops, IV infusion should be stopped or the nitropaste wiped off.

Hypotension resulting from cardiac tamponade is an emergency condition that requires immediate pericardiocentesis.

Management of Refractory Myocardial Ischemia and Hemodynamic Instability

Transient ischemia and coronary artery occlusion can be caused by catheter-induced spasm, cannulation of a severely diseased coronary artery, or a severe ostial lesion. Initial intervention is removal of the catheter from the coronary ostium. Continued myocardial ischemia should initially be treated with pharmacologic therapy beginning with nitrates, either sublingual nitroglycerin (0.4 mg every 5 minutes), or IV or intracoronary nitroglycerin

(100-mcg boluses repeated every 5 minutes as necessary). Nitroglycerin can be used, provided that the patient does not have hypotension. For patients with tachycardia, negative inotropic therapy with a β-blocker, such as metoprolol (5 mg IV every 5 minutes), or a calcium channel blocker, such as verapamil (2.5 to 5 mg IV every 5 minutes), should be considered if the patient is otherwise hemodynamically stable.

When ischemia persists after optimal medical treatment, or when it is associated with significant hemodynamic instability including pulmonary edema or hypotension or both, mechanical circulatory support should be considered.

Circulatory Support Devices

Circulatory support devices can be used either prophylactically or after occurrence of a complication during CTO PCI.[2] Four devices are currently available in the United States for providing percutaneous left ventricular hemodynamic support: the intraaortic balloon pump (IABP), the Impella (2.5, CP, and 5.0, Abiomed Inc., Danvers, MA), the TandemHeart (Cardiac Assist Inc., Pittsburgh, PA), and venoarterial extracorporeal membrane oxygenator (VA ECMO) (Fig. 8.4, Table 8.3).

Determining the need for prophylactic or urgent insertion of a hemodynamic support device depends on the patient's clinical condition (hemodynamic status, left ventricular systolic function and end-diastolic pressure), procedural risk (for example retrograde chronic total occlusion [CTO] PCI through the last remaining vessel), and local device availability and expertise.[11]

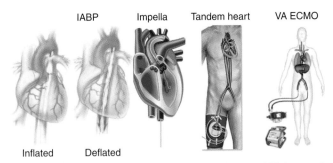

IABP   Impella   Tandem heart   VA ECMO

Inflated   Deflated

Fig. 8.4 Currently available circulatory support devices. *IABP,* Intraaortic balloon pump; *VA ECMO,* venoarterial extracorporeal membrane oxygenator. (From Brilakis ES. *Manual of Coronary Chronic Total Occlusion Interventions. A Step-By-Step Approach.* 2nd ed. Elsevier; 2017.)

Table 8.3

Hemodynamic Support Devices.

	IABP	Impella	TandemHeart	VA ECMO
Feasibility				
Availability	+++	++	+	+
Arterial access size required	7–8 F	12 F (Impella 2.5) 14 F (Impella CP) 21 F (Impella 5.0)	15–17 F arterial 21 F venous	14–17 F arterial 18–21 F venous
Contraindications	• High bleeding risk • Severe aortic regurgitation • Thoracic or abdominal aorta aneurysm	• High bleeding risk • Severe aortic regurgitation • Severe PAD[a] • Left ventricular thrombus • Mechanical aortic valve • Ventricular septal defect	• High bleeding risk • Severe aortic regurgitation • Severe PAD[a]	• High bleeding risk • Severe aortic regurgitation • Severe PAD[a]
Efficacy				
Cardiac output increase (L/min)	0.3–0.5	≈2.5 (Impella 2.5)[b] ≈4.0 (Impella CP) ≈5.0 (Impella 5.0)	4–5[b]	4–5[b]
Affected by arrhythmias	Yes	No	No	No
Requires adequate right ventricular function	Yes	Yes	Yes	No
Can correct respiratory failure	No	No	Yes[c]	Yes

Continued on following page

Table 8.3

Hemodynamic Support Devices. (Continued)

	IABP	Impella	TandemHeart	VA ECMO
Complications				
Risk for lower limb ischemia	+	++	+++	+++
Transseptal puncture required	No	No	Yes	No
Risk for bleeding	+	++	++	++
Risk for hemolysis	+	++	++	++

IABP, Intraaortic balloon pump; *PAD*, peripheral arterial disease; *VA ECMO*, venoarterial extracorporeal membrane oxygenator.
[a]Transcaval access can be used for placing the arterial cannula in case of severe peripheral arterial disease
[b]Depending on arterial cannula size
[c]Adding an oxygenator to the TandemHeart circuit

Intraaortic Balloon Pump

The IABP is the smallest circulatory support device, but it also provides the least hemodynamic support (0.5 L/min of blood flow). The IABP is usually inserted percutaneously through a 7-F or 8-F femoral arterial sheath. The IABP mechanism of action is inflation of a balloon with helium in the aorta during diastole, displacing blood peripherally and increasing cardiac output, while reducing left ventricular end diastolic pressure. Indications and contraindications for IABP use are summarized in Box 8.2.

IABP counterpulsation increases diastolic pressure and coronary blood flow and decreases myocardial oxygen demand (i.e., reduces afterload). Balloon inflation in diastole (at the dicrotic notch on the central arterial pressure tracing) increases diastolic pressure, which increases coronary artery pressure and coronary flow. Deflation of the balloon just before systole (at end diastole, at the upstroke of arterial pressure tracing) results in decreased ventricular afterload, which decreases myocardial oxygen consumption and increases cardiac output (Fig. 8.5).

Box 8.2 Indications and Contraindications for Intraaortic Balloon Counterpulsation.

Indications

Refractory unstable angina
Cardiogenic shock
Postoperative hemodynamic compromise
Acute myocardial infarction with mechanical impairment as a result of mitral regurgitation or ventricular septal defect
Intractable ventricular tachycardia as a result of myocardial ischemia
Patients with left main coronary stenosis or severe three-vessel disease undergoing anesthesia for cardiac surgery
High-risk PCI
Maintenance of vessel patency after PCI with slow flow

Contraindications

Anatomic abnormality of femoral-iliac artery
Iliac or aortic atherosclerotic disease impairing blood flow runoff
Moderate or severe aortic regurgitation
Aortic dissection or aneurysm
Patent ductus (counterpulsation may augment the abnormal pathway of aortic-to-pulmonary artery shunting)
Bypass grafting to femoral artery
Bleeding diathesis
Sepsis

PCI, Percutaneous coronary intervention; *PTCA,* percutaneous transluminal coronary angioplasty.

Diastole: Balloon inflation
Augmentation of diastolic pressure
• Coronary perfusion ↑

Systole: Balloon inflation
Decreased afterload
• Cardiac work ↓
• Myocardial oxygen consumption ↓
• Cardiac output ↑

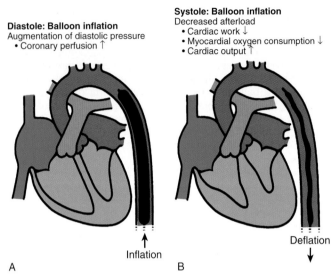

A   Inflation   B   Deflation

Fig. 8.5 Schematic representations of **(A)** balloon inflation during diastole and **(B)** balloon deflation just before the onset of systole. Diastolic augmentation increases coronary artery perfusion, and balloon deflation just before the onset of systole decreases afterload, which results in decreased myocardial oxygen demand, decreased cardiac workload, and increased cardiac output.

Technique

Before percutaneous insertion of an intraaortic balloon (IAB), the operator assesses the iliofemoral arteries and aorta for vascular disease. Significant peripheral vascular disease is a relative contraindication. An abdominal aortogram helps identify the course and disease of iliac and femoral vessels before IABP insertion.

Complications of IAB placement most commonly result from a puncture site that is too low, perforation of the superficial femoral artery, or forceful artery dissection caused by advancement of the guidewire. The puncture site should be located similar to or slightly more cranial than a standard femoral puncture for diagnostic catheterization. A low puncture may involve the superficial femoral artery, which is often too small to accept the IABP, and this may result in subsequent leg ischemia.

The IABP balloon sheath (or sheathless IABP catheter) is inserted into either groin using the modified Seldinger technique. Before IABP catheter insertion, a negative vacuum to the balloon is applied using a large syringe and the one-way valve provided in the IABP insertion kit. The catheter is loaded with the 0.018-inch or 0.025-inch guidewire provided in the IABP kit. The assembly is inserted through the sheath with the guidewire leading. The marker at the tip of the IABP catheter should be 1 to 2 cm below the top of the aortic arch at the level of the carina of the trachea. The guidewire is then removed. The central lumen is carefully flushed and connected to a pressure transducer. Fluoroscopic observation of the balloon inflation above the renal arteries confirms optimal placement.

After the catheter is positioned, the IABP tubing is connected to the IABP console and counterpulsation is initiated. In short patients, pumping may not begin if the distal end of the balloon catheter remains in the sheath. Partial withdrawal of the sheath from the femoral artery may remedy this problem. The balloon catheter is secured with sutures. The position of the balloon is rechecked before the patient is moved. After the patient has been returned to the intensive care unit, the position of the IABP is checked again with a chest radiograph.

The timing cycle of IABP inflation should begin at 1:2 pumping (one inflation for every two beats). Balloon inflation timing is adjusted to optimize the augmented diastolic pressure waveform (Fig. 8.6). The rate of central aortic pressure through the IABP lumen is used to assess hemodynamic effects.

Optimal balloon timing is guided by direct pressure readings. If no pressure wave is available, the electrocardiogram may be used for timing the balloon; however, this practice is not recommended. The electrocardiogram is used to trigger the balloon. IABP inflation should occur at the aortic dicrotic notch (T wave on electrocardiogram), and deflation should occur immediately before systole (at or before the R wave) to provide maximal diastolic flow and maximal reduction of presystolic pressure. After proper adjustment of balloon inflation and deflation, the timing cycle is set at 1:1 pumping. The factors affecting the ability of the pump to augment properly a patient's hemodynamic status are shown in Box 8.3. Care should be taken to achieve the optimal hemodynamics by adjusting the timing of inflation and deflation and location of the balloon. Box 8.4 shows possible issues occurring with improper timing of balloon inflation and deflation.

Impella

The Impella (ABIOMED, Inc., Danvers, MA) is a nonpulsatile axial flow pump that is advanced through the aortic valve and moves blood from the left ventricle into the aorta (Fig. 8.7). Use of the

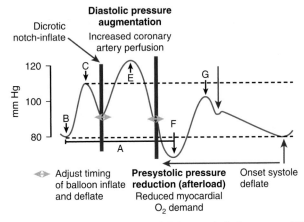

Fig. 8.6 Arterial waveforms during 1:2 intraaortic balloon pump (IABP) counterpulsation. *A,* One complete cardiac cycle; *B,* unassisted aortic end-diastolic pressure; *C,* unassisted aortic systolic pressure; *D,* dicrotic notch (balloon inflation); *E,* diastolic augmentation; *F,* assisted aortic end-diastolic pressure; *G,* assisted systole. Diastolic augmentation occurs during balloon inflation, which results in increased coronary artery perfusion. Reduction in the presystolic pressure (afterload) occurs with balloon deflation and reduces myocardial oxygen demand. Assisted systolic pressure *(G)* should be lower than unassisted aortic systolic pressure *(C)* because of a reduction in the aortic end-diastolic pressure *(F).*

Box 8.3 Factors Affecting Diastolic Augmentation

Patient Hemodynamics

Heart rate
Stroke volume
Mean arterial pressure
Systemic vascular resistance

Intraaortic Balloon Mechanical Factors

IAB in sheath
IAB not unfolded
IAB position
Kink in IAB catheter

Intraaortic Balloon Leak

Low helium concentration

Intraaortic Balloon Pump Console Factors

Timing
Position of IAB augmentation dial

IAB, Intraaortic balloon.

**Box 8.4   Issues with Improper Timing of Balloon Inflation
and Deflation.**

**Poor Intraaortic Balloon Pump Augmentation Caused by
Poor Inflation-Deflation Timing**

*Early Inflation: Inflation of the Intraaortic Balloon Before
Aortic Valve Closure*

Waveform Characteristics

Inflation before the dicrotic notch
Diastolic augmentation encroaches onto systole

Physiologic Effects

Potential premature closure of the aortic valve
Potential increase in left ventricular end-diastolic volume and pressure
Increased left ventricular wall stress (afterload)
Aortic regurgitation
Increased myocardial oxygen demand

*Late Inflation: Inflation of the Intraaortic Balloon After
Closure of the Aortic Valve*

Waveform Characteristics

Inflation of the IAB after the dicrotic notch
Absence of sharp V wave
Suboptimal diastolic augmentation

Physiologic Effects

Suboptimal coronary artery perfusion

*Early Deflation: Premature Deflation of the Intraaortic
Balloon During Diastole*

Waveform Characteristics

Deflation of the IAB seen as a sharp drop after diastolic augmentation
Suboptimal diastolic augmentation
Assisted aortic end-diastolic pressure may be less than or equal to
    unassisted aortic end-diastolic pressure
Assisted systolic pressure may rise

Physiologic Effects

Suboptimal coronary perfusion
Potential for retrograde coronary and carotid blood flow
Angina as a result of retrograde coronary blood flow
Suboptimal afterload reduction
Increased myocardial oxygen demand

Late Deflation

Waveform Characteristics

Assisted aortic end-diastolic pressure may be less than or equal to unas-
    sisted aortic end-diastolic pressure

Continued on following page

Box 8.4   Issues with Improper Timing of Balloon Inflation and Deflation. (Continued)

Prolonged rate of assisted systole rise
Diastolic augmentation may appear widened

Physiologic Effects

Afterload reduction essentially absent
Increased myocardial oxygen consumption caused by left ventricle ejecting
   against greater resistance
Prolonged isovolumic contraction phase
IAB impedes left ventricular ejection and increases afterload

**Poor Intraaortic Balloon Pump Augmentation Caused
by Arrhythmias**

Atrial Fibrillation

Use auto timing and ECG trigger

Ectopics

To ensure triggering, select the lead that minimizes the amplitude difference
   between normal QRS and ectopic QRS

Cardiac Arrest or Defibrillation

Use ECG or pressure trigger during cardiopulmonary support
If ECG or pressure trigger cannot be used, internal trigger may be used
Must stand clear of the IABP during defibrillation
The IAB should not remain immobile for more than 30 minutes in situ

---

ECG, Electrocardiogram; *IAB,* intraaortic balloon; *IABP,* intraaortic balloon pump.

Impella results in left ventricular unloading with reduction in end-diastolic pressure and volume. The Impella is available in two percutaneous types (2.5 and CP) and one device that requires surgical cutdown (5.0). The Impella RP device can provide right ventricular support by pumping blood from the inferior vena cava to the pulmonary artery and consists of a 22-F motor mounted on an 11-F catheter.[11]

The Impella catheter pulls blood from the LV chamber and pumps it into the aorta. After crossing the aortic valve with a standard 0.035-inch guidewire, a catheter is advanced into the left ventricle, followed by insertion of a stiff 0.014-inch guidewire. The Impella catheter is then advanced over this 0.014-inch guidewire until it enters the left ventricle. After removal of the guidewire, pumping is initiated. In case of prophylactic use, the Impella device is removed at the end of the procedure (usually the arterial access site is preclosed using two Perclose devices while obtaining access). If continued support is needed, the large arterial sheath

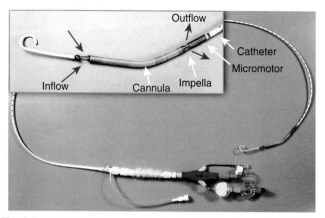

Fig. 8.7 The Impella 2.5 catheter. The tip is in the shape of a pigtail; an inflow portion is just beyond the tip; and where the rotor is housed, the cannula generates flow of blood to the outflow. This cannula portion is placed across the aortic valve so that inflow is well into the left ventricle and outflow is in the ascending aorta. The back end of the catheter hooks up to the control unit, which can monitor aortic pressure through a micrometer on the catheter and adjusts the speed of the pump. (From Valgimigli M, Steendijk P, Sianos G, et al. Left ventricular unloading and concomitant total cardiac output increase by the use of percutaneous Impella Recover LP 2.5 assist device during high-risk coronary intervention. *Catheter Cardiovasc Interv.* 2005;65:264.)

(peel-away) is removed, improving blood flow to the ipsilateral lower extremity and reducing the risk of limb ischemia.

The Impella device provides direct unloading of the left ventricle, decreased filling pressures/volumes, and increased cardiac output. Several studies have showed improved hemodynamics with the Impella catheter when compared with the IABP. The major contraindications to this device are LV thrombus, severe aortic valve stenosis, mechanical aortic valve, and peripheral arterial disease.

TandemHeart

The TandemHeart is a centrifugal pump that propels blood from the left atrium into the femoral artery. It uses a 21-F cannula placed through a transseptal puncture and a 15-F to 19-F arterial cannula. With appropriately sized arterial cannulae, full perfusion can be achieved.

The TandemHeart percutaneous ventricular assist device (pVAD) was originally used in the early 1960s to aid patients who could not be weaned from cardiopulmonary bypass (Fig. 8.8). It is a left-atrial-to-femoral artery bypass system that includes a transseptal cannula, arterial cannula, and centrifugal blood pump. This device can be left in place for several days and has been shown to significantly improve hemodynamic profiles of patients in cardiogenic shock by providing up to 4.0 L/min of blood flow. It has the benefit of unloading the left atrium and thereby improving filling pressures, workload, and oxygen demand. Major drawbacks to this system include vascular access size (22-F venous and 15-F to 17-F arterial); need for transseptal access to the left atrium, which requires a proficiency that not all interventionalists possess; and

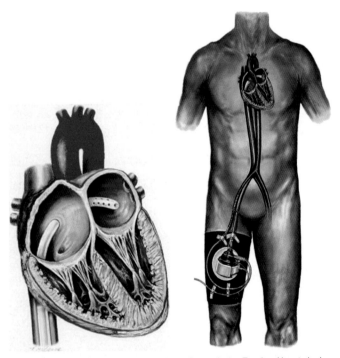

Fig. 8.8 *Left:* After a septostomy is performed, the TandemHeart device inflow cannula is placed from the inferior vena cava, across the atrial septum, and seated in the left atrium. *Right:* The pump is externally placed on the leg and pumps blood from the inflow cannula to the arterial catheter inserted into the aorta. (From TandemHeart.)

increased procedure time, which may not be possible in a hemo-dynamically unstable patient. The TandemHeart requires continuous monitoring to prevent displacement of the transseptal cannula into the right atrium. In isolation, the TandemHeart does not oxygenate the blood, but an oxygenator can be placed into the circuit to allow full cardiopulmonary support. In contrast to extracorporeal membrane oxygenation (ECMO), patients with right ventricular failure are not candidates for the TandemHeart, which also somewhat limits its use.

VA ECMO

VA ECMO consists of a centrifugal, nonpulsatile pump that circulates the blood and a membrane oxygenator. Venous blood is aspirated through a venous cannula, advanced through the oxygenator and returned to the patient through an arterial cannula.

VA ECMO can maintain systemic perfusion, but may increase myocardial oxygen demand because of increase in left ventricular end-diastolic pressure and volume, which could adversely impact myocardial recovery.[13] ECMO can cause bleeding as a result of continuous heparin administration and platelet dysfunction, thromboembolism, and vascular damage during catheter insertion.

Use of circulatory support devices can be very useful in the setting of cardiogenic shock and for prophylaxis during high-risk PCI. Determining the optimal candidates for these devices and the optimal device selection continues to evolve.

Arrhythmias
Management of Arrhythmias

Serious arrhythmias (including ventricular fibrillation, ventricular tachycardia, supraventricular tachycardia, asystole, and heart block) occur in approximately 1% of either right- or left-sided heart catheterizations. In almost all instances, the arrhythmia can be managed successfully by prompt recognition and treatment. Arrhythmias may result from intracardiac catheter manipulation, intracoronary contrast injection, or myocardial ischemia during angioplasty.

For malignant ventricular arrhythmias with hypotension, the most important determinant of short- and long-term (neurologically intact) survival of the patient is the interval from the onset of hemodynamic collapse to the restoration of effective, spontaneous circulatory and respiratory function. The following section provides suggestions for optimal treatment. These suggestions do not preclude other measures that may be indicated on the basis of specific clinical circumstances of the individual patient.

Primary Prevention of Arrhythmias

Electrocardiographic Monitoring. Continuous electrocardiographic (ECG) monitoring is essential for the performance of a safe cardiac catheterization. If a problem develops with ECG leads or equipment during the procedure, the operator must remedy it before the procedure continues.

Intravenous Access. Before the procedure is begun, a functioning peripheral IV line should be established in the patient. If peripheral venous access cannot be obtained, the operator should insert a femoral venous sheath large enough to accommodate a pacing wire and to allow rapid saline infusion. A ≥6-F femoral venous sheath should be placed in potentially unstable or acutely ill patients.

Standby Transvenous Pacing. The need for a prophylactic temporary transvenous pacemaker is determined by the patient's risk of bradyarrhythmia or heart block and ability to tolerate these arrhythmias should they occur. The use of flexible, balloon-tipped, flow-directed pacemaker wires provides the lowest risk of cardiac perforation. Risk factors for bradyarrhythmia include the following:

1. Preexisting right bundle-branch block during left-sided heart catheterization
2. Preexisting left bundle-branch block during right-sided heart catheterization, particularly when stiff catheters are used
3. Heart block greater than first degree
4. Marked sinus bradycardia
5. Coronary artery angioplasty involving the (dominant) artery supplying the atrioventricular (AV) node, especially when atherectomy or thrombus extraction devices are used (aminophylline can be used prophylactically to obviate the need for pacing).[14]

Limitation of Cardiac Catheter Manipulations. Catheter passage through the heart should be performed with caution and a smooth motion. Particular note should be made of ventricular ectopy during catheter manipulation. Vigorous stretching of the right atrium may cause atrial arrhythmias (atrial fibrillation, supraventricular tachycardia). Ventricular arrhythmias are associated with stimulation of the right ventricular outflow tract or papillary muscles by catheter contact. Removing the stimulating catheters usually terminates the arrhythmia.

Occlusive Engagement of Coronary Arteries. Engaged coronary catheter pressure should always be checked before contrast medium is injected. Figure 8.9 shows ventricularization and damping of pressure waveforms with cannulation of coronary vessels. Injection of contrast with damped or ventricularized waveforms increases the risk of dissection or arrhythmia.

Limitation of Coronary Artery Contrast. Injections of contrast medium should be sufficient to opacify the arterial tree without excessive volume or rates of injection. The operator should have the patient cough when sustained hypotension is recognized before loss of consciousness (and cardiac arrest). Forceful coughing can generate sufficient blood flow to the brain to maintain consciousness until definitive treatment can be initiated.

Defibrillation and Cardioversion. Definitive electrical treatment has the highest priority of any modality. A defibrillator should be located near the patient in each cardiac catheterization laboratory suite. Before the procedure is begun, the defibrillator should be turned on with pads easily available or conductive jelly ready to apply to the defibrillator paddles to avoid delay in defibrillation. The time to successful defibrillation is the major determinant of the patient's survival. If pulseless ventricular tachycardia or ventricular fibrillation is present, defibrillation should be performed at once. An algorithm for treatment of ventricular fibrillation with cardiopulmonary resuscitation (CPR) is provided in Figure 8.10.

Treatment for Specific Arrhythmias

The following sequences are useful for treating a broad range of patients with arrhythmias in the catheterization laboratory, but sequences should be modified as the clinical situation warrants.

Vasovagal reactions, which are often preceded by a slowing of heart rate before a decrease in blood pressure, respond dramatically to IV atropine (0.5 to 1 mg). Elevation of the patient's legs and infusion of saline may increase blood pressure transiently. Early signs of vasovagal reaction include pallor, nausea, yawning, sneezing, or coughing.

Bradycardia (ventricular heart rate <60 beats/min [bpm]) may be caused by autonomic influences (vagal) or intrinsic disease of the cardiac conducting system (ischemia). Atropine sulfate is the treatment of choice for symptomatic bradycardia, defined as a heart rate inappropriate for the hemodynamic state (e.g., a heart

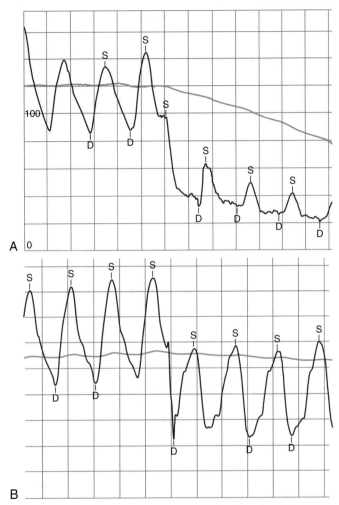

Fig. 8.9 **(A)** Hemodynamic tracing showing damping of waveform upon engagement into a coronary ostium. **(B)** Hemodynamic tracing showing damping with ventricularization of the pressure waveform. Injections with these waveforms increase the risk of vessel dissection or arrhythmia. *D,* Diastolic; *S,* systolic.

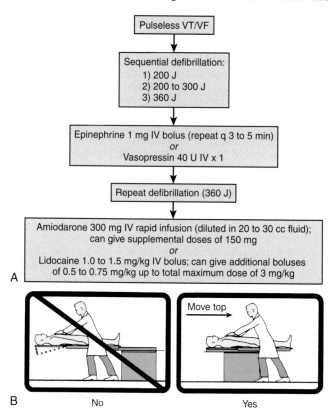

Fig. 8.10 **(A)** Advanced cardiac life support algorithm for pulseless ventricular tachycardia or ventricular fibrillation. **(B)** Cautionary illustration for cardiopulmonary resuscitation (CPR) of patient on cardiac catheterization table. Move table to base to reduce the chance of breaking table supports during cardiac compressions. *IV,* Intravenous; *J,* joule; *q,* every (Latin *quaque*); *VF,* ventricular fibrillation; *VT,* ventricular tachycardia.

rate of <80 bpm with hypotension). The initial dose of atropine to treat symptoms of bradycardia is 0.5 to 1 mg IV repeated every 5 minutes as needed to a maximum dose of 3 mg. Special care should be taken with patients who have underlying severe valvular abnormalities or coronary disease because rapid decompensation can occur during a vagal event. A transvenous pacemaker is rarely necessary to treat bradycardia but should be available if the patient is refractory to medical therapy.

Junctional rhythms and second-degree AV block (type I) often do not require specific treatment. In patients with symptoms caused by these rhythms, atropine is usually effective.

Second-degree AV block (type II) and third-degree AV block are often ultimately treated with permanent pacemaker placement. Depending on the stability of the escape rhythm, these patients frequently require transvenous pacemaker placement while awaiting permanent pacemaker placement. If bradycardia is associated with hypotension, congestive heart failure (CHF), ischemia, or infarction, transcutaneous pacing or IV atropine should be administered until a pacemaker can be inserted.

Ventricular Fibrillation. If ventricular fibrillation is present, the operator should quickly remove intracardiac catheters and perform defibrillation at once. Thereafter, the guidelines are (see Fig. 8.10):

1. Perform unsynchronized defibrillation as soon as available. For biphasic defibrillators, perform defibrillation at unsynchronized 200 J. For monophasic, the initial dose is 360 J.

2. The American Heart Association (AHA) guidelines recommend 2 minutes of quality CPR after defibrillation without stopping to assess the rhythm. For quality CPR, the rate should be ≥100/min with >2 inches (5 cm) of chest depression and complete chest recoil.

3. After 2 minutes, assess the rhythm and shock if necessary, using the maximum voltage for the device. At this time, administer epinephrine (1 mg IV every 3 to 5 minutes) or vasopressin (40 U IV one time may replace the first or second dose of epinephrine). Consider an advanced airway. The success of treatment at this point depends in large part on the adequacy of CPR. It is crucial to treat underlying abnormalities (e.g., hypokalemia, hypomagnesemia, ischemia, infarction, airway obstruction, or hypoxia) that may be causing the arrhythmia.

4. After another 2 minutes of CPR, reassess the rhythm and shock if necessary. At this time, consider amiodarone 300-mg IV bolus. If repeat dosing is necessary, administer 150 mg. If amiodarone is unavailable, lidocaine can be used (1 to 1.5 mg/kg IV, then 0.5 to 0.75 mg/kg IV every 5 to 10 minutes).

5. For persistent arrhythmia, repeat the pattern of 2 minutes of quality CPR followed by rhythm assessment and shock.

Sustained Ventricular Tachycardia. If sustained ventricular tachycardia persists after removal of intracardiac catheters, management proceeds according to the stability of the patient. In patients who are hemodynamically unstable (e.g., hypotension [systolic blood pressure <90 mm Hg], pulmonary edema, or unconsciousness), perform synchronized cardioversion at 200 J for biphasic devices and 360 J for monophasic devices. Synchronized cardioversion uses the largest R wave. If the QRS cannot be distinguished, use the unsynchronized mode. Ensure that the pads are placed properly and all personnel are clear of the patient before discharge. If paddles are used, ensure proper lubrication with conduction gel.

In patients who are hemodynamically stable, urgent or elective cardioversion is usually the appropriate initial therapy after proper patient sedation. Initial voltages are 50 to 100 J for biphasic and 100 to 200 J for monophasic. Use increased voltages for any subsequent required shocks. For persistent VT, consider antiarrhythmic therapy with amiodarone (150 mg IV bolus followed by IV drip) or lidocaine (1 to 1.5 mg/kg over 2 to 3 minutes). Lidocaine may be particularly helpful if myocardial ischemia is thought to be the etiology.

Repositioning or withdrawing intracardiac or coronary catheters can usually eliminate nonsustained ventricular tachycardia. Frequent nonsustained ventricular tachycardia caused by acute myocardial ischemia rather than catheter irritation may warrant antiarrhythmic therapy depending on the stability of the patient.

Amiodarone is the drug of choice for the management of ventricular ectopy, including ventricular tachycardia and ventricular fibrillation. Give amiodarone to stable patients as a 150-mg infusion over 10 minutes, then 1 mg/min every 6 hours, and 0.5 mg/min every 18 hours. Administer an initial dose of 300 mg to unstable or pulseless patients.

Alternatively, lidocaine should initially be given as a bolus of 1.0 to 1.5 mg/kg. Additional boluses of 0.5 mg/kg can be given subsequently (every 8 to 10 minutes) to a total dose of 3 mg/kg in the arrest setting. In the nonarrest setting, the initial bolus should be reduced by half if any of the following conditions are present: CHF, shock, hepatic dysfunction, or age older than 70 years. After successful resuscitation, a constant infusion of lidocaine at a rate of 2 to 4 mg/min should be initiated if lidocaine has been used successfully during resuscitation. Note: Wide-complex tachycardia of uncertain cause (i.e., ventricular tachycardia vs. paroxysmal supraventricular tachycardia [PSVT] with aberrancy) should be treated as ventricular tachycardia until proven otherwise. Verapamil is contraindicated.

Asystole is usually the result of extensive myocardial ischemia. Atropine is no longer recommended in the guidelines for asystole. Because it may be difficult to distinguish between asystole and fine ventricular fibrillation, asystole should be confirmed in two leads. If the diagnosis is unclear, the physician should assume that fine ventricular fibrillation is present and treat the patient accordingly. Patients in asystole should receive high-quality CPR for 2 minutes before rhythm reassessment. If no shockable rhythm is present, continue CPR and give epinephrine (1-mg IV push) every 3 to 5 minutes. Metabolic abnormalities, including hyperkalemia or severe preexisting acidosis, may cause the arrhythmia and may respond to bicarbonate.

Pulseless Electrical Activity. Pulseless electrical activity (PEA) is a heart rhythm disturbance that is fatal unless the underlying cause can be identified and treated at once. Causes of PEA in the cardiac catheterization laboratory include:

1. Hypovolemia: Treatment includes aggressive volume repletion and blood transfusions for bleeding. If anticoagulation was given, consider reversal if possible.
2. Pericardial tamponade, especially in patients with acute infarction, recent cardiac biopsy, recent endocardial pacer insertion, recent coronary intervention, or uremia: If tamponade is suspected, pericardiocentesis is warranted.
3. Massive pulmonary embolism: On rare occasions, the embolus may break up during prolonged resuscitative efforts. Some patients survive long enough for the operator to treat with thrombus aspiration catheters or thrombolytics.
4. Tension pneumothorax may occur in patients after internal jugular or subclavian venous access is obtained. Fluoroscopy may visualize air in the patient's chest. If the operator suspects that tension pneumothorax is present, he or she should carefully insert a small-bore needle attached to a syringe into the pleural space. If a tension pneumothorax is present, air under pressure is expelled.
5. Hypoxia, especially if the patient was given sedation: The operator may need to consider using reversal agents for the sedatives.

Supraventricular Arrhythmias. The hemodynamic stability of the patient determines how PSVT and atrial fibrillation should be treated.

1. In patients who are unstable (e.g., hypotension, chest pain, CHF, acute ischemia, or infarction), use synchronized cardioversion at once. As long as it does not delay the procedure, sedation with a rapid-acting IV agent (e.g., diazepam [Valium] or midazolam [Versed]) can be used for patients who are conscious and do not have hypotension. The initial discharge for atrial fibrillation is 120 J biphasic or 200 J monophasic. Initial discharge

voltage for narrow complex regular rhythm is 50 to 100 J. If conversion does not occur, increase energy levels and repeat cardioversion. If these maneuvers fail, consider antiarrhythmic therapy with amiodarone and repeat cardioversion afterward. Digitalis toxicity is a relative contraindication to cardioversion because severe bradycardia or asystole can occur after cardioversion.

2. The ventricular response can be controlled with β-blockers or IV diltiazem in patients who have atrial fibrillation and are hemodynamically stable.

3. For stable PSVT without atrial fibrillation, vagal maneuvers (Valsalva) or carotid massage in the absence of a carotid bruit can be attempted. If unsuccessful, administer adenosine at a 6-mg rapid IV push with subsequent doses of 12-mg rapid IV pushes if necessary. If no effect is seen after the adenosine push, consider larger IV access closer to the heart and a faster IV push. If the arrhythmia persists, elective cardioversion may be performed after adequate sedation. IV nondihydropyridine calcium channel blockers or IV β-blockers can also be used.

Adenosine is a naturally occurring agent that produces AV nodal blockade and increases coronary blood flow. It is 90% to 100% effective in terminating reentrant supraventricular or AV nodal tachycardia in 6- to 12-mg IV bolus doses. It has a 30-second onset of action and a 60-second offset of action. Transient flushing is the only major side effect.

To control recurring episodes of PSVT, β-blockers (including metoprolol at a 5-mg IV push) can be used. The use of β-blockers may be hazardous when cardiac dysfunction is present. The dosage for propranolol is 1 mg every 5 minutes IV, up to a total of 0.1 mg/kg. Short-acting β-blockers (esmolol) are administered in 5- to 15-mg boluses and have 5- to 10-minute half-lives.

Box 8.5 lists medications for the treatment of arrhythmias that develop during high-risk cardiac catheterization.

Tamponade

Cardiac tamponade is usually the result of coronary perforation and requires emergent pericardiocentesis. Reinfusion of the aspirated blood can minimize blood losses. Intravenous fluids and pressors are commonly administered to maintain systemic blood pressure while pericardiocentesis is being performed. If pericardial bleeding continues after balloon inflation, use of a covered stent and fat or coil embolization are usually used for achieving hemostasis (Fig. 8.3)

Box 8.5 Medications and Dosage Regimens for Arrhythmias That Develop During High-Risk Cardiac Catheterization.

Stable Ventricular Tachycardia

Amiodarone: Administer in one of two regimens, as dictated by clinical setting:

Regimen 1: 150 mg over 10 minutes, followed by infusion rate of 1 mg/min

Regimen 2: 300-mg IV rapid infusion after dilution in 20 to 30 mL of fluid; additional 150-mg rapid infusions in similar manner as indicated

Lidocaine: 1- to 1.5-mg/kg IV bolus; additional boluses of 0.5 to 0.75 mg/kg IV as indicated, up to 3 mg/kg

Pulseless Ventricular Tachycardia or Ventricular Fibrillation

Epinephrine: 1-mg IV bolus; can repeat every 3 to 5 minutes

Vasopressin: 40-U IV bolus (administer either epinephrine or vasopressin after three unsuccessful defibrillation attempts)

Amiodarone: 300-mg IV rapid infusion after dilution in 20 to 30 mL of fluid; additional 150-mg rapid infusions in similar manner as indicated

Lidocaine: 1- to 1.5-mg/kg IV bolus; additional boluses of 0.5 to 0.75 mg/kg IV as indicated, up to 3 mg/kg

---

Vascular Access Complications and Bleeding

The management of vascular access complications is discussed in detail in Chapter 2. Use of radial access and state-of-the-art techniques for obtaining femoral access (ultrasound and fluoroscopic guidance, micropuncture needle, femoral angiography after obtaining access) can minimize the risk of access-related complications.[15]

To minimize the risk of bleeding and its consequences, anemia and bleeding tendencies should be identified and etiologies known before performing the procedure. This is especially true for those patients who require PCI and may be on multiple anticoagulant and antiplatelet agents. Vitamin K and intravenous clotting factors may be administered to patients with high INR who need emergent catheterization.

Thrombocytopenia (low platelet count) is a troublesome finding on preprocedural laboratory work. For elective procedures, thrombocytopenia should be identified and its underlying cause treated before proceeding. Depending on the etiology of the thrombocytopenia and platelet count, platelet transfusions may be necessary before and during the procedure. For patients at high risk of bleeding, one should consider radial artery access; of course, nonaccess site bleeding risks remain the same.

Thromboembolic Complications

Arterial thromboembolism can occur in any vascular bed in the body manifesting as stroke, TIA, intestinal ischemia, or peripheral emboli. Treatment options depend on the vascular bed involved and presence of symptoms. Most concerning is development of neurological symptoms consistent with a stroke following cardiac catheterization. Any patient with these symptoms should receive urgent evaluation by a stroke team or transfer to a stroke center for evaluation of thrombolytics or mechanical thrombectomy. In patients receiving anticoagulants in the laboratory, intracranial hemorrhage must be ruled out. Cortical blindness is a rare event that can be caused by ionic and nonionic contrast agents. It usually manifests initially as blurry vision and progresses to total blindness. It is usually transient, resolving in 1-2 days, and requires no definitive treatment.

Contrast Media Related Complications

Contrast-induced nephropathy (CIN), the number one cause of acute renal failure in hospitalized patients, and increases morbidity and mortality. The pathogenesis is not completely understood but is felt to involve acute tubular necrosis (ATN). Hypotheses regarding the cause of ATN include direct toxic effects of contrast and renal vasoconstriction leading to medullary hypoxia.

Multiple contrast agents are currently available, and differentiating between them requires knowledge of their characteristics and recognition of their chemical and trade names (Table 8.4). Low-osmolar and nonionic contrast agents are associated with a lower incidence of bradycardia, hypotension, and myocardial ischemia, and these agents are now routinely used during cardiac catheterizations in most labs.

Several risk factors have been identified in patients at higher likelihood of developing CIN (Table 8.5). Unfortunately, many of these parameters are not modifiable and therefore do not lend themselves to modifying to avoid CIN. A risk score, devised to identify patients at higher risk of CIN, is shown in Figure 8.11. Three prophylactic strategies to decrease the risk of CIN center include

Table 8.4

Types and Characteristics of Contrast Media.		
Generic Name	**US Trade Name**	**Osmolality (mOsm/kg H$_2$O)**
Iodixanol	Visipaque 270	290
Iopromide	Ultravist 150	328
Ioversol 34%	Optiray 160	328
Iodixanol	Visipaque 320	290
Iohexol	Omnipaque 180	388
Iopamidol 40.8%	Isovue 200	413
Iopromide	Ultravist 240	483
Ioversol 51%	Optiray 240	502
Iohexol 51.8%	Omnipaque 240	520
Iopamidol 51%	Isovue 250	524
Ioxilan 62.3%	Oxilan 300	607
Iopromide	Ultravist 300	607
Iopamidol 61.2%	Isovue 300	616
Ioversol 64%	Optiray 300	651
Iohexol 64.7%	Omnipaque 300	672
Ioxilan 72.7%	Oxilan 350	695
Ioversol 68%	Optiray 320	702
Iopromide	Ultravist 370	774
Ioversol 74%	Optiray 350	792
Iopamidol 75.5%	Isovue 370	796
Iohexol 75.5%	Omnipaque 350	844

Table 8.5

Risk Factors for Development of Contrast-Induced Nephropathy.		
Patient Related	**Extrinsic**	**Possible**
Existing renal insufficiency (estimated GFR <60/mL/min/1.73 m^2)	Contrast volume administered	Metabolic syndrome
CHF	High-osmolar contrast	Diabetes
Diabetes with existing renal insufficiency	IABP used	Impaired glucose tolerance
Age >70 years	Nephrotoxic drugs	Hyperuricemia
Volume depletion	Multiple contrast administrations (within 72 h)	ACE-I or ARB
Hypotension	Urgent/emergent PCI	Female gender
Anemia		Multiple myeloma
Hypertension		Cirrhosis
Peripheral vascular disease		

Modified from Klein LW, Sheldon MW, Brinker J, et al. The use of radiographic contrast media during PCI: a focused review. *Catheter Cardiovasc Interv.* 2009;74:728.

ACE-I, Angiotensin-converting enzyme inhibitor; *ARB,* angiotensin receptor blocker; *CHF,* congestive heart failure; *GFR,* glomerular filtration rate; *IABP,* intraaortic balloon pump; *PCI,* percutaneous coronary intervention.

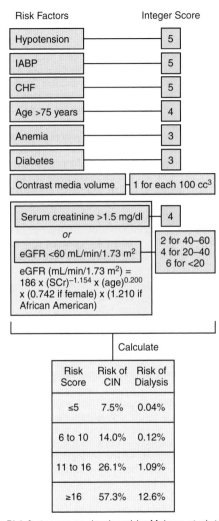

Fig. 8.11 Risk-factor scores developed by Mehran et al. to predict the likelihood of contrast-induced nephropathy *(CIN)* after percutaneous coronary intervention (PCI). Adding up all of the points for any given patient calculates the total risk score. Estimated risk for CIN and dialysis. *CHF,* Congestive heart failure; *eGFR,* estimated glomerular filtration rate; *IABP,* intraaortic balloon pump. (From Mehran R, Aymong ED, Nikolsky E, et al. A simple risk score for prediction of contrast-induced nephropathy after percutaneous coronary intervention: development and initial validation. *J Am Coll Cardiol.* 2004;44:1393-1399.)

maintaining adequate intravascular volume, limiting amount of contrast delivered, and avoiding medications that could exacerbate renal dysfunction.

Many protocols have been published that outline how to ensure adequate hydration. For high-risk patients, American College of Cardiology/Society for Cardiovascular Angiography and Interventions (ACC/SCAI) guidelines currently recommend normal saline infusion at 1 to 1.5 mL/kg/min for 3 to 12 hours before and 6 to 12 hours after the procedure. Sodium bicarbonate and N-acetylcysteine administration provide no benefit over normal saline.[16]

To minimize the chance of CIN, use the lowest amount of contrast necessary to perform the study. Measures such as minimizing contrast puffs (test shots), increasing frame rates to lessen contrast injection, avoiding ventriculography and aortography, and decreasing the number of angiograms performed can reduce the amount of contrast used. There are currently devices (Dyevert, Osprey, Minnetonka, MN) that can reduce the amount of contrast that back flows into the aorta. Iso-osmolar contrast may be beneficial in high-risk patients, such as diabetics with renal insufficiency.[17]

Medications such as angiotensin receptor blockers (ARBs), angiotensin-converting enzyme inhibitors (ACE-Is), and nonsteroidal antiinflammatory drugs (NSAIDs) can be discontinued for 1 to 2 days before catheterization. Withholding them for 3 to 4 days following the procedure is also common. However, it has never been shown that the use of ACE-Is or ARBs, in the absence of renal artery stenosis, truly increases the risk of renal insufficiency.

Allergic reactions to contrast are discussed in Chapter 1. It is worth remembering that these reactions are characterized as anaphylactoid, i.e., they do not require previous exposure to contrast (and, thus, to circulating reaginic [immunoglobulin E] antibody), but they do occur as a result of mast cell degranulation. A patient with a history of multiple food and drug allergies and those who have had previous reactions to contrast are at especially high risk. The perception that patients with a seafood or shellfish allergy are also at higher risk has never been shown to be true and should not be used as a reason to administer prophylaxis for contrast reactions.

Prophylaxis for patients who are at risk of reactions to contrast media should include prednisone and diphenhydramine (Fig. 8.12). Figure 8.13 depicts treatment algorithms for mild and severe reactions.

Radiation Injury

Preventing radiation skin injury (for the patient and the operator) is often neglected, as it is not immediately apparent. Several steps

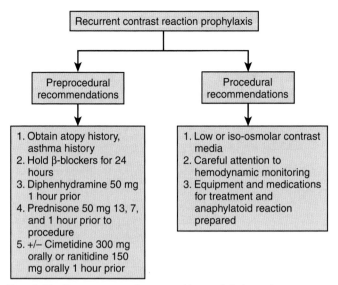

Fig. 8.12 Treatment paradigm to guide prophylaxis against contrast-induced allergic reactions. From Klein LW, Sheldon MW, Brinker J, et al. The use of radiographic contrast media during PCI: a focused review: a position statement of the Society of Cardiovascular Angiography and Interventions. *Catheter Cardiovasc Interv*. 2009;74:731.)

can be taken to minimize the risk of radiation skin injury and to detect it promptly if it occurs (Table 8.6).[18]

Medication-Related

Many medications can affect a patient's catheterization risk (Box 8.6).

Anticoagulants

Warfarin (Coumadin) should be held for at least 72 hours before the procedure, and the INR should be <1.6 for femoral access and <3.0 for radial access before the procedure to reduce the bleeding risk. Understanding why the patient has been taking warfarin is important because high-risk patients may require bridging therapy with heparin. Bridging should be considered for patients taking

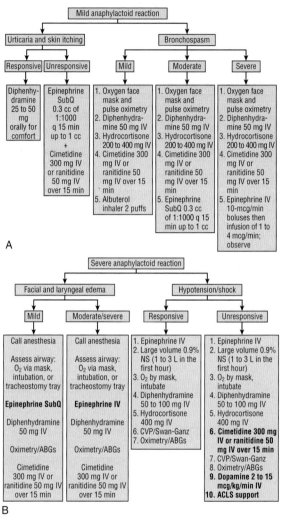

Fig. 8.13 Treatment protocols for allergic reactions to contrast. **(A)** For mild reactions; **(B)** for severe reactions. *ABG,* Arterial blood gas; *ACLS,* advanced cardiovascular life support; *CVP,* central venous pressure; *IV,* intravenously; *NS,* normal saline; *q,* every; *SubQ,* subcutaneously. (From Klein LW, Sheldon MW, Brinker J, et al. The use of radiographic contrast media during PCI: a focused review: a position statement of the Society of Cardiovascular Angiography and Interventions. *Catheter Cardiovasc Interv.* 2009;74:731.)

Table 8.6

Procedure-Based Case Management of Radiation Dose.

I. Preprocedure

A. Radiation safety program for catheterization laboratory
   1. Dosimeter use, shielding, training/education
B. Imaging equipment and operator knowledge
   1. On screen dose assessment (air kerma, DAP)
   2. Dose saving: store fluoroscopy, adjustable pulse and frame rate and last image hold
C. Preprocedure dose planning
   1. Assess patient and procedure, including patient's size and lesion(s) complexity. Examine patient for potential skin injury from prior high dose cases.
D. Informed patient with appropriate consent

II. Procedure

A. Limit fluoroscopy: step on pedal only when looking at screen
B. Limit cine: store fluoroscopy when image quality not required
C. Limit magnification, frame rate, steep angles
D. Use collimation and filters to fullest extent possible
E. Vary tube angle when possible to change skin area exposed
F. Position table and image receptor: x-ray tube too close to patient increases dose; high image receptor increases scatter.
G. Keep patient and operator body parts out of field of view
H. Maximize shielding and distance from X-ray source for all personnel
I. Manage and monitor dose in real time from beginning of case

III. Postprocedure

A. Document radiation dose in records (fluoroscopy time, $K_{a,r}$, P_{KA})
B. Notify patient and referring physician when high dose delivered
   1. $K_{a,r}$ >5 Gray, chart document; inform patient; arrange follow-up
   2. $K_{a,r}$ >10 Gray, qualified physicist should calculate skin dose
   3. PSD >15 Gray, Joint Commission sentinel event
C. Assess and refer adverse skin effects to appropriate consultant

Modified from Chambers CE. Radiation dose in percutaneous coronary intervention: OUCH . . . did that hurt? *JACC Cardiovasc Interv.* 2011;4:344-346.

DAP, Dose area product; $K_{a,r}$, total air kerma at reference point; P_{KA}, air kerma area product; *PSD*, peak skin dose.

warfarin for atrial fibrillation with a CHADS$_2$ score of 5 or 6, recent stroke within 3 months, or rheumatic heart disease. Patients on warfarin for mechanical heart valve with any mitral valve, older mechanical aortic valve (ball in cage, tilting disc), or recent stroke or transient ischemic attack (TIA) are considered as high risk, as are patients taking warfarin for venous thromboembolism with any recent stroke or high-risk thrombophilia (protein C, protein S, or antithrombin deficiencies; antiphospholipid; homozygous factor V Leiden or prothrombin genes).

Box 8.6   Medications That May Affect Cardiac Catheterization Risk.

Oral anticoagulants
Furosemide
Metformin
Insulin (especially long acting)
Sildenafil, vardenafil, tadalafil
ACE-Is (lisinopril, ramipril, enalapril)
ARBs (losartan, candesartan)
NSAIDs (ibuprofen, naproxen)

ACE-I, Angiotensin-converting enzyme inhibitor; *ARB,* angiotensin receptor blocker; *NSAID,* nonsteroidal antiinflammatory drug.

Direct oral anticoagulants (DOACs) such as dabigatran (Pradaxa), rivaroxaban (Xarelto), apixaban (Eliquis) and edoxaban (Savaysa) are now more widely used for anticoagulation, but they can increase procedural bleeding risk. Guidelines for duration of discontinuation before cardiac catheterization are shown in Table 8.7.

Generally, diuretics should not be taken on the morning of the procedure because dehydration may decrease renal flow and increase the risk of contrast nephropathy and hypotension.

Table 8.7

How Long to Stop a Direct Oral Anticoagulant before Cardiac Catheterization.	
	Days to Hold
Direct Factor Xa Inhibitors	
Apixaban (Eliquis)	2 days
Edoxaban (Savaysa)	
Creatinine clearance: 50–95	2 days
Creatinine clearance: 15–49	3 days
Rivaroxaban (Xarelto)	
Creatinine clearance: >50	2 days
Creatinine clearance: 15–49	3 days
Direct Thrombin Factor IIa Inhibitor	
Dabigatran (Pradaxa)	
Creatinine clearance: >80	2 days
Creatinine clearance: 50–79	3 days
Creatinine clearance: 30–49	4 days
Creatinine clearance: 15–29	5 days

Creatinine clearance calculator: http://www.mdcalc.com/creatinine-clearance-cockcroft-gault-equation

On the morning of the procedure, patients with diabetes should not take short-acting insulin. To avoid the risk of hypoglycemia, administer one-half to two-thirds of the daily total (for once-daily-dosing patients) or morning insulin dose (for twice-daily-dosing patients) in the form of long-acting insulin. Oral antiglycemic agents should also be held on the morning of the procedure. Metformin poses a slight but real risk of lactic acidosis and should be held both before the procedure and 48 hours after contrast administration. Creatinine levels should be checked 2 to 3 days after the procedure, and metformin can be restarted if there is no evidence of decrement in renal function.

Because of sedation during the procedure, it is difficult to monitor the diabetic patient for signs/symptoms of hypoglycemia or hyperglycemia. One should check blood sugar before initiation of the procedure and as needed throughout the case to minimize risk. If appropriate, the patient should have dextrose or insulin infusion maintained during the periprocedure period in an attempt to avoid hypoglycemia or hyperglycemia.

Erectile dysfunction medications can also cause significant harm in the catheterization laboratory. When combined with nitrate therapy, there can be a precipitous drop in blood pressure that does not respond well to volume or vasopressor resuscitation. Therefore, sildenafil (Viagra) and vardenafil (Levitra) should be withheld for a minimum of 24 hours before the procedure. Tadalafil (Cialis) has a half-life of 17.5 hours and must be withheld for 4 days before the procedure.

Treating Other Risk Factors

Systemic Hypertension

Poorly controlled hypertension increases risks throughout the procedure. In addition to the increased risk of cerebrovascular accident and respiratory insufficiency in the presence of diastolic dysfunction, elevated blood pressure increases the risk of vascular access complications. Elective procedures may need to be postponed to allow for improved blood pressure control for levels >180/100. Closure devices are relatively contraindicated in patients with significant hypertension. Attempts should be made to lower the blood pressure safely before sheath removal. To control blood pressure, the patient can be given their home medications orally or with intravenous (IV) pushes of hydralazine, metoprolol, or labetalol. It is important to continue hemodynamic monitoring of the patient postcatheterization, because high blood pressure–related complications can be detected early with continued reassessment of the patient's status.

Other Comorbidities

If possible, other comorbidities should be stabilized before the patient is sent to the catheterization suite. Patients with decompensated congestive heart failure, in whom catheterization can be delayed, should be diuresed to improve the safety and comfort of the procedure.

Chronic obstructive pulmonary disease is another illness often coexisting with cardiovascular disease, and patients who are experiencing acute exacerbations of this problem should have their procedure postponed if possible. An underdiagnosed problem in medicine is obstructive sleep apnea. These patients often become hypoxic with sedation and should have their noninvasive ventilation devices (continuous positive airway pressure [CPAP] or bi-level positive airway pressure [BiPAP]) with them during the procedure to minimize the risk of worsening their baseline respiratory insufficiency.

References

1. Dehmer GJ, Weaver D, Roe MT, et al. A contemporary view of diagnostic cardiac catheterization and percutaneous coronary intervention in the United States: a report from the CathPCI Registry of the National Cardiovascular Data Registry, 2010 through June 2011. *J Am Coll Cardiol*. 2012;60:2017-2031.
2. Kirtane AJ, Doshi D, Leon MB, et al. Treatment of higher-risk patients with an indication for revascularization: evolution within the field of contemporary percutaneous coronary intervention. *Circulation*. 2016;134:422-431.
3. Brennan JM, Curtis JP, Dai D, et al. Enhanced mortality risk prediction with a focus on high-risk percutaneous coronary intervention: results from 1,208,137 procedures in the NCDR (National Cardiovascular Data Registry). *JACC Cardiovasc Interv*. 2013;6:790-799.
4. Rao SV, McCoy LA, Spertus JA, et al. An updated bleeding model to predict the risk of post-procedure bleeding among patients undergoing percutaneous coronary intervention: a report using an expanded bleeding definition from the National Cardiovascular Data Registry CathPCI Registry. *JACC Cardiovasc Interv*. 2013;6: 897-904.
5. Tsai TT, Patel UD, Chang TI, et al. Validated contemporary risk model of acute kidney injury in patients undergoing percutaneous coronary interventions: insights from the National Cardiovascular Data Registry Cath-PCI Registry. *J Am Heart Assoc*. 2014;3:e001380.
6. Yeh RW, Normand SL, Wolf RE, et al. Predicting the restenosis benefit of drug-eluting versus bare metal stents in percutaneous coronary intervention. *Circulation*. 2011;124:1557-1564.
7. Wasfy JH, Rosenfield K, Zelevinsky K, et al. A prediction model to identify patients at high risk for 30-day readmission after percutaneous coronary intervention. *Circ Cardiovasc Qual Outcomes*. 2013;6:429-435.
8. Sawaya FJ, Lefèvre T, Chevalier B, et al. contemporary approach to coronary bifurcation lesion treatment. *JACC Cardiovasc interv*. 2016;9:1861-1878.
9. Prasad A, Banerjee S, Brilakis ES. Images in cardiovascular medicine. Hemodynamic consequences of massive coronary air embolism. *Circulation*. 2007;115:e51-e53.

10. Ellis SG, Ajluni S, Arnold AZ, et al. Increased coronary perforation in the new device era. Incidence, classification, management, and outcome. *Circulation*. 1994;90:2725-2730.
11. Brilakis ES. *Manual of Coronary Chronic Total Occlusion Interventions. A Step-By-Step Approach*. 2nd edition: Elsevier; 2017.
12. Brilakis ES, Best PJ, Elesber AA, et al. Incidence, retrieval methods, and outcomes of stent loss during percutaneous coronary intervention: a large single-center experience. *Catheter Cardiovasc Interv*. 2005;66:333-340.
13. Tomasello SD, Boukhris M, Ganyukov V, et al. Outcome of extracorporeal membrane oxygenation support for complex high-risk elective percutaneous coronary interventions: a single-center experience. *Heart Lung*. 2015;44:309-313.
14. Megaly M, Sandoval Y, Lillyblad MP, Brilakis ES. Aminophylline for preventing bradyarrhythmias during orbital or rotational atherectomy of the right coronary artery. *J Invasive Cardiol*. 2018.
15. Sandoval Y, Burke MN, Lobo AS, et al. Contemporary arterial access in the cardiac catheterization laboratory. *JACC Cardiovasc Interv*. 2017;10:2233-2341.
16. Weisbord SD, Gallagher M, Jneid H, et al. Outcomes after angiography with sodium bicarbonate and acetylcysteine. *N Engl J Med*. 2018;378:603-614.
17. Eng J, Wilson RF, Subramaniam RM, et al. comparative effect of contrast media type on the incidence of contrast-induced nephropathy: a systematic review and meta-analysis. *Ann Intern Med*. 2016;164:417-424.
18. Chambers CE. Radiation dose in percutaneous coronary intervention: OUCH… did that hurt? *JACC Cardiovasc Interv*. 2011;4:344-346.

Special Techniques

CHAD A. KLIGER • PAUL SORAJJA

Transseptal Heart Catheterization

Transseptal heart catheterization is used for direct access to the left atrium (LA) and its associated structures (e.g., LA appendage and pulmonary veins) and antegrade approaches for the left ventricle (LV) and mitral valve. In the majority of patients, hemodynamic assessment of the left-sided chambers can be performed with antegrade right-heart catheterization (i.e., pulmonary capillary wedge measurement) and retrograde aortic catheterization for LV pressure. However, optimal hemodynamic assessment of the left-sided chambers requires transseptal catheterization in important subsets of patients (e.g., those with mitral stenosis or obstructive hypertrophic cardiomyopathy). New percutaneous therapies for structural heart interventions also require operator expertise in the techniques of transseptal heart catheterization.

Indications

The indications for transseptal heart catheterization are:

1. Direct hemodynamic assessment of the LA and LV for patients in whom such data cannot be obtained using retrograde aortic techniques, antegrade right-heart catheterization, or noninvasive imaging evaluations.
2. Access for percutaneous, structural heart interventional therapies. These therapies include balloon mitral valvuloplasty, transcatheter mitral valve replacement, LA appendage closure, transcatheter mitral valve repair, mitral valve-in-valve therapy, and treatment of mitral paravalvular prosthetic regurgitation.

Contraindications

The contraindications for transseptal heart catheterization are:

· patient cannot be in a supine position;
· LA or right atrial (RA) thrombus;

- atrial myxoma;
- absence of right femoral venous access to the RA as a result of masses, thrombus, or other causes of obstruction.

Consider transseptal left-sided heart catheterization carefully for patients with distorted cardiac anatomy resulting from congenital heart disease, dilated aortic root, marked atrial enlargement, or thoracic skeletal deformity. As an alternative approach, transseptal heart catheterization using right internal jugular access has been performed in select cases.

Technique

Equipment

Figure 9.1 shows the transseptal sheath with a curved dilator and a long hollow needle that are used to cross the atrial septum. The transseptal sheath is frequently 7 F or 8 F, often with a side arm that facilitates hemodynamic assessment of multiple sites with a single transseptal access (e.g., end-hole measurement for LV; side-arm port for LA pressure). The curved dilator and transseptal sheath assembly accepts a 0.032-inch guidewire that is passed from the femoral vein into the superior vena cava (SVC). The modified transseptal needle has a 21-gauge needle tip to reduce the hazard of accidental puncture of the aorta or atrial wall. Several different shapes and sizes of the transseptal needle curve are available, with the appropriate selection depending on the patient's specific anatomy (Fig. 9.2). The transseptal needle system is gently curved and attached to a pressure transducer with a rotating adapter for free movement of the long needle as it travels in the venous system through the catheter and for its manipulation toward the atrial septum.

Procedural Steps

Transseptal catheterization can be performed using fluoroscopy alone, although adjunctive imaging with either transesophageal or intracardiac echocardiography has been increasingly used to facilitate safety and accuracy of the puncture site. Such accuracy is mandated for certain interventional procedures (e.g., MitraClip, Watchman) and can increase the success of other percutaneous therapies (e.g., posterior puncture for medial paravalvular defect closure). Fusion imaging with overlay from computed tomography (CT) has also been described for transseptal catheterization (see Fusion Imaging to Facilitate Cardiac Catheterization). The following steps describe the procedure when relying on fluoroscopy

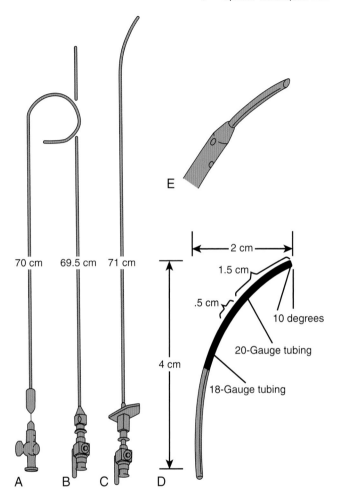

Fig. 9.1 For insertion of the curved transseptal catheter **(A)** from the femoral vein into the right atrium (RA), the straight stylet **(B)** is used. The modified transseptal needle **(C)** has a 21-gauge needle tip to reduce hazard from accidental puncture of the aorta or atrial wall, and the catheter **(E)** has side holes (to enhance injection of contrast medium) and a tapered tip to facilitate entry into the femoral vein and traversal of the atrial septum. **(D)** Detail of transseptal needle tip. (From Ross J, Jr. Transseptal left heart catheterization a 50-year odyssey. *J Am Coll Cardiol.* 2008;51:2107-2115.)

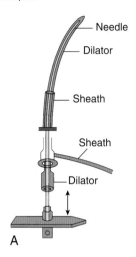

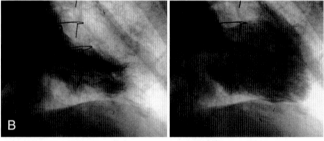

Fig. 9.2 **(A)** Transseptal catheter assembly. The distance between the transseptal needle and dilator hub *(arrow)* is set so that the needle lies just inside the dilator. **(B)** Frames of left ventricular (LV) cineangiogram using transseptal sheath and Berman catheter in LV. *Left,* Systolic frame; *right,* diastolic frame. Note ring of prosthetic aortic valve. (Fig. 9.2A from Weiner RI, Maranhao V. Development and application of transseptal left heart catheterization. *Cathet Cardiovasc Diagn.* 1988;15:112-120.)

alone, with additional comments for incorporating adjunctive echocardiography.

1. The transseptal catheter must be measured against the transseptal needle to identify the position at which the needle extends outside the catheter (Fig. 9.3). This measurement is made before inserting the catheter-needle assembly. The operator places the catheter over the needle, notes at which point the

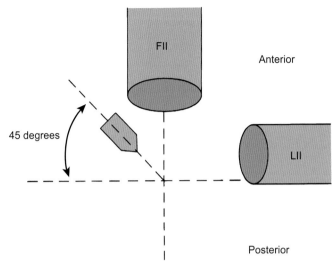

Fig. 9.3 The transseptal *arrow* is oriented approximately 45 degrees posteriorly. *FII*, Frontal image intensifier; *LII*, lateral image intensifier. (From Weiner RI, Maranhao V. Development and application of transseptal left heart catheterization. *Cathet Cardiovasc Diagn.* 1988;15:112-120.)

needle leaves the catheter end, and marks this distance with the right thumb. The right thumb position is used to keep the needle inside the catheter and protect from inadvertent needle damage.

2. To mark the aortic valve level as an anatomic reference point, place a pigtail catheter in the sinus of Valsalva at the aortic valve. For patients with an aortic valve prosthesis visible on fluoroscopy or when echocardiography is used, a pigtail catheter is not needed. In all cases, monitor the aortic or systemic arterial pressure during transseptal puncture.

3. Use fluoroscopy to determine landmarks for puncture. Figure 9.4 shows a right anterior oblique (RAO) projection, at which a horizontal line is drawn from the lower end of the pigtail catheter that intersects with the vertical line of the RA border. The fossa ovale is typically 1 cm below this line at its midpoint. If a left anterior oblique (LAO) projection is available, the operator can help to ensure a posterior orientation of the needle trajectory. In this view, the location of the fossa ovale is typically one-half to two-thirds of the distance from the aorta to the posterior wall of the LA (Fig. 9.5).

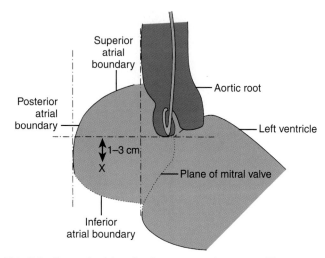

Fig. 9.4 The optimal location for transseptal puncture. Diagrammatic representation of the structures visualized in 40-degree right anterior oblique (RAO) projection. Limits of the atria are depicted behind the aorta. The pigtail catheter positioned in the noncoronary aortic cusp defines the posterior boundary of the aortic root. *X*, The point of intended atrial septal puncture. (From Croft CH, Lipscomb K. Modified technique of transseptal left heart catheterization. *J Am Coll Cardiol.* 1985;5:904-910.)

4. Advance a 0.032-inch guidewire to the SVC via the right femoral vein.

5. Advance the transseptal catheter (and sheath) over the guidewire to the SVC. It is important to have the end of the catheter in the SVC before removing the guidewire, because this position minimizes the need for superior movement of the assembly. Withdraw the wire and then aspirate the catheter.

6. Advance the transseptal needle through the catheter. As the transseptal needle is passed through the transseptal catheter to the SVC, rotate it at three points along its course to facilitate movement through the pelvic vessels. The first is at the iliac crest, the second over the spine near the renal vein, and the third at the inferior junction of the cardiac silhouette. The needle should rotate freely over these three segments and slide smoothly up through the transseptal catheter. Damage to the catheter or injury to the patient can occur if the needle does not rotate freely.

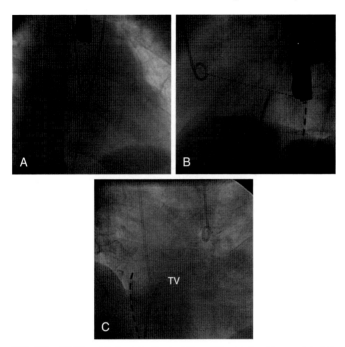

Fig. 9.5 **(A)** The pigtail marks the location of the aortic valve on anterior-posterior imaging, with the tip of the transseptal catheter inferior and medial to the aortic valve. **(B)** On the lateral projection, the transseptal puncture site is at approximately two-thirds of the distance from the aortic valve to the posterior wall of the left atrium (LA). **(C)** In the right anterior oblique (RAO) view, the transseptal dilator engages the fossa ovalis posterior to the pigtail catheter (aortic valve) but anterior to the right atrial (RA) silhouette *(dashed line)*. *TV*, Tricuspid valve. (From Babaliaros VC, Green JT, Lerakis S, et al. Emerging applications for transseptal left heart catheterization old techniques for new procedures. *J Am Coll Cardiol.* 2008;51:2116-2122.)

7. Position the needle in the SVC with the needle tip kept within the catheter, whose position was previously noted by the finger separation of the hub from the sheath. Connect the needle to a pressure transducer for continuous observation of atrial pressure during septal crossing.

8. Withdraw the catheter and needle assembly, now held fixed together, downward (caudally) from the SVC into the RA with a clockwise rotation of the metal arrow indicator of the needle angle pointing posterior-medially between a 4 o'clock and 5 o'clock position (see Fig. 9.3).

9. On withdrawal downward into the RA, pass the catheter assembly over the aortic knob with a forward motion and, on further withdrawal, pass under the superior limbus into the fossa ovale. Slightly advance the catheter-needle assembly until making secure contact with the atrial septum. Approximately 20% of patients have a patent foramen ovale, which allows unobstructed passage of the catheter assembly into the LA without needle puncture.

10. After the catheter and needle assembly makes secure contact with the atrial septum, maintain firm pressure on the sheath and catheter and advance the needle into the septum while continuously monitoring pressure waveforms. When echocardiography is used, perform imaging to demonstrate indentation of the atrial septum by the needle and a posterior orientation of the assembly (Fig. 9.6).

11. Clockwise rotation of the entire assembly leads to posterior positioning of the needle on the atrial septum and counterclockwise rotation will move it anteriorly. The atrial septum courses anteriorly from inferior to superior. Thus, movement of the assembly to a superior position will also result in slight anterior positioning and inferior movements will result in relatively posterior positioning.

12. Observe the LA pressure waveforms to note entry of the needle into the LA. If the operator is in doubt about the location of the needle tip, aspirate blood to determine oxygen saturation (which should be arterial) or inject a small amount of contrast material under fluoroscopy. After confirming the proper positioning of the needle in the LA, advance it slightly and advance the catheter over the needle with a counterclockwise rotation of the needle, which permits the transseptal catheter to turn anteriorly toward the mitral valve. The operator can give small amounts of contrast during manipulation across the septum to help avoid injury of the posterior or superior walls of the atrium.

13. The operator can advance the sheath over the transseptal catheter. This advancement can be performed with or without removal of the needle, by fixing the catheter. During the advancement of the sheath, the relatively abrupt transition between the catheter and sheath can cause the assembly to be pushed off the atrial septum back into the RA with loss of transseptal access. To help minimize this error, use gentle forward pressure taking care to avoid inadvertent forward movement of the assembly. This forward pressure can be applied after withdrawing the needle and reinserting a preshaped guidewire (e.g., Inoue wire).

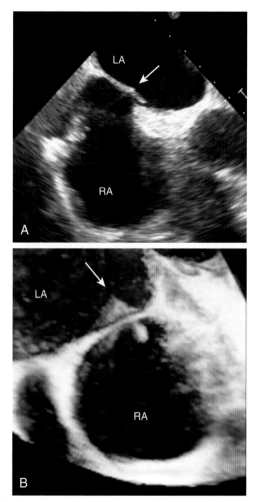

Fig. 9.6 **(A)** Two-dimensional and **(B)** three-dimensional echocardiography shows tenting of the atrial septum *(arrow)* with the catheter pointed posteriorly and away from the aortic valve. *LA,* Left atrium; *RA,* right atrium. (From Babaliaros VC, Green JT, Lerakis S, et al. Emerging applications for transseptal left heart catheterization old techniques for new procedures. *J Am Coll Cardiol.* 2008;51:2116-2122.)

14. To access the LV, insert a guidewire into the transseptal catheter or sheath and advance across the mitral valve and into the
LV. Do not turn the sheath without a wire or dilator in place,
because it is thin-walled and easily kinked. Pass a balloon
catheter (filled with carbon dioxide to minimize risk in the
event of balloon rupture) through the transseptal sheath and
float the catheter into the LV. The operator can transduce the
balloon catheter for ventricular pressure or use it as a rail for
passing the transseptal catheter into the LV.

15. The timing of heparin administration is at the preference of the
operator. Some operators prefer administering prior to transseptal puncture, others prefer after. Regardless, full heparinization (100U/kg IV) should occur once transseptal access has
been successfully obtained.

The fossa ovale is located in the middle third of the atrial
septum and is concave toward the LA in a normal heart. Valvular
disease may significantly alter the location of the fossa ovale. In
aortic valve disease, a dilated ascending aorta may displace
the fossa superiorly and anteriorly. In mitral valve disease, the LA
usually enlarges posteriorly and inferiorly and displaces the fossa
ovale inferiorly. In severe mitral disease, the fossa may become
everted and displaced into the lower third of the septum.
This makes the fossa difficult to locate on catheter descent and
transseptal puncture technique must be modified accordingly. In
general, left atrial enlargement leads to horizontal displacement,
which usually requires a shallow needle trajectory (~50 degrees).
Right atrial enlargement leads to vertical displacement, which
requires a more aggressive needle shape (~70 to 90 degrees).

In some patients, the atrial septum can be thickened and
difficult to cross with the transseptal needle or catheter assembly.
A transseptal method using radiofrequency energy to ablate the
atrial septum has been developed. A needle, which is fully insu-
lated excepted for the 21-gauge tip, is connected to a generator
that creates monopolar output to deliver 10 W of energy for
2 seconds (Baylis Medical Company, Quebec, Canada). Comparing
the radiofrequency method with conventional transseptal needle
techniques, a randomized trial showed a shorter time to transseptal puncture (2.3 min vs. 7.3 min) and a higher rate of success
(100% vs. 72.2%) with radiofrequency.

When there is concern about the forward pressure needed to
advance a transseptal needle or catheter assembly, the atrial
septum can be initially crossed with a low-profile guidewire. In this
technique, the catheter assembly and needle is used to indent
the septum, followed by advancement of a 135-cm long 0.014-inch
diameter nitinol wire (SafeSept, Pressure Products, San Pedro, CA).

Box 9.1   Risks Related to Transseptal Catheterization

- Cardiac perforation
  - RA
  - Posterior LA
  - LA appendage
  - Pulmonary vein
  - LV
- Puncture into the aortic root
- Pericardial tamponade[a]
- Embolus from the LA

LA, Left atrium; *LV,* left ventricle; *RA,* right atrium.
[a]Almost all deaths related to transseptal catheterization are a result of tamponade.

The tip of this wire is sharp to allow relatively easy passage across the septum; once across, the preshaped configuration helps to prevent inadvertent injury from forward advancement of the catheter assembly into the LA.

Risks of Transseptal Catheterization

Punctures of the aortic root, the coronary sinus (CS), or the posterior free wall of the atrium are potentially lethal complications (Box 9.1). In patients who have not been given anticoagulants, the 21-gauge tip of the needle rarely causes a problem. However, if the large transseptal catheter assembly is advanced into these spaces, cardiac tamponade can easily occur. The catheter-needle combination should not be advanced if the operator is not satisfied with the position of the transseptal catheter in the right atria. If the catheter assembly is not in the correct position, the operator must remove the transseptal needle, reinsert the guidewire to the SVC, and reposition the assembly toward the fossa ovale, as indicated earlier.

Direct Left Ventricular Puncture

The development of retrograde arterial catheterization and transseptal techniques has enabled clinicians to access the LV without direct puncture in the vast majority of patients. Nonetheless, there remain diagnostic and therapeutic indications for this technique, mainly in patients with double left-sided mechanical prostheses or certain therapies (e.g., paravalvular leak closure). Because of the high potential for complications, only experienced operators should perform direct LV puncture.

Indications

The indications for direct left ventricular puncture are:

1. Direct hemodynamic assessment of the LV and left ventriculography, when diagnostic data cannot be obtained using other vascular access or from noninvasive imaging evaluations. This indication occurs mainly in patients who have undergone replacement of the mitral and aortic valves with mechanical prostheses.

2. Structural heart interventions whose therapies are either delivered through the LV apex or require the creation of transcatheter heart rails for delivery. These therapies include mitral valve placement and percutaneous closure of paravalvular prosthetic regurgitation.

Direct LV puncture should be avoided in patients with intracardiac thrombus and in those on therapeutic anticoagulation.

Technique

Direct LV puncture is most commonly performed with echocardiographic guidance. Recently, techniques with guidance from CT overlay in the catheterization laboratory also have been developed (see Fusion Imaging to Facilitate Cardiac Catheterization).

When relying on echocardiography, the LV apex is imaged from the apical window to determine the direction of the long axis of the LV at a position that is superior to the rib margin. The operator memorizes this angle and marks the position in the chest with an indelible pen. Following sterile prepping of the puncture area, an 18-gauge needle with a Teflon sheath is inserted. Some operators prefer needles with stylets to avoid coring the myocardium, whereas others choose to connect the needle to a pressure transducer for hemodynamic monitoring during insertion. Once the needle enters the LV, it is advanced 2 to 3 mm further to ensure that the outer Teflon sheath is fully advanced into the LV. The needle is then removed, leaving the sheath in place for diagnostic use or therapeutic interventions. Note that after its removal, the needle should not be reintroduced into the Teflon sheath in the patient. Figures 9.7 and 9.8 illustrate a typical case of direct LV puncture and associated hemodynamics.

Following completion of the procedure, the apical access site can be closed with placement of an occlude device. Currently, there are no FDA-approved devices for closure of the LV apex, but several devices (AMPLATZER Muscular VSD Occluder, AMPLATZER Duct Occluder, and AMPLATZER Vascular Plug II, St. Jude Medical, St. Paul, MN) have been used. Following reversal of anticoagulation,

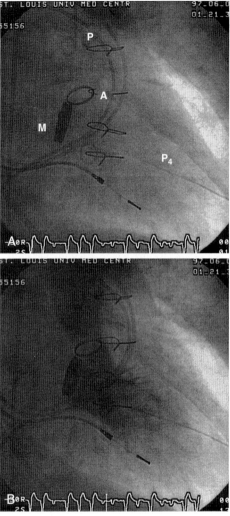

Fig. 9.7 Cineangiographic frames before **(A)** and during **(B)** left ventriculography through the pigtail catheter *(P₄)* positioned from the left ventricular apex. The supravalvular pigtail catheter *(P)* is positioned above the aortic ring *(A)*, which is adjacent to the mitral ring *(M)*. Multiple pacing leads and two pulmonary artery catheters are positioned near the supraaortic pigtail catheter. Contrast injection during ventriculography shows no mitral regurgitation.

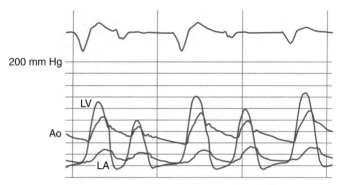

Fig. 9.8 Left ventricular *(LV)*, left atrial *(LA)*, and aortic *(Ao)* pressures (0- to 200-mm Hg scale) showing aortic and mitral prosthetic valve gradients. Note the influence of the paced beats on the valve gradients.

the distal disk of the closure device is withdrawn until secured to the endocardial surface of the LV. Positioning can be identified by landmarks on adjunctive imaging and confirmed by contrast injection through the sheath. The entire device is then uncovered, such that the proximal disk is on the epicardial surface. At that time, elongation and systolic compression of the device should be noted through the cardiac cycle to confirm correct placement.

Complications

The patient should be observed carefully for hemopericardium, hemothorax, or pneumothorax. Should any of these complications occur, they can be treated with direct aspiration or surgery as needed. A vasovagal reaction with bradycardia and hypotension may be encountered. Bleeding complications may result from laceration of the left anterior descending, its branches, or intercostal arteries. Patients who have had previous cardiac surgery usually have obliterated pericardial space, which decreases the likelihood of cardiac tamponade.

Fusion Imaging to Facilitate Cardiac Catheterization

When performing cardiac catheterization, fusion imaging, which merges two or more imaging sources (e.g., echocardiography, CT, and fluoroscopy), helps to overcome the spatial limitations of a single imaging source. This integration, made possible through the use of proprietary software, leads to benefits of individualized planning and guidance to improve procedural accuracy and safety.

Computed Tomography Angiography–Fluoroscopy Fusion Imaging

Fusion imaging using computed tomography angiography (CTA) and fluoroscopy imaging provides a three-dimensional (3D) model that allows important cardiac and surrounding structures to be identified, while preserving the temporal resolution of fluoroscopy. All patients undergo a preprocedural CTA (preferably ≥256-slice) with retrospective electrocardiogram (ECG)-gating. DICOM (Digital Imaging and Communications in Medicine) data for a single phase, typically diastolic, 75% of the R–R interval, are subsequently uploaded to the fusion workstation. These preprocedural two-dimensional (2D) images are volume-rendered in 3D, followed by segmentation to identify the ventricles, valves, ribs, coronary arteries, and great vessels, with optimization depending on information needed (Figs. 9.9 and 9.10). Landmarks are placed for each site-specific access approach. The CTA images are registered by markers (e.g., bronchi/carina, prosthetic valve frame, pacemaker wires, aorta, and coronary arteries) in two views taken ≥30 degrees apart. For live overlay, volume-rendered, 3D images are replaced with an outlined view of the segmented cardiac structures. During the procedure, 3D-rendered images are displayed in real time with the same perspective as the synchronized fluoroscopic C-arm.

For transapical access, required cardiac structures include the ribs, left lung, and left anterior descending artery. Preselected landmarks are placed to identify skin entry, LV epicardial entry site, and structural defect. A safe path or cylinder is generated, connecting the landmarks, such that a direct line is made into the LV away from lung parenchyma, coronary arteries, and papillary muscles (Fig. 9.11). The skin is entered with the needle trajectory confirmed in RAO and LAO views. The LAO view is en face such that the landmarks and cylinder are completely in line, generating a target into the LV. With CTA-fluoroscopic fusion imaging, the accuracy of transapical puncture is usually within 5 mm of intended entry.

For transseptal puncture using CTA-fluoroscopic fusion imaging, a landmark is placed on the interatrial septum typically at the fossa ovalis (Fig. 9.12). Standard transseptal puncture techniques, as described earlier, can then be used.

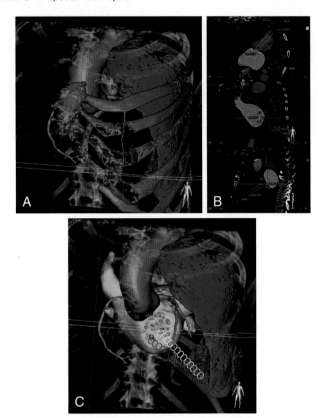

Fig. 9.9 Images showing three-dimensional (3D) volume-rendering, segmentation, and placement of landmarks. Preprocedural two-dimensional (2D) computed tomographic angiography (CTA) images are 3D volume-rendered and automatically segmented to identify cardiac structures including the left ventricle *(LV; red)*, left atrium *(green)*, and aorta *(orange)*. Additional structures that can be manually segmented include the coronary arteries *(purple;* extending from the aortic root), mitral annular calcification/prosthetic valve *(yellow)*, lung *(purple)*, and ribs *(orange)*. Landmarks are then placed to identify skin, LV entry, center of mitral prosthesis *(MV)*, paravalvular leak *(PVL)*, and transseptal entry *(blue circle; TRSEPT)*. A "safe path" is generated, connecting the skin and LV entry landmarks toward the PVL *(red cylinder)* or MV *(yellow cylinder)* for transapical access. **(A)** Full-volume view; **(B)** axial, coronal, and sagittal planes; **(C)** cutplane view with the LV removed. *AV,* Atrioventricular node.

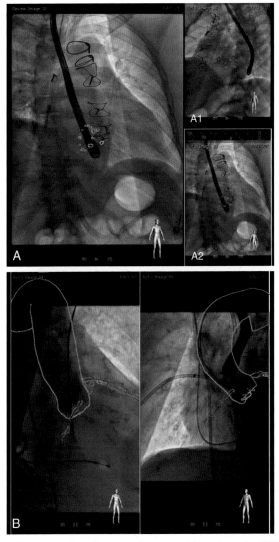

Fig. 9.10 Registration of computed tomographic angiography (CTA) with fluoroscopy. CTA images are registered using internal markers **(A)** such as mitral annular calcification/prosthetic valve *(yellow outline)* in two different views performed at least 30 degrees apart *(A1,* left anterior oblique [LAO] 30 degrees; *A2,* right anterior oblique [RAO] 30 degrees). When internal markers are not available, aortography can be performed **(B)**.

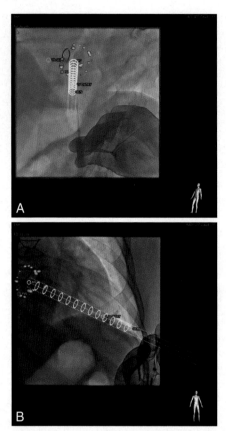

Fig. 9.11 Overlay of computed tomography angiography (CTA) onto fluoroscopy for transapical access. Once registered, the volume-rendered three-dimensional (3D) image is replaced with an outlined view of the cardiac structures and is overlayed, together with landmarks, onto fluoroscopy. CTA images are displayed in the same perspective as the C-arm and move with C-arm rotations. **(A)** For transapical access, the C-arm is in the left anterior oblique (LAO) view, where the landmarks (skin entry, left ventricle [LV] entry, and mitral prosthetic valve center) are lined up. The safe path *(yellow cylinder)* becomes a bull's-eye for 21-gauge micropuncture needle entry. **(B)** The right anterior oblique (RAO) view confirms needle trajectory and angulation before puncture. The mitral annular calcification/prosthetic valve *(yellow)* and paravalvular leak *(red)* can also be visualized.

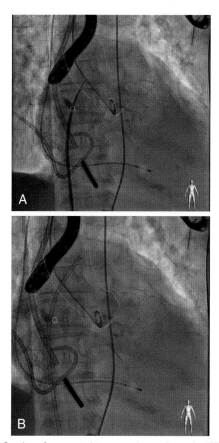

Fig. 9.12 Overlay of computed tomography angiography (CTA) onto fluoroscopy for transseptal access. Outlined view of the aorta and coronary arteries *(orange)*. Their positioning is confirmed by the presence of a pigtail catheter placed into the aortic root. **(A)** The transseptal needle/sheath is visualized crossing the interatrial septum at the site of landmark placement *(blue circle)*, with contrast staining of septum noted. **(B)** Once needle positioning is confirmed by imaging and hemodynamics, the sheath is advanced into the left atrium (LA). The site of sheath passage can be visualized at the site of intended puncture.

Transesophageal Echocardiography–Fluoroscopy Fusion Imaging

Transesophageal echocardiography (TEE)–fluoroscopy fusion imaging merges live echocardiography and fluoroscopy in a volumetrically fused image dataset. This type of imaging does not require contrast and overcomes some limitations of CTA, including lack of motion compensation and nonsimultaneous data acquisition. Nonetheless, imaging with TEE-fluoroscopy is restricted to the echocardiographic field of view. In TEE-fluoroscopy, 2D and 3D images are obtained using the IE33 echocardiographic system with an X7-2t TEE probe (Philips Healthcare, Andover, MA). The fluoroscopy table is placed with the echocardiographic probe tip at the center of the registration window with the entire TEE faceplate well visualized. Landmarks are placed and subsequently overlayed onto fluoroscopy. Changes in position or angulation of the TEE probe are immediately registered and updated on the live fluoroscopic image. Four viewing windows are available: (1) echo view, which mimics the display of traditional echocardiographic images; (2) C-arm view, which displays the echocardiographic images in reference to the C-arm orientation; (3) free view, which allows the interventionalist and echocardiographer to move the echocardiographic image freely while keeping track of virtual C-arm orientation; and (4) x-ray view, the traditional fluoroscopic 2D image with overlayed landmarks (Fig. 9.13). For transseptal access, a landmark is placed on the interatrial septum at an appropriate site on the septum in x-plane and confirmed in a 3D view. These views can then be used to guide transseptal access.

Pressure Sensor Guidewire to Assess Pressure Across Mechanical Prosthetic Valves

An alternative method to obtain LV pressure across mechanical prosthetic valves is to use a 0.014-inch pressure sensor guidewire. The use of a catheter to cross a mechanical prosthetic valve is generally prohibited because of the potential for catheter entrapment. However, a fine-diameter (0.014-inch) guidewire with a high-fidelity pressure sensor has been used safely in several cases. It is important to note that there can be error in pressure measurement because of the inability to zero the electronic pressure transducer once it has been placed into the LV. Caution should be used when passing the guidewire through the mechanical valve and retrieving it. An example of a pressure guidewire used to cross an aortic prosthetic valve is shown in Figure 9.14.

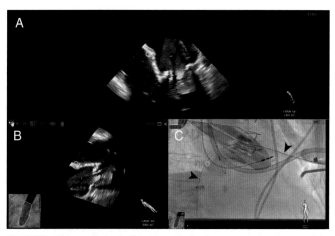

Fig. 9.13 Echocardiography-fluoroscopy fusion for percutaneous transseptal–transapical mitral valve-in-valve implantation. **(B)** The transesophageal echocardiography (TEE) probe is automatically registered to fluoroscopy in reference to the faceplate *(green probe)*. **(C)** The landmark is placed at the site of directed transseptal puncture *(blue circle)*, visualized on the echo view **(A)**. Free **(B)** and x-ray **(C)** views are displayed with the C-arm angulations **(B** and **C**, *bottom right)*. In the x-ray view, the three-dimensional (3D) volume space is overlayed directly onto fluoroscopy showing successful valve-in-valve implantation with trivial paravalvular regurgitation. *Arrowheads* indicate arteriovenous rail from the transseptal and transapical access points.

Endomyocardial Biopsy

Indications, Contraindications, and Complications

Monitoring cardiac transplant rejection and determining anthracycline cardiotoxicity are the only two definitive indications for endomyocardial biopsy (Box 9.2). Other indications include evaluation for infiltrative cardiomyopathy, myocarditis that may benefit from immunosuppressive therapy, and occasionally, differentiation between restrictive and constrictive cardiomyopathies. Relative contraindications to endomyocardial biopsy are anticoagulation and anatomic abnormalities.

Complications of endomyocardial biopsy can be access-site related (3%), valvular regurgitation (3%), arrhythmia (1%), conduction abnormalities (1%), cardiac perforation (0.7%), and death

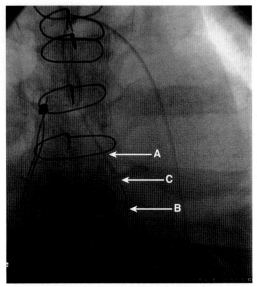

Fig. 9.14 The cineframe shows a St. Jude valve with a Radi 0.014 pressure wire across the valve, advanced through a multipurpose catheter. The tilting disk valve (DV) in the mitral position made a transseptal approach impossible. *A,* 6-F multipurpose catheter; *B,* Radi pressure wire; *C,* leaflet of St. Jude valve.

Box 9.2   Indications for Endomyocardial Biopsy

Definitive

- Cardiac transplantation follow-up
- Monitoring of anthracycline cardiotoxicity

Possible

- Viral myocarditis
- Secondary cardiomyopathies (sarcoidosis, hemochromatosis, and amyloidosis)
- Differentiation of restrictive versus constrictive cardiac disease
- Endocardial fibrosis
- Hypereosinophilic syndrome
- Malignancies involving the heart

Table 9.1

Major Complications of 2505 Retrospective and 543 Prospective Endomyocardial Biopsy Procedures.		
	Retrospective (Absolute/%)	**Prospective (Absolute/%)**
Pericardial tamponade with pericardiocentesis	2/0.08	0/0
Permanent complete AV block with permanent pacemaker required	1/0.04	0/0
Urgent cardiac surgery	0/0	0/0
Advanced cardiac life support	0/0	0/0
Hemothorax or pneumothorax	0/0	0/0
Death	0/0	0/0

From Holzmann M, Nicko A, Kuhl U, et al. Complication rate of right ventricular endomyocardial biopsy via the femoral approach: a retrospective and prospective study analyzing 3048 diagnostic procedures over an 11-year period. *Circulation* 2008;118:1722-1728.
 AV, Atrioventricular.

(0.4%). Complication rates are higher for patients with cardiomy-opathy than for heart transplant recipients (Table 9.1).

Biopsy Devices

There are two basic types of bioptomes: (1) stiff shaft (preshaped) devices (Konno, Kawai, and Stanford bioptomes; Fig. 9.15) and (2) floppy shaft devices (King and Cordis bioptomes; Fig. 9.16) that are positioned with the aid of a long sheath. The femoral sheath dilator is 94 cm long and the long sheath is 85 cm long. Biopsy sheaths come in 5-cm and 7-cm curves (for hearts with large right atria or transplanted hearts).

Technique

Endomyocardial biopsy can be performed under fluoroscopic or echocardiographic guidance from the femoral or internal jugular approach.

Femoral Approach

After the patient is given local anesthesia, the right or left femoral vein is punctured using the modified Seldinger technique and a 0.038-inch guidewire is advanced into the femoral vein. A 7-F biopsy sheath with a 7-F dilator is advanced over the guidewire.

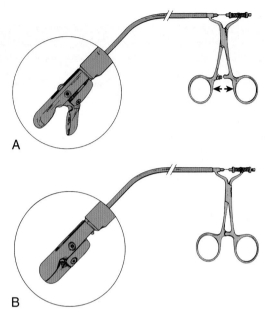

Fig. 9.15 Scholten bioptome. **(A)** Open; **(B)** closed. (From Tilkian AG, Daily EK. *Cardiovascular Procedures: Diagnostic Techniques and Therapeutic Procedures.* St Louis; Mosby: 1986.)

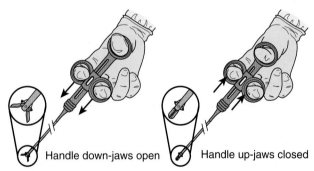

Handle down-jaws open   Handle up-jaws closed

Fig. 9.16 Disposable biopsy forceps with formable tip, pivoting jaws, clear wire–braided body, stainless-steel cutting jaws, stainless-steel wire coil, and a spring-loaded, three-ring plastic handle that controls the operation of the jaws. The thumb ring of the handle is flexible and rotates to accommodate any thumb position, reducing manual stress.

A large-curve (7-cm) sheath is used when the atrium is dilated, as in cardiac transplantation. In some systems, the dilator is not completely radiopaque. The sheath and dilator are advanced into the RA. The dilator is withdrawn into the sheath. With the help of the guidewire, the sheath is advanced across the tricuspid valve and into the right ventricle (RV). The biopsy sheath is equipped with a valve and side arm for flushing. The sheath is flushed and connected to the pressure monitor, and a RV pressure tracing is identified. A floppy shaft biopsy forceps is advanced through the sheath and into the RV. The sheath is pointed horizontally toward the intraventricular septum, which should be confirmed in the LAO projection to ensure that the bioptome has not inadvertently entered the CS. The RV outflow tract (upward sheath angle) and (usually) the inferior (downward sheath angle) and RV free wall should be avoided.

To reduce the chance of perforation, the operator opens the bioptome jaws inside the sheath before the bioptome exits the sheath (Fig. 9.17). The bioptome is carefully advanced with the

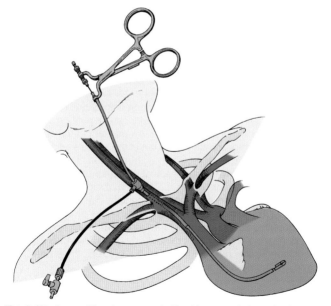

Fig. 9.17 Internal jugular approach. The bioptome tip is in the right ventricular (RV) apex, pointing toward the ventricular septum. (From Tilkian AG, Daily EK. *Cardiovascular Procedures: Diagnostic Techniques and Therapeutic Procedures.* St Louis; Mosby: 1986.)

jaws fully open until contact with the ventricular wall is made and the bioptome shaft is slightly bent. The bioptome jaws are then closed. After 2 to 3 seconds, to permit tissue excision, the bite is slowly withdrawn into the sheath as the sheath is advanced. A tugging sensation is often felt by the operator on full extraction of the bioptome into the sheath. After the bioptome is removed from the patient, the sheath should be aspirated and flushed to eliminate air bubbles. (Flushing can be minimized if saline is free to flow into the sheath as the bioptome is being withdrawn. Otherwise, air fills the negative space of the bioptome through the valve.) The procedure is repeated until an adequate number of specimens (usually four to six) are obtained. RV pressures are measured before and after the biopsy. The biopsy sheath is removed and hemostasis is secured.

For heterotopic heart transplantation (i.e., piggyback hearts), the RA of the donor's heart is located in the right hemithorax. Its connection to the atrium of the recipient's heart may be marked with a radiopaque ring. The biopsy sheath is advanced over the guidewire and into the RV of the donor's heart, and biopsy samples are taken as described.

Internal Jugular Approach

Extensive experience in performing endomyocardial biopsies under echocardiographic guidance and fluoroscopy has been reported (Figs. 9.17 and 9.18). An 8-F short sheath is inserted into the right internal jugular vein using the standard Seldinger technique. A rigid, curved bioptome is inserted through the venous sheath and into the RA. A counterclockwise (anterior) rotation helps guide the bioptome past the tricuspid valve. Further counterclockwise rotation straightens the curve and orients the bioptome toward the central ventricular septum. The operator should readily target the apical septum to avoid trauma to the tricuspid valve, which is abundant in chordae. On fluoroscopy, the RAO view facilitates apical placement, whereas the LAO view ensures positioning against the ventricular septum. When biopsy of other segments is desired, echocardiography can be used to target those segments to increase the diagnostic yield of the procedure. Some operators use echocardiography alone, which allows portability for performance of biopsies at the bedside and also avoids exposure to radiation. Following completion of the biopsies, the sheath is removed, and hemostasis is secured.

Pericardiocentesis

Pericardiocentesis may be required for the diagnosis and management of acute and chronic pericardial effusions. In cardiac

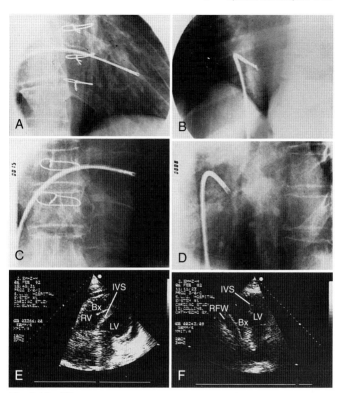

Fig. 9.18 **(A)** Anteroposterior cineangiographic image of femoral endomyo-cardial bioptome location. **(B)** Corresponding left anterior oblique (LAO) view. **(C–D)** Same views in another transplant recipient show nearly identical angiographic location but positioning of bioptome and sheath against the RV free wall *(RFW)*. Bx, Bioptome; *LV,* left ventricle. E-F, Simultaneous two-dimensional (2D) echocardiographic image shows position of bioptome against the right ventricular *(RV)* side of the interventricular septum *(IVS)*. (Figs. 9.18A–C: From Bell CA, Kern MJ, Aguirre FV, et al. Superior accuracy of anatomic positioning with echocardiographic over fluoroscopic-guided endomyocardial biopsy. *Cathet Cardiovasc Diagn.* 1993;28:291-294.)

tamponade, this is a lifesaving technique. Pericardiocentesis is usually preceded by echocardiographic confirmation of the pericardial effusion. In cases in which a pericardial effusion is known or suspected with acute hemodynamic compromise, echocardiographic assessment should not delay the performance of pericardiocentesis.

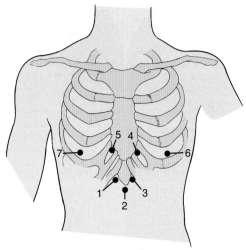

Fig. 9.19 Locations for pericardiocentesis. *1–3,* Xiphoid approaches; *4,* fifth left intercostal space at sternal border; *5,* fifth right intercostal space at the sternal border; *6,* apical approach; *7,* approach for major fluid accumulation on the right side. (Modified from Spodick DH. *Acute Pericarditis.* New York; Grune & Stratton: 1959.)

Approach

The most common approach is subxiphoid, but other access routes are acceptable depending on the depth from the skin and the location and volume of the pericardial effusion (Fig. 9.19). The advantage of the subxiphoid approach is a decreased likelihood of laceration of the coronary and internal thoracic arteries. Placement of the needle approximately a finger width below the edge of the rib is necessary to avoid difficulty in advancing the catheter through fibrous tissue near the xiphoid process.

Setup and Positioning

The patient is positioned at a 30- to 45-degree, head-up angle to permit pericardial fluid to pool on the inferior surface of the heart. Local anesthetic is given at the needle puncture site and more is instilled through the pericardial needle as it is advanced perpendicularly to the skin initially, then lowered to an angle nearly parallel with the floor moving under the xiphoid process toward the left shoulder. If the patient is obese, a larger needle and some force may be required to tip the syringe under the subxiphoid process toward the heart (Fig. 9.20).

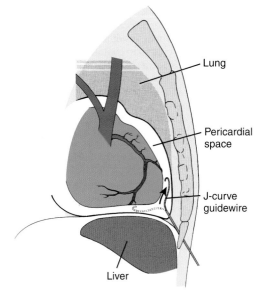

Fig. 9.20 Passing a flexible J tip of the guidewire through the pericardial needle into the pericardial space. (From Tilkian AG, Daily EK. *Cardiovascular Procedures: Diagnostic Techniques and Therapeutic Procedures.* St Louis; Mosby: 1986.)

For elective procedures, right-heart pressures are measured with a balloon-tipped catheter positioned in the pulmonary artery to assess equalization of diastolic right-sided pressures (and to document the change with intervention) and then withdrawn into the RA for continuous monitoring of RA pressure during pericardial puncture and effusion drainage. A peripheral arterial line (e.g., radial line or 5-F sheath placed in a femoral artery) is often used for monitoring systemic pressure.

Puncture of the Pericardium

Either a micropuncture needle or a long 16- or 18-gauge needle connected to a stopcock, and tubing to a pressure transducer, can be used. When using a hollow needle, it is important to note that aspiration during passage through the skin may block the needle with subcutaneous tissue. Thus, some prefer use with a stylet or an alternative access needle, such as the Angiocath (14 to 24 gauge; Becton, Dickinson and Company, Franklin Lakes, NJ), which contains an inner stylet that is removed once puncture of the pericardium has been performed. The pericardial puncture feels similar to a lumbar puncture. The operator should exercise care when advancing the needle. Excessive forward pressure may result in crossing suddenly through the pericardium and into a cardiac chamber or laceration of an epicardial vessel. Chronic effusions are often clear yellow, occasionally serosanguineous, or less commonly, dark brown. Acute effusions resulting from trauma, cancer, or artery perforation are frankly bloody.

To confirm passage into the pericardial space, the stopcock can be turned for transduction of pressure. In this manner, inadvertent ventricular puncture can be recognized at once. In cases of tamponade, pericardial pressure resembles atrial pressure. For further confirmation, agitated saline can be injected through the needle or catheter with simultaneous echocardiographic imaging to demonstrate location in the pericardial space (Fig. 9.21). If the needle or catheter is in a cardiac chamber (e.g., RV or LV), the bubbles will be seen in the cavity and then dispersed rapidly by ventricular ejection. Electrocardiographic guidance has been used historically, with the current of injury seen on contact with the epicardium (Figs. 9.22 and 9.23). Hemodynamic monitoring and echocardiography is now the favored approach for pericardiocentesis.

When the needle or catheter is in the pericardial space, a guidewire is passed under fluoroscopy high into the pericardial space (transverse pericardial sinus) followed by an exchange for a multiple side-hole catheter (e.g., pigtail) or sheath. Pericardial and atrial pressures are measured, effusion is aspirated, and pressures are measured again after the pericardial space is empty (Fig. 9.24). Large syringes (>50 cc) or a vacuum jar can be used to facilitate rapid removal of pericardial fluid. In the event of effusion resulting from cardiac perforation, the removed blood can be

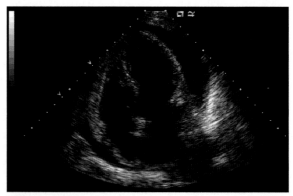

Fig. 9.21 Echocardiogram with large amount of fluid in the pericardial space.

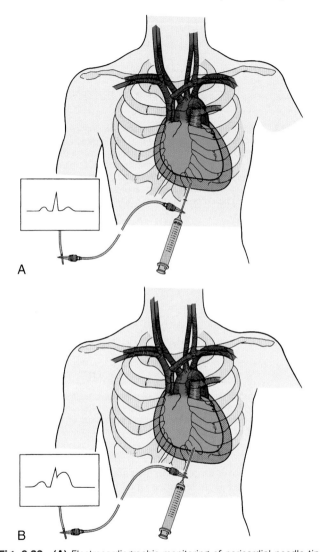

Fig. 9.22 **(A)** Electrocardiographic monitoring of pericardial needle tip. Note the normal ST segment when the tip is not touching the epicardium. **(B)** When the needle tip touches the epicardium, the current of injury (the contact current) with an elevated ST segment is seen. (From Tilkian AG, Daily EK. *Cardiovascular Procedures: Diagnostic Techniques and Therapeutic Procedures.* St Louis; Mosby: 1986.)

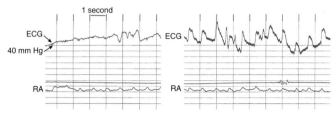

Fig. 9.23 Electrocardiogram (ECG) method during pericardiocentesis. *Left,* The ECG shows normal tracing; the ECG clip is attached to the pericardial needle. *Right,* On advancement of the needle through the pericardium, contact is made with the heart, as shown by the ECG injury current. *RA,* Right atrial pressure. (From Kern MJ, Aguirre FV. Interpretation of cardiac pathophysiology from pressure waveform analysis: pericardial compressive hemodynamics, Part III. *Cathet Cardiovasc Diagn.* 1992;26:152-158.)

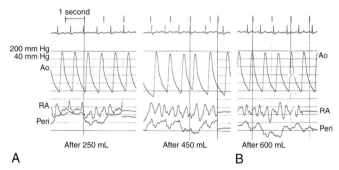

Fig. 9.24 Hemodynamic results of pericardiocentesis. **(A)** Aortic *(Ao)* pressure. **(B)** Right atrial *(RA)* pressure before and after withdrawal of pericardial fluid. Note the elimination of pulsus paradoxus of aortic pressure and the return of y-descent of the RA waveform after pericardiocentesis.

placed in a cell saver for return to the patient. If the position of the needle or catheter is uncertain, a small amount of radiographic contrast medium or agitated saline under echocardiographic guidance can be injected. Contrast medium pools in the dependent portion of the pericardial space but rapidly washes out of a vascular space if a cardiac chamber has been entered inadvertently.

Samples of the pericardial fluid should be sent to the laboratory for appropriate chemistries, cultures, and cytology, as indicated by clinical presentation. The multiple side-hole catheter or sheath is left in place with a sterile dressing until serial echocardiography demonstrates no recurrent effusion. Catheter placement can cause residual chest discomfort that can be treated with systemic analgesia or periodic injection of local anesthesia directly into the pericardial space.

Intravascular Foreign Body Retrieval

Catheter fragments can result from injudicious insertion or removal of catheters from the subclavian, jugular, peripheral (portacaths), or rarely, inferior vena caval approaches. Guidewire fragmentation, coronary stent loss, and embolization of structural devices (e.g., AMPLATZER occluders) can also occur in the systemic arterial circulation during interventional procedures. Several catheter and wire loop systems have been designed to retrieve intravascular foreign bodies. Snares can have single (e.g., AMPLATZ GooseNeck, Covidien, Plymouth, MA) or multiple (e.g., EN Snare, Hatch Medical, Atlanta, GA; Multi-Snare Bi-Plane Design, B. Braun Interventional Systems, Inc., Bethlehem, PA) loop configurations, with a range of sizes and steerability (Fig. 9.25). An intracoronary guidewire fragment can be retrieved from the coronary artery with the use of a loop passed through a small intracoronary guiding catheter. When performing such retrieval, it is important to note that the size of the vascular access sheath should be generous and based on the largest diameter of the foreign body, regardless of its orientation, that is expected to occur during removal. If the sheath is too small, severe vascular injury will occur during foreign body retrieval. A delivery catheter is advanced to the snaring site over a 0.035- or 0.038-inch wire. Tightening of the snare occurs with retrieval into the delivery catheter; this backward tension needs to be maintained to avoid loss of capture of the foreign body. Examples of foreign body retrieval are shown in Figures 9.26 and 9.27.

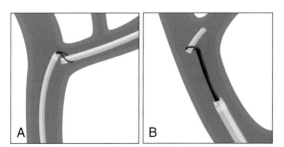

Fig. 9.25 **(A)** A loop snare is used to capture a catheter end. **(B)** The loop snare can be used to capture catheter fragments. (Reproduced with permission of Covidien.)

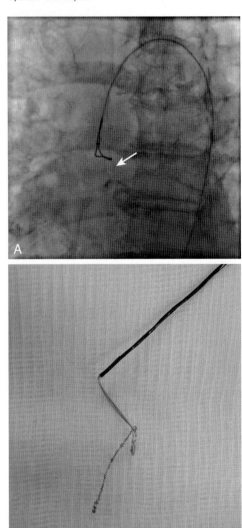

Fig. 9.26 A coronary stent is retrieved using a 15-mm GooseNeck snare. **(A)** Stent loss during percutaneous coronary intervention of the right coronary artery *(arrow)*. A 15-mm GooseNeck snare is used to capture the stent. **(B)** The captured stent can be seen within the snare after removal.

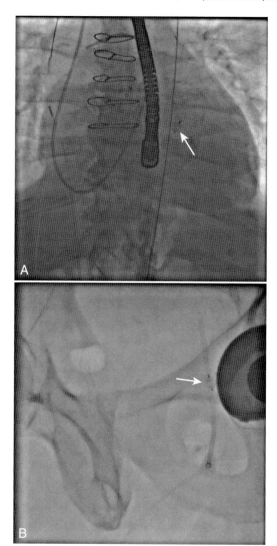

Fig. 9.27 Retrieval of an embolized AMPLATZER Vascular Plug II. **(A)** Embolization of the 6-mm vascular plug *(arrow)* into the left ventricle (LV) occurs during paravalvular leak closure. **(B)** The embolized occluder becomes embedded in the left femoral artery *(arrow)*.

Continued

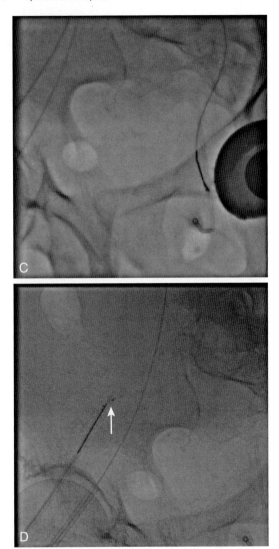

Fig. 9.27, cont'd (C) Through a right femoral artery sheath, a 10-mm GooseNeck snare is placed antegrade into the left femoral artery to retrieve the embolized plug. **(D)** The plug is removed via the contralateral femoral artery *(arrow)*.

Suggested Readings

Bell CA, Kern MJ, Aguirre FV, et al. Superior accuracy of anatomic positioning with echocardiographic- over fluoroscopic-guided endomyocardial biopsy. *Cathet Cardiovasc Diagn.* 1993;28:291-294.

Brockenbrough EC, Braunwald E. A new technique for left ventriculography and transseptal left heart catheterization. *Am J Cardiol.* 1960;6:1062-1064.

Croft CH, Lipscomb K. Modified technique of transseptal left heart catheterization. 1985; *J Am Coll Cardiol.* 5:904-910.

Holzmann M, Nicko A, Kühl U, et al. Complication rate of right ventricular endomyocardial biopsy via the femoral approach: a retrospective and prospective study analyzing 3048 diagnostic procedures over an 11-year period. *Circulation.* 2008; 118:1722-1728.

Hsu JC, Badhwar N, Gerstenfeld EP, et al. Randomized trial of conventional transseptal needle versus radiofrequency energy needle puncture for left atrial access (the TRAVERSE-LA study). *J Am Heart Assoc.* 2013;2:e000428.

Kern MJ, Deligonul U. *The Interventional Cardiac Catheterization Handbook.* St Louis: Mosby; 1996.

Mason JW, O'Connell JB. Clinical merit of endomyocardial biopsy. *Circulation.* 1989;79:971-979.

Miller LW, Labovitz AJ, McBride LA, et al. Echocardiography-guided endomyocardial biopsy. A 5-year experience. *Circulation.* 1988;78(suppl 3):99-102.

Ross J, Jr. Transseptal left heart catheterization a 50-year odyssey. *J Am Coll Cardiol.* 2008;51:2107-2115.

Wadehra V, Buxton AE, Antoniadis AP, et al. The use of a novel nitinol guidewire to facilitate transseptal puncture and left atrial catheterization for catheter ablation procedures. *Europace.* 2011;13:1401-1405.

Research Techniques

BARRY A. BORLAUG • JOERG HERRMANN •
MORTON J. KERN

Research techniques have been and continue to be of great value for understanding common problems in cardiology. Moreover, many of these techniques, once solely limited to the research arena, have been incorporated into routine diagnostic cardiac catheterization, such as fractional flow reserve (FFR) and intravascular ultrasound (IVUS). This chapter is an overview of commonly used research procedures in the cardiac catheterization laboratory (Tables 10.1 and 10.2).

Attitude Toward Research in the Catheterization Laboratory

The support staff in the cardiac catheterization laboratory may view research studies as unnecessary, unimportant, or dangerous to the patient. These commonly held misconceptions should be dispelled and the use and safety of the procedure advocated. It is to be emphasized, however, that only skilled physicians, with directed goals and institutional research board approval, should apply these research techniques. Discoveries that are to be made are invaluable in identifying new therapies and advancing the frontiers of treatment for cardiac disease. It is most helpful for nurses and catheterization laboratory physicians to appreciate these aspects and convey a sense of confidence and enthusiasm to the patient in reaching a common goal, that is, to improve the care and outcome of patients with heart disease.

Quantitative Coronary and Left Ventricular Angiography

Although visual estimation is universally used during angiography in the clinical setting, significant observer variability is the rule. Quantitative coronary angiography (QCA) and ventriculography are used to help overcome the subjective limitations of angiographic

Table 10.1

Research Techniques.	
Objective	**Method**
I. Ventricular Function	
1. Systolic function	Ventricular P-V relationship (simultaneous LV pressure with LV volume by echocardiogram, contrast angiogram, nuclear angiogram, or impedance catheter)
	Variables derived: end-systolic P-V slope, intercept; contractility (+dP/dt)
2. Diastolic function	Ventricular P-V relationship (as above)
	Variables derived: end-diastolic P-V slope, intercept; relaxation (−dP/dt, τ, K)
3. Exercise studies	
4. Combined hemodynamic and echocardiographic studies	
II. Myocardial Blood Flow (Coronary Vasodilatory Reserve, Effects of Drugs)	
	Indicator dilution; inert gas (xenon, nitrogen); thermodilution
	Doppler flow velocity
	Digital radiographic studies
III. Endothelial Function	
1. QCA	
2. Doppler flow	
3. QCA	
IV. Electrical Function (Abnormal Conduction, Excitation)	
	Electrophysiologic studies
	His bundle
	Atrial and ventricular refractory periods
	Conduction abnormalities
	Inducible ventricular ectopy
	Bypass tracts

dP/dt, Derivative of pressure (dP) with respect to time (dt); *LV,* left ventricular; *P-V,* pressure-volume; *QCA,* quantitative coronary angiography.

interpretation. Because of time constraints, these methods are typically performed off-line after data acquisition.

Quantitative Coronary Angiography

QCA can be performed using digital (or hand-held) calipers or, more commonly, computer-generated automated edge detection

Table 10.2

Additional Research Techniques in the Catheterization Laboratory.

Left Ventricular Function	Methods
Pressure-Volume Relationships	
End systole	High-fidelity pressure
End diastole	LV volume
	LV gram (cineangiographic, digital)
	RV gram
	2D echocardiogram
	Impedance catheter
Wall Stress	
LV mass	Quantitative ventriculography
Diastolic function	High-fidelity pressure
	Doppler mitral inflow
Ventricular interaction	RV/LV high-fidelity pressures
Aortic impedance	Aortic flow velocity, high-fidelity pressure
Coronary Physiology	
Coronary blood flow, coronary reserve, coronary vasodilation (response to drugs)	Pharmacologic studies with papaverine, adenosine, acetylcholine
	Physiologic flow responses during interventional procedures, such as angioplasty or hemodynamic studies
Ischemia Testing	
Induced tachycardia	Electrophysiologic study
Isoproterenol, dopamine	Pharmacologic infusion
Transient coronary occlusion	Coronary angioplasty

2D, Two-dimensional; *LV,* left ventricular; *RV,* right ventricular.

systems. For exact measurements, image calibration is required from an object with known dimensions, most commonly a contrast-filled coronary catheter. The catheter image is enlarged for measurement of its diameter to generate a calibration factor (millimeters/pixel) that is used to calculate vessel lumen size. QCA software then examines brightness values in the area of interest and uses digital algorithms to calculate vessel diameter from automatic border detection from operator-selected centerlines.

Commonly measured parameters from QCA are minimal lumen diameter (MLD), reference vessel diameter, acute lumen gain (final MLD–baseline MLD) after percutaneous coronary

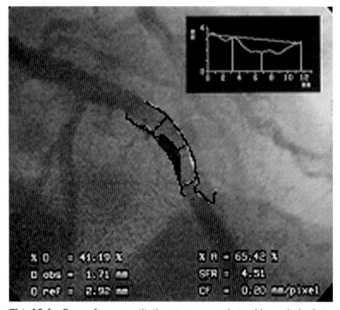

Fig. 10.1 Frame from quantitative coronary angiographic analysis. Automatic edge and center line are performed and dimensions calibrated against object (guide catheter) of known size.

intervention (PCI), late lumen loss (follow-up MLD–final MLD) after PCI, and percent diameter stenosis (Fig. 10.1).

Limitations of QCA, which can lead to data variability, include inconsistencies in image acquisition (e.g., vessel foreshortening, different imaging planes or magnification) and frame selection and differences in vessel tone among measurements. Significant discrepancy in distances from x-ray generator to calibration device (i.e., catheter) and to coronary vessel also leads to underestimation or overestimation of measurements. Precision can be improved with use of intracoronary (IC) vasodilators for maximal vasodilatation, complete contrast filling of the artery, and identical imaging equipment and planes among measurements.

Quantitative Ventriculography

Quantitative ventriculography is best performed with biplane imaging using a 60-degree straight left anterior oblique (LAO) projection and a 30-degree right anterior oblique (RAO) projection.

End-diastolic and end-systolic frames of a completely opacified ventricle during a normal sinus rhythm beat are examined using the centerline chord method. In this method, chords perpendicular to a centerline in a frame halfway between end-systolic and end-diastolic images are created and then normalized to the end-diastolic perimeter. Regional wall motion is quantified based on the degree of local chord shortening (positive values = hyperkinesis; negative values = hypokinesis) (Fig. 10.2).

Quantitative Coronary Flow
Doppler Coronary Flow Velocities

Coronary flow reserve (CFR; maximal coronary blood flow/resting coronary blood flow) is a global measure of coronary vasodilator circulatory capacity and is affected by epicardial and microvascular circulatory abnormalities (Fig. 10.3). It was historically measured by coronary sinus (CS) blood flow with the use of a continuous thermodilution technique. Currently, coronary flow is determined from IC arterial flow velocity using 0.014-inch Doppler-tipped sensor guidewires. In the Doppler technique, quantitative measurement of coronary flow is obtained from the use of pulsed sound waves (12 to 15 MHz) and measurement of the returning signal reflecting off moving red blood cells. The Doppler guidewire can also be coupled with a pressure sensor (Fig. 10.4) to measure simultaneous poststenotic coronary pressure and flow.

A pressure-temperature sensor-tipped guidewire also can be used to simultaneously measure FFR (by coronary pressure) and CFR (by coronary thermodilution) with calculation of the index of microvascular resistance (IMR). Measurement of physiologic response of coronary circulation to various drugs, maneuvers, and interventions, as well as assessment of the significance of coronary obstructive lesions before and after revascularization are examples of useful applications (Box 10.1). Measurement of volumetric changes in coronary blood flow can be combined with measurement of myocardial oxygen consumption (arterial and CS blood) to identify whether increases in blood flow are caused by increased myocardial oxygen demand (i.e., metabolic regulation) or pharmacologic changes independent of myocardial demand (e.g., primary artery vasodilation or constriction).

Doppler Methodology and Setup

Setting up the Doppler wire system usually takes less than 10 minutes. Timing of the reflected sound waves is used to measure blood flow velocities from moving red blood cells in a sample area that

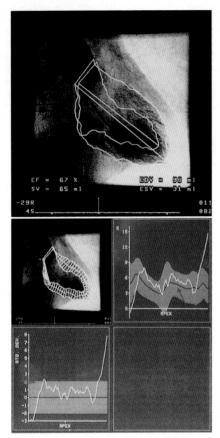

Fig. 10.2 Quantitative left ventriculographic wall motion analysis. Normal left ventricular (LV) wall motion shows concentric inward motion of all LV wall segments. *Bottom:* Chords and deviation from midline. The centerline method of regional wall motion analysis uses end-diastolic and end-systolic LV endocardial contours. *Bottom, lower panel:* A centerline is constructed by the computer midway between the two contours. Motion is measured along 100 chords constructed perpendicular to the centerline. Motion at each chord is normalized by the end-diastolic perimeter to yield a shortening fraction. Motion along each chord is plotted for the patient *(single red arrow)*. Mean motion in the normal ventriculogram group *(double red arrow)* and one standard deviation *(STD. DEV.)* above and below the mean *(dotted line)* are shown for comparison. Wall motion also is plotted as the difference in units of standard deviations from the normal mean *(right panel)*. The normal ventriculogram group mean is represented by the horizontal zero line *(below left)*. *EDV,* End-diastolic volume; *EF,* ejection fraction; *ESV,* end-systolic volume; *SV,* stroke volume.

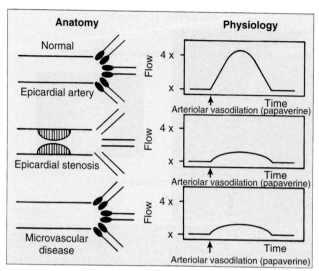

Fig. 10.3 Normal epicardial coronary artery and microvascular bed and coronary vasodilatory reserve (CVR) responses. When both components are normal, CVR is normal. CVR can be abnormal as a result of epicardial artery narrowing or microvascular disease. (From Wilson RF. Assessment of the human coronary circulation using a Doppler catheter. *Am J Cardiol.* 1991;67:44D-56D.)

is 5 mm from the tip of the wire (and 2 mm across)—far enough away so that blood velocity is not affected by the wake of the wire. The returning signal is transmitted in real time to the display console. A gray-scale spectral scrolling display shows velocities of all red blood cells within the sample volume. Key parameters are derived from automatically tracked peak blood velocities, making them less sensitive to position (Fig. 10.5).

The Doppler guidewire has a forward-directed ultrasound beam that diverges in a 27-degree arc from the long axis (measured in the −6-dB round-trip points of the ultrasound beam pattern). A pulse repetition frequency of >40 Hz, pulse duration of +0.83 seconds, and sampling delay of 6.5 seconds are standard for clinical use. The system is coupled to a real-time spectrum analyzer, videocassette recorder, and video page printer. The spectrum analyzer uses online fast Fourier transformation to process the Doppler audio signals. Simultaneous electrocardiographic and arterial pressure data are also displayed (Fig. 10.6). In vivo testing has demonstrated excellent correlation of the Doppler

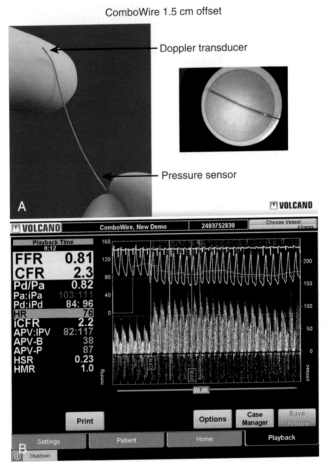

Fig. 10.4 **(A)** Combination pressure and flow sensor guidewire. The pressure sensor is located at the junction between the soft radiopaque portion and the stiff portion of the guidewire. The Doppler crystal is at the distal tip of the wire. **(B)** Panel from display for simultaneous coronary pressure flow recordings. *APV,* Average peak velocity; *APV-B,* average peak velocity base; *APV-P,* average peak velocity peak; *CFR,* coronary flow reserve; *FFR,* fractional flow reserve; *HMR,* hyperemic microvascular resistance; *HR,* heart rate; *HSR,* hyperemic stenosis resistance; *Pa,* aortic pressure; *Pd,* distal coronary pressure; *Pd/Pa,* pressure ratio. (Courtesy Volcano Corporation, Rancho Cordova, CA.)

Box 10.1   Uses of the Doppler FloWire.[a]

CVR assessment
   Syndrome X
   Transplant coronary arteriopathy
Collateral flow studies
Coronary flow research studies
   Pharmacologic and endothelial function studies
   Intraaortic balloon pumping
   Coronary physiology of vascular disease
   Ischemic test correlation

CVR, Coronary vasodilatory reserve.
[a]FloWire Doppler Guide Wire (Volcano Corporation, Rancho Cordova, CA)

guidewire–measured velocity with electromagnetic measurements of flow velocity and volumetric flow.

Proper engagement of the coronary ostium with a guiding catheter is key to assure the administration of the entire specified amount of any drug to be given. Before the Doppler guidewire is placed into an artery, the patient should be given intravenous (IV) heparin (40 to 60 U/kg with target activated coagulation time >200 seconds). After diagnostic angiography or during angioplasty, the Doppler guidewire is passed through a standard angioplasty Y connector attached to a guiding catheter. The guidewire is advanced into the artery and beyond the target location (e.g., stenosis) by a distance equal or greater than 5 to 10 times the arterial diameter (~2 cm). Avoid placement in any side branches. Obtain distal flow velocity data at rest and during hyperemia (Figs. 10.7 and 10.8).

It is important to note that Doppler coronary velocity measures only relative changes in velocity. Volumetric coronary flow is calculated as velocity (cm/s) multiplied by vessel area (cm²). For measurement of absolute blood flow, the following assumptions must be made:

1. The cross-sectional area of the vessel being studied remains fixed during hyperemia.
2. The vessel lumen is cylindrical with a velocity profile that is not distorted by arterial disease.
3. The angle between the crystal and sample volume remains constant and <30 degrees from the horizontal flow stream.

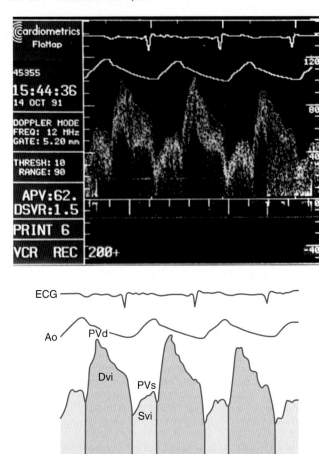

Fig. 10.5 Normal coronary flow velocity spectra showing small systolic and large diastolic velocity components. *Bottom:* Diagram of measurements shows a darkly hatched diastolic velocity integral *(Dvi)*, lightly hatched systolic velocity integral *(Svi)*, and peak systolic and diastolic velocities *(PVs and PVd,* respectively). The means of diastole and systole and total cycle variables can be computed. *Ao,* Aortic pressure; *APV,* average peak velocity (mean); *DSVR,* diastolic-to-systolic velocity ratio; *ECG,* electrocardiogram. (From Ofili EO, Kern MJ, Labovitz AJ, et al. Analysis of coronary blood flow velocity dynamics in angiographically normal and stenosed arteries before and after endolumen enlargement by angioplasty. *J Am Coll Cardiol.* 1993;21:308-316.)

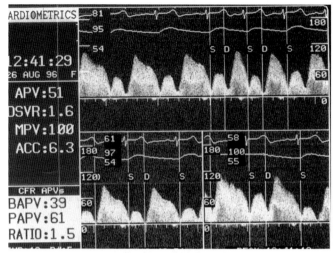

Fig. 10.6 Doppler flow velocity screen is split into continuous phasic signals *(top)* and base and hyperemic signal storage areas *(below)*. Electrocardiogram and aortic pressure are at the top of each signal area. Scale is 0 to 120 cm/s *(far right)*. *Upper left corner:* Numbers in dark boxes are heart rate and systolic and diastolic blood pressure. *ACC,* Acceleration; *APV,* average peak velocity; *BAPV,* base of average peak velocity; *CFR,* coronary flow reserve; *D,* diastolic marker; *DSVR,* diastolic-to-systolic velocity ratio; *MPV,* maximal peak velocity; *PAVP,* peak of average peak velocity; *S,* systolic marker.

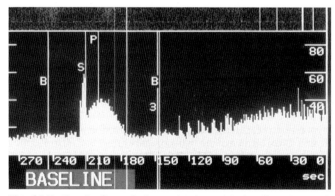

Fig. 10.7 Doppler flow velocity continuous trend plot of average peak velocity panel. Baseline value *(B)* is obtained. Intracoronary (IC) adenosine is injected (note artifact before search *[S]*). Hyperemia is stimulated and peak *(P)* hyperemia is captured and stored.

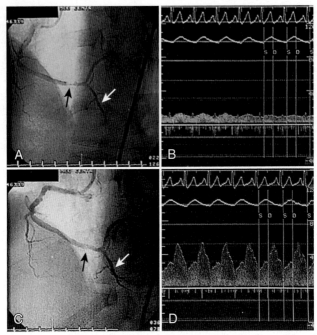

Fig. 10.8   Distal coronary flow velocity before **(A)** and after **(C)** successful percutaneous transluminal coronary balloon angioplasty of the distal right coronary artery (90% stenosis). **(B)** Distal prepercutaneous transluminal coronary balloon angioplasty flow velocity is 12 cm/s with reduced phasic pattern. **(D)** After percutaneous transluminal coronary balloon angioplasty, the mean flow velocity is 35 cm/s with a normal phasic pattern. *Black arrows:* Percutaneous transluminal coronary balloon angioplasty sites. *White arrows:* Doppler guidewire sample volume location.

Coronary Flow Reserve

Hyperemic measurements are obtained by IC injections of adenosine (30 to 50 mcg in the right coronary artery and 50 to 100 mcg in the left coronary artery). It is important to give doses high enough to induce complete vasodilation. Some protocols use ultra-high doses of adenosine (>200 mcg); however, the incremental benefit of these larger doses is unproven. Guide catheter position (i.e., avoid suboptimal selective engagement into the coronary artery and disengagement with very forceful manual injection) is critical to accuracy.

Table 10.3

Physiologic Criteria Associated with Clinical Applications.				
Indication	CFR	iFR	HSRv[a]	FFR
Ischemia detection	<2.0	<0.89	>0.8	<0.75
Deferred angioplasty	>2.0	<0.89	—	>0.80
Endpoint of angio- plasty	>2.0 to 2.5[b]	—	—	>0.90
Endpoint of stenting	—	—	—	>0.90

From Kern MJ, Lerman A, Bech JW, et al: Physiological assessment of coronary artery disease in the cardiac catheterization laboratory: a scientific statement from the American Heart Association Committee on Diagnostic and Interventional Cardiac Catheterization, Council on Clinical Cardiology. *Circulation.* 2006;114:1321–1341.
  iFR, instantaneous wave free ratio; *FFR,* fractional flow reserve; *HSRv,* hyperemic stenosis resistance index; *rCFR,* relative coronary vasodilatory reserve.
  [a]Measured in mm Hg/cm/s.
  [b]With <35% diameter stenosis.

CFR is computed as the ratio of hyperemic and basal mean flow velocities. A normal CFR is >2.0. Comparisons of CFR and FFR for detection of ischemia based on noninvasive testing as a gold standard are shown in Table 10.3.

Measurement of Collateral Circulation

Coronary collateral flow can be measured with the use of the Doppler-tipped flow wire (Fig. 10.9) and pressure wire. Before placing the wire in the patient, a 0.014-inch pressure wire is set at 0 (atmosphere), calibrated, and advanced through a balloon catheter, and positioned in the vessel of interest. Collateral flow is measured by simultaneous measurement of mean aortic pressure (PAo; mm Hg), coronary occlusion pressure (Poccl; mm Hg), and central venous pressure (CVP; mm Hg). Collateral flow is calculated as (Poccl–CVP)/(PAo–CVP).

Translesional Hemodynamics

Although the hemodynamics of coronary flow can be assessed by Doppler flow velocity as described earlier, there are instances in which it is also important to examine translesional pressure at rest and at hyperemia.

Fractional Flow Reserve

In clinical practice, the ischemic potential of a questionable or intermediate (40% to 70%) stenosis can be determined by FFR.

LAD with collaterals

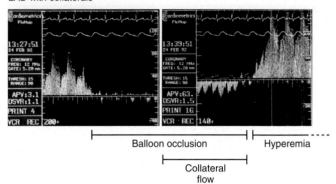

| Balloon occlusion | Hyperemia |

Collateral flow

Fig. 10.9 Time sequence of flow velocity during coronary balloon occlusion in a patient with a left anterior descending *(LAD)* coronary artery filled with collaterals originating from the right coronary artery. Note the retrograde collateral flow velocity below the baseline in a phasic pattern, appearing after 15 seconds of coronary occlusion. On release of balloon occlusion, immediate anterograde hyperemia can be observed in the distal bed with a loss of the retrograde flow pattern, corresponding with successful angioplasty. *APV,* Average peak velocity (mean); *DSVR,* diastolic-to-systolic velocity ratio. (From Kern MJ, Donohue TJ, Bach RG, et al. Quantitating coronary collateral flow velocity in patients during coronary angioplasty using a Doppler guidewire. *Am J Cardiol.* 1993;71:34D-40D.)

FFR is computed as the ratio of aortic pressure (from the guide catheter) to poststenotic pressure measured from a pressure guidewire placed beyond the stenosis at rest followed by hyperemia (adenosine IV infusion or IC bolus). The technique of FFR for clinical practice is described in detail in Chapter 6.

For research into coronary hemodynamics, note that FFR can be subdivided into three components describing the flow contributions by the coronary artery, myocardium, and collateral supply. FFR of the coronary artery (FFR_{cor}) is defined as the maximum coronary artery flow in the presence of a stenosis divided by the theoretic normal maximum flow of the same artery (i.e., the maximum flow in that artery if no stenosis were present). Similarly, FFR of the myocardium (FFR_{myo}) is defined as maximum myocardial (artery and bed) flow distal to an epicardial stenosis divided by its value if no epicardial stenosis were present. Stated another way, FFR represents that fraction of normal maximum flow that remains despite the presence of an epicardial lesion. Note that at maximal hyperemia, FFR_{cor} is about equal to FFR_{myo} because myocardial bed resistance is minimal. The difference between FFR_{myo} and FFR_{cor} is FFR of the collateral flow.

The following equations are used to calculate the FFR of a coronary artery and its dependent myocardium:

$$FFR_{cor} = (P_d - P_w)/(P_a - P_w)$$

$$FFR_{myo} = (P_d - P_v)/(P_a - P_v)$$

$$FFR_{collateral} = FFR_{myo} - FFR_{cor}$$

where P_a, P_d, P_v, and P_w are pressures of the aorta, distal artery, venous (or right atrial), and coronary wedge (during balloon occlusion) pressures, respectively. Because FFR_{cor} uses P_w, it can be calculated only during coronary angioplasty. In most clinical circumstances, P_v is negligible relative to aortic pressure and is omitted from calculations. P_v may be included when right atrial pressure is >10 mm Hg and may influence FFR ±0.02 units in patients with elevated right atrial pressure.

Microcirculatory Resistance

The IMR is defined as the ratio of distal coronary pressure to the inverse of mean transit time during maximal hyperemia. It is a quantitative index that is unique to the microcirculation and independent of epicardial coronary artery disease. IMR uses distal pressure and thermodilution flow obtained from a single pressure wire (St. Jude Medical, St. Paul, MN), as assessed by the inverse of the arrival (transit) time of a room-temperature saline bolus to the distal coronary artery segment (Fig. 10.10). By measuring the mean transit time at rest and comparing it with the mean transit time at peak hyperemia, a thermodilution CFR can be calculated. Although CFR has been studied in microvascular dysfunction, IMR is superior to CFR, because it is not affected by resting hemodynamics, making it more reproducible, even after hemodynamic perturbations. When measured immediately after primary PCI for ST-segment elevation myocardial infarction (STEMI), IMR predicts the amount of myocardial damage and left ventricular (LV) recovery better than other indices, such as CFR, ST-segment resolution, or Thrombolysis in Myocardial Infarction (TIMI) Study Group myocardial perfusion grade, and is an independent predictor of long-term clinical outcomes including death and rehospitalization for heart failure.

Another calculation of coronary hemodynamics, hyperemic microvascular resistance (HMR), is defined as the ratio of mean distal coronary pressure to flow velocity at hyperemia. When

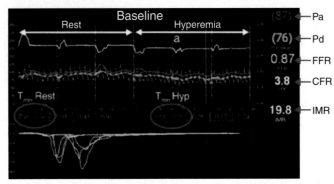

Fig. 10.10 Simultaneous measurement of pressure and flow (by thermodilution). *Top:* Proximal *(Pa)* and distal *(Pd)* pressures at rest *(left)* and during hyperemia *(right)*. *Bottom:* Thermodilution curves at rest and during hyperemia, with associated average transit times at baseline and hyperemia circled. These values are used to calculate coronary flow reserve *(CFR)* and the index of microcirculatory resistance *(IMR)* (right). *FFR*, Fractional flow reserve. (From Martin KC, Yeung AC, Fearon WF. Invasive assessment of the coronary microcirculation. Circulation 2006;113:2054-2061.)

compared with actual microvascular resistance, HMR is overestimated in the presence of coronary stenosis because of the absence of coronary collateral flow input. HMR is reflective of an increase in actual myocardial resistance, identifying a pertinent pathophysiologic alteration in microvasculature. The status of coronary microcirculation plays a role in determining susceptibility toward periprocedural myocardial infarction (MI) during elective PCI and may guide adjunctive preventive therapies.

Nonhyperemic Indices

Use of an adenosine-free or adenosine-independent pressure-derived index of coronary stenosis severity is a desirable feature among those working in the cardiac catheterization laboratory. The assessment of stenosis severity by FFR requires that coronary resistance is stable and minimal, usually achieved by the administration of adenosine. Sen et al. used wave-intensity analysis to identify a period in the cardiac cycle during which equilibration or balance between pressure waves moving forward and reflecting back from the aorta and distal microcirculatory ceased in a portion of diastole called the *wave-free period*. This wave-free period begins at 75% of diastole and ends immediately before systole. The microvascular resistance in this period is fixed and potentially has

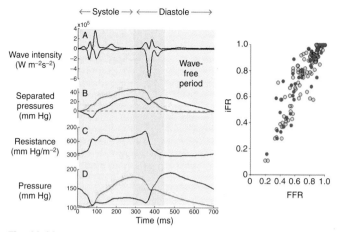

Fig. 10.11 Wave-intensity analysis *(A)* demonstrates proximal and micro-circulatory (distal) originating waves generated during the cardiac cycle. A wave-free period can be seen in diastole when no new waves are generated *(left panel, shaded, most right).* This corresponds to a time period in which there is minimal microcirculatory (distal)-originating pressure *(B),* minimal and constant resistance *(C),* and a nearly constant rate of change in flow velocity *(D).* (Separated pressure above diastole is the residual pulsatile separated pressure component after subtraction of diastolic pressure.) *FFR,* Fractional flow reserve; *iFR,* instantaneous wave-free ratio. *Right panel*: comparison of FFR vs. iFR. (Data from Davies JE, et al. *Circulation.* 2006;113:1767-1778; Sen S, Escaned J, Malik IS, et al. Development and validation of a new adenosine-independent index of stenosis severity from coronary wave-intensity analysis: results of the ADVISE [ADenosine Vasodilator Independent Stenosis Evaluation] study. *J Am Coll Cardiol.* 2012; 59:1392-1402.)

the ability to differentiate mild from severe lesions hemodynamically. Like FFR, the ratio of proximal to distal coronary pressures during the wave-free period, called the *instantaneous wave-free ratio (iFR)*, provides a measure of lesion significance (Fig. 10.11). In several studies (ADVISE, REVISE, and RESOLVE), the iFR and resting distal coronary pressure (Pd)/aortic pressure (Pa) ratio have been shown to correlate closely with FFR ($r = 0.90$) and thus may obviate the need for hyperemic stimulus in selected patients. In the RESOLVE study, which examined 1974 lesions, the optimal iFR to predict an FFR <0.8 was 0.92, with accuracy of 80%. For the resting Pd/Pa ratio, the cutpoint was 0.92, with an overall accuracy of 92% and no significant differences between iFR and Pd/Pa. Both measures have 90% accuracy in predicting positive or negative FFR in 65% and 48% of lesions, respectively (Fig. 10.12). These data

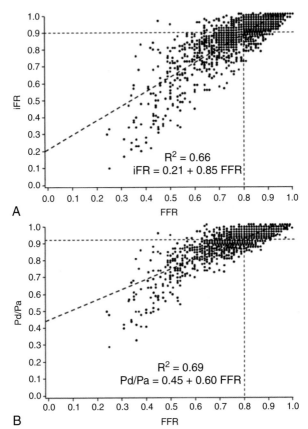

Fig. 10.12 Scatter plots show the relationship between instantaneous wave-free ratio *(iFR)* and fractional flow reserve *(FFR)* and distal coronary pressure *(Pd)*/aortic pressure *(Pa)* ratio and FFR. *Dashed lines:* Lines of best fit. **(A)** *Horizontal dashed line:* Optimal iFR cutoff of 0.90 on the basis of receiver-operating characteristic (ROC) analysis. **(B)** *Horizontal dashed line:* Optimal Pd/Pa cutoff of 0.92. R_2 regression value. The wave-free period was calculated using a fully automated algorithm. The iFR, calculated by dividing the mean Pd by Pa during the wave-free period under basal conditions, was found to agree closely with the FFR (r = 0.9, P = 0.001). **(A)** and **(B)** *Right, dotted lines:* Threshold cutoff values for the iFR and FFR. R^2, Ratio squared. (From Jeramias A, Maehara A, Genereux P, et al. Multi-center core laboratory comparison of the Instantaneous wave-free ratio and resting Pd/Pa with fractional flow reserve: the RESOLVE study. *J Am Coll Cardiol.* 2014;63:1253-1261.)

suggest that resting indices of lesion severity demonstrated an overall accuracy, with an FFR of approximately 80%, which can be improved to 90% in a subset of lesions. Clinical outcome studies, currently in progress, are required to determine whether use of iFR or Pd/Pa might obviate the need for hyperemia in selected patients.

Endothelial Function Assessment

The endothelium is the innermost lining of all blood vessels, composed of a single layer of endothelial cells that fulfill a number of important functions for vascular biology. Normal endothelial function is responsible for control of coronary blood flow through appropriate signaling to the arterial vascular smooth muscle to dilate or to constrict and has a second function of regulating vascular thrombosis through release of antithrombin and antiplatelet factors to deter inappropriate clot formation on the vessel walls. Dysfunction of the endothelium resulting in pathologic vasomotion and thrombus formation is a result of multiple etiologies, many of which also are implicated in the pathogenesis of atherosclerosis. The presence of endothelial dysfunction has been associated with increased risk for cardiac events, even in the presence of angiographically normal-appearing coronary arteries.

The assessment of status of endothelial function requires an infusion catheter containing the Doppler wire. This system is placed in the artery using standard techniques (usually the proximal left anterior descending [LAD] artery). Following baseline measurements of flow (i.e., velocity via the Doppler wire multiplied by area via the quantitative measurement of the coronary diameter), graduated infusions of acetylcholine (10^{-6} M to 10^{-4} M) are administered directly into the coronary artery.

In patients with normal endothelial function, acetylcholine infusion causes endothelial-dependent production of nitric oxide and results in vasodilatation (i.e., epicardial vasodilatation and/or increase in Doppler flow velocity; Fig. 10.13). Conversely, in patients with dysfunctional endothelia, coronary flow either fails to increase or decreases because of vasoconstriction, which manifests either as blunting of the rise or an actual fall in Doppler flow velocity. Changes in the Doppler flow pattern can also be caused by vasoconstriction of the epicardial vessel, which would be an equally abnormal (paradoxical) response. QCA is used to differentiate between epicardial and microvascular endothelial dysfunction. Nitroglycerin is given at the end of the procedure to reverse any constriction of the larger vessels. It may not, however, reverse profound vasoconstriction of the distal vasculature, which may require nitroprusside. Administering calcium channel blockers

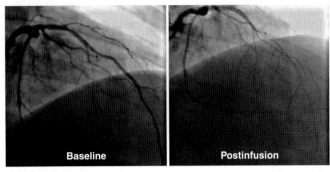

Fig. 10.13 Assessment of endothelial function with acetylcholine infusion. *Left:* Baseline angiography of the left coronary artery. *Right:* Severe vasoconstriction of the left anterior descending (LAD) artery following infusion of acetylcholine (usual dose 10^{-6} to 10^{-4} mol/L).

(usually verapamil) can also be an alternative for refractory vasoconstriction.

The most commonly used agent to determine endothelium-independent vasorelaxation is adenosine, which is given before administration of acetylcholine (alternatives include dipyridamole and papaverine). In the past, additional agents to test endothelium-dependent vasorelaxation included bradykinin, substance P, and calcium ionophore.

Other techniques to study vasoreactivity involve complex neurovascular mechanisms, such as cold pressure and mental stress testing. Atrial pacing and exercise can also be used to study the endothelium-dependent, flow-related response to increase in myocardial oxygen demand. All of these studies can be combined with other tests (such as blood sampling for metabolic parameters, multilead electrocardiograms, or [speckle tracking] echocardiograms) to assess, for instance, the association among vasoreactivity, myocardial ischemia, and symptoms.

As indicted earlier, with specific catheters, IMR can be calculated as the distal coronary pressure divided by the inverse of the hyperemic mean transit time measured simultaneously. This index was validated in experimental models but limitations need to be entertained if this technique is applied. For instance, any collateral blood flow has to be incorporated into the calculations (by multiplying IMR by the ratio of coronary FFR and myocardial FFR), because IMR will otherwise progressively increase with increasing degrees of epicardial coronary artery stenoses (as seen with studies using Doppler-derived FFR).

For any of these functional studies, cessation of drugs and stimulants (e.g., coffee) that might influence the results is important, especially for the validity of research protocols. Anxiety and sedation can also have an effect, which needs to be taken into consideration.

Invasive Coronary Imaging for Research

Intravascular Ultrasound

High-frequency, two-dimensional (2D) IVUS imaging uses catheters of ≤2.9 F with either mechanically or electronically rotating 20- to 40-MHz echo crystals that produce cross-sectional images of the artery (Fig. 10.14). (See Chapter 6 for additional information about IVUS.) Ultrasound catheters are introduced over guidewires in a monorail fashion, followed by image acquisition during manual or automated (0.5 to 1.0 mm/s) pull back. In mildly diseased or normal arteries, a characteristic three-layered image is usually observed. These images are more accurate than those using angiography for characterizing the amount of atherosclerosis as well as identifying other characteristics, such as lipid pool and calcium. IVUS can also reveal remodeling patterns, in which there is either an increase or a decrease in vessel size with atherosclerotic plaque growth. Indeed, the technique has revealed important differences among patient groups, such as between diabetics and nondiabetics. For patients who have undergone or are planning to undergo placement of IC stents, IVUS can be used to assess reference vessel diameter and stent expansion. Nowadays, research studies using this tool are investigating the in vivo characterization of atherosclerotic plaque, progression and regression of atherosclerosis, responses to new pharmacologic agents, and results of percutaneous interventional techniques.

Gray-scale IVUS can characterize the extent and distribution of atherosclerotic plaques. However, the low echo frequency of tissue representing the composition of lipid-containing and mixed plaque is not well defined by gray-scale IVUS.

Using spectral analysis and Fourier transforms of the radiofrequency (RF), ultrasound backscatter signals produce images known as *virtual histology (VH)*, which permit tissue level assessment of plaque composition. VH IVUS technology (Volcano Corporation, Rancho Cordova, CA) has been shown to have an 80% to 92% in vitro accuracy to identify the four different types of atherosclerotic plaques (e.g., fibrous, fibrofatty, dense calcium, and necrotic core). Validation of atherosclerotic coronary plaques by

Normal LAD transplant

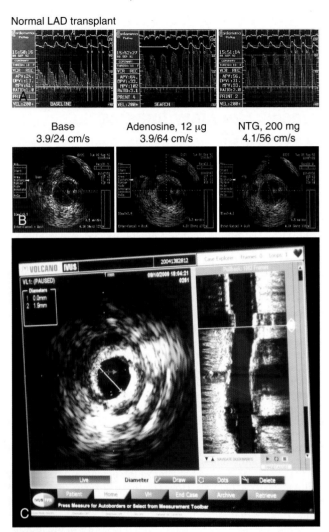

| Base
3.9/24 cm/s | Adenosine, 12 µg
3.9/64 cm/s | NTG, 200 mg
4.1/56 cm/s |

Fig. 10.14 Simultaneously obtained Doppler guidewire flow velocity signals **(A)** and IVUS coronary lumen dimensions **(B)**. **(B)** Cross-sectional artery images show a normal lumen with a diameter of 3.9 mm and minimal changes to adenosine or nitroglycerin *(NTG)*. **(C)** Intravascular ultrasound *(IVUS)* display screen in catheterization laboratory. *APV,* Average peak velocity; *DPVi,* diastolic peak velocity integral; *LAD,* left anterior descending artery; *MPV,* maximal peak velocity; *Ratio,* coronary reserve ratio; *VEL,* velocity scale.

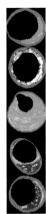

1. Fibrotic

2. Fibrocalcific

3. Pathological intimal thickening

4. Thick cap fibroatheroma

5. VH–thin cap fibroatheroma
   (presumed to be high risk)

Fig. 10.15 Images of virtual histology *(VH)* by intravascular ultrasound (IVUS) for five atherosclerotic pathologies.

VH is based on mathematical autoregressive spectral analysis of IVUS backscattered data. The presence of fibrous, fibrofatty, necrotic core, and dense calcium areas are assessed within the histologic region of target plaque using RF data collection scans. Fibrous areas are designated as green, fibrofatty as yellow, dense calcium as white, and necrotic core as red. The predicted plaque composition is displayed as a color-coded tissue map. IVUS signals, processed by discrete Fourier transforms, result in high resolution of spectral estimates. Figure 10.15 shows VH images and the corresponding histology of coronary atherosclerosis.

Optical Coherence Tomography

Optical coherence tomography (OCT) is a catheter-based imaging system that uses near-infrared (NIR) light (wavelengths of 1250 to 1350 nm) to produce high-resolution, in vivo, real-time images of coronary arteries. In this technique, a fiberoptic wire (0.019-inch diameter) emits light and records reflection during rotation and pull back within the artery. The glass fibers that transmit the light for imaging constitute a fiberoptic array with a distal lens that serves to focus the transmitted light. Advantages of OCT are high axial (12 to 18 μm) and lateral (20 to 90 μm) resolution in comparison with IVUS (150 to 300 μm) as well as relatively faster pull back capability (20 to 40 mm/s) with newer-generation systems. OCT requires a blood-free zone, which can be accomplished with

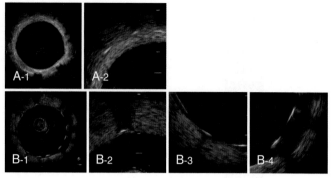

Fig. 10.16 Images from optical coherent imaging system after drug-eluting stent implantation. **(A-1)** Optical coherence tomography (OCT) image immediately after stent implantation. Struts are visible with shadows at 4 o'clock and 6 o'clock positions. **(A-2)** Magnified view of stent strut covered by endothelium. **(B-1)** Stent malapposed to vessel with evident struts at distance from vessel wall at 3 o'clock to 6 o'clock positions. **(B-2, B-3,** and **B-4)** Magnified sections of **B-1** showing apposed and unopposed struts. (From Kubo T, Imanishi T, Kitabata H, et al. Comparison of vascular response after sirolimus-eluting stent implantation between patients with unstable and stable angina pectoris: a serial optical coherence tomography study. *JACC Cardiovasc Imaging.* 2008;1:475-484.)

either balloon occlusion and saline infusion or, in systems with faster pull back, brief contrast bolus injections (~4 mL/s) (Fig. 10.16).

Current OCT systems allow tissue penetration of 1.5 to 3.5 mm (versus 4 to 8 mm with IVUS). OCT can be used to identify and to delineate thin fibrous caps, calcium, vessel dissection, and thrombus with high resolution. For PCI patients, the high resolution of OCT also allows detailed imaging of stent apposition and the degree of neointimal tissue coverage of stent struts (see Fig. 10.16). In fact, this technique has yielded important new insight in this regard.

Angioscopy

Coronary angioscopy (Fig. 10.17), which allows direct visualization of the internal surface of a vessel, provides information about the pathology of coronary lesions and the pathophysiology of acute coronary syndromes. The coronary angioscope (Vecmova, Clinical Supply Co., Gifu, Japan) uses a fiberoptic core advanced through a delivery catheter over a wire to the coronary artery. A soft atraumatic latex balloon on the delivery catheter is inflated to occlude

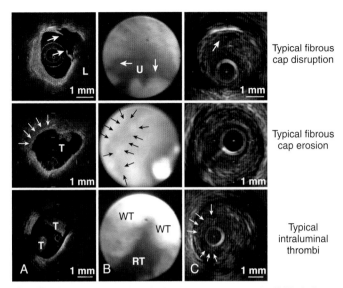

Typical fibrous cap disruption

Typical fibrous cap erosion

Typical intraluminal thrombi

Fig. 10.17 Corresponding optical coherence tomography (OCT) *(column* **A**), angioscopy *(column* **B**), and gray-scale intravascular ultrasound (IVUS) *(column* **C**). *Top row* shows typical fibrous cap disruption *(arrows)*, *middle row* shows plaque (surface) erosion *(arrows)*, and *bottom row* shows intraluminal thrombi *(arrow)*. (From Kubo T, Imanishi T, Takarada S, et al. Assessment of culprit lesion morphology in acute myocardial infarction: ability of optical coherence tomography compared with intravascular ultrasound and coronary angioscopy. (L = lipid-rich plaque, U = ulceration, WT = white thrombus, RT = red thrombus) *J Am Coll Cardiol.* 2007;50:933-939.)

blood flow. Blood is then cleared away from view with injection of 5 to 10 mL saline. Angioscopy has been demonstrated to be safe and feasible in human coronary arteries during cardiac catheterization. It provides a full color, three-dimensional (3D) image of the coronary artery internal vessel surface and can be used to assess plaques that have ruptured or are involved with thrombus. The current generation of angioscopes has excellent image resolution and increased flexibility, allowing better examination of complex and vulnerable lesions. However, several limitations to performing angioscopy exist. Angioscopy can only visualize the surface of the vessel without imaging below the very thin intima. Plaque composition can only be inferred from the intensity of the yellow color. The yellow plaque is confirmed indirectly by histology to be lipid-rich vulnerable plaque. Visualization of proximal blood vessel segments is limited because of the need for a sufficient landing zone beyond the left main artery for the occluding balloon. Distal vessel segments are also not readily visualized. Finally, balloon occlusion can lead to myocardial ischemia.

Near-Infrared Spectroscopy Coronary Imaging System

Invasive imaging of the coronary artery with IVUS provides a detailed anatomic quantitative description. VH can be produced by the analysis of RF backscatter signals applying Fourier transforms and statistical validations for four tissue histologies. Color-coding the VH signals permits identification of thin cap fibroatheroma as well as other more stable plaque types (Fig. 10.18).

In a manner similar to VH, NIR wavelength light can be used to detect cholesterol content in a vessel, another component intimately associated with vulnerable coronary plaques. The NIR LipiScan catheter uses the basic principle of spectroscopy, a technique used by chemists to identify molecules based on their distinct spectroscopic signature. Using this principle, the catheter has a fiberoptic core reflecting laser light at a specific wavelength trained at linoleic acid, the major chemical constituent of cholesterol within plaques. The fiberoptic core transmits NIR light and is used in a manner analogous to an IVUS catheter. An automatic pull back device pulls the infrared catheter within the artery from distal to proximal during the scanning for cholesterol. As the spectrum of light goes through the blood and into the vessel wall, its reflection is collected and analyzed. Because the vessel wall absorbs some of the spectra, the spectroscopic signature is a function of the light sent out and light returned (the difference is the absorbed light). Cholesterol signal is designated as yellow and nonlipid as red or black. No signal is white. The LipiScan console performs several functions. In brief, it provides (1) NIR light source for spectroscopy, (2) data-processing system that analyzes the signals returned from the pull back interface, (3) user interface to the system, (4) means of data storage, and (5) communication to the pull back interface that drives the automated scanning of the LipiScan coronary imaging catheter core. The console consists of the following major components: laser and laser delivery system, computer system and software, and power module.

This technique provides a "chemographic" map of cholesterol deposits within the artery, displayed as if the artery had been laid open and spread out from distal to proximal. The chemogram is based on an algorithm that quantitates the likelihood of a lipid-core plaque in any particular 2-mm block of vessel. The chemogram is color-coded, with bright yellow indicating a greater than 90% likelihood of a lipid-core plaque and red indicating no evidence of lipid-core plaque. The chemogram approach was

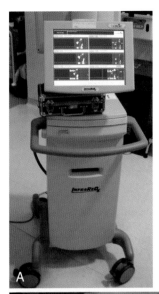

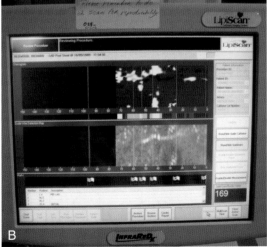

Fig. 10.18 **(A)** LipiScan console with display screen, enclosed computer, and attached cable to the automatic pull back interface device, which transmits near-infrared (NIR) catheter signals into the console for analysis. **(B)** Close-up of LipiScan display screen showing low-cholesterol *(red)* and high-cholesterol *(yellow)* content inside vessel. (Reproduced with permission from Infraredx, Inc.)

validated in an autopsy study. The Food and Drug Administration (FDA) has approved the LipiScan catheter for the detection of lipid-core plaques. The risks and limitations of the LipiScan catheter are similar to those of the IVUS catheter.

Combined Hemodynamic and Echocardiographic Modalities

Although cardiac catheterization provides gold-standard data regarding intracardiac pressures, essential data regarding chamber volumes are lacking in commonly used catheter systems. Simultaneous 2D echocardiography can provide volumetric data, in addition to tissue Doppler imaging for characterization of ventricular motion. An advantage of echocardiography is the potential for continuous observation of LV chamber size, geometry, wall motion, and beat-to-beat changes in flow during study interventions without additional radiation.

Some echocardiographic machines used for studies in the cardiac catheterization laboratory can be modified to accept pressure and other signals from the physiologic recorder (Figs. 10.19 and 10.20). Specialized input amplifiers for echocardiographic

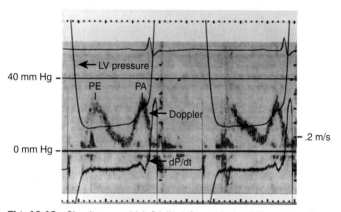

Fig. 10.19 Simultaneous high-fidelity left ventricular *(LV)* pressure (0- to 40-mm Hg scale) superimposed on Doppler echocardiogram, showing peak early *(PE)* and peak atrial *(PA)* filling waves of mitral valve inflow. Superimposed is the dP/dt signal from LV pressure tracing and the electrocardiogram. These combined methods permit analysis of function that is not available with a single technique. *dP/dt,* Derivative of pressure (dP) with respect to time (dt).

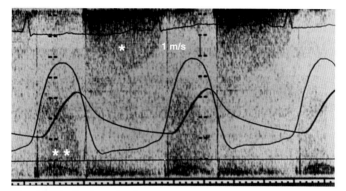

Fig. 10.20 Aortic and left ventricular (LV) pressure superimposed on Doppler aortic flow velocity showing aortic stenosis and insufficiency characterized by the Doppler waveform. Aortic stenosis is superimposed on the systolic ejection gradient *(**)*, and aortic insufficiency can be observed over the diastolic period with reversed diastolic velocity observed *(*)*.

machines are available, facilitating the recording of pressures simultaneously with echocardiographic parameters. Use of Doppler echocardiography and simultaneous hemodynamics has advanced the understanding of cardiac function and provides a means of examining questions previously unanswered with the use of other techniques.

Myocardial Metabolism
Measurement of Specialized Blood Products

Transmyocardial (proximal aorta/coronary ostium and CS) blood sampling is used to study myocardial metabolism. Measurements of pyruvate, lactate, and oxygen extraction are the most common outputs. The transmyocardial extraction of drugs after systemic delivery can also be determined. Under normal circumstances, lactate is actively taken up in the myocardium and converted to pyruvate for subsequent oxidative metabolism, such that the gradient of lactate from CS to artery is positive. With ischemia, this gradient is reversed, and lactate accumulates in the CS blood.

Specialized collection tubes for various substances and heparinized syringes for oxygen blood samples should be prepared in advance so that the physician can pass the drawn blood quickly to the technicians for insertion into the collecting tubes. In addition to sample tube preparation, ice, a centrifuge, or a series of dilutional tubes may be required. These techniques are not complicated, but correct labeling and anticipation of which samples will be obtained at which point in the procedure reduce errors without unnecessarily prolonging the study.

Coronary Sinus Catheterization

CS catheterization can be performed with a superior or inferior central venous approach. The ostium of the CS is located inferior and posterior to the tricuspid valve. Suitable for cannulation of the CS are Amplatz left catheters or multipurpose coronary catheters. After careful insertion in the right atrium, the catheter is directed toward the tricuspid valve and in a posterior direction. Gentle medial advancement with a 1- to 2-mL flush of contrast medium enables the physician to know when the catheter has entered the CS. Ventricular ectopy indicates contact with the right ventricular wall or septum, which is corrected with withdrawal and advancement after slight rotation. The CS catheter is usually positioned in the anteroposterior view, with the catheter seen passing upward across the tricuspid valve and spine. In the LAO position, the catheter appears to be coming directly in plane toward the observer. In the RAO position, it should pass posterior and away from the ventricular apex (i.e., not into the right ventricle). Care should be taken not to cannulate the inferior cardiac vein and to avoid perforation of the CS, right ventricle, or atrium. Historically, dedicated CS thermodilution catheters were used to measure myocardial blood flow to solve for myocardial oxygen consumptions using the Fick method. However, these catheters are no longer available, and flow may be best assessed using a Doppler flow wire in an epicardial vessel.

High-Fidelity Micromanometers

Pressure data from standard fluid-filled catheter systems are sufficient for most clinical hemodynamic studies but suffer from well-recognized artifacts and suboptimal frequency-response to accurately assess ventricular properties in research studies. When high-fidelity data are required for hemodynamic assessment, micromanometer transducer-tipped catheter measurements are used. High-fidelity pressure measurements are useful for studies of cardiac contractility, diastolic relaxation, compliance, afterload reduction, and myocardial metabolism. High-fidelity pressures also may be combined with quantitative volume measurements to examine chamber function. Volumetric data can be acquired using ventricular angiography, simultaneous echocardiography, or, in specialized centers, a conductance catheter system.

Assessment of Systolic Function

Contractility represents the ability of the myocardial muscle to shorten or thicken against a load. Although ejection fraction (EF) is the most common clinical assessment of contractility in practice, it is highly dependent on ventricular afterload. For example, at the same level of contractility, EF steeply declines as afterload increases. Robust measures of chamber contractility must account for both afterload and preload.

The peak rate of pressure increase during isovolumic contraction (dP/dt_{max}, Fig. 10.21) is relatively afterload independent and

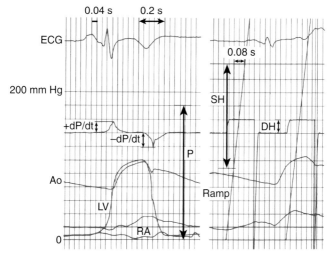

Fig. 10.21 High-fidelity, micromanometer-tipped hemodynamic tracings of aortic and left ventricular *(LV)* pressures with differentiated dP/dt signal showing method of calculation of dP/dt. See text for details. To compute dP/dt:
1. Slope height *(SH)*: mm deflection from ramp over 80 ms
2. Derivative height *(DH)*: mm deflection of square box of derivative
3. Compute K = (12.5 × SH)/DH
4. Scale factor P = mm paper deflection of 200 mm Hg
5. Compute dP/dt:

$$dP/dt = \frac{200 \text{ mm Hg}}{P}(K)$$

Peak dP/dt positive or negative deflection; normal value range: 1500 to 1800 mm Hg/s. *Ao*, Aortic pressure; *dP/dt*, derivative of pressure (dP) with respect to time (dt); *ECG*, electrocardiogram; *P*, paper height for 200 mm Hg; *RA*, right atrial pressure; *Ramp*, ramp from differentiator.

readily measured using a high-fidelity micromanometer, by taking the first derivative of pressure (dP) with respect to time (dt). dP/dt_{max} varies directly with preload, which limits its use during interventions that alter chamber filling volume, but it is very useful in detecting acute changes in chamber contractility where preload is relatively constant, such as with acute administration of cardiac resynchronization therapy. The preload sensitivity of dP/dt_{max} can be mitigated by indexing to instantaneous pressure, and an advantage of this parameter is the lack of a requirement for simultaneous volume assessment. dP/dt_{max} should not be estimated from fluid-filled catheters given their poor frequency response.

Other load-independent measures of contractility include stroke work index (SWI), preload-recruitable stroke work (PRSW), and end-systolic elastance (Ees; see Fig. 10.21). Stroke work is defined by the area subtended by the pressure-volume loop, quantifying the hydraulic work performed by the LV with each beat. This is often estimated in practice by the product of mean blood pressure and stroke volume. Similar to dP/dt_{max}, stroke work varies directly with preload, and dividing by left ventricular end-diastolic volume (LVEDV) makes SWI a relatively load-independent ejection measure of inotropy.

Conductance catheter systems are required for measurement of Ees and PRSW. These systems combine a high-fidelity pressure micromanometer with electrodes that measure the conductance of a small voltage difference between the tip of the catheter and specified proximal electrodes. The conductance between these sites varies with chamber volume, and, after calibration, it provides real-time measures of LV volume. Use of these methods requires specialized catheters and analysis systems but provides accurate data regarding ventricular systolic and diastolic function.

Measurement of Diastolic Function

In routine diagnostic catheterization, an elevated left ventricular end-diastolic pressure (LVEDP) in a normal-sized heart is often assumed to indicate a stiff ventricle from diastolic dysfunction. Although this assumption may often be true, it must be remembered that increased intrathoracic pressure, right-heart pressures, and pericardial restraint may each contribute to observed increases in LVEDP, particularly in patients with heart failure.

The gold-standard index of early diastolic relaxation is the time constant tau (τ) of LV pressure decay, which can be readily obtained during isovolumic relaxation (the time between aortic valve closure and mitral opening) using micromanometer catheters (Fig. 10.22). τ is typically <40 to 45 ms in a normal LV and is prolonged in patients with heart failure, cardiomyopathy, or

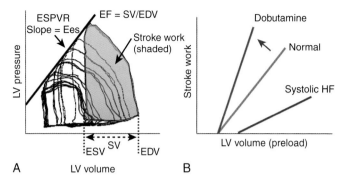

Fig. 10.22 Ventricular contractility in the pressure-volume plane is expressed by end-systolic elastance *(Ees)*, defined by the slope and intercept of the end-systolic pressure-volume relationship *(ESPVR)*. **(A)** Stroke work performed by the ventricle is represented by the area of the pressure-volume loop *(shaded area)*. Indexing stroke work to preload (end-diastolic volume *[EDV]*) provides a measure of contractility. The slope of the relationship between stroke work and EDV (preload-recruitable stroke work [PRSW]) is higher in normal hearts than in hearts of patients in systolic heart failure. **(B)** Adrenergic stimulation with dobutamine increases this slope, indicative of an increase in contractility. *EF,* Ejection fraction; *ESV,* end-systolic volume; *HF,* heart failure; *LV,* left ventricular; *SV,* stroke volume. (Modified from Borlaug BA, Kass DA. Invasive hemodynamic assessment in heart failure. *Heart Fail Clin.* 2009;5:217-228.)

hypertensive heart disease. The maximal rate of pressure drop (dP/dt$_{min}$) during isovolumic relaxation can be determined in a manner similar to that of dP/dt$_{max}$, as another measure of early relaxation. These indices should not be calculated from fluid-filled pressure data.

The so-called passive stiffness of the LV is more difficult to measure, because it requires simultaneous assessment of chamber pressure and volume to plot the curvilinear end-diastolic pressure-volume relationship (EDPVR; Figs. 10.22 and 10.23). An EDPVR that is shifted up and to the left indicates increased diastolic stiffness. The EDPVR from a single heartbeat may differ markedly from the curve measured at different preloads, and gold-standard measurement of the EDPVR ideally requires measuring pressure and volume during diastasis (where transmitral flow is zero), under a number of different preload states using a conductance catheter. This is usually performed with an inferior vena cava (IVC) occlusion catheter and is only done in highly specialized research protocols.

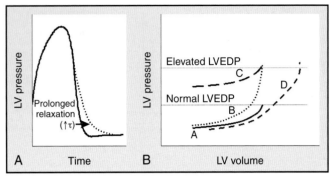

Fig. 10.23 **(A)** Kinetics of left ventricular *(LV)* relaxation are quantified by rate of pressure decay during isovolumic relaxation (the period between aortic valve closure and mitral valve opening). With prolonged relaxation (increased time constant τ), LV pressure remains elevated longer in early diastole. **(B)** The gold standard for assessing diastolic LV compliance relies on measuring curvilinear slope of the end-diastolic pressure-volume relationship (EDPVR). A steeper slope *(dotted line)*, shifted up and to the left, indicates decreased diastolic compliance compared with a normal EDPVR *(curve A)*. Elevated left ventricular end-diastolic pressure *(LVEDP)* may exist if the ventricle is stiffer *(curve B)*, overly filled with blood as in systolic heart failure *(curve D)*, or with enhanced external pressure as in pericardial constriction *(curve C)*. In most heart failure patients, some combination of each of these factors contributes. (Modified from Borlaug BA, Kass DA. Invasive hemodynamic assessment in heart failure. *Heart Fail Clin.* 2009;5:217-228.)

Exercise in the Catheterization Laboratory

Heart failure may be broadly defined as an inability of the heart to pump blood to the body commensurate with its metabolic needs or to do so only with elevated filling pressures. However, in patients without apparent volume overload (particularly with a normal EF), it is often difficult to discern whether symptoms of dyspnea or fatigue are caused by cardiovascular pathologies or other mechanisms, such as pulmonary disease, obesity, or deconditioning. Dynamic exercise can discern cardiac versus noncardiac sources of symptom limitation. Exercise evaluations help relate symptoms to hemodynamic changes reflective of cardiac dysfunction and can point toward noncardiac causes of dyspnea when hemodynamic responses are normal. Exercise may be dynamic or isometric—the former being more representative of activities of daily life and the latter being more feasible to perform in most catheterization laboratories.

In healthy young humans, upright exercise is associated with an increase in LV preload (end-diastolic volume [EDV]) with no change in LV filling pressure and decreases in end-systolic volume (ESV; increase in contractility). Enhanced diastolic filling is achieved by creation of a suction gradient during early diastole from LV apex to base, favoring rapid filling. In patients with coronary artery disease or heart failure, these reserve mechanisms may be insufficient to cope with stress, and LV filling pressure then increases with exercise. Although the definition of abnormal LV filling pressure with exercise has not been clearly agreed on, pulmonary capillary wedge pressures, left atrial pressures (in the absence of mitral stenosis), or LVEDPs of more than 25 mm Hg are considered by most to be elevated. The upper limit of normal probably varies with age, because prior studies of healthy elderly men without cardiovascular disease reported increases in pulmonary capillary wedge pressures during exercise to 17 ± 5 mm Hg in the absence of symptoms. Ideally, pressures are reported at end-expiration, where there is equalization between intrathoracic and atmospheric pressure, but automated systems generally use the mean of inspiration and expiration. The latter can disagree substantially with end-expiratory values in patients with morbid obesity or parenchymal lung disease, for which intrathoracic pressure swings are dramatic.

During exercise, cardiac output (CO) should increase in tandem with oxygen consumption. When oxygen delivery is insufficient to meet metabolic needs, increased extraction occurs, such that the arterial-venous difference increases and pulmonary artery saturation drops. The Dexter index has been suggested as one method to quantify what constitutes a "normal" CO response to exercise, where the predicted cardiac index (CI) is equal to $2.99 + 0.0059 \times$ (measured oxygen $[O_2]$ consumption index with exercise). This equation was derived from seven healthy volunteers studied by Dexter and colleagues. An abnormal CI response is present if the observed peak CI is $<80\%$ of that predicted by the Dexter formula. A related scheme relies on the "exercise factor": for every 100-mL/min increase in oxygen consumption with exercise, the CO should increase by at least 600 mL/min; thus, the normal exercise factor is ≥ 6. Numerous studies since those of Dexter have confirmed that the normal increase in CO relative to oxygen consumption is 6:1. A limitation for many laboratories is that this method requires simultaneous assessment of oxygen consumption, which is not available in most laboratories.

Dynamic Physical Exercise

Exercise hemodynamics may be measured in supine or upright positions depending on equipment availability and vascular access. There are a number of important differences between upright and supine exercise.

1. Ventricular EDV, EDP, and stroke volume are lower at rest when upright. Preload EDV is maximal at rest in the supine position and does not increase further with exercise. In contrast, with upright exercise, EDV does increase, with enhanced venous return.

2. Resting heart rate and diastolic arterial pressure are both higher when upright, whereas pulmonary artery and intracardiac filling pressures are lower.

3. Stroke volume increases 1.4-fold to twofold with maximal upright exercise and tends to increase proportionally more compared with supine because preload (EDV) starts from a lower rest level. Stroke volume increases less with supine exercise.

4. Exercise pulmonary artery and wedge pressures and stroke volumes are lower in the upright position, but the total exercise changes (i.e., exercise-baseline) are similar between upright and supine exercise.

The supine cycle ergometry exercise protocol used in the Mayo Clinic Catheterization Laboratory is as follows:

1. Resting hemodynamic data recordings are obtained with the patient supine and feet flat. A tight-fitting mask coupled to a metabolic cart with expiratory gas analyzer is used to measure ventilation, oxygen consumption, and carbon dioxide production. The metabolic measurements allow quantification of exercise capacity and CO by the Fick method.

2. Exercise begins at 20 Watts, followed by 10- to 20-Watt increases every 3 minutes until maximum tolerated workload. Heart rate is recorded continuously; and pressures in the pulmonary artery, wedge, and right atrium are recorded halfway through each stage. We use a 7-F catheter introduced through a 9-F sheath, with the side arm of the sheath transducing central venous right anterior pressures continuously. If expired gas analysis is performed, the CO may be determined by the Fick method. If oxygen consumption cannot be measured, thermodilution CO should be used, because the Fick method cannot be used during exercise without simultaneous gas analysis (oxygen consumption increases several-fold during exercise). It is often difficult to obtain reproducible and accurate thermodilution outputs during exercise. Patient-reported symptoms of dyspnea and fatigue are quantified by Borg Scales at each stage.

3. When the patient is near maximum tolerated workload, based either subjectively or on a respiratory quotient of >1.0, peak pressures are recorded with repeat assessment of CO.

4. Additional measures may be required based on the specifics of the case (e.g., assessment of transvalvular gradients in mitral or aortic stenosis; ventriculography or echocardiography for dynamic mitral regurgitation).

5. A final set of recovery measurements are recorded and the feet are removed from the cycle.

If leg ergometry is not possible, exercise may be performed using an arm ergometer or by lifting weights. Increases in heart rate and CO are less marked with arm exercise because smaller muscles are recruited, but increases in filling pressures can still be detected. During arm exercise, patients often perform a Valsalva maneuver that can spuriously increase all intracardiac pressures owing to the increase in intrapleural pressure. Therefore, to obtain diagnostic quality data, patients must be coached to avoid engaging this maneuver.

Interpretation of hemodynamic findings encompasses examination of absolute pressure levels and their proportionality to determine origin of elevation (e.g., left sided or pulmonary) and changes in stroke volume and CO. Pulmonary resistance and transvalvular gradients should be calculated. Patients with heart failure display abnormal increases in LV filling pressure and pulmonary artery pressure, with inadequate vasodilation and a depressed CO and heart rate response. Patients with pulmonary vascular disease have pulmonary hypertension (mean pulmonary artery pressure >30 mm Hg), no significant change in LV filling pressure, and thus an elevated pulmonary resistance (i.e., >2.5 Wood units $\times$ m^2).

Isometric Exercise

Isometric exercise (skeletal muscle contraction without shortening) also may be performed using a handgrip with a graded hand dynamometer. Measurements of hemodynamic data and ventricular function are obtained during sustained handgrip at a predetermined range (30% to 50% of the maximal handgrip contraction) for 3 to 4 minutes. The size of the involved muscle group is unimportant, provided that maximal voluntary contraction is maintained to increase oxygen demand during the isometric exercise period. Isometric exercise does not involve body motion that may interfere with hemodynamic measurements and is feasible in a larger number of laboratories. Isometric exercise increases heart rate and CO without significant effects on vascular resistance. As with arm weights, an involuntary Valsalva maneuver during straining may occur during unsupervised isometric exercise; and thus, respiratory patterns should be observed. Careful monitoring, patient cooperation, and practice in use of the handgrip dynamometer minimize false hemodynamic information.

Other Physiologic Maneuvers

Valsalva Maneuver

The Valsalva maneuver is performed by having the patient forcibly expire against a closed glottis and strain as if having a bowel movement. This increases intrathoracic pressure, which initially reduces afterload (transmural wall stress) in the strain phase, and then subsequently reduces venous return and stroke volume in ensuing phases (Fig. 10.24). Shortly after Valsalva release, venous return increases, causing an increase in stroke volume and blood pressure with reflex bradycardia (overshoot phase). The magnitude of the Valsalva maneuver can be quantified by measuring the pressure against which the patient expires. An adequate maneuver requires maintenance of approximately 20- to 30-mm Hg positive intrathoracic pressure for 10 to 15 seconds. The Valsalva maneuver can be performed safely and without complications by almost any patient. The blood pressure response to the Valsalva maneuver can be used to assess LV filling pressures, because the normal drop in systolic arterial pressure is lost in patients with elevated pulmonary wedge pressure; pulmonary venous congestion is so extreme that they cannot drop EDV (Figs. 10.24 and 10.25). In addition, hemodynamic findings of hypertrophic cardiomyopathy and different types of valvular lesions may be more pronounced during the Valsalva maneuver because of changes in ventricular load and ejection (see Chapter 3).

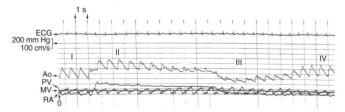

Fig. 10.24 Valsalva maneuver showing the effects on aortic (Ao) pressure, mean coronary velocity (MV), phasic coronary velocity (PV), and right atrial (RA) pressure. The four phases of the Valsalva maneuver (see text) are enumerated I, II, III, and IV. ECG, Electrocardiogram.

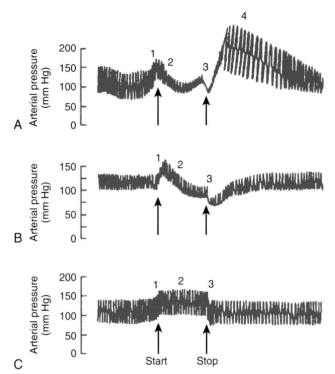

Fig. 10.25 Changes in arterial blood pressure in response to the Valsalva maneuver. The initial strain phase of the Valsalva *(1)* produces an increase in pressure related to the increase in intrathoracic pressure. During ongoing forced expiration against a closed glottis *(2)*, preload declines in the normal heart **(A)** reducing blood pressure. Valsalva release *(3)* causes an immediate decrease in pressure as a result of loss of increased intrathoracic pressure. Release is then followed by an overshoot phase *(4)* related to enhanced venous return and increased stroke volume. **(C)** In patients with heart failure and markedly elevated left-heart filling pressures, Valsalva does not result in a sufficient drop in preload to reduce stroke volume (because of marked congestion), so pressure remains elevated until release. This is termed the "square wave" response and is indicative of pulmonary capillary wedge pressure (PCWP) of >25 mm Hg. Response **(B)** (termed "absent overshoot") is intermediate between normal and the square wave and is reflective of modestly elevated filling pressures. (From Zema MJ, Restivo B, Sos T, et al. Left ventricular dysfunction—bedside Valsalva manoeuvre. *Br Heart J.* 1980;44:562.)

Muller Maneuver

The patient performs the Muller maneuver by inspiring against a closed glottis; thus, this maneuver is essentially the opposite of the Valsalva. The subject inhales, reducing intrathoracic pressure to -30 to -60 mm Hg for 30 seconds. This enhances venous return to the right side of the heart while also increasing LV afterload (increased transmural wall stress). Increases in LV EDVs and ESVs are noted with diminished stroke volume, reduced CO, and reduced EF. This maneuver is used to augment right-sided heart murmurs and to decrease the physical findings of obstructive cardiomyopathy by a reduction in LV outflow gradient. Right-to-left shunting is enhanced during the Muller maneuver and also acutely during strain release in the Valsalva maneuver.

Cold Pressor Testing

Cold pressor testing stimulates the sympathetic nervous system, mediated by cold-induced pain receptor activation in the forearm, hand, or forehead. Hemodynamic findings occurring with cold pressor testing include increases in heart rate (5% to 15%), systolic and mean arterial pressure (15% to 20%), and CO. These responses usually occur within 2 minutes of application of the cold stimulus. In normal subjects, cold pressor testing increases coronary blood flow and reduces coronary vascular resistance, possibly through enhanced flow-mediated vasodilation. Cold pressor testing in some patients with coronary artery disease causes coronary vasoconstriction, which may be potentiated by a β-adrenergic blockade. Angina is rarely precipitated, although changes in regional LV function may occur.

Hyperventilation

Hyperventilation has been used to induce coronary spasm. Deep breathing (30 breaths/min for 5 minutes) is a commonly used method. Ischemia is rarely precipitated during hyperventilation but may commonly occur at the termination of rapid breathing. Heart rate, oxygen consumption, arteriovenous oxygen difference, and arterial pH increase during hyperventilation, whereas arterial pressure, pulmonary artery pressure, and arterial PCO_2 fall. Peripheral vascular resistance, CO, and LV stroke volume are unchanged with the increase in LVEF seen in normal patients. These abnormalities may not be observed in patients with stable or variant angina.

Pharmacologic Stress

Pharmacologic stresses are used to assess alterations of ventricular function.

Nitrates

Nitrates decrease systolic and mean arterial pressure and produce a reflex increase in heart rate in patients who do not have congestion at rest. Nitroglycerin is a predominant venodilator and thus serves to reduce preload preferentially, although afterload reduction may also be seen, particularly in patients with elevated arterial impedance at rest. Nitrates do not have direct effects on LV performance, except indirectly through reflex autonomic stimulation. Nitroglycerin relieves coronary vasospasm and ischemia, which may indirectly lead to improved LV function in some patients.

Amyl nitrite, usually given as an inhalation, acts in a fashion similar to that of nitroglycerin but is much more rapid in action. This acute preload reduction makes amyl nitrate useful for detecting dynamic obstruction in hypertrophic cardiomyopathy.

Nitroprusside is a balanced arterial and venous dilator and can potently reduce LV preload and afterload. Because of enhanced afterload sensitivity, patients with systolic heart failure may derive marked benefit from nitroprusside, with improvements in CO, reduction in filling pressure, and mild or no drop in blood pressure. In contrast, elderly patients and especially those with heart failure and preserved EF display much more dramatic reductions in blood pressure with nitroprusside. Nitroglycerin and nitroprusside are commonly used to reduce left-heart pressures and determine reversibility of pulmonary hypertension in heart failure patients. Nitroprusside may also be used in low-gradient, low-output aortic stenosis to discern whether true severe valvular stenosis is present.

β-Adrenergic Stimulation

Dobutamine and isoproterenol are synthetic catecholamines that increase contractility and heart rate and reduce vascular resistance. IV infusions and 2D echocardiographic examination of LV wall motion are used to screen for ischemia. These agents are also given in patients with low-gradient, low-output aortic stenosis to determine true severity and evaluate for provocable LV outflow gradients in patients with hypertrophic cardiomyopathy. Isoproterenol is generally preferred for the latter type of patient because dobutamine can induce significant gradients even in nondiseased hearts.

Pacing

Temporary transvenous pacing may be used in the catheterization laboratory to increase myocardial oxygen demand and blood flow or to examine relationships between heart rate and contractility (force-frequency response) or relaxation (rate-relaxation response). Pacing may also be used to regularize heart rate in patients with atrial fibrillation (e.g., for studies examining ventricular interdependence in pericardial constriction, which require a normalized rate). In contrast with exercise and β-adrenergic agonists, pacing does not increase CO or enhance venous return, and it cannot be considered a physiologic stressor enough to simulate physical exertion.

Rapid Volume Loading

Bolus infusion of saline is often performed to unmask diastolic dysfunction or pericardial constriction in patients with normal right atrial pressures at baseline. Under normal circumstances, the heart can accommodate this increase in filling volume and enhance output by the Frank-Starling mechanism. With diastolic dysfunction and/or pericardial restraint, this ability is compromised, and pressures or signs of constriction may become more evident. A simpler alternative involves performing measurements during a straight leg raise, which also enhances venous return. Approximately 20% of healthy volunteers will develop a pulmonary wedge pressure of >15 mm Hg with rapid saline infusion, but values >18 mm Hg are strong evidence of abnormal LV diastolic compliance properties. Like pacing, volume loading cannot be considered to be an adequate substitute for exercise because the changes in heart rate, preload, afterload, wall stress, contractility, and myocardial oxygen demand are quite different between the two stressors.

Nurse and Technician Viewpoint

The nursing and technical staff should be presented with a clear, concise project protocol, which should include:

1. Overview of the project with clearly delineated objectives
2. Patient safety
3. Special equipment if necessary
4. Additional staffing if required
5. Data sheets (prepared to facilitate study periods)

   If additional sterile equipment is necessary, a "protocol pack" with all additional equipment aids should be included with setup. Many research techniques require the use of special catheters that must be interfaced with various flow meters, computers, and other equipment. Personnel must be careful not to contaminate the sterile field when connecting the catheter to the interface cable. There are two ways to approach this situation. One is to sterilize all interface cables. The other is to wrap the nonsterile cable in a sterile drape. If the latter technique is used, the physician must be careful not to pull the nonsterile cable into the sterile field. If medications are involved, dose calculation worksheets aid the staff in drug preparation.

Suggested Readings

Andersen MJ, Borlaug BA. Invasive hemodynamic characterization of heart failure with preserved ejection fraction. *Heart Fail Clin*. 2014;10:435-444.

Bezerra HG, Costa MA, Guagliumi G, Rollins AM, Simon DI. Intracoronary optical coherence tomography: a comprehensive review clinical and research applications. *JACC Cardiovasc Interv*. 2009;2:1035-1046.

Borlaug BA, Kass DA. Invasive hemodynamic assessment in heart failure. *Heart Fail Clin*. 2009;5:217-228.

Borlaug BA, Nishimura RA, Sorajja P, Lam CS, Redfield MM. Exercise hemodynamics enhance diagnosis of early heart failure with preserved ejection fraction. *Circ Heart Fail*. 2010;3:588-595.

Chapman CB, ed. Physiology of muscular exercise. *Circ Res*. 1967;20(suppl 1):I1-I255. (Also available as Monograph 15 from American Heart Association.)

den Heijer P, Foley DP, Hillege HL, et al. The 'Ermenonville' classification of observations at coronary angioscopy—evaluation of intra- and inter-observer agreement. European Working Group on Coronary Angioscopy. *Eur Heart J*. 1994;15:815.

Dexter L, Whittenberger JL, Haynes FW, Goodale WT, Gorlin R, Sawyer CG. Effect of exercise on circulatory dynamics of normal individuals. *J Appl Physiol*. 1951;3:439.

Fearon WF, Balsam LB, Farouque HM, et al. Novel index for invasively assessing the coronary microcirculation. *Circulation*. 2003;107:3129-3132.

Fujimoto N, Borlaug BA, Lewis GD, et al. Hemodynamic responses to rapid saline loading: the impact of age, sex, and heart failure. *Circulation*. 2013;127(1):55-62.

Gibson CM, Cannon CP, Murphy SA, et al. Relationship of TIMI myocardial perfusion grade to mortality after administration of thrombolytic drugs. *Circulation*. 2009; 101:125-130.

Jeremias A, Maehara A, Généreux P, et al. Multicenter core laboratory comparison of the instantaneous wave-free ratio and resting Pd/Pa with fractional flow reserve: the RESOLVE study. *J Am Coll Cardiol*. 2014;63:1253-1261.

Jiangping S, Zhe Z, Wei W, et al. Assessment of coronary artery stenosis by coronary angiography: a head-to-head comparison with pathological coronary artery anatomy. *Circ Cardiovasc Interv*. 2013;6:262-268.

Kass DA, Maughan WL. From 'Emax' to pressure-volume relations: a broader view. *Circulation*. 1988;77:1203-1212.

Kern MJ, Samady H. Current concepts of integrated coronary physiology in the catheterization laboratory. *J Am Coll Cardiol*. 2010;55:173-185.

Kern MJ, Dupouy P, Drury JH, et al. Role of coronary artery lumen enlargement in improving coronary blood flow after balloon angioplasty and stenting: a combined intravascular ultrasound Doppler flow and imaging study. *J Am Coll Cardiol*. 1997; 29:1520-1527.

Lerman A, Zeiher AM. Endothelial function: cardiac events. *Circulation*. 2005;111:363-368.

McLaurin LP, Grossman W. Dynamic and isometric exercise during cardiac catheterization. In: Grossman W, ed. *Cardiac Catheterization and Angiography*. Philadelphia, PA: Lea & Febiger; 1974.

Meijboom WB, Van Mieghem CA, van Pelt N, et al. Comprehensive assessment of coronary artery stenoses: computed tomography coronary angiography versus conventional coronary angiography and correlation with fractional flow reserve in patients with stable angina. *J Am Coll Cardiol.* 2008;52:636-643.

Mirsky I. Assessment of diastolic function: suggested methods and future considerations. *Circulation.* 1984;69:836-841.

Mitchell JH, Harris MD. Exercise and the heart: physiologic and clinical considerations. In: Willerson JT, Sanders CA, eds. *Clinical Cardiology.* New York, NY: Grune & Stratton; 1977.

Nair A, Kuban BD, Tuzcu EM, et al. Coronary plaque classification with intravascular ultrasound radiofrequency data analysis. *Circulation.* 2002;106:2200-2206.

Nallamothu BK, Spertus JA, Lansky AJ, et al. Comparison of clinical interpretation with visual assessment and quantitative coronary angiography in patients undergoing percutaneous coronary intervention in contemporary practice: the Assessing Angiography (A2) project. *Circulation.* 2013;127:1793-1800.

Nasu K, Tsuchikane E, Katoh O, et al. Accuracy of in vivo coronary plaque morphology assessment: a validation study of in vivo virtual histology compared with in vitro histopathology. *J Am Coll Cardiol.* 2006;47:2405-2412.

Nolte F, van de Hoef TP, Meuwissen M, et al. Increased hyperaemic coronary microvascular resistance adds to the presence of myocardial ischaemia. *EuroIntervention.* 2014;9:1423-1431.

Ofili EO, Kern MJ, Labovitz AJ, et al. Analysis of coronary blood flow velocity dynamics in angiographically normal and stenosed arteries before and after endolumen enlargement by angioplasty. *J Am Coll Cardiol.* 1993;21:308-318.

Pijls NH, van Son JA, Kirkeeide RL, De Bruyne B, Gould KL. Experimental basis of determining maximum coronary, myocardial, and collateral blood flow by pressure measurements for assessing functional stenosis severity before and after percutaneous transluminal coronary angioplasty. *Circulation.* 1993;87:1354-1367.

Sagawa K, Suga H, Shoukas AA, Bakalar KM. End-systolic pressure/volume ratio: a new index of ventricular contractility. *Am J Cardiol.* 1977;40:748-753.

Seiler C, Fleisch M, Garachemani A, Meier B. Coronary collateral quantitation in patients with coronary artery disease using intravascular flow velocity or pressure measurements. *J Am Coll Cardiol.* 1998;32:1272-1279.

Sen S, Escaned J, Malik IS, et al. Development and validation of a new adenosine-independent index of stenosis severity from coronary wave-intensity analysis: results of the ADVISE (Adenosine Vasodilator Independent Stenosis Evaluation) study. *J Am Coll Cardiol.* 2012;59:1392-1402.

Sheehan FH, Schofer J, Mathey DG, et al. Measurement of regional wall motion from biplane contrast ventriculograms: a comparison of the 30 degree right anterior oblique and 60 degree left anterior oblique projections in patients with acute myocardial infarction. *Circulation.* 1986;74:796-804.

Kubo T, Imanishi T, Takarada S, et al. Assessment of culprit lesion morphology in acute myocardial infarction: ability of optical coherence tomography compared with intravascular ultrasound and coronary angioscopy. *J Am Coll Cardiol.* 2007;50:933-939.

Tolle JJ, Waxman AB, Van Horn TL, Pappagianopoulos PP, Systrom DM. Exercise-induced pulmonary arterial hypertension. *Circulation.* 2008;118:2183-2189.

van't Hof AW, Liem A, Suryapranata H, Hoorntje JC, de Boer MJ, Zijlstra F. Angiographic assessment of myocardial reperfusion in patients treated with primary angioplasty for acute myocardial infarction: myocardial blush grade. Zwolle Myocardial Infarction Study Group. *Circulation.* 1998;97:2302-2306.

Weiss JL, Frederiksen JW, Weisfeldt ML. Hemodynamic determinants of the time-course of fall in canine left ventricular pressure. *J Clin Invest.* 1976;58:751-760.

Optimization of Quality in the Cardiac Catheterization Laboratory

CHARLES CHAMBERS • JOAQUIN E. CIGARROA

Every percutaneous coronary intervention (PCI) program must have a quality improvement committee that routinely performs the following: (a) a review of quality processes and outcomes with risk adjustment, (b) peer review of difficult or complicated cases, and (c) individual operator assessment including random case reviews. This 2011 PCI Guidelines class I recommendation from the American College of Cardiology (ACC)/American Heart Association (AHA)/Society for Cardiovascular Angiography and Interventions (SCAI) has been recognized as essential by providers and administrators for nearly two decades. However, variations in program implementation may impact effectiveness. All facilities should have an independent catheterization laboratory quality program and not just perform quality assurance (QA) as a subset of a hospital-wide program; physician participation, essential to the QA process, should be mandatory; administrative support must be adequate to support data collection/entry. Without requirements for "how to do quality" and limited methods for assessing an individual QA program, assuring quality in one's catheterization laboratory QA program can be challenging. This chapter will review the necessary steps for effective QA implementation. In concert with prior editions, the assurance of quality as it relates to documentation and patient safety will also be reviewed in this chapter.

Quality Improvement/Assurance

Quality care in the cardiac catheterization laboratory requires each program to evaluate its performance through a meaningful continuous quality improvement (CQI) process providing program evaluation, deficiency identification, methods for remediation, and final reassessment. SCAI has been a leader in this area, publishing its first guidelines on quality nearly 25 years ago. SCAI's quality efforts have continued since with position papers and the living document, *2011 Catheterization Laboratory Quality Improvement Tool Kit* (SCAIQIT), designed to assist individual laboratories in this quality effort.

CQI is an iterative method to evaluate operational approaches and to remedy deficiencies beyond the isolated assessment of adverse outcomes; peer review is an essential component of this process. CQI requires a dedicated physician champion, a staff champion, a quality improvement committee specific to the catheterization laboratory, and full support from hospital administration. Increasingly recognized, the interconnectivity of quality of care, cost effectiveness, and reimbursement ramifications require this integral partnership. However, only through active, nonpartisan, nonpunitive physician participation will this process be beneficial to the operator, staff, hospital administration, and ultimately the patient by continually improving processes and efficiencies, which will, in turn, improve outcomes.

Six elements for a CQI program include (1) establishing the Quality Committee, (2) identifying quality indicators, (3) systematic data collection using standard definitions, (4) benchmarking of data with appropriate analysis and peer review, (5) implementation of a plan to correct deficiencies with follow-up, and (6) appropriate use of conferences for case review and education. (Table 11.1)

Quality Committee

The QI process starts with a committee of physicians, staff, and hospital administration. This should be established just for the cardiac catheterization laboratory to address issues specific to the laboratory. Although it is essential that this committee interact with other committees within the hospital, the cardiac catheterization laboratory director should chair this committee with specific QA staff from the catheterization laboratory. Physician and staff "champions" are required for this process to be effective.

In addition to the interventional cardiologists, the composition of a PCI CQI committee may include noninvasive cardiologists, primary care physicians, catheterization laboratory nurses, technologists, and hospital administrators. Rotation of members and lead should be in conjunction with department chairs or the hospital medical director. In small PCI programs, all active staff interventionists may be included. In larger laboratories, a formal and fair process for selecting and replacing members must be devised. An expert in interventional cardiology with established credibility, often the catheterization laboratory director, should

Table 11.1

Essential Components to the Catheterization Laboratory Quality Process.

1. Quality Committee
   a. Catheterization laboratory medical director
   b. QA staff/catheterization laboratory quality champion
2. Identification of Quality Indicators
   a. Structure
   b. Process
   c. Outcomes
3. Data Collection
   a. Appropriate number of trained staff required
4. Benchmarking with Data Analysis and Peer Review
   a. Participation in large/national database
   b. Risk adjustment required
   c. Physician assessment: nonpunitive and without bias
5. Implementation and Follow-up
   a. Goals required
   b. Tools created
6. Conferences
   a. Morbidity and mortality
   b. Challenging cases
   c. Educational topic review

chair this committee with a dedicated staff lead. Interaction with hospital risk management is required to assure appropriate confidentiality. However, this is an independent group whose goal is quality in the laboratory. Interaction with all subspecialties should be established to assure all aspects of patient care within the laboratory are covered.

The CQI Committee's responsibilities are outlined in Table 11.2. Patient safety is the central purpose of the CQI process. The quality program should monitor clinical outcomes, complication rates, compliance with policies and procedures both internal as well as those from external regulatory and/or accrediting bodies, and patient satisfaction. The committee must be nonpunitive and behave equitably and transparently to ensure fairness to the operator, quality for the patient, and credibility for the committee. The CQI committee should meet at regular intervals but be available for ad hoc meetings if necessary. External reviews should be requested when deemed appropriate.

Identification of Quality Indicators

The key to assessing quality is to identify appropriately and measure quantitatively and qualitatively indicators directly and

Table 11.2

Responsibilities of a Catheterization Laboratory Quality Committee.

1. Regular meetings (monthly).
2. Identify metrics of care to be monitored (from NCDR reports).
3. Review all serious adverse events (e.g., death, emergency CABG, stoke).
4. Perform random film audits for appropriateness, adequate imaging, and outcomes.
5. Review data on process and outcome metrics.
6. Identify quality issues. (e.g., any hospital complication with frequency >90th percentile of peer hospitals as well as any physician with outlier incidence of complications).
7. Develop remediation plans, oversee implementation, check results (i.e., plan/do/check/act cycle).
8. Refer larger issues for appropriate intervention. (e.g., disruptive physician behavior referred to department director.

Modified from: Bashore TM, Balter S, Barac A, et al. 2012 American College of Cardiology Foundation/Society for Cardiovascular Angiography and Interventions expert consensus document on cardiac catheterization laboratory standards update: A report of the American College of Cardiology Foundation Task Force on Expert Consensus documents developed in collaboration with the Society of Thoracic Surgeons and Society for Vascular Medicine. *J Am Coll.* Cardiol. 2012;59:2221-305.
 CABG, Coronary artery bypass grafting; *NCDR,* National Cardiovascular Data Registry.

indirectly involved in the delivery of patient care. Three indicators will be discussed for organizational purposes: Structural, Process, and Outcomes.

Structural indicators are objective, easy to collect, and often established beyond the confines of the catheterization laboratory. Structural indicators are considered by hospital privileging or staff credentialing/recredentialing and include: medical training, licensure, board certification, procedure volume, and participation in conferences/continuing medical education. The method for credentialing and the ongoing assessment of proficiency must be developed in accordance with local governance policies and professionally developed standards. The granting of privileges by healthcare systems is within the legal and ethical purview of these institutions. Establishing a minimum standard limits confrontation when physicians are either inadequately trained or fail to maintain required qualifications. Operator procedural volume is a weak and inconsistent measure of quality and should not be used as a quality indicator in isolation. Institutional volume is a better programmatic predictor of outcomes but does not supersede actual outcomes.

Process indicators reflect patient evaluation and management, appropriateness of a procedure, and treatment adherence to guidelines (Table 11.3). The key to the quality assurance program

Table 11.3

Examples of Process Indicators.

Direct Patient Care-Related Indicators

Quality of angiographic studies
Report generation/quality of interpretation

System Specific Indicators

Patient transport/lab turnover/bed availability
Preprocedure assessment
Emergency response time
CT/anesthesia/respiratory care/perfusion
Door-to-balloon time

Guidelines Driven Indicators

Infection control/radiation safety
Treatment protocols (contrast, drugs)
Procedure indications/new devices
Appropriateness criteria

Cost Related Indicators

Length of stay pre/post procedure
Disposables-quality of supplies
Personnel/staffing

is to evaluate the environment leading up to a specific outcome and not merely to react to the metric. Because of the qualitative component of these measures, they are more challenging to assess, less objective, and prone to potential observer bias. However, these indicators are helpful in working through the entire process from protocols, to staffing, to turnover of the room, and to patient length of stay. Assessing these indicators allows a more complete analysis of outcomes in the QA process.

Outcome is a measure/indicator of what happened to the patient and provides a reflection of how the patient was managed. Since patient care outcomes are now publicly available, they are the most recognizable. Quality assurance programs are challenged by the assessment of specific adverse events particularly in both the low and high volume operator, because events are proportional to case number. Risk adjustment provided through database participation is an essential component to this process. The variables inherent in comparing high volume and low volume institutions and/or operators by the use of whisker plots provided by these national registries require careful identification of many variables and statistical validity. While both individual physician and hospital scorecards provide information on performance, they are not sufficient when used alone. The outcome data derived in this process should not be used to punish the practitioner but rather guide the identification of processes for improvement through performance improvement projects.

Data Collection

Since data are pivotal to this process, accurate data collection and entry are mandatory. Effective data collection requires a data repository, effective utilization of the electronic health record, development of a structured cardiac catheterization laboratory report, and dedicated/trained personnel for data acquisition. Because adequate knowledgeable staff are required, hospital administration must be actively involved in providing the required support, referred to as fulltime equivalents (FTEs). Random audits are needed to assure data authenticity. System cross-talk between hospital, catheterization laboratory, and database entry systems is essential for both demographic data and procedural findings. Decreasing repeated same data set entry decreases staff time and the potential for error. Information technology systems for the cardiac catheterization laboratory and the hospital should be integrated to allow seamless information transfer. Data access must be restricted for both patient privacy and potential medical-legal concerns. The Health Insurance Portability and Accountability Act (HIPAA) of 1996 established rules for patient anonymity, which must be followed.

Benchmarking with Data Analysis and Peer Review

Participation in regional and or national databases is required for risk adjustment. In assessing quality, adverse outcomes are often equated to (lack of) quality and, in turn, related to performance. However, it is well established that adverse events do occur, even in the best hands and at the best centers. The frequency of these events is, in large part, related to the condition of the patient and inherent risk of the procedure; this may be impacted by the experience and skill of the operator and the center. Although volume is often considered a surrogate for quality, this may not always be the case.

Benchmarking against national standards is a valuable means to understand high variances in low incidence adverse events. Such analyses and collection of many of these variables are captured in ACC-NCDR Cath PCI Registry as well as in other recognized regional registries. Not only have registry data been shown to be effective in predicting outcomes, they provide quarterly reports with benchmarking and risk-adjusted outcomes. Version 5 of NCDR-PCI will even have an option for 30-day follow-up. The registries use standardized definitions to collect patient demographics, clinical variables, and outcomes on each procedure. These evidence-based data elements are combined with process and performance measures that are linked to current ACC/AHA/SCAI clinical practice guidelines and appropriate use criteria. Collaboration with Centers for Medicare and Medicaid Services (CMS) is ongoing in a variety of projects to measure and to assess quality. There are limitations in the registries because of the lack of long-term follow-up, self-reporting with limited mandated periodic auditing, voluntary participation, and cost.

Data analysis requires a review of both the specific adverse events and the risk adjusted event rates for the facility and the operator. Specific adverse events should be identified and individual case review performed. A sample case report form is provided in Table 11.4. Results should be reviewed and discussed at the CQI meetings. In the case of possible litigation, the cardiac catheterization laboratory CQI process should work with hospital risk management but not be driven by them.

The peer review component for case review applies both to index cases identified as adverse outcomes and to randomly selected cases. This must be nonpunitive and unbiased. Index case assessment may not identify issues with an operator's standard practice of patient selection and case performance. Random case review can provide this and should include approximately 10% of the laboratory volume. An external review should be considered if an adequate internal review is not possible because of potential conflicts or overall manpower issues. Appropriate Use Criteria (AUC) compliance and its assessment is a responsibility of the Quality Committee. As AUC has evolved in both definition and application, processes must be in place to assess AUC and review cases where issues arise regarding procedure appropriateness.

Implementation and Follow-up: "Closing the Loop"

Interventions to improve performance should be the goal of the CQI process focusing on benchmarks below the median, as deemed appropriate by the committee. Once performance variance has been identified, the CQI committee must investigate the cause and devise a solution. Illustrative examples may include an excessively high rate of access site complications, contrast-induced nephropathy, excessive radiation doses, etc. In recent years, the importance of appropriate behavior has been identified with distinctions such as the Joint Commissions "disruptive physician." As this is a quality issue, quality committees are now appropriately being charged with coordinating interventions in these cases. Nonpunitive programs should be established to correct identified variances and to address specific issues to improve the

Table 11.4

Data Quality Event Review Form.

Patient Data

Patient Name:_____ Age:_____ ID#:_____

Procedure:_____ Physician:_____ Date:_____

Reason for Review:

Potential for Patient Safety:_____; Sentinel Event:_____

Mortality: In Lab_____; In Hospital_____ 30 Day _____

Morbidity: Neuro:_____; Vascular:_____; Coronary:_____;

Arrhythmia:_____; Renal:_____; Radiation:_____

Other:_____

Case Summary:

_____

Risk Group:	Average/Low	High	Salvage
Clinical	_____	_____	_____
Cath	_____	_____	_____

Process Review:

	Appropriate	Uncertain	Inappropriate
Indication:			
Technique:			
Management:			

Related to: Disease:_____; Provider:_____; System:_____;

*Preventable:*_____; Not Preventable:_____; Comments:_____

Recommendation by Reviewer: _____

_____ Reviewer:_____

Recommendation by Committee: _____

_____

Patient Safety/Risk Management Review: Y N; *Hospital/Department Review:* Y N; *Corrective Action:* Y N; Education_____; Proctor_____;

Other:_____

Date:_____ Signature:_____

Modified from Heupler FA, Chambers CE, Dear WE, et al. Guidelines for peer review in the cardiac catheterization laboratory. *Cathet Cardiovasc Diagn.* 1997;40:21-32.

total laboratory performance. Neutral, nonpartisan reviews are essential with the removal of all potential conflicts of interest among individuals and or competing groups. The goal is quality improvement for better patient care and safety to improve outcomes.

When the CQI process identifies a systemic problem requiring remediation, the tools available for this process improvement are implemented. Establishing practice protocols and order sets will standardize practice and should limit variation in individual performance. Scorecards benchmark performance and can provide feedback allowing outliers to see potential areas for improvement. Identifying the need for intervention is a clear component of this process. Education, either with in-laboratory proctoring or outside continuing medical education (CME), can allow for any potential knowledge gaps to be narrowed. Laboratory surveys provide feedback for both individual and overall laboratory performance. Positive reinforcement created by working with hospital administration to provide incentives, such as enhanced educational opportunities, may prove beneficial in performance improvement. For the disruptive physician, counseling may be required with confidential but swift correction of behavior issues. Safeguards must be in place to assure proper behavior and to protect the identified physician from unfair or punitive targeting.

Penalties or sanctions, e.g., suspension of privileges, should be considered only after other methods of correction have failed. The seriousness of the sanction should fairly mirror the seriousness of the problem and the responsiveness of the operator. If it is concluded that the operator has a deficiency in knowledge or skill, the CQI Committee or outside reviewer can recommend an appropriate educational approach and/or mentorship and consider limiting privileges until defined expectations have been met. When all appropriate measures to improve performance are unsuccessful, the committee may recommend further action, such as suspension or revocation of an operator's privileges. All institutions have a policy for this situation including reporting to state regulatory bodies.

Conferences

Cardiac catheterization conferences should be held routinely and include: challenging cases, topic review, and Morbidity and Mortality. An attendance threshold for maintenance of privileges should be established and enforced. In these conferences, it is rewarding to review and to discuss clinical and technically challenging cases, including those with complications and unexpected developments during a PCI. Topic updates in interventional cardiology, with CME as appropriate, are important for maintaining operator and staff proficiency. Separation of peer review from teaching activities is essential because of the legal issues surrounding potential discovery for nonprotected conferences. Federal and state regulations shield participants from litigation in peer review activities. Proceedings of peer review activities are protected against subpoena and are not discoverable in most situations. Admixing peer review proceedings in other settings should not occur.

The Morbidity and Mortality (M&M) Conferences are a traditional key component in the catheterization laboratory quality process, because adverse events are frequently the emphasis of QA. (Table 11.5) Most academic programs have well developed M&M conferences. These not only assess quality but also provide memorable educational opportunities for all participants while satisfying ACGME requirements for fellowship training. Despite the ubiquity and importance of M&M, the literature has been lacking in specifics on "how to do" an M&M conference. These specifics can help to prevent inappropriate or punitive case selection and/ or a lack of impartiality in scoring/assessing performance. Recent publications have addressed this with recommendations for more universal standardization (Table 11.5).

Application of CQI

There are numerous challenges in applying PCI CQI processes in a constructive and impartial manner. In 2011, the Society of Cardiovascular Angiography and Intervention (SCAI) created the Quality Improvement Tool Kit (SCAI QIT) to help catheterization laboratories with the process. Catheterization Laboratory Accreditation may offer an opportunity to obtain an external assessment utilizing uniform standards and site reviews to assess and to assure

Table 11.5

Morbidity and Mortality Conference.
• **Leadership:** Physician Catheterization Laboratory Director or Quality Chairperson for the Laboratory should lead. All efforts to create a nonpunitive environment must be taken in settings where competition may be involved. Bias must not be perceived.
• **Attendance:** M&M should occur regularly, at least quarterly if not monthly, and should be attended by all Interventional Physicians. Teaching hospitals use this as a teaching tool. Physician extenders, laboratory staff, administration attendance should be decided locally. Attending physician/fellow should present case.
• **Case selection:** Triggers for case selection must be established with the following considered: In-laboratory death, cardiac arrest with CPR, defibrillation, intubation, perforation with or without tamponade requiring RX, prolonged acute closure/major dissection, unplanned circulatory support, cerebral event, major vascular event/ bleeding.
• **Outcomes and confidentiality:** Review sheet (Table 11.4) completed by chairperson after discussion and consensus reached. Results referred to Quality Committee for review as appropriate. Discussions are protected per Peer Review statute.

quality. SCAI was founded, and then partnered with the American College of Cardiology (ACC), to create the first catheterization laboratory accrediting organization, Accreditation for Cardiovascular Excellence (ACE). In recent years, ACC has formed its own catheterization laboratory accreditation service. Similarly, SCAI has separated from ACE, joining the Intersocietal Accreditation Commission (IAC). Both internal assessment through the SCAI QIT and external assessment with accreditation are available to assist laboratories in assuring the required quality measures are in place.

Challenges arise with CQI and must be addressed. Use of these data for nonquality purposes, e.g., developing marketing strategies or improving operating margin, must be cautioned if not discouraged. Conflicts of interest are common among competing physicians who may perceive a financial advantage to adjudicate adversely another physician's care. Operator outcomes must be presented with absolute confidentiality maintained. Physicians whose activities are being investigated must be protected, and the use of confidential information to target an individual physician must be considered a breach of this process. Sanctions for such behavior should be formalized in the Medical Staff Bylaws and applied to violators.

The CQI process may be best implemented by incorporating clinical practice guidelines and appropriateness criteria. Specific quality measures to improve constructively patient selection for PCI, operator performance, team proficiency, and overall care systems should be selected carefully by the CQI committee. With proper implementation of the CQI process, physician and laboratory performance will improve and quality patient care provided.

Documentation

Documentation in the cardiac catheterization laboratory involves preprocedure documentation of the patient history/physical as well as the informed consent, in laboratory documentation of events, and postprocedure report generation with findings and recommendations. In an era of increased litigation, careful scrutiny of procedure appropriateness, expanding electronic medical records/informatics, and the importance of appropriate documentation cannot be understated.

The Centers of Medicare and Medicaid Services (CMS), state regulations governing hospitals and other health care facilities, professional organizations, and results of lawsuits and local policy, all influence standards for medical record documentation. Each organization must develop internal policies that govern medical record documentation and retention of documents. The process for corrections, revisions, and/or addendums in the medical record is governed by this organizational policy.

Preprocedure: History/Physical and Informed Consent

Preprocedure documentation of pertinent information relevant to the cardiac catheterization is required and outlined in several Standards and Best Practice documents. The history should include prior cardiac procedures (catheterization/PCI/CABG), specific allergies (contrast reaction), and medications (anticoagulants/antiplatelet agents). Physical examination should include access to specific findings with documentation of pulses, bruits, asymmetric blood pressures, ABI, etc. Lab work appropriate to an invasive procedure with contrast administration should be recorded. The physician and patient should discuss potential use of dual antiplatelet therapy, risks of bleeding, and implications for potential timing of noncardiac surgery for patients who are considering noncardiac surgery in the future. The clinician should assess the bleeding risk for the patient and address pertinent bleeding risk avoidance strategies.

Informed consent recognizes the cardiologist's duty to provide the patient or responsible party with adequate information about the planned procedure(s) to include why it is being recommended, the potential benefits/ risks as well as the risks and alternatives of refusing the recommended procedure. The patient must be given the opportunity to ask questions and to have them answered and understood with an interpreter provided if language barriers are present. The consent discussion must be documented in the medical record. Each facility will have organizational policies governing consents for treatment.

Procedure Documentation

Intraprocedure documentation begins with the time-out, mandated for all invasive procedures. Performed with all staff and operators present, this verifies the correct patient is undergoing the correct procedure with essential information (allergies, medications, etc.) shared with everyone. For documentation during the procedure, a chronologic procedure log is the standard for this essential information. Containing documentation of the time-out, procedure times, medications, equipment used, vital signs, in-lab complications, radiation, contrast, etc., this log is generated by the nurses/staff and is retained in the patient's permanent medical record.

The Cardiac Catheterization Report

In 2014, ACC/AHA/SCAI published a Health Policy Statement (HPS) on structured reporting in the cardiac catheterization laboratory. This HPS recognizes that the final report is an essential component of every cardiovascular test and procedure that involves imaging. This vital document records key data used to assess indications and appropriateness of care, details technical aspects of the procedure, describes findings and observations, lists results and calculations, provides the interpretation of the study, and conveys patient care recommendations when appropriate. In addition to providing essential information to the care providers, the final report should be utilized in billing and inventory management, process and performance improvement, outcomes analysis, teaching and education, and data registry participation. The final report is a legal medical record document and should be of the highest quality to optimize patient outcomes and institutional operational efficiencies.

The final report should be clear, concise, organized, consistent, reproducible, understandable, and in a format that is flexible to accommodate evolutionary procedural changes and documentation requirements with prose limited to allow database interactions. The HPS statement presents a prototype report for reference and is divided into three sections. The first section, the front page, should be a single page that contains the highest value clinical information. The second section is dedicated to the graphical representations of the findings and possibly images imported into the report. The third section contains all of the remaining data presented ideally as a series of structured, formatted tables. Contained within this HPS are procedure-specific content outlined for diagnostic cardiac catheterization, coronary intervention (PCI), peripheral vascular and cerebral vascular procedures, valvular heart disease including TAVR, structural/congenital heart disease, and combination procedures.

The cardiologist is responsible for reporting the medical procedure. When immediate report generation is not possible, a brief procedure should be generated with the full report ideally available within 24 hours. The final report should contain all the relevant information about the indication for the procedure, the access site(s) used, the catheter and sheath sizes used, and the specific procedures performed (e.g., right heart/ left heart catheterization, left ventriculography, and selective coronary arteriography). Hemodynamic data requires personal review of the tracings. The final report should detail any and all complications occurring during the procedure. Some physicians conclude reports with therapeutic recommendations. When provided, care must be taken to recognize legitimate differences of clinical management strategies to avoid potential confusion amongst multiple care providers.

Patient Safety

Patient safety is defined as being free from accidental harm as a result of a health care encounter. The cardiac catheterization laboratory leadership must create and nurture a culture of personal safety in which each individual team member is free to address concerns without fear of criticism. The Joint Commission requires accredited organizations to have a patient safety program to limit/ prevent patient errors with a response program in the event that harm does occur.

There are 15 published goals that an organization must meet with six applicable to the cardiac catheterization laboratory: (1) improve the accuracy of patient identification by using two unique identifiers and preventing transfusion errors related to misidentification; (2) improve communication effectiveness among the health care team; (3) improve the safety of medication use with proper labeling of all medications, medication containers, and solutions, off and on the sterile field, in all invasive settings and reduce the likelihood of patient harm from anticoagulant therapy; (4) reduce the risk of health care–associated infections; (5) accurately and completely reconcile medication across the continuum; and (6) use of universal protocol for preventing wrong site, wrong procedure, or wrong patient by conducting preprocedure verification process with time-out.

Risk Management and Medical Malpractice

Adverse or unexpected outcomes will occur in the cardiac catheterization laboratory. Patients, families and/or responsible parties should be informed as soon as possible of an adverse or unexpected outcome. Initial communication should include only the available information and avoid speculation. Continued communication is then required with the patient and family to understand the event and its implication for the patient's health. The best approach to avoiding litigation is to keep the lines of communication always open. Documentation of events and interactions is essential to this process.

The clarity of a health care provider's entry into a patient's record is essential, validating the increased use of electronic medical records, personal data assistants, and medical software to identify drug interactions. Although written communication in the medical record is important, open verbal communication between the health care provider and the patient and family is equally essential. Letting the patient know they are important to the health care provider is an integral part of good health care.

Medical malpractice frequently occurs as a result of unresolved anger and frustration of the patient and family, which is lessened by personal interactions. Statements such as "no one would answer my questions," "no one took time to explain anything," and "no one returned my calls" often indicate the underlying motivation that provoked the patient to become a plaintiff. The plaintiff, after the initiation of the lawsuit, sits confident in the expectation that "they'll answer my questions now," "they'll explain it all to me now," or "they'll return this call."

The type of adverse or unexpected outcome may dictate that a root cause analysis be conducted by the cardiac catheterization laboratory. The risk management, quality management, or patient safety departments within the organization usually facilitate this process. The purpose of conducting a root cause analysis is to identify systems and processes that may have contributed to the adverse or unexpected outcome. Not all adverse outcomes are the result of an error and not all health care errors cause adverse outcomes. Changing procedures, rather than focusing on human error, helps to ensure that the procedures practitioners follow prevent medical errors from continuing to occur.

Conclusion

The cardiac catheterization laboratory is a highly specialized and sophisticated unit. Quality assurance is the key to success in this environment. Risks are inherent to any invasive procedure with best quality assured through strong leadership, a culture of safety, sound policies and procedures, compliance with those policies and procedures, and well-trained, dedicated professionals.

Suggested Reading

Bashore TM, Balter S, Barac A, et al. 2012 American College of Cardiology Foundation/Society for Cardiovascular Angiography and Interventions expert consensus document on cardiac catheterization laboratory standards update: A report of the American College of Cardiology Foundation Task Force on Expert Consensus documents developed in collaboration with the Society of Thoracic Surgeons and Society for Vascular Medicine. *J Am Coll Cardiol*. 2012;59(24):2221-2305. Available at: https://www.ncbi.nlm.nih.gov/pubmed/22575325.

Chambers CE. Morbidity and mortality and beyond: assuring quality in cardiac catheterization laboratories quality program. *Circ Cardiovasc Qual Outcomes*. 2017. https://doi.org/10.1161/CIRCOUTCOMES.117.004001

Klein LW, Uretsky BF, Chambers CE, et al. Quality assessment and improvement in interventional cardiology. A position statement of the Society of Cardiovascular Angiography & Interventions. Part I. Standards for quality assessment & improvement in interventional cardiology. *Catheter Cardiovasc Interv*. 2011;77:927-935.

Levine, GL, Bates ER, Blankenship JC, et al. 2011 ACCF/AHA/SCAI guidelines for percutaneous coronary intervention. *J Am Coll Cardiol*. 2011;58:44-122.

Naidu AA, Aronow HD, Box LC, et al. SCAI expert consensus statement: 2016 best practices in the cardiac catheterization laboratory: (endorsed by the Cardiologic Society of India and Sociedad Latino Americana de Cardiologia Intervencionista; Affirmation of Value by the Canadian Association of Interventional Cardiology-Association Canadienne de Cardiologie d'intervention). *Catheter Cardiovasc Interv*. 2016;88:407-423.

Sanborn TA, Tcheng JE, Anderson HV, et al. *J Am Coll Cardiol*. 2014;63(23):2591-2623.

APPENDIX A

Invasive Cardiovascular Examination and Procedures

Catheter Size Specifications.			
French Size	**Inches**	**Millimeters**	**Centimeters**
1.0	0.013	0.33	0.03
2.0	0.026	0.67	0.07
3.0	0.039	1.00	0.10
4.0	0.053	1.33	0.13
5.0	0.066	1.67	0.17
6.0	0.079	2.00	0.20
7.0	0.092	2.33	0.23
8.0	0.105	2.67	0.27
9.0	0.118	3.00	0.30
10.0	0.131	3.33	0.34
11.0	0.144	3.67	0.37
12.0	0.158	4.00	0.40

Note: 1.0 F = 0.33 mm; 2.0 F = 0.67 mm; 3.0 F = 1.00 mm.

APPENDIX B

Heart Diagrams

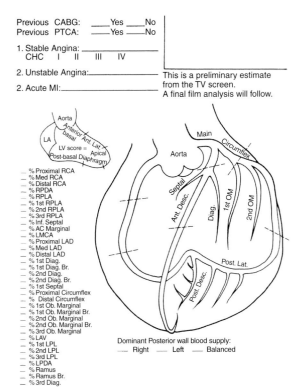

Fig. B.1 Diagram of heart and its branches, which can be used for the patient and family to indicate location of stenoses and state of the LV wall motion. *AC,* Acute circumflex; *Ant.,* anterior; *Br.,* branch; *CABG,* coronary artery bypass graft; *CHC,* Canadian heart class; *Desc.,* descending; *Diag.,* diagonal branch; *Inf.,* inferior; *LA,* left atrium; *LAD,* left anterior descending; *Lat.,* lateral; *LMCA,* left main coronary artery; *LPDA,* left posterior descending artery; *LPL,* left posterior lateral; *LV,* left ventricle; *MI,* myocardial infarction; *Ob.,* obtuse; *OM,* obtuse marginal; *Post.,* posterior; *PTCA,* percutaneous transluminal coronary angioplasty; *RCA,* right coronary artery; *RPDA,* right posterior descending artery; *RPLA,* right posterior lateral artery.

Name: _____   Date: _____

Age: _____   Cath #: _____

WT: _____

HT: _____

BSA: _____

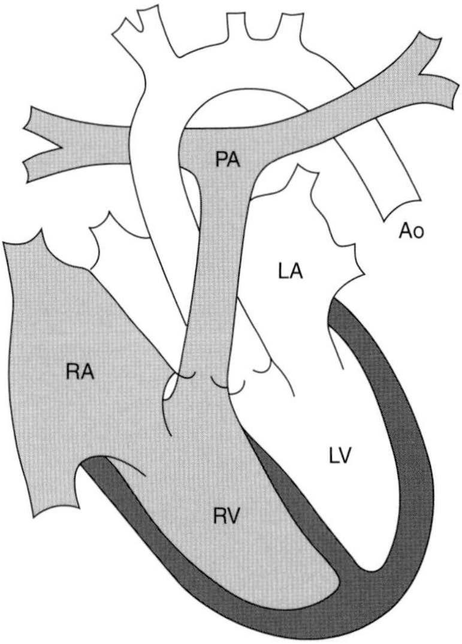

<u>TD:</u>

CO = _____ L/min

CI = _____ L/min/m^2

<u>Fick:</u>

CO = _____ L/min

CI = _____ L/min/m^2

SVR = _____ dynes/s/cm^{-5}

PVR = _____ dynes/s/cm^{-5}

TPG = _____ mm Hg

Fig. B.2 *Ao,* Aorta; *BSA,* body surface area; *CI,* cardiac index; *CO,* cardiac output; *HT,* height; *LA,* left atrium; *LV,* left ventricle; *PA,* pulmonary artery; *PVR,* pulse-volume recording; *RA,* right atrium; *RV,* right ventricle; *SVR,* systemic vascular resistance; *TD,* thermodilution; *TPG,* transpulmonary gradient; *WT,* weight.

APPENDIX C

Functional Anatomy of the Heart

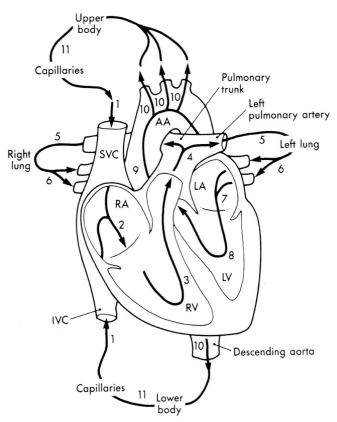

Fig. C.1 Blood flow through the heart and peripheral circulatory system. *AA,* Aortic arch; *IVC,* inferior vena cava; *LA,* left atrium; *LV,* left ventricle; *RA,* right atrium; *RV,* right ventricle; *SVC,* superior vena cava.

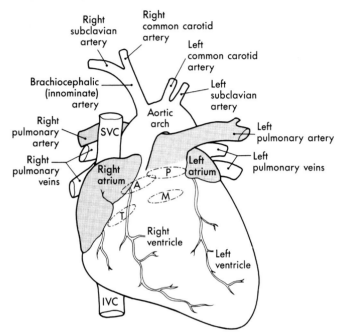

Fig. C.2 Anterior view of the heart and major vessels. *A,* Aortic; *IVC,* inferior vena cava; *M,* mitral; *P,* pulmonic; *SVC,* superior vena cava; *T,* tricuspid.

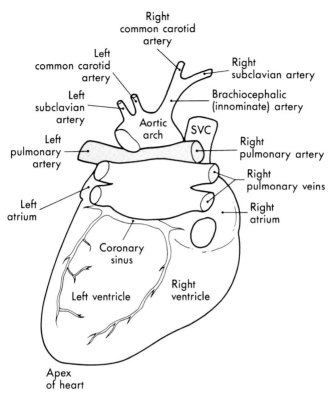

Fig. C.3 Posterior view of the heart and major vessels. *SVC*, Superior vena cava.

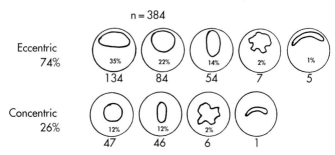

Fig. C.4 Distribution and configuration of coronary stenoses. (From Santamore WP, Corin WJ. New concepts regarding constriction within a stenosis Influence of intraluminal pressure changes. WP Santamore, WJ Corin. *Trends Cardiovasc Med*. 1992;2:189-196.)

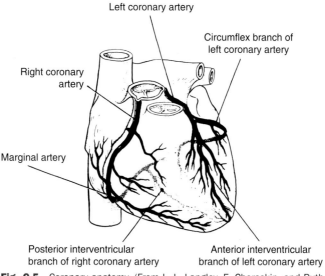

Fig. C.5 Coronary anatomy. (From L. L. Langley, E. Cheraskin, and Ruth Sleeper. *Dynamic Anatomy and Physiology*. 5th ed. New York: McGraw-Hill; 1980.)

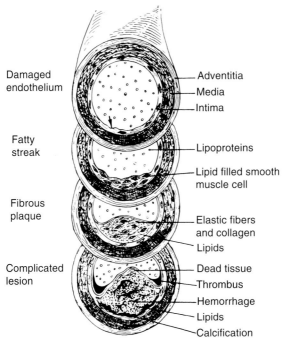

Fig. C.6 Evolution of an atherosclerotic coronary plaque. (From Lewis SM, Collier IC. *Medical-Surgical Nursing: Assessment and Management of Clinical Problems*. St Louis: Mosby; 1996.)

APPENDIX D

Tables of Units, Calculations, and Conversions

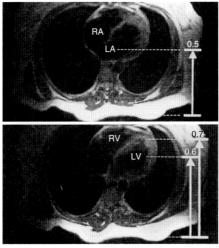

Fig. D.1 Computed tomography of chest demonstrating position of heart chambers. *LA,* Left atrium; *LV,* left ventricle; *RA,* right atrium; *RV,* right ventricle. (From Brown LK, Kahl FR, Link KM, et al. Anatomic landmarks for use when measuring intracardiac pressure with fluid-filled catheters. *Am J Cardiol.* 2000;86:121.)

Table D.1

Guidelines for Location of Catheter Tip for Zero Leveling.	
Fraction of Anteroposterior Distance (From Back to Front)	**Catheter Tip Location Within the Chest**
0.75	Right ventricle and apex of the left ventricle
0.70	Anterior wall of the left ventricle
0.65	Middle of the left ventricle and right atrium
0.60	Posterior wall of the left ventricle
0.55	Mitral valve, superior vena cava, pulmonary trunk
0.50	Left atrium

Table D.2

Normal Left Ventriculogram Ejection Phase Indices.			
	Average	**Standard Error**	**Range**
Sinus Beat			
Ejection fraction[a]	0.71	0.01	0.64–.77
Ejection fraction[b]	67.3	1.0	62–72
Ejection vector[a]	1.19	0.03	1.28–1.07
End-diastolic volume (mL/m^2)	70.4	3.9	54–89
End-systolic volume (mL/m^2)	20.3	0.7	17–24
Postextrasystolic Potentiation Beat			
Ejection fraction[a]	0.82	0.01	0.76–0.85
Ejection fraction[b]	69.9	1.9	64–79
Ejection vector[a]	1.39	0.03	1.26–1.50
End-diastolic volume (mL/m^2)	78.5	3.2	68–90
End-systolic volume (mL/m^2)	14.2	0.7	11–17

From Pujadas G. *Coronary Angiography in the Medical and Surgical Treatment of Ischemic Heart Disease.* New York: McGraw-Hill; 1980.
[a]As fraction of end-diastolic volume.
[b]Percentage of total stroke output is 50.

Table D.3

Oxygen Consumption per Body Surface Area in (mL/min)m² by Sex, Age, and Heart Rate.

Age (years)	Heart Rate (bpm)												
	50	60	70	80	90	100	110	120	130	140	150	160	170
Male Patients													
3				155	159	163	167	171	175	178	182	186	190
4			149	152	156	160	163	168	171	175	179	182	186
6		141	144	148	151	155	159	162	167	171	174	178	181
8		136	141	145	148	152	156	159	163	167	171	175	178
10	130	134	139	142	146	149	153	157	160	165	169	172	176
12	128	132	136	140	144	147	151	155	158	162	167	170	174
14	127	130	134	137	142	146	149	153	157	160	165	169	172
16	125	129	132	136	141	144	148	152	155	159	162	167	
18	124	127	131	135	139	143	147	150	154	157	161	166	
20	123	126	130	134	137	142	145	149	153	156	160	165	
25	120	124	127	131	135	139	143	147	150	154	157		
30	118	122	125	129	133	136	141	145	148	152	155		
35	116	120	124	127	131	135	139	143	147	150			
40	115	119	122	126	130	133	137	141	145	149			

Continued on following page

Table D.3

Oxygen Consumption per Body Surface Area in (mL/min)m² by Sex, Age, and Heart Rate. (Continued)

Age (years)	Heart Rate (bpm)												
	50	60	70	80	90	100	110	120	130	140	150	160	170
Female Patients													
3					153	157	161	165	169	172	176	180	183
4					149	152	156	159	163	168	171	175	179
6		130	141	150	142	146	149	153	156	160	165	168	172
8		125	134	145	136	141	144	148	152	155	159	163	167
10	118	122	129	137	133	136	141	144	148	152	155	159	163
12	115	119	125	133	130	133	137	141	145	149	152	156	160
14	112	116	122	129	127	131	134	133	143	146	150	153	157
16	109	114	120	126	125	128	132	136	140	144	148	151	
18	107	111	118	123	123	127	130	134	137	142	146	149	
20	106	109	116	121	121	125	128	132	136	140	144	148	
25	102	106	114	119	118	121	125	128	132	136	140		
30	99	103	109	118	115	118	122	125	129	133	136		
35	97	100	106	114	111	116	119	123	127	130			
40	94	98	104	110	109	112	117	121	124	128			

From LaFarge CG, Meittinen OS. The estimation of oxygen consumption. *Cardiovasc Res.* 1970;4:23-30.

Table D.4

Dimensions and Units of Some Commonly Used Physical Quantities.

Physical Quantity	Definition	Common Units	Dimensions
Mass	Not defined	gram (g)	M
Length	Not defined	centimeter (cm)	L
Time	Not defined	second (s)	T
Area	Length squared	cm^2	L^2
Volume	Length cubed	cm^3	L^3
Density	Mass per unit of volume	g/cm^3	ML^{-3}
Velocity	Length per unit of time	cm/s	LT^{-1}
Acceleration	Velocity per unit of time	cm/s^2	LT^{-2}
Flow	Volume per unit of time	cm^3/s	L^3T^{-1}
Force	Mass times acceleration	dyne or $g/cm/s^2$	MLT^{-2}
Pressure	Force per unit of area	$dyne/cm^2$ or $g/cm/s^2$	$ML^{-1}T^{-2}$
Resistance to flow	Pressure drop across a hydraulic segment per unit of flow	$dyne/s/cm^{-5}$	$ML^{-5}T$
Work	Force times distance	erg or dyne/cm or $g/cm^2/s^2$	ML^2T^{-2}
Power	Work per unit of time	dyne/cm/s or $g/cm^2/s^3$	ML^2T^{-3}

From Yan SS. *From Cardiac Catheterization Data to Hemodynamic Parameters.* 3rd ed. Philadelphia: FA Davis; 1987.

Table D.5

Conversion Factors and Constants (Decimal Factors).

Multiples	Designation	Symbol	Submultiples	Designation	Symbol
10^{12}	tera-	T	10^{-12}	pico-	p
10^9	giga-	G	10^{-9}	nano-	n
10^6	mega-	M	10^{-6}	micro-	μ
10^3	kilo-	K	10^{-3}	milli-	m
10^2	hecto-	h	10^{-2}	centi-	c
10		dk	10^{-1}		d

Length

1 meter (m) = 10 decimeters = 100 centimeters (cm) = 1000 millimeters (mm) = 1.0936 yards (yd) = 3.2808 feet (ft) = 39.37 inches (inch)
1 kilometer (km) = 1000 m = 0.6214 mile (mi)
1 cm = 0.3937 inch
1 in = 2.54 cm
1 ft = 30.48 cm = 0.3048 m
1 mi = 1.6093 km = 1609.3 m = 1760 yd = 5280 ft
1 micron (m) = 0.000001 m = 10^{-6} m
1 millimicron = 0.000000001 m = 10^{-9} m

Pressure

1 atmospheric pressure (atm) = 760 mm Hg = 14.6 pounds/inch^2
1 cm $H_2O \times 0.735$ = 1 mm Hg
1 cm Hg $\times 1.36$ = 1 cm H_2O

Weight

1 pound (lb) = 0.454 kilogram (kg)
1 kg = 2.204 lb

Temperature, Degrees Celsius (C) and Fahrenheit (F)

$$C = \frac{5°(F - 32°)}{9}$$

$$F = \frac{(C \infty 9) + 32°}{5}$$

C, Celsius; F, Fahrenheit.

Table D.6

Normal Pressures in the Heart and Great Vessels.[a]		
Pressure (mm Hg)	**Average**	**Range**
Right Atrium		
Mean	2.8	1–5
a wave	5.6	2.5–7
c wave	3.8	1.5–6
x wave	1.7	0–5
v wave	4.6	2–7.5
y wave	2.4	0–6
Right Ventricle		
Peak systolic	25	17–32
End diastolic	4	1–7
Pulmonary Artery		
Mean	15	9–19
Peak systolic	25	17–32
End diastolic	9	4–13
Pulmonary Artery Wedge		
Mean	9	4.5–13
Left Atrium		
Mean	7.9	2–12
a wave	10.4	4–16
v wave	12.8	6–21
Left Ventricle		
Peak systolic	130	90–140
End diastolic	8.7	5–12
Brachial Artery		
Mean	85	70–105
Peak systolic	130	90–140
End diastolic	70	60–90

[a]Reference level = 10 cm above the spine of a recumbent subject.

Table D.7

Normal Average Values for Left Ventricular Parameters by Angiocardiography.

Angiographic Method	No. Patients	Age Group	End-Diastolic Volume (mL/m²)	End-Systolic Volume (mL/m²)	Ejection Fraction	Wall Thickness (mm)
Biplane modified Arvidsson	3	Adults	95	36	0.63	7.7
Biplane Dodge area-length	16	Adults	70	24	0.67	10.9
Biplane Dodge area-length	6	Adults	79	29	0.67	8.5
Biplane modified Dodge	6	Adults	71	30	0.58	
Single plane cineangiogram (right anterior oblique)	5	Adults	104	31	0.70	
Biplane Arvidsson	9	Children	88	32	0.64	
Biplane cineangiographic	19	Children younger than 2 years	42		0.68	
Biplane cineangiographic	37	Children older than 2 years	73		0.63	

APPENDIX E

Radiologic Configuration of Prosthetic Heart Valves

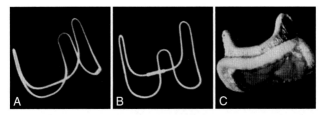

Fig. E.1 Carpentier-Edwards supraannular bioprosthesis, aortic position. **(A)** Posteroanterior radiograph; **(B)** and **(C)** left lateral view radiograph and photograph. One continuous narrow wireform outlines each of the three stents and the portion of the base ring between stents. Although superficially similar to the radiographic silhouettes of the Carpentier-Edwards bioprosthesis, in the supraannular model the change of shape of the wireform as it shifts from base ring to stent is more gradual, giving the wire a gently curving appearance rather than a right-angle appearance. (From Mehlman DJ. A guide to the radiographic identification of prosthetic heart valves: an addendum. *Circulation.* 1984;69:102-105.)

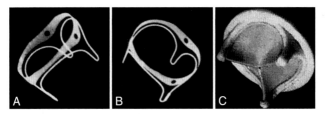

Fig. E.2 Carpentier-Edwards pericardial valve prosthesis, mitral position. **(A)** Posteroanterior radiograph; **(B)** and **(C)** left lateral radiograph and photograph. The base ring is marked by a flattened circular ring with three holes. The flattened ring does not extend into the stents as is seen in the Ionescu-Shiley xenograft. In addition, a narrow wireform outlines each of the three stents and the base ring between the stents. The wire curves gently between stent and base ring, similar to the Carpentier-Edwards supraannular bioprosthesis. (From Mehlman DJ. A guide to the radiographic identification of prosthetic heart valves: an addendum. *Circulation.* 1984; 69:102-105.)

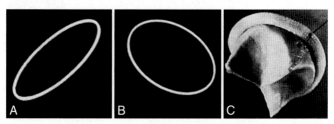

Fig. E.3 Hancock pericardial heart valve, mitral position. **(A)** Posteroanterior radiograph; **(B)** and **(C)** left lateral radiograph and photograph. The base ring is a narrow, circular, wirelike form. The remainder of the valve is radiolucent. The radiographic silhouette is similar to that of the Hancock porcine xenograft. (From Mehlman DJ. A guide to the radiographic identification of prosthetic heart valves: an addendum. *Circulation* 1984;69:102-105.)

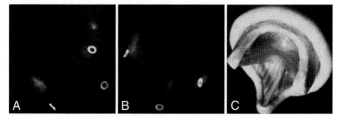

Fig. E.4 Hancock II porcine xenograft, mitral position. **(A)** Posteroanterior radiograph; **(B)** and **(C)** left lateral radiograph and photograph. The base ring and stents are radiolucent. Three tiny circular rings mark the distal external aspects of the three stents. (From Mehlman DJ. A guide to the radiographic identification of prosthetic heart valves: an addendum. *Circulation*. 1984;69:102-105.)

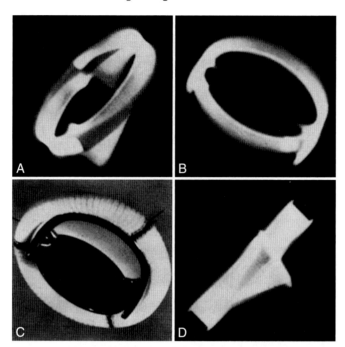

Fig. E.5 Omniscience prosthetic heart valve, mitral position. **(A)** Postero-anterior radiograph; **(B)** and **(C)** left lateral radiograph and photograph; **(D)** oblique radiograph demonstrating disc on edge. Emerging from the wide base ring are two low-profile struts that are fastened to the base ring along their length. Although reminiscent of the silhouette of the Lillehei-Kaster prosthesis, the struts are shorter and form a much lower profile. On routine chest radiographs, the disc is likely to be radiolucent. The disc of the Omniscience prosthesis (unlike the Lillehei-Kaster) is radiopaque when viewed on edge. (From Mehlman DJ. A guide to the radiographic identification of prosthetic heart valves: an addendum. *Circulation.* 1984;69:102-105.)

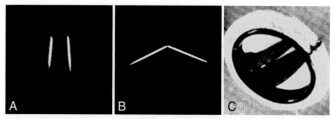

Fig. E.6 St. Jude Medical valve, mitral position. **(A)** Oblique radiograph demonstrating both discs on edge in the open position; **(B)** oblique radiograph demonstrating both discs on edge in the closed position; **(C)** left lateral photograph. On routine chest radiographs, the St. Jude Medical valve is likely to be radiolucent. When viewed on edge, the discs are radiopaque. The base ring is radiolucent. (From Mehlman DJ. A guide to the radiographic identification of prosthetic heart valves: an addendum. *Circulation.* 1984;69:102-105.)

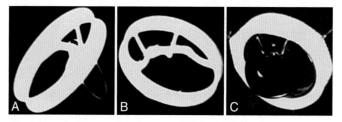

Fig. E.7 Bjork-Shiley cardiac valve prosthesis with convexoconcave disc, mitral position: **(A)** Posteroanterior radiograph; **(B)** and **(C)** radiograph and photograph. The radiographic silhouette is essentially the same as the Bjork-Shiley prosthesis with straight disc and incorporated disc marker. The flattened base ring is encircled by a groove. Emerging from the base ring toward its center are two eccentrically located U-shaped structures of unequal size. The radiolucent disc contains a narrow circular radiopaque disc marker that is seen from any projection. (From Mehlman DJ. A guide to the radiographic identification of prosthetic heart valves: an addendum. *Circulation.* 1984;69:102-105.)

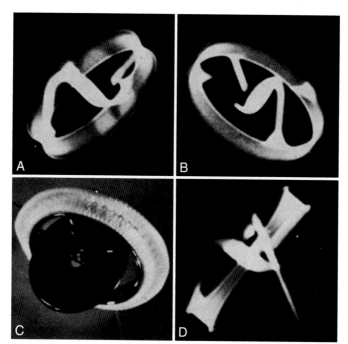

Fig. E.8 Medtronic Hall (formerly called Hall-Kaster) prosthetic heart valve, mitral position. **(A)** Posteroanterior radiograph; **(B)** and **(C)** left lateral radiograph and photograph; **(D)** oblique radiograph demonstrating disc on edge. Four projections emerge from the base ring toward the center of the ring. Two short straight projections of equal size are on opposing sides of the base ring. A longer straight projection is perpendicular to the short projections. A large hooklike projection is opposite the long straight projection. On routine chest radiographs, the disc is likely to be radiolucent. When viewed on edge, the disc is radiopaque. (From Mehlman DJ. A guide to the radiographic identification of prosthetic heart valves: an addendum. *Circulation.* 1984;69:102-105.)

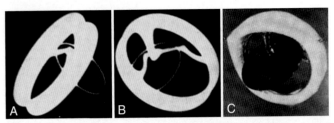

Fig. E.9 Bjork-Shiley integral monostrut cardiac valve prosthesis, mitral position. **(A)** Posteroanterior radiograph; **(B)** and **(C)** left lateral radiograph and photograph. The radiographic silhouette is similar to that of the Bjork-Shiley convexoconcave and straight disc valves. The flattened base ring is encircled by a groove. Emerging from the base ring toward its center is a wide U-shaped structure. Perpendicular to the flattened portion of the U is a short straight projection with a very small hook or bulge on its end. The radiolucent disc contains a narrow circular radiopaque disc marker that is seen from any projection. (From Mehlman DJ. A guide to the radiographic identification of prosthetic heart valves: an addendum. *Circulation.* 1984; 69:102-105.)

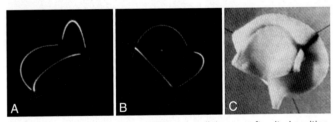

Fig. E.10 Ionescu-Shiley low-profile pericardial xenograft, mitral position. **(A)** Posteroanterior radiograph; **(B)** and **(C)** left lateral radiograph and photograph. The base ring consists of three narrow wireform arcs, each length approximately one-third the circumference of the base ring. Adjoining arcs are separated by small radiolucent areas. The stents are radiolucent. (From Mehlman DJ. A guide to the radiographic identification of prosthetic heart valves: an addendum. *Circulation.* 1984;69:102-105.)

APPENDIX **F**

Basic Electrocardiography

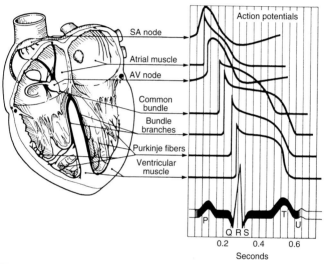

Fig. F.1 Genesis of electrocardiogram and pathways through the heart. *AV*, Atrioventricular; *SA*, sinoatrial. (Modified from the CIBA Collection of Medical Illustrations, Vol. 5.)

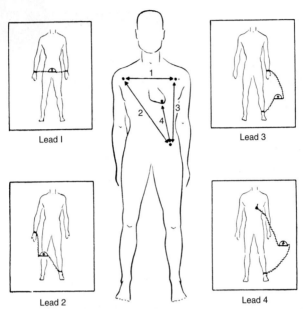

Fig. F.2 Standard limb leads and one precordial lead. (From Marriott HLJ. *Practical electrocardiography.* 7th ed. Baltimore: Williams and Wilkins; 1983.)

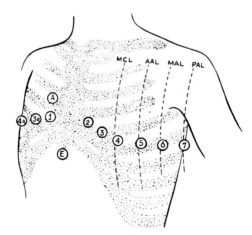

Fig. F.3 Precordial points for chest leads. *AAL,* anterior axillary line; *MAL,* mid axillary line; *MCL,* mid clavicular line; *PAL,* posterior axillary line. (From Marriott HLJ. *Practical Electrocardiography.* 7th ed. Baltimore: Williams and Wilkins; 1983.)

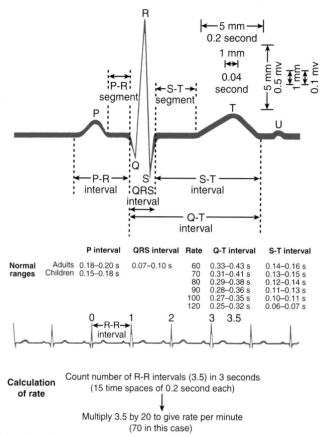

Fig. F.4 Components of the electrocardiogram (ECG) demonstrating normal intervals. (Modified from the CIBA Collection of Medical Illustrations, Vol. 5.)

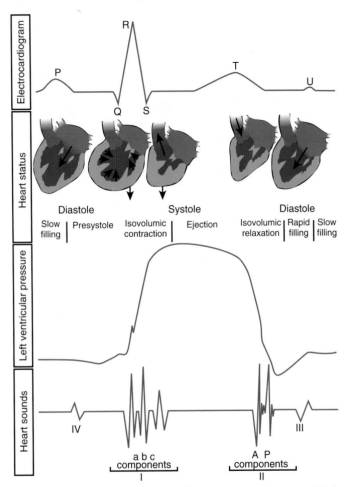

Fig. F.5 Electrical and mechanical activity sequence of the heart. (Modified from the CIBA Collection of Medical Illustrations, Vol. 5.)

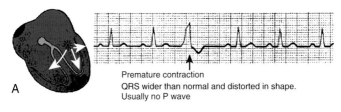

Premature contraction
QRS wider than normal and distorted in shape.
Usually no P wave

A

Rate >120: ventricular tachycardia

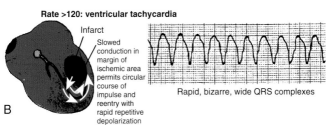

Infarct

Slowed
conduction in
margin of
ischemic area
permits circular
course of
impulse and
reentry with
rapid repetitive
depolarization

Rapid, bizarre, wide QRS complexes

B

Ventricular fibrillation

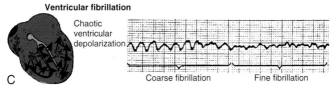

Chaotic
ventricular
depolarization

Coarse fibrillation   Fine fibrillation

C

Fig. F.6 **(A)** Rhythm strip demonstrating a premature ventricular contraction (PVC). **(B)** Rhythm strip demonstrating a run of monomorphic ventricular tachycardia. **(C)** Rhythm strip demonstrating ventricular fibrillation. (Adapted from Scheidt S. *Clinical Symposia.* 1983;35:37; 1984;36:29.)

INFARCTION

1. Injury = elevated ST segment

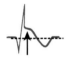
Elevation

- Signifies an acute process; ST returns to baseline with time.
- If T wave is also elevated off baseline, suspect pericarditis.
- Location of injury may be determined similar to infarction location.
- If ST depression, suspect digitalis effect or subendocardial infarction.

2. Ischemai = inverted T wave

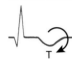
T

- Inverted T wave is symmetrical.
- T waves are usually upright in leads I, II, and V_2–V_6, so check these leads for T wave inversion.

3. Infarction = Q wave

Q

- Small Qs may be normal in V_5 and V_6.
- Abnormal Q must be one small square (.04 s) wide.
- Also abnormal if Q wave depth is greater than one-third of QRS height in lead III.

Anterior infarction

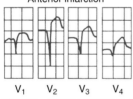
V_1 V_2 V_3 V_4

1. ST elevation with/without abnormal Q wave.

2. Usually associated with occlusion of the left anterior descending branch of the left coronary artery.

Fig. F.7 Electrocardiogram (ECG) changes seen during myocardial injury, ischemia, and infarction. (Courtesy Genentech, South San Francisco, CA.)

Inferior infarction

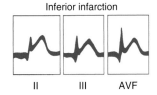

II   III   AVF

1. ST elevation with/without abnormal Q wave.

2. Usually associated with right coronary artery (RCA) occlusion.

Lateral infarction

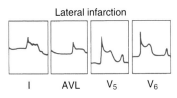

I   AVL   V$_5$ V$_6$

1. ST elevation with/without abnormal Q wave.

2. May be a component of a multiple site infarction.

3. Usually associated with obstruction of left circumflex artery.

Posterior infarction

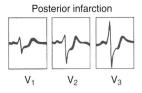

V$_1$ V$_2$ V$_3$

1. Tall R wave and ST depression in V$_1$ and V$_2$ (reciprocal changes).

2. May be a component of a multiple site infarction.

3. Usually associated with obstruction of RCA and/or left circumflex coronary artery.

Fig. F.8 Electrocardiogram (ECG) changes in which acute inferior, lateral, and posterior infarction are demonstrated. (Courtesy Genentech, South San Francisco, CA.)

Methods for Common Drugs

Box G.1 Converting Infusion Rates.

Converting desired dose (mcg/min) to infusion rate (mL/min or mL/h):

$$\frac{\text{Desired dose}\left(\dfrac{\text{mcg}}{\text{min}}\right)}{\text{Drip concentration}\left(\dfrac{\text{mcg}}{\text{mL}}\right)} = \text{mL/min}$$

If using a volume infusion pump that uses a mL/h format, such as an IVAC Model 560, convert μg/min to mg/h:

$$\frac{\text{Desired dose}\left(\dfrac{\text{mcg}}{\text{min}}\right)}{\text{Drip concentration}\left(\dfrac{\text{mcg}}{\text{mL}}\right) \times 60} = \text{mL/h}$$

Automatic Infusion Pump, IVAC Corporation, Minneapolis, MN.

Box G.2 Infusion Methods of Potent Drugs.

Drug Doses Given in Different Units

mg/min	mcg/kg/min	mcg/min	U/h
Lidocaine	Dopamine	Nitroprusside	Heparin
Procainamide	Dobutamine	Nitroglycerin	
Bretylium	Amrinone		
Aminophylline	Norepinephrine		
Hydralazine			
Amiodarone			

Common Concentrations

Nitroprusside (50 mg/250 mL) = 200 mcg/mL
Nitroglycerin (50 mg/250 mL) = 200 mcg/mL
Norepinephrine (8 mg/250 mL) = 32 mcg/mL

Continued on following page

Box G.2 Infusion Methods of Potent Drugs. (Continued)

Dobutamine (1 g/250 mL) = 4000 mcg/mL
Dopamine (800 mg/250 mL) = 3200 mcg/mL
Hydralazine (100 mg/100 mL) = 1 mg/mL
Lidocaine (2 g/250 mL) = 8 mg/mL
Heparin (2500 U/250 mL) = 100 U/mL

Converting desired dose in mcg/kg/min to infusion rate in mL/h:

1. Weight (in kg) $\times$ desired dose/kg/min = mcg/min

2. $\dfrac{mcg/mL}{60} = mcg/mL/min$

3. $\dfrac{mcg/min}{mcg/mL/min} = mL/h$ infusion rate

Example: Dopamine (assume 70 kg at 3 µg/kg/min)

1. Compute dose for weight:

$$70 \times 3 = 210 \text{ mcg/min}$$

2. Compute drug concentration per minute (from common concentrations):

$$\frac{320 mcg/mL}{60^*} = 53.3 \text{ mcg/mL/min}$$

3. When using IVAC delivery in mL/h, compute dose of IVAC:

$$\frac{210 \text{ mcg/min}}{53.3 \text{ mcg/mL/min}} = 3.9 \times mL/h$$

[a]Round off to nearest whole number when setting infusion pump.

Converting infusion rates (mL/h) to dose (µg/min):

$$\frac{\text{Rate}\,(mL/h) = mcg/mL}{60} = mcg/min$$

Converting infusion rate (mL/h) to dose for weight (µg/kg/min):

$$\frac{\text{Rate}\,(mL/h) = mcg/mL}{60 = mcg/min} = mcg/min$$

$$\frac{mcg/min}{kg\ weight} = mcg/kg/min$$

Automatic Infusion Pump, IVAC Corporation, Minneapolis, MN.

Box G.3   Quick Millereau Method.

1 μg/kg/min = 1 mL/h
Drug dose: mg = 3 × body weight kg in 50-mL solution

Example 1: Dobutamine for 50-kg Patient

$$3 \times 50 \text{ kg} = 150 \text{ mg in } 50 \text{ mL}$$
$$= 1 \text{ mL/h}$$
$$= 1 \text{ mcg/kg/min}$$

(If 0.1 μg/kg/min is needed, use 0.3 × body weight.)

Example 2: Norepinephrine for 80-kg Patient

If you need range of 0.1 to 3 μg/kg/h, use 0.3 × body weight.

$$0.3 \times 80 \text{ kg} = 24 \text{ mg in } 50 \text{ mL}$$
$$= 0.1 \text{ mcg/kg/min}$$
$$= 1 \text{ mL/h}$$

If infusion rate = 2.5 mL/h, dose infused = 0.25 μg/kg/min.

From Millereau M. Dilution of potent drugs. *Am J Cardiol.* 1991;68:418.

Index